D0934185

REHABILITATION OF THE PHYSICALLY DISABLED ADULT

REHABILITATION OF THE PHYSICALLY DISABLED ADULT

Edited by C. John Goodwill
and M. Anne Chamberlain

London and Sydney
CROOM HELM

SHERIDAN MEDICAL BOOKS

Croom Helm Ltd, 11 New Fetter Lane,
London, EC4P 4EE

Croom Helm Australia, 44-50 Waterloo Road,
North Ryde, 2113, New South Wales

British Library Cataloguing in Publication Data

Rehabilitation of the physically disabled
adult.
1. Physically handicapped – Rehabilitation
I. Goodwill, C. John II. Chamberlain, M. Anne
615'.8 RD797

ISBN 0-7099-3874-8
ISBN 0-7099-3883-7 Pbk

Published in the USA in 1988 by
Sheridan Medical Books, Sheridan House Inc.,
145 Palisade Street, Dobbs Ferry, NY 10522

Printed and bound in Great Britain at the
University Press, Cambridge

Contents

Part Six: Care and Treatment

Part Seven: Equipment

Preface and Acknowledgements

Good care of disabled people is not easy: it is a complex matter involving a variety of professionals, doctors, nurses, therapists and Social Service department staff. The needs of patients may change considerably over time and it may be difficult for those treating the disabled person to find the information they need when they need it.

This book is designed to help in just this situation, to fill a gap by bringing together much information and practical advice not available elsewhere. The joint authors have worked in the rehabilitation field for many years. They have gathered together acknowledged experts whose wisdom and expertise have been given generously in the hope that the lives of many disabled people may be enhanced and improved and their carers' burden lightened.

We express our grateful thanks to all who have written so ably for us, to those who have commented on contributions, and to those who have helped in many other ways. We believed that this book needed to be written and we hope its usefulness will be some recompense to our loving and long-suffering families.

The book would not have been produced without the sustained and invaluable work of our secretaries, Mrs Barbara O'Sullivan in London and Mrs Jackie Packter in Leeds. We also acknowledge with pleasure the help of the photographic departments of Kings College Hospital and the General Infirmary at Leeds. We are grateful to John Rowley for the original design on which the cover of this book is based. M.A.C. is grateful to Dr John Young who, whilst working with her in Leeds, shouldered many of her clinical responsibilities to release her to write. She also wishes to record her thanks to all the staff at the National Demonstration Centre at the Ida Hospital in Leeds who developed rehabilitation there with her, and in doing so taught her much that has been incorporated in this book.

John Goodwill
Anne Chamberlain
January 1988

Contributors

R. Cairns B. Aitken, MD FRCP, Professor of Rehabilitation Studies, University of Edinburgh

Elizabeth M. Badley, DPhil MSc, Deputy Director Epidemiology Research Unit, University of Manchester Medical School, Manchester

Christine Budden, BSc SRN, Continence Adviser, The Incontinence Clinic, St Pancras Hospital, London

Edward G. Cantrell, MD FRCP, Senior Lecturer in Rehabilitation, Consultant Rheumatologist, Southampton General Hospital

M. Anne Chamberlain, BSc FRCP, Consultant Physician in Rehabilitation Medicine, General Infirmary at Leeds; Honorary Senior Lecturer, School of Medicine, University of Leeds; Director of the National Demonstration Centre in Rehabilitation, Leeds

Roger L. Coakes, MB BS FRCS, Consultant Ophthalmic Surgeon, Kings College Hospital, London

George M. Cochrane, MA MB BS FRCP, Consultant Physician in Rehabilitation Medicine, Mary Marlborough Lodge, Nuffield Orthopaedic Centre, Oxford

Anthony K. Coughlan, PhD, Principal Clinical Psychologist, St James's University Hospital, Leeds

Rosemary Curry, DipCOT, Formerly Senior Occupational Therapist, National Demonstration Centre in Rehabilitation, Ida and Robert Arthington Hospital, Leeds

Simon O'N Daunt, MB MRCP, Consultant in Rheumatology and Rehabilitation, Colchester General Hospital

Brian Meredith Davies, MD(Lond) FFCM DPH, Formerly Director of Social Services City of Liverpool, Lecturer in Public Health and Clinical (Preventive) Paediatrics, University of Liverpool

Mary Davies, BSc PhD, Former Education and Training Officer, The Association to aid the Sexual and Personal Relationships of People with a Disability (SPOD), London

Christine Dowding, MSc SRN, Clinical Teacher, Salisbury School of Nursing

Peter Eames, MB BCH DPM, Consultant Neuropsychiatrist, The Burden Neurological Hospital, Bristol

Pamela Enderby, PhD MSc FCST, Chief Speech Therapist, Frenchay Hospital, Bristol

Mandy Fader, SRN, Continence Adviser, The Incontinence Clinic, St Pancras Hospital, London

Elizabeth Fanshawe, OBE DipCOT, Director, Disabled Living Foundation, London

Jillian Fisher, MCSP SRP, Previously Superintendent Physiotherapist, National Demonstration Centre in Rehabilitation, Ida and Robert Arthington Hospital, Leeds

C. John Goodwill, MB BS FRCP, Consultant Physician in Rheumatology and Rehabilitation, Kings College Hospital, London

Helga Hanks, BSc MSc Dip Psych ABPsS, Principal Clinical Psychologist, St James's University Hospital, Leeds; Honorary Lecturer, University of Leeds

Magdi Hanna, FFARCS, Consultant Anaesthetist and Consultant to the Pain Clinic, Kings College Hospital, London

John F. Harrison, MB BS FRCP, Consultant Geriatrician with responsibility for Younger Disabled Unit, Mosely Hall Hospital, Birmingham

Peter N. Hirschmann, MSc(Lond) FDS RCS DDR RCR, Consultant Dental Surgeon, Dental Hospital at Leeds

David Hughes, DipCOT, Disability Officer, Social Services Department, Leeds City Council

John A.A. Hunter, MD FRCP(Ed), Consultant Physician in Rehabilitation Medicine, Astley Ainslie Hospital, Edinburgh

Graham Jackson, MB BS FRCP, Consultant Cardiologist, Lewisham and King's College Hospitals, London

Mary Jackson, MSCP, Superintendent Physiotherapist, The General Infirmary at Leeds

Peggy Jay, FCOT SROT, Occupational Therapist, London

Alastair Kent, MA MPhil Dip CG, Formerly Principal, Banstead Place, Queen Elizabeth's Foundation for the Disabled, Banstead, Surrey

R. Langton Hewer, MB BS FRCP, Consultant Neurologist, Bristol; Clinical Lecturer, University of Bristol; Director, Bristol Stroke Unit

Robin L. Luff, BSc MB BS FRCS, Medical Officer, DHSS Limb Fitting Centre, Queen Mary's Hospital, Roehampton, London

James Malone-Lee, MB BS MRCP, Senior Lecturer and Consultant, The Incontinence Clinic, St Pancras Hospital, London

Helen March, DipCOT, Community Occupational Therapist, Social Services Department, Leeds City Council (previously Head, OT National Demonstration Centre in Rehabilitation, Leeds)

C. David Marsden, FRS MSc MB BS FRCP, Professor of Neurology, Institute of Neurology, National Hospital for Nervous Diseases, London

Carol Martin, BA MSc DipPsych ABPsS, Principal Clinical Psychologist, Halifax General Hospital, Halifax, W. Yorks

Michael R. Masser, MB BS FRCS MRCP, Senior Registrar in Plastic Surgery, Wessex Regional Plastic Surgery Unit, Odstock Hospital, Salisbury

D. Lindsay McLellan, MB FRCP, Europe Professor of Rehabilitation, Southampton General Hospital

Frederick R. Middleton, BA MB MRCP DPhys Med, Consultant in Disability Medicine, Medical Rehabilitation Centre, Camden Road, London

Mary Moore, MSc, Senior Psychologist, Manpower Services Commission, Sheffield

Timothy R. Morley, MB BCh FRCS, Consultant Orthopaedic Surgeon, Kings College Hospital, London

John Moxham, MD MRCP, Consultant Physician, Kings College Hospital, London

Vera Neumann, MRCP, Senior Registrar in Rheumatology and Rehabilitation, The General Infirmary at Leeds

Jolyon R. Oxley, MB BChir MRCP, Senior Physician, Chalfont Centre for Epilepsy, Gerrards Cross, Bucks

Philippa Perkins, MGrad Dip Phys MCSP, Superintendent Physiotherapist, National Demonstration Centre in Rehabilitation, Ida and Robert Arthington Hospital, Leeds

David Porter, BSc MSc, Research Rehabilitation Engineer, King's College School of Medicine and Dentistry, London

V. Colin Roberts, PhD FIEE, Professor of Medical Engineering, Kings College School of Medicine and Dentistry, London

James C. Robertson, FRCP DCH, Consultant in Rheumatology and Rehabilitation, Salisbury and Southampton; Director, Wessex Regional Rehabilitation Unit, Odstock, Wilts

Ragai M. Shaban, MB DPhysM, Locum Senior Registrar in Rheumatology and Rehabilitation, Salisbury General Hospital

S. Dafydd G. Stephens, MB BS MRCP, Consultant in Audiological Medicine, Welsh Hearing Institute, University Hospital of Wales, Cardiff

Janet Stowe, DipCOT, Senior Research Occupational Therapist, Rheumatology and Rehabilitation Research Unit, School of Medicine, 36 Clarendon Road, Leeds

Ian Swain, BSc PhD SEng MIEE, Principal Medical Physicist, Salisbury General Hospital

Christine Tarling, DipCOT SROT, Team Leader (Specialist Services), Social Services Department, Metropolitan Borough of North Tyneside,

Derick T. Wade, MD MRCP, Consultant Physician in Neurological Disability, Rivermead Hospital, Oxford

Philip H.N. Wood, FRCP FFCM, Director of the Arthritis and Rheumatism Council Epidemiology Research Unit, and Honorary Professor of

Community Medicine, University of Manchester Medical School; Honorary Regional Specialist in Community Medicine, North Western Regional Health Authority

Verna Wright, MD FRCP, ARC Professor of Rheumatology, School of Medicine, University of Leeds

Part 1

Definition and Assessment of the Problem

1

Aims of Rehabilitation

John Goodwill and Anne Chamberlain

AIMS OF REHABILITATION

Medicine has not always concerned itself with dramatic cures: indeed it is not so long ago that the physician was unable to intervene in what would now seem mundane, lobar pneumonia: he watched and prayed that the patient weathered the crisis. Not until the 1930s and 1940s did he have the chance of changing such events with any regularity. Yet the face of modern medicine continues to change fast. Health services of the last quarter of the twentieth century are concerned with diseases and operations that differ from those found at its inception. Then, there was much infectious disease, including tuberculosis, a great deal of maternal and child morbidity and the management of arthritis had barely begun. There was no provision for younger patients who were chronically ill, dependency from osteoarthritis of the hip could not be relieved by arthroplasty nor angina by coronary artery bypass. Rheumatic heart disease caused much morbidity; polio was feared for its ability to kill and maim the young.

We now have a different picture: tuberculosis is no longer a threat, the old infectious diseases produce few fears but the emergence of a new one, AIDS, has produced dramatic new ones. The management, if not the cure, of arthritis, is vastly improved and arthroplasties of the hip enable many to live alone well into old age, or extreme old age! There are new problems, for we have seen the incidence of cerebral palsy due to birth injury and anoxia decline, yet are aware that many smaller babies survive. Surgical intervention in spina bifida peaked in the early 1970s and has declined; the cohort of sufferers rendered phocomelic due to thalidomide have all reached their early twenties.

The caring tradition is old. The first evidence that early man exhibited compassion is some 60,000 years old, and comes from Northern Iraq. The bones of an old man with severe arthritic changes and a congenital abnormality which would have rendered his right arm useless, lie beside those of another with a recent injury. Both these and five other skeletons are surrounded by pollen, indicating that floral tributes had been paid to the dead (Passmore, 1979). Sometimes admirable traditions become insidiously inappropriate. The wheelchair and limb fitting centres of the UK were designed for the young fit veterans of the First World War, not the elderly arteriopaths who now commonly use these services, and the McColl report (1986) would suggest that changes are required.

Many of the advances in rehabilitation practice have arisen as a result of experience gained in wars, such as the Second World War and that in Vietnam. However, we have to acknowledge what many would prefer to forget — that we are in a nuclear age. Rehabilitation is about tertiary response to insult or disease and all would desire to ease the unhappy lot of any survivors of a nuclear blast who might survive, albeit temporarily, to inhabit a nuclear winter. However, it is extremely doubtful whether any techniques of modern rehabilitation would have relevance to this situation, where communications would have been disrupted and where for all but a few, living conditions would be primitive, at best perhaps approximating to mediaeval. None with paraplegia, or pressure sores or severe disability could survive for long. In the past, rehabilitation has enhanced the survival of the war-wounded. But, given the known scenario, the most appropriate medical response to nuclear war would seem to be primary and preventative (BMA, 1983).

Patterns of rehabilitation in the late twentieth century are only now emerging in the UK, though various models are in existence elsewhere (e.g. Sweden, USA and Australia). It is becoming clearer that many doctors in a wide range of disciplines require a body of knowledge and ready access to information which will speed their patients through the process of recovery, or at least help to maximise the potential they still have after trauma, surgery or disease. Too often doctors and other health or Social Services professionals do not assess the potential for improving the function of the patient, and are not prepared to seek advice from those with expertise in the field.

It is of great importance that patients should have access to sufficient help to ensure that they live life to the best level they are able. Yet patients despair at the complexity of support services, and access to them. Doctors also despair when they are poorly prepared and unable to give help. This is partly because rehabilitation and supporting services for disabled people have grown up in a disorganised manner. It is also because of the difficulty in linking health services and social services. Too often we settle for less than the best. The result is predictable, and is exemplified by the huge national bill for pressure sores. Great costs are engendered but care remains patchy; patients are poorly served; carers are worn out; the employment of both carers and patients is lost too readily, and both suffer empty and lonely lives.

Many of the writers in this book have broken new ground: their findings have not always been fully appreciated. Many have realised over recent decades that although they have been dealing with ostensibly different topics (perhaps head injury or motor neurone disease), their philosophies, their approach and their methods of calling up resources have much in common. The editors hope that a new generation of doctors and other professionals will build on these writings. Whilst the details of organisation of services, or of hardware, will vary from country to country, perhaps philosophies will not. We hope, too, that those using this book and studying for qualifications such as the Diploma in Medical Rehabilitation, who come from other countries, will take back to their own countries some useful ideas. We would welcome readers' comments.

REFERENCES

McColl Report (1986) *Review of the Artificial Limb and Appliance Centre Services*, vol. 1, HMSO, London

Passmore, R. (1979) The declaration of Alma-Ata and the future of primary care. *Lancet*, 10 Nov.

Report of the British Medical Association's Board of Science Education (1983) Medical Effects of Nuclear War. John Wiley, Chichester

2

The Epidemiology of Disablement

Philip Wood and Elizabeth Badley

An epidemiological appraisal of disablement contributes to the activities of clinicians in various ways. Information on the frequency and characteristics of occurrence of specific conditions giving rise to disability provides the background for diagnostic assessment. Knowledge of the natural history and outcome enlighten management and guide development of prognosis. Clinicians are also concerned to secure the resources needed to assist individuals with disabilities, a group that has generally fared not that well in obtaining an equitable share of medical services and technology, nor of social welfare provisions either. This takes one more into the field of policy and planning. Different types of information are needed for these various purposes. In this chapter we shall try to cover these different aspects, so far as available data allow.

With our aim specified in that way, a series of questions needs to be considered:

(1) *Why is an appraisal being undertaken?* If the emphasis is to be placed on understanding the origins of disablement, then the clinical picture has to be completed by information on the occurrence of mild as well as severe involvement. On the other hand if the concern is with the outcomes or consequences of illness and their amelioration, i.e. with the service needs of disabled individuals, only those with degrees of severity requiring special services have to be taken into account.

(2) *Who is disabled?* This question may be answered by documenting the characteristics of affected individuals in terms such as age, sex and ethnicity. If only particular subgroups of the population are affected, light may be shed on the origins of the problem, and such findings will also indicate vulnerable subgroups on whom attention may be preferentially focused (such as by screening).

(3) *How are people affected?* This calls for measurement of the extent

or severity of the problem, of the needs that ensue, and of associated phenomena — including the consequences of various actions by physicians, and the responses by people with disabilities to their own circumstances.

(4) *Where are the affected?* Identifying the situations in which disablement is encountered may reveal geographical variations, for example, which in turn could draw attention to influences on expression of the problem, whilst more localised variations may indicate the role of environment in determining handicap.

(5) *When does the problem get recognised?* This calls for review of trends in variation of disability-related phenomena, as well as considering the sensitivity of their detection at various levels of health and social services organisation.

(6) *What is the impact of disablement?* In other words, quantification of the size of the problem, which establishes its scale and is helpful when trying to resolve conflicts in priorities.

NATURE OF DISABLEMENT

Before proceeding further it is necessary to clarify the nature of the phenomena being considered. For this purpose we shall draw on the usage of WHO's *International Classification of Impairments, Disabilities, and Handicaps* (ICIDH; WHO, 1980), on which we have enlarged elsewhere (Wood, 1980; Wood and Badley, 1980). In its simplest form this may be represented as a sequence:

disease or disorder → impairment → disability → handicap

where → should be read as implying 'may lead to'. For those unfamiliar with these terms their meanings are, briefly:

Impairment: any disturbance of the normal structure and functioning of the body, including the systems of mental function. It is characterised by a permanent or temporary psychological, physiological or anatomical loss or abnormality, and includes the occurrence of an abnormality, defect or loss in a limb, organ, tissue or other structure of the body, or in a functional system or mechanism of the body.

Disability: the loss or reduction of functional ability and activity consequent upon impairment. It is characterised by excesses and deficiencies of behaviour and other functions customarily expected of the body or its parts, and represents objectification of impairments in everyday life and activity.

Handicap: the disadvantage experienced as a result of impairment or disability. It is characterised by a discordance between the individual's performance or status and the expectations of the particular group of which he or she is a member, including the individual's own expectations. Handicap thus represents the social and environmental consequences of impairments and disabilities.

Disablement: a generic term referring to any experience identified variously by the terms impairment, disability and handicap.

In ideal circumstances one ought to be able to document the frequency of each of the different states in the sequence, but unfortunately the necessary data are rarely available. In practice all one can usually do is take account of disablement at two levels. Measures of the overall burden are provided by estimates of impairment of any degree. These can be used as a proxy for the population at risk of being disabled. Those with considerable current needs are better indicated by people with severe disabilities; such individuals may generally be regarded as handicapped. Wherever possible data on the two levels will be presented, and distinction will be made between the three major classes of medical disorder giving rise to disablement:

(a) emotional and intellectual impairments, due to mental retardation and mental illness;

(b) sensory impairments including the special senses of vision and hearing — data specific to other functions of communication, notably speech, are not readily available;

(c) physical impairments (congenital, the result of trauma, or due to other conditions).

FREQUENCY OF OCCURRENCE

Much tends to be made of whether information is up to date. Regrettably there is no regular representative source of information on types of disablement, and the results of *ad hoc* surveys usually offer the most reliable guide. Inescapably the latter may not be very recent, but their quality generally outweighs this drawback. The best data available from Great Britain refer back to the early or mid 1970s, and it is on these we have had to draw. The Government Social Survey is repeating its definitive study of the impaired, but results will not be available until mid-1988.

Table 2.1 shows estimates for the frequency of the three major classes of medical disorder giving rise to disablement in adults in Great Britain at the two levels of severity. This gives an impression of the overall picture. The rates quoted may be converted into the numbers affected by multiplying

Table 2.1: Approximate estimates of the frequency of impairment and severe disability in adults in Great Britain (from Wood and Badley, 1978a) (relevant home population of Great Britain aged 15+ years: 41,779 thousand)

Class of impairment	ICD rubrics (8th revision)	Frequency of occurrence (per thousand population) Impairment (all degrees)	Severe disability	Age group on which based (years)	Source of estimate (*i* = impairment, *sd* = severe disability)
Mental (total)		*100.7*	*11.6*		
retardation	310–315	22.4	2.2	15+	*i* = IQ <70 from distribution (mean 100, SD 15); *sd* from DHSS, 1971
illness	290–300.4, 301–304	78.3	9.4	15+	*i* from GP psychosis consulting rates (OPCS, 1974); *sd* from DHSS, 1975
Sensory (total)		*159.8*	*5.4*		
visual	370–379	102.4	3.9	15+	*i* from lenses supplied 1973; *sd* from registered blind, etc. (DHSS, 1976)
hearing	388, 389	57.4	1.5	16+	*i* and *sd* from DHSS, 1977
Physical (total)		*82.6*	*18.0*		
congenital	286.0, 330, 343, 344, 740–759	1.0	0.2	16+	mainly Harris, 1971
trauma	N800–N999	9.6	1.0	16+	mainly Harris, 1971
other	remainder	72.0	16.8	16+	mainly Harris, 1971
All classes		*343.1*	*35.0*		

the former by the population figure cited at the head of the table. It can be seen that 34 per cent of all adults manifest some degree of impairment. Visual, mainly refractive, errors are much the commonest problem, followed closely by mental illness and physical impairments arising from disease rather than trauma or congenital conditions.

One-tenth of the impaired are severely disabled, so the latter comprise 3.5 per cent of the adult population. It is striking, though, that there are marked differences between the classes in the relationship between the two levels of disablement. One in four or five of those impaired by congenital or other physical conditions are severely disabled, whereas less than one in 25 of those with sensory impairment are affected severely.

Interpretation

The estimates for impairment obviously reflect disturbances of normal structure and functioning of the body. However, in a large proportion of individuals the impairment does not significantly interfere with functional ability, so that these people are not necessarily disabled. Moreover, although the order of magnitude of the estimates is daunting, it has to be recalled that the bodies of very few individuals are without some abnormality of structure or function. What such figures offer is a measure of those who may be in need of help to minimise the deviation, as well as indicating those at risk of deterioration to a more severe state of disablement.

We should perhaps also draw attention to what amounts to a misuse of such data. Emotive claims on behalf of different groups of disabled people are often encountered. Estimates of the frequency of particular classes of impairment tend to be quoted in isolation. High rates are usually cited and, as Todd (1978) noted, the worst aspects of the condition are generally emphasised. In the mind these two pieces of information can become fused together, so that a sense of urgency is created. The urgency may often be justifiable, but two difficulties result.

The first is that an unduly unfavourable impression of the condition can be created, which often adds to the fears of those newly diagnosed as suffering from the underlying disorder. The selective quality of individual clinical experience by doctors often serves to exacerbate this aspect. Thus there has tended to be exaggeration of the overall severity of multiple sclerosis or, on a different plane, of the lethality of systemic lupus erythematosus.

The second difficulty is that the urgency has tended to give rise to responses by society that are piecemeal and confined to particular disabilities; what may be regarded as preferential treatment of the blind is an obvious example. The net result has usually been medical services, social policies and research programmes, all of which are neither adequate nor appropriate to the overall problem.

The latter difficulty then spills over to those with severe disabilities, for whom relevant support is often lacking. For instance, what view of disablement experience can justify the implicit notion that assistance, such as in the form of a mobility allowance, is no longer needed after an individual reaches retirement age? What emerges, then, is an inadequate comprehension of the experience of disablement by society as a whole, and sadly this is frequently shared by many of the professionals concerned to help people with disabilities.

Prevalence and incidence

The material presented in Table 2.1 could be assembled only by making a number of assumptions, the justification for which we have discussed elsewhere (Wood and Badley, 1978a). Perhaps the most serious problem is that, of the figures set out side by side in Table 2.1, some are true prevalence measures whereas others, notably the service utilisation data, relate to incidence (i.e. to events happening to people, rather than indicating the frequencies of the underlying conditions). This was unavoidable because satisfactory prevalence estimates were not available for some impairments.

Because of the extended time spans over which people are affected, estimates of the incidence of chronic conditions are generally lower than measures of their prevalence; this is in contrast to the situation with acute disorders. The use of incidence ratios in regard to certain recurring or chronic states, such as visual impairments or various forms of mental illness, can thus be justified. If anything, measures such as patient consulting rates tend to underestimate the prevalence of this type of disorder.

CHARACTERISTICS OF PEOPLE WITH DISABILITIES

There have tended to be two perspectives on disablement. One has generally focused on disability, giving emphasis to dissimilarities between affected individuals. We shall begin by summarising information relevant to this approach, to provide a background, whilst recognising that highlighting differences is unhelpful to efforts seeking more general solutions that could be incorporated in future policy.

Specific medical conditions

Although there have been understandable attempts to demedicalise the situation of individuals who have to live with chronic disorders, by almost rejecting medical labels, the nature of the specific conditions from which people suffer still accounts for the largest part of the variance in the occurrence of disablement. Thus, for example, the everyday problems differ quite appreciably between someone who has had a stroke and someone else with rheumatoid arthritis.

Table 2.2 shows estimates for the principal classes of condition occurring in people with impairments, together with an indication of the frequency of severe disability. Due to the nature of the survey from which these figures were derived, they are not fully representative; they are based largely on persons with locomotor disabilities, individuals with mental or sensory impairments being included only if they were severely disabled, and people in institutions were also not taken into account. Estimates for the latter have been offered in Badley *et al.* (1978).

Other features of disablement

Much thinking on disablement is still dominated by the stereotype of a young adult in a wheelchair, suffering perhaps from paraplegia or multiple

Table 2.2: Principal classes of condition occurring in impaired adults in Great Britain (from Badley *et al.*, 1978, after Harris, 1971)

Severity and underlying medical cause*	Prevalence of impairment (per 1000 population)	Severely and very severely disabled					
		Proportion of impaired (%)	Estimated frequency (per ¼ million)†	Proportion in age group (%)			Female to male ratio
				16–44	45–64	65+	
Very severe (>50%)							
Stroke	3.31	51.9	427 (240)	1.5	24.5	74.0	1.8
Multiple sclerosis	0.60	64.3	96 (49)	28.3	59.0	12.7	1.7
Parkinsonism	0.56	51.4	72 (31)	2.1	50.6	47.2	0.9
Severe (25–40%)							
Rheumatoid arthritis	3.43	38.0	323 (83)	5.5	41.0	53.5	4.8
Geriatric conditions	3.11	27.6	211 (110)	0.3	2.0	97.7	3.1
Neoplasm	0.70	30.1	52 (18)	7.6	18.2	74.1	1.6
Paraplegia	0.54	33.4	45 (17)	13.0	36.3	50.7	1.2
Moderate (15–24%)							
Other arthritis (arthrosis)	18.67	16.3	751 (136)	1.2	21.3	77.6	4.7
Infancy and youth	2.60	16.4	102 (55)	59.8	31.2	9.0	1.1
Blind	1.80	15.0	66 (24)	7.0	4.7	88.4	1.5
Genitourinary	0.86	22.4	48 (20)	0	7.8	92.2	4.5

Mild (<15%)							
Circulatory	10.93	11.6	309 (98)	0.2	20.9	78.9	2.8
Respiratory	7.59	7.8	144 (29)	3.2	34.5	62.3	0.8
Trauma	6.32	12.6	197 (46)	6.5	30.0	63.5	1.9
Other special senses	5.22	7.6	93 (14)	0	6.6	93.4	5.5
Other rheumatic disorders	4.92	11.3	134 (28)	11.3	40.6	48.0	3.1
Coexistent conditions	3.30	11.5	92 (14)	2.3	11.3	86.3	6.6
Amputations	3.23	6.6	52 (15)	19.8	33.7	46.5	0.5
Miscellaneous	2.75	17.9	120 (33)	9.0	34.7	56.3	2.1
Digestive	1.52	10.3	39 (11)	0	8.0	92.0	11.5
Metabolic	1.30	8.9	28 (14)	0	16.7	83.3	7.9
Poliomyelitis	0.93	9.8	23 (9)	29.3	60.0	10.7	2.3
Mental illness	0.84	14.7	29 (19)	18.9	34.7	46.3	3.0
All conditions	*85.02*	*16.6*	*3453 (1113)*	*6.0*	*25.9*	*68.1*	*2.6*

* Figures in parentheses after severity indicate the proportions of the impaired who are severely or very severely disabled. Most of the diagnostic groups are self-explanatory, although amplification is provided in Badley *et al.*, 1978. The two that may give rise to uncertainty are as follows:

(1) 'Infancy and youth': conditions mainly manifesting themselves in this age period, including mental subnormality, cerebral palsy, congenital heart disease and other malformations, birth injuries, haemophilia, epilepsy, rheumatic fever, muscular dystrophy and osteomyelitis.

(2) 'Coexistent conditions': relatively 'minor' conditions by no means exclusively associated with the presence of other diseases, although this tended to be the general pattern of their occurrence, and including hernia, varicose veins, vertigo, debility, etc.

† Figures in parentheses indicate estimated frequency of the very severely disabled (special care group) per 250,000 population, i.e. an average health district population in the UK.

sclerosis. Some groups of people with disabilities tend to reinforce this image when claiming their rights to better support. However, the second most important influence on disablement experience, age, reveals the inappropriateness of these views. As can be seen in Table 2.2, two-thirds of the severely disabled are over retirement age, and only one in 16 are under 45 years, observations that have profound implications for the types of policy that may be appropriate to ameliorate the difficulties and even for the policy areas likely to be of relevance.

Two features deserve to be emphasised. First, what are thought of as the chronic disabling conditions of later life, such as arthritis, stroke and circulatory disorders, are certainly the main problems in the elderly. Nevertheless an appreciable proportion of individuals with these conditions are under the age of 65 years. Stroke, for instance, is the number three cause of severe disability in those aged 45–64 years, being exceeded only by rheumatoid arthritis and other arthritis (the latter being predominantly osteoarthritis), and it takes the top place among the very severely disabled in this age group.

The second feature is somewhat complementary. To avoid 'contamination' of the problems of the disabled with those of the elderly, social policy initiatives are often directed towards what are referred to as the young chronic sick, i.e. excluding those over retirement age from consideration (this is what led to anomalies such as that already noted, termination of entitlement to mobility allowance). However, if those in Table 2.2 aged 65 and over are excluded the mean age of the remainder of impaired persons is 50.8 years, just over half being 55–64 and a further quarter in the immediately preceding decade.

Overall there is an excess of women among the disabled, although at ages up to 65 years the prevalence ratios for all degrees of impairment tend to be slightly higher in men — preferential mortality in this sex probably precludes them from dominating the picture at all ages. The prevalence of impairment also shows quite marked regional differences, and variations in population age distributions by no means account for all the differences. Variations in the occurrence of all causes of morbidity and of industrial accidents contribute to the differences, as does the influence of social status. Finally, in a small minority of individuals, concentrated predominantly among the more severely disabled, a powerful influence is the presence of multiple impairments, particularly those resulting from conditions affecting more than one system of the body.

Experience of disadvantage

At the beginning of this section we remarked that there have been two perspectives on disablement. The second of these considers the disadvantages or handicap that result from disability. An indication of such experiences helps one to perceive that people with disabilities are also notable for the disadvantages they have in common. The shared nature of many of their problems reflects the fact that much of the disadvantage is generally imposed on individuals with disabilities by the manner in which society organises itself. Realisation of this source of influence assists the quest for social remedies capable of fairly wide application.

A full profile of the disadvantages that result cannot be established because the relevant data have not been collected. The best approximation is offered in Table 2.3, which indicates handicap experience in adults. Again one would expect variations in living conditions and social circumstances to lead to geographical differences, but the source data were insufficiently robust to justify pursuing this aspect. Over and above limitations in available information, the attempt to marshal data in Table 2.3 has also been constrained within the limits of the ICIDH — i.e. attention has been confined to expressions of disadvantage that can be conceived of in terms of more universal experience.

One of the problems with most work so far is that it has tended to concentrate on the material circumstances of disabled people, which can readily lead to the assumption that such individuals are responsible for the amelioration of their status to a greater extent than it is realistic to suppose. For example, fairly central to much rehabilitation thinking has been appreciation of dependence, particularly in relation to physical functions. Such ideas have certainly tended to be individualistic, insufficient regard often being paid to the many things that are quite outside an individual's control. For instance, how independent is any person in finding a job, when the availability of work opportunities in one's locality is determined by much wider social and economic circumstances?

On the other hand, attention has been drawn to constraints imposed by the physical environment in the form of architectural barriers and the like, yet social policy development has been slow, in the UK at least, to accommodate such insights. Social support is generally inadequate, and is often additionally tarnished with confusing attitudes about 'charity', although the latter can scarcely account for the poverty of policies to assist the helpers. The social climate is also relevant, particularly such factors as the difficulty in developing self-regard in the face of stereotyping and stigma.

Formal systems of assessment of disablement, including the ICIDH, have at times been criticised for being too individualistic. However, one has to start by studying the experience of individuals with disabilities before one can appraise the problems in a broader context and seek common elements that might illuminate extraneous determinants of disablement. The criticism can perhaps be understood by realising that part of what is being taken issue with is the attitude and conduct of organised services devoted to helping people with disabilities. The latter reflect the heritage

Table 2.3: Indications of disadvantage (handicap) in five dimensions in physically impaired adults (from Wood and Badley, 1978b, after Harris, 1971)

Dimension of handicap	Accomplishment or state	Proportion of all impaired (%)
*Physical independence**	Difficulty in:	
	washing hands and face	7 (3% impossible)
	getting to and using WC	17 (3% impossible)
	washing all over	27 (12% impossible)
	having a bath (excl 8.5% lacking a bath)	53 (22% impossible)
Mobility	Confined to house:	
	bedfast	1
	chairfast	2
	otherwise housebound	10
	Able to get out of house:	
	only if accompanied	11
	on own but with difficulty	23
	without undue difficulty	53 (may take longer getting around)
Occupation	Ceased employment (because of disability):	
	prematurely retired	24
	now a housewife	7
	Otherwise not employed:	
	other retired	19
	housewives†	26
	temporarily sick	3
	In employment:	
	in occupation centre	0.4
	at school or university	0.3
	other	20
*Social integration**	Living alone:	21 (cf. only 5% of general population)
	of those living alone:	
	do not have television	25 (cf. 6% of those living with others)
	do not watch television	2 (cf. 4% of those living with others)
	Recreations interfered with (by disability)‡:	
	unable to go to clubs	18
	unable to go to other places	15 (e.g. shops, parks, etc.)
	have had to give up hobbies	59
	not had holiday in previous 4 years	34 (cf. 60% of very severely disabled)
*Economic self-sufficiency**	*Extra expenses incurred* (because of disability):	
	for living accommodation	3 (for adaptation or maintenance)
	for laundry	15
	for other things (e.g. heating, diet)	
	one extra	25 (NB extra expense
	two extra	9 impossible for those
	three extra	3 on very low incomes)

Weekly income:§	
of those living alone, less than £10	85 (age-standardised, cf. 75% in general population)
median weekly income	£9 (cf. £18 in general population)

* Proportions not exclusive.
† Housewives may be unable to take up paid work, or may have difficulty with household tasks; 28 per cent of all housewives in the sample were unable to do more than one task connected with housework, cooking, or shopping.
‡ Strictly interpreted, recreations are an aspect of occupation, but they are used here to illustrate loss of contact with the outside world.
§ The survey was carried out in1969; present incomes are higher because of effect of inflation, but there is no evidence the relativities have changed.

from a somewhat paternalistic and prescriptive approach, and what is being challenged is arrangements that appear to compromise the autonomy and freedom to express opinions of people with disabilities — those the services are supposed to exist to help. In fact the whole notion of handicap, which endeavours to set experience in its social context, should serve as an antidote to many of these difficulties.

At the same time it is noteworthy that services are often complained about because they are not sufficiently individualised. This might also be thought to apply to attempts at describing universal experience, such as by systematised collection of information, as if more individual and personal concerns have not been taken into account. The latter include needs in regard to communication with health professionals, problems encountered in the expression of sexuality, and difficulties in obtaining insurance cover — all topics covered in papers in the journal *International Disability Studies.*

A BROADER PERSPECTIVE

Before one can explore the basis on which various of these difficulties might be overcome, some thought has to be given to other dimensions of the problem. This is necessary if one is to avoid developing 'remedies' that fail to take into account often competing influences. Such an exercise can also be regarded as providing opportunities to falsify or refute any insights that might emerge from a more limited appreciation of the situation.

Time trends

It is not possible to say anything direct about changes over time in disablement experience, because there were no adequate studies to document the situation on earlier occasions. Moreover, three important changes have to be acknowledged. The first concerns what might be termed underlying risks. Over the past 40 years there have been marked changes in the pattern of morbidity, and hence in the consequential disablement. The community burden has increasingly come to be dominated by chronic and generally non-fatal illnesses, with their much bigger and more persistent toll of disability.

The second change has been demographic. An increasing proportion of the population is elderly (over 65 years) and particularly very elderly (over 75 years). The marked increase in disability phenomena with age has already been noted, so that a growing burden of disablement is scarcely surprising — which has implications for what policy initiatives may be feasible.

The third influence has been rather more complex. On the one hand there have been changes in societal attitudes and expectations, with which have been associated demands for more sensitive responses to the problems of chronic illness. Such forces have provoked more enlightened social policies, one expression of which was the pressure which led to production of the ICIDH. However, this trend towards enlightenment now seems to be threatened in the wake of economic stagnation and adaptation to zero growth, because superficially more emotive imperatives in the form of medical technology compete for scarce resources. On the other hand these attitudes have also been assimilated by people with disabilities themselves, and they, in turn, have sought a greater say in the determination of their situation. In its most radical form this development has echoed the appraisals of oppressed female and black groups, leading to emergence of the movement for independent living and further challenge to restrictive notions of rehabilitation.

The global burden

Statements about disablement in other countries have to be more circumspect because good data are lacking. However, all the indications are that experience in other western countries, the so-called developed part of the world, resembles that in Great Britain. The variations that may be encountered appear to be largely attributable to differences in demographic structure, such as the notably younger population of Australia and, less so today, the United States of America, and these are compounded by differences in ascertainment related to legislative provisions specifying different thresholds of eligibility for assistance and other benefits.

As far as numbers are concerned the World Health Organization has estimated that throughout the world 450–500 million people are disabled, representing a prevalence ratio of one in ten. The precision of this estimate, and the level of disability implied, are understandably open to some question. It is probably more appropriate to recognise that about a third of the world population is impaired in some way, a third of those with impairments are disabled to some degree (which is close to the one in ten estimate), and a third of the latter experience sufficiently severe restriction in activity as to be handicapped. Although such estimates may be crude, the evidence is nevertheless quite sufficient to provide a basis for developing policies to begin confronting this toll.

An approximation to the situation in the world as a whole is offered in Figure 2.1, which shows the underlying causes of disability. The marked difference from the situation in the UK, indicated in Table 2.1, is due to the predominant distribution of the world's population in less developed countries. In fact one-third of those affected are children, and four-fifths of the disabled live in developing countries.

IMPLICATIONS

It can be seen that the total burden in Figure 2.1 is subdivided into three groups of roughly similar size — developmental, acute and chronic conditions, the two former accounting for 64 per cent of the total. A large part

Figure 2.1: Classes of disorder giving rise to disability in the world (from Wood, 1983). (WHO estimate of population affected: 450–500 million)

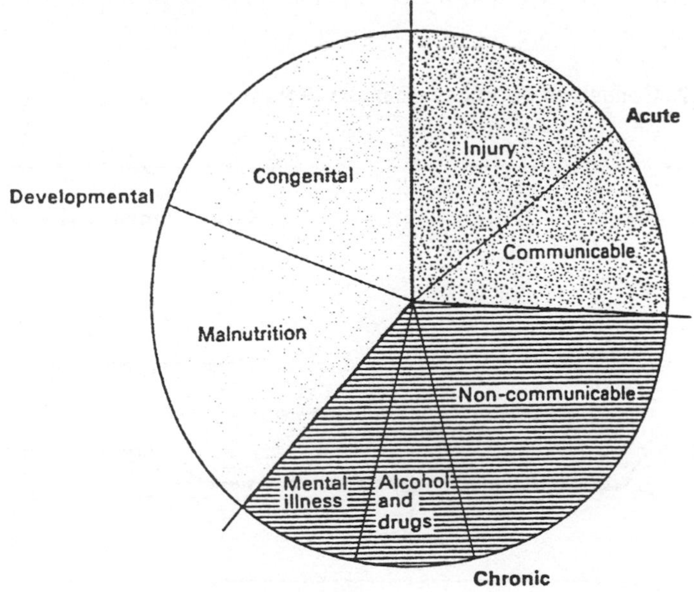

of the developmental and acute conditions could be prevented by application of conventional public health insights, and particularly by immunisation and improved nutrition. Much the biggest challenge, therefore, is to learn more about why what is possible is not put into effect, a conclusion that probably applies with almost as much force to controlling chronic disorders and their consequences in Great Britain as it does to other conditions elsewhere in the world. It is to the possibilities for such control that we shall now turn.

Control of disablement

Individual measures to improve the situation of people with disabilities will be described elsewhere in this book. What is appropriate at this juncture is to appreciate that control of the overall problem can be approached systematically. In order to do this there is one point that requires further clarification. Although the simple sequential model presented earlier might be taken as implying that handicap comes about as a direct result of impairment or disability, the situation is not quite like this.

Impairment and disability give rise to handicap only by the interaction of other influences (Figure 2.2). One of these is the physical environment in which the individual lives. This includes the structure of the dwelling, such as the existence of steps and stairs, as well as more universal features such as the local terrain (e.g. presence of steep hills) and architectural barriers in public buildings. A second is the resources available to the individual, not only in terms of income and material possessions but also personal qualit-

Figure 2.2: Genesis of handicap or disadvantage

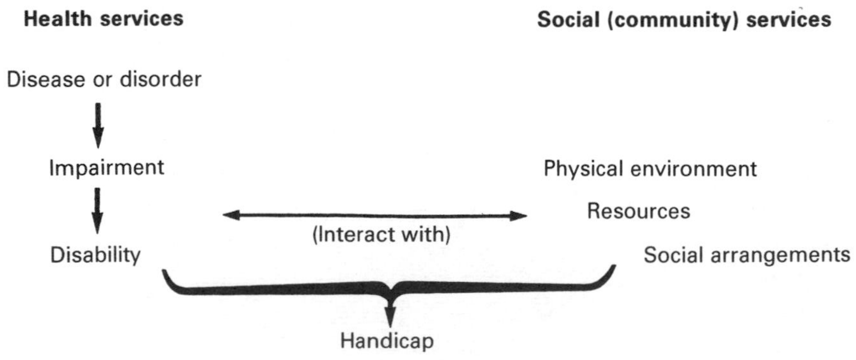

Health services | **Social (community) services**

Disease or disorder
↓
Impairment
↓
Disability

(Interact with) ⟷

Physical environment
Resources
Social arrangements

↓
Handicap

ies, attainments (including occupation), and self-regard, and, in addition, assistance by aids, and support by the family and wider friendship networks. A third class of influence is represented by social arrangements, which include formal services and intangibles such as the attitudes of others (e.g. stigma and stereotyping) and the values of both the immediate and the wider social groupings to which the individual belongs, which influence the expectations of people with disabilities and those who come into contact with them.

Display of such factors (Figure 2.2) promotes identification of alternatives to be considered when appraising control. We have discussed a model for this in its most general form elsewhere (Wood and Badley, 1985), and Table 2.4 presents selective examples relevant to the present context. Health may be promoted in non-specific ways by measures that benefit those without illness as much as the sick. Policies that minimise social disadvantage include broad areas such as urban design, educational and employment opportunities, transport policies and initiatives directed at public attitudes.

In more conventional vein, the most proximal opportunity for control of disablement arises in connection with control of the underlying disorders, an elaboration of which is provided in Table 2.4. This serves to highlight the dependence of 'preventing' disablement on disease prevention and, failing that, on cure or appropriate arrest or medical amelioration of the pathological process. The word 'preventing' has been enclosed in quotation marks because, even though the World Health Organization endorses such usage, to conceive of prevention (in effect, pre-event) once a disease has developed is surely a contradiction in terms.

Figure 2.2 helps to bring out another very important point. The traditional focus of health services has been on individual-oriented measures, ranging from medication (to arrest disease progression) and reconstruction (e.g. hip replacement surgery for someone disabled by coxarthrosis) to functional rehabilitation by means such as remedial therapy. The limitation of this approach is that most serious chronic maladies are not amenable to dramatic and efficacious intervention in this manner, whilst the other options, through welfare services and social policy, have generally tended to be undervalued and neglected — and yet these opportunities have a great potential to minimise disadvantage, even in the face of incurable conditions.

These social initiatives, too often regarded as being beyond medical purview, are admittedly somewhat complex in their organisation, responsibility being split between different agencies. In fact one important source of difficulty is itself the administrative separation from health service arrangements. Moreover, the level of operation is also more varied. For example, there are individual-oriented options, such as provision of an aid, or undertaking adaptation of a dwelling. In addition there are more collect-

Table 2.4: Selected examples from a strategy for the control of disablement (from Wood, 1983)

Primary control (to prevent) — largely a function of social policy, particularly through such means as development of appropriate services

(i) *Health promotion,* which may be:

(a) handicap-oriented (enablement), through urban design (re. isolation), educational and employment opportunities, transport policies, social attitudes, etc.

(b) disease-oriented, through family planning, antenatal care, breast feeding, immunisation, adequate diet, prophylactic replacement (e.g. salt for workers under thermal stress), and physical activity

(ii) *Protection* (hazard containment), which may be:

(a) collective, by repression (e.g. clean water), reduction (speed limits), restriction (sanitation), regulation (alcohol), evasion (pedestrianisation), separation (surgeon's gloves), modification (product design, such as cot slats), and awareness (e.g. domestic illumination) — fuller examples are given in Wood (1983)

(b) individual, by limiting access (such as to domestic fires) and by genetic counselling, contact tracing, avoiding ototoxic drugs, prophylaxis (e.g. penicillin for rheumatic fever), and identification of risk factors

Secondary control (to arrest)

(i) *Reaction* — identifying damage, which is largely a function of social policy

(a) prompt response, such as automobile seatbelts and emergency (rescue) services

(b) screening, for early detection and treatment

(ii) *Stabilisation* — countering damage, related to the availability of health services

(a) cure — many conventional medical initiatives (e.g. hormone replacement)

(b) amelioration — avoiding impairment and disability by arrest of disease progression (part of WHO's first level 'disability prevention')

Tertiary control (to repair) — control of disablement

(i) *Restoration* — control of disability (WHO's second level 'disability prevention'), a function of the availability of health and remedial care

(a) reconstruction (e.g. total hip replacement)

(b) rehabilitation (e.g. remedial services, provision of aids)

(ii) *Maintenance* — control of handicap (WHO's third level 'disability prevention'), largely a function of social policy

(a) continuing care (e.g. monitoring for deterioration)

(b) enablement (e.g. extension of opportunities, vocational resettlement)

(c) support (e.g. welfare provision, assistance, aid to family)

ively arranged options, such as the availability of disability pensions or initiatives to improve town planning or other social policy areas.

If what we have written is seen as a criticism of the orientation of a large part of medical activity, so be it. However, the responsibility can also be seen to rest more squarely on other shoulders, those of the policy-makers and administrators or managers in the different spheres of organisation and government. One of the obstacles to greater enlightenment on the part of these latter individuals has been the confusion in appreciation contributed by concerned physicians. The result has tended to be *ad hoc* collective responses that have been insensitive to the totality of the challenge, ones which at the same time have often promoted inequity between different groups — and inequity can hardly ever be the route to overcome disadvantage. The antidote to all these difficulties must be a framework for comprehending the nature and extent of the challenge, and it is in the spirit of contributing to this endeavour that our appraisal should be seen.

REFERENCES

Badley, E.M., Thompson, R.P. and Wood, P.H.N. (1978) The prevalence and severity of major disabling conditions — a reappraisal of the Government Social Survey of the handicapped and impaired in Great Britain. *Int. J. Epidemiol.*, *7*, 145–51

Harris, A.I. (1971) *Handicapped and impaired in Great Britain*, part 1. Office of Population Censuses and Surveys, Social Survey Division. HMSO, London

Todd, J.W. (1978) Consultant physician to outpatients. *Br. Med. J.*, *1*, 417–20

Wood, P.H.N. (1980) The language of disablement — a glossary relating to disease and its consequences. *Int. Rehabil. Med.*, *2*, 86–92

Wood, P.H.N. (1983) Prospects for control. In J. Wilson (ed.), *Disability prevention, the global challenge.* Leeds Castle Foundation and Oxford University Press, Oxford, chapter 7 (pp. 87–97)

Wood, P.H.N. and Badley, E.M. (1978a) Setting disablement in perspective. *Int. Rehabil. Med.*, *1*, 32–7

Wood, P.H.N. and Badley, E.M. (1978b) An epidemiological appraisal of disablement. In A.E. Bennett (ed.), *Recent advances in community medicine*, no. 1. Churchill Livingstone, Edinburgh, chapter 9 (pp. 149–73)

Wood, P.H.N. and Badley, E.M. (1980) People with disabilities — toward acquiring information which reflects more sensitively their problems and needs. Monograph No 12. World Rehabilitation Fund, New York

Wood, P.H.N. and Badley, E.M. (1985) The origins of ill-health — an appraisal of strategy for health for all and its implications. In A. Smith (ed.), *Recent advances in community medicine*, no. 3. Churchill Livingstone, Edinburgh, chapter 2 (pp. 11–37)

World Health Organization (WHO) (1980) *The international classification of impairments, disabilities, and handicaps — a manual of classification relating to the consequences of disease.* WHO, Geneva

3

Social Factors in Disability

Brian Meredith Davies

It is now widely accepted that social factors play an increasing role in the lives of everyone. But if an individual happens to be disabled, their effect is far more marked. Social factors may produce a great variety of effects in patients who apparently have the same diagnosis and even the same disability. An example is given by anyone who suddenly loses his or her sight as a young adult. Here the disability is constant loss of vision, yet the result in different people will vary considerably. Some will be able to return to work and eventually become totally independent again; but there will be others in whom the result will be totally devastating, they will never work again and their lives will have become completely changed and limited.

The identification of adverse social factors is important because if they can be changed, and their effect diminished, this may well represent the individual's best chance to improve his/her quality of life. Social factors often hold the key to relative success or failure.

Many social factors can have an effect on disability and this is influenced by:

(1) The age of the patient at the onset of disability.

(2) The type of disability, whether it is physically disfiguring, life-threatening, progressive or static, multiple or single. Other important features include whether it involves the special senses or intelligence, or is the result of an accident or illness.

(3) The section of the community to which the individual belongs (social class).

(4) The type of family of the disabled person.

(5) Any features which increase uncertainty are likely to be detrimental.

(6) Various forms of stigma experienced or imagined by the patient and family.

(7) Environmental circumstances — housing, isolation and lack of social life.

SOCIAL FACTORS AND DIFFERING CIRCUMSTANCES

(1) The age of the patient when the disability starts

This is important because it may raise serious doubts as to whether the individual can cope with his/her immediate responsibilities. Equally, disability starting during further education is likely to produce more serious effects than the same starting after the completion of training. A particularly damaging time for any serious disability to start is *early in parenthood*, for the birth and care of young children emphasises how dependent the child is on his/her parents, especially the mother. This can produce an acute feeling of guilt in any mother who suddenly becomes ill and disabled. Such a reaction is not uncommon when rheumatoid arthritis suddenly starts in a woman in the middle or late 20s, by which time she may well have one or two young children. Her problem is well illustrated in the book *Stigma* (Hunt, 1966), where one such patient wrote:

> here I am, a child and husband to care for and starting an incurable disease. I was told to go home and learn to live with it! I went home and quite simply refused to recognise the facts; I was put on steroid treatment, got a measure of relief and pressed on with my household duties, disregarding medical orders to rest.

Later she described how her condition deteriorated so much that she had to be admitted to hospital. This is often a special problem following diagnosis of a serious chronic disability, before the patient has accepted and adjusted to the problem.

To develop any disability in middle age can seem to be 'the last straw' to someone facing many other problems (teenage children, marital problems, menopause, etc.). Again, in retirement, the onset of a disability can seem worse as, in many, the motivation to get back to a normal life is often diminished.

(2) The type of disability

This can be a factor which increases or diminishes social problems. A disability that is physically disfiguring, especially to the face, is always especially difficult. Most of us depend much in our personal relationships on being able to recognise a familiar face. Therefore to a husband or wife it can be an extra problem if your spouse suddenly becomes unrecognisable due to serious scarring after burns. This is especially so when such a disability occurs early in marriage.

Social problems are often greater in a progressive disease (as often occurs in multiple sclerosis) and these are heightened if, in addition, the disease is life-threatening. Part of the social problem is the uncertainty which progressive diseases evoke (see (5) below). *A multiple disability* usually adds to social problems; indeed it may be difficult to identify the main problem, e.g. after a head injury is impairment of mental function or lack of physical coordination the greater drawback?

A special problem follows *accidents, especially if there is a question of compensation.* The same type of disability caused by an illness (i.e. paraplegia) will often lead to fewer problems than one caused by an accident. Indeed, until the compensation question has been resolved it may be impossible to assess accurately the final degree of improvement.

(3) The section of the community the disabled person belongs to (social class)

This can have a bearing on the social problems. In the Black report, 'Inequalities in Health (DHSS, 1980), social class analysis is used extensively to demonstrate the effect of social class on health. Blaxter (1976) showed that the resultant social problems (financial and other), as well as the ability to find solutions, are affected by social class. In elderly disabled patients social class has an even greater effect, particularly in the way they perceive the need for assistance. Townsend and Wedderburn (1965) showed that

> nearly half those in social Class I and II ... already had privately paid for local authority domestic help, and nearly half the others said they needed help. But only a sixth of those in Social Class V who were severely incapacitated had such help and only a fifth of the remainder felt the need of it.

The ability to adjust following severe disability seems greater in Social Class I and II compared with IV and V. Indeed in all aspects those in Social Class I and II are in an advantageous position. The Black report emphasised that the longer the period of incapacity the less likely it is that the sick person will be able to return to the same type of work with the same employer. Skilled manual workers are more likely to have their jobs kept open for them than are semi-skilled or unskilled workers. The conclusion reached was 'Clearly, in considering the needs of the disabled long term sick, and aged infirm, *financial problems and problems of subsequent re-employment are both pertinent and class related.*'

(4) The family of any disabled person is always a crucial factor

To have an understanding family is a tremendous asset, but a caring family is not always the one which best understands the problems of disability. Indeed a very caring family may overprotect the disabled person, and that can be a serious disadvantage. Such overprotection is commonly seen at the onset of any disabling condition, and especially when disability starts in late middle life or in retirement. Overprotection is also a problem with the young person who has been disabled since childhood, and where no effort has been made to ensure the child has mixed with normal children during education. In the middle-aged adult a particular problem can be a suggestion from relatives that the disabled person now should be considered elderly when actually he/she is in the 40s or 50s!

When the main wage-earner of the family becomes disabled, social problems usually increase. The family in which both husband and wife work are less at risk compared with the family with only one wage-earner. *One-parent families are always at special risk.*

It is always important to look upon the family as a single unit for the social problems will often involve all members of the family. *Children can become handicapped by the disability of a parent, but equally by the birth of a disabled child*, or the development in a child of a disabling condition, can quickly lead to serious problems for the parents and even to the breakup of a marriage. Tew and Laurence (1973), in their controlled survey in Bristol with families with spina bifida, found there was a marked increase in marital breakdowns in families with an affected child. Only one in four of such families were free from marital difficulties, and relationship between the parents tended to deteriorate over the years. *The divorce rate was twice that in the control group.*

(5) Social factors

Any social factor *which increases uncertainty* will make it more difficult to overcome the adverse effects of disability, for uncertainty about employment or financial matters can be very damaging. This is especially so if the medical prognosis is doubtful, i.e. multiple sclerosis. It is important that any natural anxiety and apprehension are brought to the surface, and the only effective way to do this is to discuss such matters with the patient. *One should never be afraid of too much communication with a disabled person*, for this is a lifeline to the insecure, and any disabled individual fearful and apprehensive about his/her future is certainly insecure.

Stigma

Many different forms of stigma are still felt by a number of people and their families. This stigma is felt or assumed and even when exaggerated, as may often be the case, will quickly provide a barrier between the disabled person and the rest of the community, leading to isolation and bitterness, both serious problems in themselves.

Environmental social factors

Environmental and social factors such as inadequate housing and consequent lack of mobility are insidious problems, for so often they begin as minor inconveniences and eventually become major problems as the patient gets older and frailer. They may determine the patient's eventual lifestyle. Many people in their 80s who have even minor disabilities find that it is the combination of adverse housing conditions and their disability which makes it impossible for them to remain in their own home. This means they have to enter some residential home or nursing home when they would much prefer to remain in their own home. It is most important to realise that the *best chance of overcoming adverse environmental conditions lies early in the disability* for, if delay occurs, *options contract* and the person gradually becomes more resistant to change.

CONSEQUENCES OF SOCIAL FACTORS IN DISABILITY

Barriers to recovery are usually increased by adverse social factors. If total recovery is not possible, social factors can be particularly important for, if they can be improved, the quality of life of the disabled person will be enhanced; but the reverse is equally true. However, the problem is rarely a simple one, for *the attitude of the individual is all-important.* It is all too easy to accept defeat in the face of adverse social factors when a more positive approach would succeed. Too often *self-pity, social isolation or overprotection* dominate and these, in the end, can be more damaging than the original poor environmental or other social factors.

EFFECT OF DISABILITY ON DISABLED PERSONS

It is important to consider the interplay between social factors and their personal effect on those who are disabled. The following are crucial;

(1) Confidence in the future

It is not always easy for a disabled person to feel confident about the future, but to achieve anything in life one first must implicitly believe it is possible. Hence a belief in one's ability to overcome problems is always an advantage.

Another way of expressing this is to emphasise that optimism and enthusiasm are prerequisites to success or, at the other end of the scale, pessimism is often a harbinger of failure.

In practice, confidence in the future can quickly evaporate unless the disabled person realises three factors:

(a) that minor setbacks are inevitable, and an ability to overcome them must be developed;

(b) success is usually a slow process and only comes after many failures;

(c) that recovery and rehabilitation are rarely steady and continuous. A far more usual pattern is a long period of slow gradual improvement in function, often punctuated by minor setbacks, until quite suddenly there is a dramatic advance in the disabled person's function.

(2) Motivation

Motivation is so important in any disabling condition, and can help reduce discomfort and improve function. It is also important for the disabled person to understand as much as possible about the disabling condition, the reasons for symptoms and how to diminish them. Many disabled people never understand the principles of care, and how much depends on achieving the right balance between rest and activity. Too many individuals, particularly if they are retired, do not realise that, although rest may be essential in the acute or early stages of a disability, it can be overdone. Consequential limitation of function can be the result. It is rarely sensible for such an old person to give up all forms of activity or recreation which have in the past been enjoyed, just because now some pain or discomfort is experienced. It is far better to prescribe a simple analgesic, and explain to the patient that the recreation can do no permanent damage and will help to maintain physical function.

It is often helpful if the disabled person is both determined and even obstinate in insisting on keeping going, even to the extent of rejecting any unhelpful professional advice concerning the restriction of various activities.

(3) Social isolation

Social isolation can easily follow any disability, and can produce as many or more problems than the original condition. There are many insidious ways this can develop:

(a) The physical problems of caring for the disabled person can become all-absorbing and time-consuming, so that the husband and wife looking after their disabled spouse now have no time or energy left to meet people or to carry out their normal social functions. Any such household quickly becomes very isolated, particularly if there is no close family living nearby to insist on sharing the problem. Various forms of '*respite care*', where sitters-in can help or where the patient goes into some temporary respite home for a short period, can be a great help.

(b) Feelings of guilt and shame can be important causes of social isolation. It is curious how embarrassed many patients feel when the cause of their disability is an illness rather than an accident. Margaret

Mayson, who developed rheumatoid arthritis when aged 26, writing in the book *Stigma*, described how sensitive she became to comments about her crutches.

When an acquaintance, completely uninhibited herself, called out 'Whatever is the matter with you?' I muttered 'It's just arthritis', feeling thoroughly ashamed. I would have felt quite happy to be able to say I'd broken a leg ski-ing or riding, because a healthy body temporarily maimed is very different from a body affected by a progressively crippling disease. A child's remark, 'Why is that lady in a push-chair?' did not worry me, but my son at 8 years old was embarrassed. 'Silly nit', was his terse comment. I sought to mollify his feelings at being singled out as a child whose mother was 'different' and, in doing so, became myself less sensitive to my disabilities.'

The value of bringing problems to the surface is obvious, and day care can be useful in this respect. To be forced to meet many different people is always helpful in maintaining a balanced and, if possible, humorous view of life. It can be of value to meet the occasional person who is more seriously disabled than oneself, for it helps to reduce *self-pity*, which can be so destructive;

(c) *One factor which quickly leads to social isolation is limitation of mobility*, and everything must be done early in any disability to combat immobility. In particular, anticipation of future difficulties is essential. Any patient having *mobility problems will be at greater risk as they grow older*, therefore environmental factors such as housing should be carefully considered at an early stage. This means either ground floor accommodation or a flat reached by a lift. A house will be all right if the ground floor has an extra room which can serve as a bedroom, and has a downstairs w.c. and at least a shower. It is also an advantage if a car can reach the front door, so that friends and family can take out the disabled person much more easily. This is particularly important with elderly disabled people.

(4) Family problems

Human relationships, especially within the family, are very important to a disabled person. One hears so many professionals advising 'independence', yet what is really more valuable is 'interdependence', where the disabled person becomes a useful contributing member of the family. It is therefore always helpful to search for ways in which *the disabled person can actively help*, for example babysitting, taking messages (being on call), book-keeping, etc. It is balance between caring and independence which is difficult to get right; far too many families smother the disabled person with overprotection.

(5) The importance of a positive attitude

Reference has already been made to the adverse effect of uncertainty which results in a negative attitude: if the future is so uncertain why bother to train for some job or to take up some new recreation or even start an adult education course, for what use will it be? Although such an attitude is understandable, there is little justification for such a negative view. The expectation of life for many disabled people may be little different from anyone else. Everything should be done to encourage a positive approach, particularly early in the disability, and it is always of value to discuss this aspect with the patient at an early stage.

Political overtones enter into this field. Because of the inequality and stigma there is a tendency for all radicals in politics to champion the cause of the disabled as the underdog. This is not always helpful, as it tends to increase the division in society to confirm that disabled people are different and shoud be prepared to accept a lower standard of life. Many of the most damaging aspects of disability would probably still be present even if political changes were to introduce some overall benefit or pension for disabled people. This would certainly help in many instances, although even if financial difficulties could be eased, many other serious social problems would remain. *It is the lack of choice* (which so often is the result of shortage of money) that is most damaging, for to be unable to make choices emphasises that one is not as independent as others. It is for this reason that professionals should always *search for ways which will encourage disabled persons to make choices.*

SOCIAL FACTORS AND THE DOCTOR TREATING THE DISABLED PERSON

It is when radical treatment of the underlying cause of the patient's disability comes to an end that some doctors adopt a wrong attitude. In an attempt to be realistic, the patient is told 'Well, there is little more that I can do for you, you'll just have to get used to living with your disability'. This is most unhelpful to disabled people and their families, as well as being untrue. Every doctor must know where specialist medical rehabilitation advice is available in the area, and where to contact other Health and Social Services for help.

It is impossible to overemphasise that doctors are always responsible not only for arranging the appropriate medical treatment but for ensuring that the patient is helped to overcome adverse social factors.

IMPORTANCE OF APPROACH AND ATTITUDE OF THE DOCTOR

The approach and attitude of any doctor towards the disabled person is crucial, especially at their first meeting. It is at this stage that it is so important for the doctor to listen to what the patient has to say, for what is required is not only an accurate assessment of the various signs and symptoms, and the making of a diagnosis, but identification of the main fears and worries of the individual and family. This process takes time, and it is here that many doctors working in primary health care fail.

The next stage is for a *plan of action* to be drawn up by the doctor and other professionals working with the patient and family. It is here that every effort should be made to leave final choices of the various options open to the disabled person, for if he/she feels the plan has been developed with his/her help, success is far more likely. The various social problems which must be overcome are usually complex, and it always helps to remember that disability is a continuum, as so correctly emphasised in the Warnock report of 1978. This really means that it is only possible to plan properly the care of any disabled person if future problems and difficulties are anticipated. The young adult disabled will gradually become a middle-aged person, and eventually an elderly one. Consequently new problems will occur, and *the best way of reducing them is by advice, early in their development.*

IMPORTANCE OF CHOICE AND ANTICIPATION OF FUTURE PROBLEMS

It is always of value to encourage the disabled person and family to anticipate new problems and then to choose the best solutions. Take the example of trying to find the ideal accommodation for any disabled person with a mobility problem. A specially built bungalow may not turn out to be the best solution if it is situated in the wrong area and is cut off from family and friends. The disabled person must make the final choice without any undue pressure. The patient will be motivated to ensure it becomes a success. It is always easier to criticise and resent other people's choices rather than one's own.

Although this book is about disabled adults, a few will have been handicapped from childhood. In these people there is a marked tendency for the parents, especially the mother, to continue to adopt a very protective attitude even when they become adults. Although this is natural initially, it becomes more and more restrictive and impractical as the disabled person reaches adult life. If no steps are taken to alter such a parental attitude, new social problems will eventually emerge. Because of the differences in age between the disabled young adult and his/her parents (usually between 25 and 35 years), as the years slip by, it becomes increasingly obvious that the parents will not be able always to go on looking after their son/daughter. A number of dedicated parents fall into this trap and, as they reach the age of 70-plus, become increasingly anxious about the future care of their disabled son or daughter, who is probably aged between 30 and 45 years. *Such a problem can only be prevented by anticipation, and by doing everything possible to encourage the young disabled person to become independent when he/she is aged between 20 and 30.* Various forms of specially designed or sheltered housing can enable the young persons to set up their own home, either alone or with a friend, especially if day care services also assist by training and helping to support the individual (see Chapter 37). Such a move is very helpful as it emphasises normality; many able-bodied young people move away from home at this time of life and it allows the young disabled person to mature and develop in a more normal way, as well as ensuring there will never be an acute crisis to solve as an ageing parent suddenly becomes ill or infirm and can no longer cope.

If nothing is done the inevitable result will be a sudden emergency admission of the young disabled person to some home or even chronic hospital, which is probably the very last thing the parents or son/daughter wanted, and such a move often results in an embittered disabled person.

PROFESSIONAL COORDINATION

One of the best ways to ensure that careful anticipation of future problems takes place is to arrange *regular professional coordination meetings,* and not to wait for a crisis situation. The case conference can be of particular value in continuing-care situations, in anticipating problems and in finding solutions. This is because all of the professionals attending tend to concentrate on different aspects. Such meetings are also most helpful in demonstrating to other professionals (including doctors) the various social aspects of disability. As wide a group of professionals as possible should attend — consultant or registrar, doctor in primary health care, health visitor, district nurse, hospital and district occupational therapist, physiotherapist, hospital and district social worker.

Lack of coordination results in much misery to which professionals may unknowingly contribute by failing to play their part in coordination. This is the crucial mistake, for even when dealing with the most severely disabled person, whose mobility is grossly limited and who may be suffering from an irreversible disability such as tetraplegia, much can be done to reduce the social problems the individual and the family have to face. Many of the solutions may not be medical ones, but *their effect upon the disabled person can be very important in determining quality of life.* It is for this reason that all doctors, whether working in primary health care or in hospital, should always seek the help of other professionals, such as social workers, who can be of help to these patients and their families.

REFERENCES

Blaxter, M. (1976) *The meaning of disability*, Heinemann, London

DHSS (1980) *Inequalities in health* (Black report), HMSO, London

Hunt, P. (1966) *Stigma — the experience of disability*, Geoffrey Chapman, London

Mayson, Margaret (1966) *Essay in stigma*, Geoffrey Chapman, London

Tew, B. (1974) Special education, *Forward Trends*, *1* (2) (June)

Tew, B. and Laurence, K.M. (1973) Mothers, brothers and sisters of patients with spina bifida. *Developmental and Medical Neurology*, (Suppl.) *29*, 69-76

Townsend, P. and Wedderburn, D. (1965) The aged in the Welfare State, *Bell Occasional Papers on Social Administration*

Warnock report (1978) *Special educational needs*, Cmnd 7212, HMSO, London

4

Psychological Aspects of Disability

Anthony Coughlan

INTRODUCTION

The way in which people react to acquiring a disability, and the extent to which they adjust to it (i.e. feel that they continue to lead a reasonably worthwhile and fulfilling life) varies enormously from person to person. This chapter attempts to outline the major factors that influence people's reactions and their abilities to adjust. These will be considered under the following headings:

Nature of the disability:
- (a) type
- (b) severity
- (c) mode of onset, knowledge and expectations
- (d) progression

Personality:
- (a) coping style
- (b) self-image and self-esteem

Brain damage (if applicable):
- (a) personality change
- (b) cognitive change
- (c) denial/neglect

Reaction of others
Supportive network
Financial security
Quality of professional care

NATURE OF THE DISABILITY

The nature of the disability comprises four components: (a) type — e.g. blindness, paraplegia, ataxia; (b) severity; (c) mode of onset — acute or gradual; (d) progression — improvement, static, intermittent decline or steady decline. These components will each have an effect on how the person reacts and copes. Different conditions involve these components to differing degrees, so it is not possible here to give anything other than broad accounts of their effects.

(a) Type

Each type of disability brings its peculiar hindrances to everyday life and gives rise to frustration with the consequent likelihood of irritability, impatience and outbursts of anger or tearfulness. Over time, as the person learns new ways of carrying out old tasks or adopts routines that circumvent some of the difficulties, these reactions will subside, though some particular difficulties may always remain irksome and a cause of irritation. In addition to the general frustrations specific occupational or recreational activities will be precluded by particular disabilities, leading possibly to a sense of loss of fulfilment, loss of self-esteem and feelings of isolation. For some people there may also be a strong interaction between the type of disability and their self-esteem in that particular disabilities are intensely threatening to their views of themselves as worthwhile. In such instances problems in adjustment are likely to occur. This is further discussed in the section on personality factors.

(b) Severity

As a general rule the more severe the disablement the more frustration it will give rise to, and the greater is the likelihood that occupational or recreational activities will be affected. In some instances independent living will be rendered difficult or impossible, giving rise to a variety of adverse feelings, but particularly those of lowered self-esteem and vulnerability. Nonetheless, many people — after an initial period of shock, anger, despair and frustration — bear severe disablement with great fortitude and dignity, whilst others may seem devastated by relatively trivial handicaps and be preoccupied by them. These differences arise predominantly through the interaction of the type and severity of the condition with the robustness of the person's personality, and with his/her self-image.

(c) Mode of onset, knowledge of condition and expectations

With acute onset the sufferer is confronted with a sudden alteration in circumstances. This can produce a variety of reactions — most commonly shock, bewilderment and disbelief — and may result in a state of mental numbness akin to that experienced by people who lose a loved one through sudden bereavement. This phase is likely to be followed by one of anxiety and uncertainty when a multitude of thoughts, worries and fantasies about the future will occur: 'will I recover?', 'how will I cope with my job?', 'what will others think of me?', 'am I going to be in a wheelchair for life?', 'how will my family cope?', 'will I ever find a boyfriend if I've got this?', 'will my wife stick by me?', 'will I need an operation?'. The extent to which these anxieties can be dispelled will vary from condition to condition, and with the individual's circumstances. In the early stages prognosis may well be unclear and uncertainty unavoidable.

With gradual onset much will depend on the type and severity of the condition and the person's knowledge of the condition. There may be a period of diagnostic investigations that may give rise to optimism that a cure will be available, and/or anxiety that something dire will be revealed. If no cure is available the effect of this information may well be to produce feelings of shock similar to those in the acute conditions, although some degree of uncertainty will be alleviated. If the condition is a progressive one (e.g. multiple sclerosis or motor neurone disease) the reaction will also be influenced by the information given. If a diagnostic label is provided the person's knowledge and/or fantasies about the condition will be important. Many people harbour notions about the way a condition might progress that may be quite unrealistic. In some instances an unrealistically rosy view may serve as a defence against anxiety, and the costs and benefits of introducing realism have to be carefully considered. In other cases there will be fears about unpleasant developments that are unlikely or impossible, and these will give rise to much unnecessary anxiety. It is important to be on the lookout and probe for such fears as they are not always volunteered, especially in busy clinics.

(d) Progression

If improvement occurs the person may be left with no disability or only a residual one. In such cases the anxieties and the uncertainties following the onset will usually disappear and a return to the normal emotional state will take place. However, some people will find themselves destabilised by the event. This may take the form of a specific anxiety about a recurrence (whether or not the likelihood of this is clear from the medical evidence) or a more general neurotic disturbance, possibly arising from notions of vulnerability, reduced control over one's own fate and the threat to the self-image if there was a recurrence.

If permanent disability ensues the person is faced with having to adapt to the altered circumstances. There may be difficulties at the practical level, the social (see Reactions of Others) and the psychological. Many people will show great fortitude in making such adaptations, but even so there will almost always be periods of frustration, doubt and despair. This phase has been likened to the period of mourning that follows a bereavement, the person in this instance mourning the loss of part of his identity and having to be reconciled with continuing life without it. The duration of this 'mourning' will vary enormously from person to person but, as in normal bereavement, can often be made more constructive and less overwhelming by counselling. However, for some people a frank depressive illness may develop during the mourning phase and warrant treatment with antidepressant medication. Motivation will be variable during the mourning phase, but improve as it is passed through, and eventually a more realistic state should be reached in which the person acknowledges his limitations but is able to maintain a more positive approach to learning any necessary new skills and to preparing for an altered lifestyle. A few people will never emerge from the mourning phase despite continued efforts by family, friends and professionals, and may become locked in protracted unhappiness, self-pity, withdrawal or difficult (usually demanding or irritable) behaviour. For such people it is likely that the self-esteem is so strongly bound up in a particular rigid self-image that deviations from this image are too threatening.

For those who are faced with a *progressive condition* reaction will be influenced by the person's expectations concerning the condition (whether true or false), the stage (or severity) that the condition has reached, the rate of decline and whether it is steady or intermittent. Many of the progressive disabling conditions are neurological, and involve some cerebral deterioration in their later stages, so that reaction will also depend on organic changes in personality and emotional state. It is therefore difficult to make more than vague general statements about the course of the reaction to progressive conditions, and the following comments must be seen as such. Bouts of depression or anxiety are likely to occur throughout the course of the condition as long as insight is preserved, and will often follow a deterioration in the condition. Frustration is likely to increase with deterioration in the condition. However, a progressive condition also affords opportunity to prepare psychologically for deterioration. The expectation of decline may enable the person to prepare for increasing loss of independence and increased reliance on practical aids and assistance from others, as well as to prepare for changes in lifestyle. Imaginary rehearsal of 'what it will be like' may occur, allowing the person to work through some of the emotional discomfort in advance of the event, so that it is less acute when deterioration actually takes place. Again, here there may be a parallel with bereavement processes in that some people are able to make a reasonably swift adjustment to bereavement, having cared for the dying person and completed some of the mourning in advance. Others may cope with impending deterioration by denial or minimisation of its likelihood, believing or hoping that they will be the ones for whom the condition takes the most mild course, or for whom a cure will eventually be found. Some may go searching for cures, either trying fad treatments they hear about via friends and the media, or visiting a string of specialists in the hope of obtaining a more satisfactory prognosis.

PERSONALITY

(a) Coping style

It is to be expected that people will generally react to, and cope with, disability in accord with their usual methods of dealing with stressful situations. Thus, after the initial shock and uncertainty, those who are vulnerable to depression or anxiety are likely to lapse into depressed or anxious states; those that pride themselves on being independent or have a low tolerance to frustration may display considerable anger or irritation; those who have always tended to minimise or deny difficulties may become unrealistic about their limitations or spend considerable amounts of time unrealistically seeking cures; and those that habitually bear adversity with fortitude will on the whole show determination to overcome their new problems. For some people, however, the constitutional method of coping with stress may be unusable as regards disability, or incapable of dealing with the magnitude of the event. A tendency to ignore, deny or walk away from stressful experiences may sometimes be impossible to maintain with a disability that confronts the person 24 hours a day, and common fortitude may be defeated by the severity of disability. The result may be bursts of neurotic behaviour as the person oscillates between maintaining his normal coping style and feeling overwhelmed by a situation that cannot be escaped.

(b) Self-image and self-esteem

The extent to which disability disrupts a person's self-image, and thereby his self-esteem, is probably the most important factor in determining how the person copes with disability. Each person has a view of himself, his perceptions of his physical and cognitive attributes, of his character, of his achievements and of his relationships with others. By self-image is meant his evaluation of himself, based on these perceptions, on a multitude of dimensions. These dimensions can be considered as descriptive bipolar scales, such as 'good–bad', 'strong–weak', 'lucky–unlucky'. By self-esteem is meant that part of his evaluation that is based on the dimensions that he considers particularly important, i.e. on those dimensions that relate to his sense of intrinsic worth. Which dimensions a person considers to be important will vary from individual to individual, being a reflection of the many influences and experiences that over the years have helped shape the person's personality. However, common ones are 'attractive–unattractive', 'strong–weak', 'clever–stupid', 'masculine–feminine', 'competent–incompetent', 'interesting–dull', 'sexually desirable–sexually undesirable', 'independent–dependent', 'important–insignificant' and 'successful–unsuccessful'. The set of dimensions that contribute most to the person's self-esteem will be referred to as 'core' dimensions. It is essential to realise that how a person relates particular physical and cognitive attributes, particular aspects of character, and particular achievements and relationships to points on any dimension is an idiosyncratic matter. Thus physical strength and financial success may be associated with being highly sexually desirable, competent and clever for one person but not for another. It is also the case that a person's rating of himself on a particular dimension may bear little relationship to any objective assessment or how other people would evaluate him. Thus two people may obtain equal examination results or be equally attractive to a third person, but may well evaluate themselves very differently on the 'clever–stupid' and 'attractive–unattractive' dimensions.

Whilst being aware of some aspects of themselves they might wish to change, most people have a generally positive self-esteem, i.e. they have a sense of intrinsic worth as human beings, although the intensity and robustness of this positive self-image will vary from person to person. If particular physical or cognitive attributes, aspects of character, achievements or relationships with others are associated with strong positive evaluations on core dimensions then loss or impairment of these will probably be associated with strong negative evaluations. Such losses or impairments will then give rise to a devalued self-esteem, i.e. a devaluation of one's sense of intrinsic worth. If substantial devaluation occurs then a negative self-esteem, i.e. a loss of one's sense of intrinsic worth, will result and emotional disturbance is likely to arise. This will often take the form of depression, but may take other forms such as anger, irritability or generally difficult and erratic behaviour.

Disability can disrupt a person's self-esteem if the person holds stereotyped views about disabled people or people with particular disabilities, so that such people are generally viewed by the person as rating poorly on his core dimensions. Stereotypes get built up over the years, and will contain the person's knowledge, fears and fantasies about different disabilities as derived from experience, education, gossip and media coverage, and from society's and peer-group values. These stereotypes may differ from disability to disability, or all be rather similar, coming under an umbrella stereotype of 'disabled' with little differentiation between conditions. Many of these stereotypes may well have considerable negative connotations and so be viewed with unease or distaste by the person. If the person then acquires a disability that he has endowed with strong negative connotations it will be difficult for him to maintain a positive self-esteem.

Self-esteem is nonetheless still vulnerable to disability in persons who have no strong stereotyped notions about disabled people. Self-image will probably be altered by the disability, but whether self-esteem is affected depends on whether the disability involves those cognitive attributes that the person values most, i.e. those that are related to strong positive evaluations on his core dimensions. (The difference between this and holding a stereotype is that the person may not regard other disabled people with the same disability as himself in a negative way, but nonetheless has negative views of himself because of his disability.) As noted earlier, it is an idiosyncratic matter as to which physical and cognitive attributes contribute most to a person's sense of worth, and so individuals will vary as to how any particular disability affects the self-image and self-esteem. An important corollary of this is that a mild disability in one sphere may be more devastating to a person's self-esteem than a severe disability in another. For example, if a person places high value on verbal skills because they imply for him cleverness, competence and strength, then a mild dysphasia, causing hesitancy in speech and occasional muddling of words, will give rise to feelings of stupidity, incompetence and weakness, and may cause him more distress than loss of use of a hand. Of course, the loss of a hand is unlikely to be received lightly, but the person will come to terms with his loss more quickly, and whilst he might suffer periodic frustration because of the limitations the loss imposes, it will not devalue his sense of worth or prevent him from feeling he can lead a fulfilling life to the same extent as the dysphasia will. For another person the reverse may obtain; a substantial dysphasia will be reasonably well tolerated but partial functioning of the hand will be viewed as a major catastrophe.

The effect of disability on self-esteem may be a direct or indirect one. Some physical or cognitive attributes may be valued for their own sake; e.g. a person may associate physical mobility with independence and arithmetical ability with competence, so that loss or impairment of these attributes leads directly to a devaluation in self-esteem. Indirect effects arise when the disability interrupts some other aspect of life that contributes strongly to self-esteem. For example the person may set great store by success in business or athletic prowess, maybe associating these with masculinity, and so any disablement that prevents these achievements will lead to a devaluation in self-esteem. Of course, prevention of these achievements may have other implications, such as future financial problems or loss of social contacts which in themselves will be a cause for concern. However, it is important not to overlook the self-esteem component: it may be this which underlies any problems in long-term adjustment.

The extent to which self-esteem can remain preserved following a particular physical or cognitive disability will depend on how many other things contribute to the person's self-esteem (aspects of character, achievements, relationships and other physical and cognitive attributes) and remain intact. The more that do so, the less devastating the particular loss or impairment will be, i.e. it is helpful if the person does not have all his self-esteem 'eggs' in one basket. Counselling may assist the person to modify his self-image and to become more flexible as to those aspects that constitute self-esteem, and thereby help the person to regain some fulfilment in life. However, some people will maintain a very rigid and narrow view of what attributes make them worthwhile, and be impervious to counselling, possibly resenting any attempt to encourage them to examine their view.

Disablement may also cause disruption to a person's self-esteem by preventing the person from realising his fantasies or ambitions. Fantasies and ambitions may be dispensable for many people, in that fantasies may be accepted as unattainable dreams, and in that the goals or ambitions, although desired, do not have the status of personal necessities — i.e. if they fail to be realised they would probably not greatly detract from self-esteem. For some people, however, fantasies or ambitions may act as a defence against a weak or negative self-esteem — 'there may not be much to me at the moment, but one day . . .', i.e. self-esteem would be greatly enhanced by their realisation. If loss or impairment of a physical or cognitive attribute necessary to the realisation of such a fantasy or ambition occurs then, whether the fantasy or ambition had any chance of success or not, the person's defence against his negative self-esteem will be reduced and problems in adjustment may follow.

BRAIN DAMAGE (see Chapter 24)

Brain damage can be a direct cause of disability (e.g. head injury or stroke) or a feature of a more general condition that gives rise to disability (e.g. multiple sclerosis). In either case the brain damage may affect how the person reacts to the disability. The main ways in which the effect operates are:

(a) Personality change

Personality change can constitute a major disability in its own right, but it may also colour the reaction to other disabilities. Amongst the common changes are (1) an increase in irritability or shortness of temper resulting in the person becoming less tolerant of the frustrations of disability; (2) an increased tendency to worry or to become absorbed in one's own problems so that the person becomes preoccupied with the difficulties caused by the disability; (3) an increased disposition to depression so that in the case of progressive disability deterioration will be harder to bear; (4) rigidity of thought may occur so that the person becomes less flexible in approach to problems caused by the disability and less amenable to practical advice or counselling. In some cases, however, most noticeably those involving frontal lobe damage, the change may give rise to (5) emotional blunting or euphoria so that the person, although aware of the disability and the limitations caused by it, seems to lack appropriate concern. This could perhaps be confused with a good adjustment to the disability if it were not for the fact that the lack of concern will extend to many other problems that might confront the person, and there will be a lack of motivation to deal with them. In addition other aspects of the 'frontal-lobe syndrome' may well be present, such as contented apathy, impulsivity and disinhibition. In cases of very severe disablement lack of concern may be regarded as a blessing, but it will also mean that in instances where remedial therapy could potentially make a useful impact there will be a lack of motivation to engage. This type of personality change is often seen with head injuries. It may also occur in progressive conditions, for example in the later stages of multiple sclerosis where it sometimes supersedes an earlier depressive change.

(b) Cognitive change

It is often difficult to demarcate between the effects of cognitive impairment and personality change on reaction to disability. The more severe the brain damage the more both are likely to be present. In addition some changes occasioned by brain damage, such as lack of insight, lack of judgement and rigidity of thought, appear to lie across the personality/cognitive boundary. That being said, severe generalised cognitive impairment may be associated with lack of insight into the extent of disability, or with reduced awareness of the limitations it imposes. Nonetheless there may be considerable frustration expressed at those aspects of the disability that the person is aware of, though motivation to engage in remedial therapy may be lacking either because of personality change or the person's intellectual grasp of the situation. Severe speech or memory problems may also cause problems in remedial therapy because the person is unable to comprehend or remember instructions.

(c) Denial/neglect

Substantial cerebral lesions that involve the parietal lobes can produce a lack of awareness of contralateral paralysis or visual field impairment. In severe instances there will be denial that a paralysed limb is paralysed; confrontation will usually elicit further denial, perplexity or some excuse that the limb is only temporarily out of action. There will also be marked neglect of the half of space contralateral to the lesion (virtually always in association with a hemianopia); in the more severe cases half of the body may remain ungroomed and food on one half of the plate will remain unseen and uneaten. In most cases the denial of paralysis disappears fairly rapidly (usually within a month or so of, say, a severe stroke) but neglect of the half of space tends to be more persistent, and the person may spend some weeks or months bumping into things on the affected side, 'losing' things that have been placed there or misreading the beginnings or ends of words and sentences (depending on which is the affected side). In most cases the person gradually becomes aware of the problem and learns to compensate for the hemianopia by turning the head in the appropriate direction.

REACTIONS OF OTHERS

The reaction of family, friends and other acquaintances, e.g. work colleagues, will have an important bearing on how the person copes. Generally, the closer the relationship the more important the reaction of the other person will be. If the person is accepted by others despite his disability then this will help maintain his self-esteem, although sometimes even the most sincere and committed efforts by those with the closest relationship are insufficient to overcome a severe loss of self-esteem. However, if the person meets with rejection then self-esteem is, not surprisingly, liable to be devalued. Rejection at a sexual level may be particularly dispiriting (and frustrating). Some people find disablement in others renders them sexually unattractive, and so although they may wish to continue living with and caring for their disabled partner they feel unable or unwilling to indulge in a sexual relationship. The sexual problems that arise through disablement are dealt with in detail elsewhere in this volume (Chapter 30).

Those with close relationships to the disabled person, i.e. spouses, parents or children, are likely to be the ones that care for him if the disablement necessitates this. Mostly this care is carried out with understanding and good grace, but sometimes the carer feels overburdened or unjustly burdened. If such feelings are communicated to the disabled person he in turn is likely to feel guilty, insecure or rejected. Sometimes, however, the disabled person feels rejected despite no such communication from the carers: this can arise because the person had a low self-esteem or was prone to anxiety before the onset of disablement or has developed these features since. Overprotection or overcaring is another way in which those who care for the disabled sometimes react. This may arise through pity, a desire not to see the disabled person suffer any more, through concern that the person might become more disabled or die (e.g. if the person has suffered a heart attack or stroke), or through an attempt to assuage feelings of guilt that one's actions or negligence caused or contributed to the disability. Unless the disabled person enjoys a dependent and fussed-over existence, overprotection will tend to foster anger and irritation.

Often non-disabled people *feel uncomfortable* when talking to disabled people because they find the disability repulsive, or because they feel great pity and therefore don't know what to say, or because they are afraid they may say something which will be upsetting, such as talking about enjoyable activities that the disabled person is unable to indulge in. Some non-disabled people will deal with their feelings by avoiding disabled people, looking away from them, ignoring them in conversation or talking to them in a patronising manner. These actions are likely to give rise to feelings of rejection and anger in the disabled person. As time goes on the non-disabled person may overcome his discomfort, and interaction will be less painful for both. However, further awkward encounters may become a long-term hazard for the disabled people as they encounter new people. For some it may always rankle, whilst others will rightly interpret it as a problem of the non-disabled person, and either ignore it or actively seek to put the non-disabled person at ease.

SUPPORTIVE NETWORK

The more severe the disability the more likely the person will have to give up his occupation or leisure activities. This will considerably reduce his opportunities for social interaction and may therefore lead to social isolation. If mobility is substantially impaired then opportunities for socialising will be further reduced in that visits to relatives and friends, to shops, pubs, meetings, theatres, etc., will become difficult or impossible and the person will be reliant on the efforts of others for social contact. The existence of a supportive network of family and close friends may then be vital to preserving social contact. The visits from work colleagues and friends made through specific leisure pursuits are liable to tail off over the course of a year whilst relatives and long-standing friends, assuming they live reasonably close at hand, tend to be the more persistent visitors. People vary in how much they value social contact, but for those to whom it is important, but who unfortunately lack nearby close friends and relatives, feelings of loneliness, boredom and even worthlessness may result. Many will deal with these problems by attendance at day centres, but for some this will be an unacceptable solution as mixing with other disabled people will be seen as distasteful or second-best, and be more threatening to self-esteem than the loneliness.

Depending on the nature and the severity of disablement there may be partial or total dependence on others for the needs of everyday living such as shopping, cooking, cleaning and self-care. Those with a supportive network of family and/or close friends are likely to be more able to remain living at home, either with their family or by themselves, and so despite the dependence there will be opportunity to retain as much home comforts, community contact and independence as possible — all of which will help to preserve a sense of well-being. For those without family or friends to help out there may be no alternative but to give up their home and accept residential care within Social Services or the NHS, a move which may be strongly resented or resisted.

Reactions to dependence are likely to be mixed. Dependence may be resented because it devalues the self-esteem or because it makes the person feel a burden to others (whether or not others communicate such a message). This resentment may be expressed in various ways, such as demoralisation, guilt, and hostility to the carers. On the other hand the person may feel grateful to his carers and, because of his dependence, also concerned not to upset them in case he should be rejected by them. This may cause anxiety and the need for reassurance that the carers want him, and also may produce a state of passive compliance with the carer's wishes, with the person feeling unable to complain or express negative feelings. Not uncommonly both types of feelings will be present, i.e. resentment and concern not to upset, and this may give rise to forms of 'passive' aggression, by which is meant difficult behaviour for which the person cannot seemingly be blamed. An inexplicable worsening of physical symptoms, such as incontinence, might be an example. However, it must be emphasised that such an interpretation should not be made lightly, and should have supporting evidence from enquiry into the person's feelings.

FINANCIAL SECURITY

Despite the persisting truth of the cliché that money does not buy happiness, money is able to buy a considerable amount of comfort and thus give freedom from the demoralising effects of deprivation. For many people disablement will mean loss of employment and a prolonged existence of financial hardship. This can exacerbate frustration and social isolation, and lead to additional strain on self-esteem. Although there are State benefits for the disabled these are usually insufficient to allow more than a basic level of subsistence. There are also provisions for supplying aids for the disabled, for supplying home help or assistance from district nurses and for adapting existing accommodation to suit needs or, if necessary, for rehousing. However, there are also often shortages and waiting lists, and for many disabled people the various provisions are barely adequate. Being financially well off can allow the person to remedy the inadequacies of State provisions, and to have some control over the material aspects of life. It can also help give freedom from guilt and worry over how dependents are to be supported, and thereby help to retain self-esteem (Chapter 37, Social Services and Benefits).

QUALITY OF PROFESSIONAL CARE

From the onset of his condition the disabled person will come into contact with a variety of professional carers, such as doctors, nurses, remedial therapists, social workers, residential care staff, etc. Which particular professional groups, and with what frequency and at what stage, will depend on the nature of his condition. The person's physical and material well-being will be influenced by the competence with which they carry out their technical skills but, unless substantial negligence occurs, it is the manner in which they do so that will have the greatest bearing on his emotional well-being.

It is the person's *level of anxiety* that is most likely to be influenced by the behaviour of professionals. This is particularly important in the days or weeks following the onset of disability. At that time the person will have been faced with a sudden change in circumstances, or will perhaps be undergoing a series of seemingly mysterious investigations. He is likely to feel frightened, and to have many questions and fantasies about the future coursing through his head. He will hope that the professionals will have at least some of the answers. The willingness of the professional staff to sit and listen to his worries, to accept and understand them without censure and, if possible, to proffer information and advice, will go a long way in helping to reduce anxiety. Conversely, if professional staff appear abrupt, remote, too busy to listen, or uninterested or even dismissive of the person's worries (so that he is made to feel stupid or inadequate) then his anxiety is likely to be raised and his motivation or morale may decline. There may, of course, be many instances in which the professionals are unable to provide the information or give the reassurances that the person seeks. In such instances some professionals will prefer to be remote, in order not to appear useless or to avoid unpleasant feelings of helplessness. This remoteness is unlikely to be of benefit. It may be more helpful to sit and discuss the limitations on providing what the patient seeks in a sympathetic and unhurried manner. Even in instances where withholding information is deemed to be the most humane course of action professionals should be prepared to listen to, and acknowledge, the person's worries.

Most people will readily talk about their worries if given a secure (i.e. sympathetic and unhurried) atmosphere. Some, however, will still hold back because they fear their anxieties or fantasies will make them seem stupid. It is therefore important to enquire about the person's apprehensions in a manner that actively and sincerely reassures him that they are natural, and not a sign of stupidity. It is also important to explore and acknowledge the anxieties that anyone who will be caring for the disabled person may have and, providing there is no conflict with confidentiality, to proffer advice and information. Any reduction in the carer's anxiety will be beneficial to the person being cared for. Even if there are questions that cannot be answered, or problems that cannot be solved, the fact that the professional is prepared to listen, and shows understanding, can give comfort to both the disabled person and the carer.

5

The Doctor's Assessment of the Disabled Person

John Goodwill

The usual medical history is so structured that it begins with the presenting symptom and its duration and is followed by a full description of this and concurrent symptoms. Frequently this is followed by direct questions, which have been found by experience to be relevant to the specialty or diseases under consideration. Assessment must start with a full clinical history, examination, diagnosis and investigations where needed.

This model rarely considers the implications of the disease in terms of description of lifestyle. Frequently the patient has the same perception of the relevance of these as the doctor, and therefore the mismatch of the patient, now at dis-ease with his environment, is unexplored so that little possibility exists that this will be improved unless the disease is cured. Thus the young mother with arthritis in her wrists rarely confesses that she is terrified of dropping the baby, and the person with multiple sclerosis and frequency of urination does not say that the lack of accessible public lavatories precludes any shopping expeditions.

It should be realised that function is the final common pathway of disease expression and thus: *the history should thus be extended to include the functional implications of each symptom.*

Certain features are necessary for the diagnosis of a disease. In many cases these will have been formalised. Thus rheumatoid arthritis can be diagnosed according to ARA criteria, and Behçet's disease according to one of at least three schedules, perhaps the best of which are the Japanese which stratify the probability of diagnosis.

Nevertheless the features that are necessary for the diagnosis of disease are not necessarily those required of an assessment of the disability. If we consider again the patient with multiple sclerosis, diagnosis requires that lesions are separated anatomically in the nervous system and chronologically. But the patient's life can remain undisturbed after several minor episodes that establish diagnosis (events such as transient paraesthesiae or numbness). The onset of paraplegia, of urgency and frequency, or of severe ataxia may, however, mean that the patient loses his job, independence and ability to mix in society.

The disabled person requires time and patience in order to assess all the problems, both medical and social, arising from the illness or injury. Despite accurate diagnosis and specific medical or surgical treatment very many patients remain disabled. Any medical condition may cause temporary or permanent disability. The main groups of physical disability are:

Cardiac, e.g. myocardial ischaemia
Respiratory, e.g. chronic obstructive airways disease
Sensory deprivation; reduction of vision or hearing
Locomotor disability: arthritis; amputation; Neurological — stroke, multiple sclerosis, Parkinson's disease, cerebral palsy, spina bifida, paraplegia, etc.
Incontinence
Multiple disabilities

Many of these cause a mixture of locomotor, sensory, intellectual or other problems. *These permanent disabilities require assessment*, lack of which is a frequent cause of inadequate advice and management. Once the problems and their priority order have been found the solutions may become clearer.

WHAT DOES THE PATIENT WANT AND EXPECT?

The patient must be assessed by the doctor, and the disabilities and residual abilities consequent upon the accident or illness must be recorded, together with suggested action for further assessment and advice. The disabilities may be static, fluctuant or progressive. It is vital to find out how the patient views the problems in everyday life arising from the condition. Prompting of patients is required because too often they will suppress many of the real problems, believing that the doctor will not be interested or will not be able to help. The medical assessment will gradually disclose other problems which patients had not mentioned, or of which they have been unaware; frequently a difficult matter will be suppressed because the patient can see no answer to the problem, suppression being the easiest method to cope with it. Problems may be clinical or social; they should be listed together with the *setting of realistic goals* and methods of achieving these goals.

Patient's expectations are important

Patients have been known to come to a clinic merely for a repeat prescription for special shoes, but have found themselves examined from head to toe by an enthusiastic doctor who found a wealth of abnormalities for investigation, quite irrelevant to the patient, who has then forgotten to order the shoes.

Several expectations lie buried in a consultation: those of the patient may differ from those of the carers (markedly so in head injury) and again these may be at variance with those of the referring GP, the hospital doctor and other involved professionals. Questions such as 'What can I do for you?', 'What have you come for?' (appropriately said!) and 'What have they said about your coming to this clinic?' can yield helpful, and at times, strange or sad replies.

It is helpful if a patient does not come alone to a rehabilitation clinic, for disability rarely involves only the patient. The whole family can be considered disabled, and it is important to have some indication of their characters, strengths and weaknesses, and roles. It helps greatly to have them present with the patient when an attempt is made to explain the disease, the disability and the aims of treatment. It helps for all to agree on a priority order for these.

Personality and intellectual function

Knowledge of the previous education, work experience and recreations will help to understand what sort of person has the disability, as this will affect the patient's needs and wants. These will vary from those of the very active independent person to those of a patient who is content to sit at home doing relatively little, with very modest ambitions in life. The latter patient will appear to do less well with rehabilitation management but will be much more easily satisfied than the former, who may well set unrealistic goals and be disappointed in not achieving them. In the absence of brain damage personality does not change with the occurrence of disability, but its pre-existing features may be accentuated and behaviour may be altered. Patients may be less able to repress the undesirable features of themselves, although sometimes hidden strength is revealed to understand and cope with the disability. Often the patient's children are a better guide to previous behaviour patterns than the spouse, who may be quite unrealistic about previous abilities and the patient's likely response to disability (Chapter 4).

At the end of the interview the doctor should be in a position to make some assessment of the patient's intellect, his orientation, cognitive function, short- and long-term memory, ability to concentrate, to synthesise information, to structure it, to sort and sequence it, and to follow instruction. Affect can be appreciated: is the patient depressed (and if so, is this appropriate), anxious, lacking in confidence, unrealistic, apathetic, or unmotivated. How does he perceive himself? What are his powers of communication?

The patient's comprehension

The patient's comprehension of his condition will affect his response as much as the disability itself, this response progressing through reactions of depression, anger and rejection, in different combinations, later hopefully emerging as acceptance of the true situation. One must aim for an *active acceptance of the remaining ability* and not a passive concentration on the disability. The psychological processes of acceptance are very similar to mourning, which is now for the previously normal self and for the lost opportunities in the future. One therefore needs to know something of the previous self. Stroke, head injury and multiple sclerosis (MS) may all cause organic brain damage, with results varying from aggression in head injury to emotional outbursts in stroke, depression or euphoria in MS. Any of these may make it difficult for the patient to understand realistically how and what can be achieved. Perhaps in some severe disabilities denial is the only psychological response that makes life possible, and occasionally this must be accepted by those treating the patient. Usually honesty and full explanation of the treatment goals is essential to success. Reduction of memory and learning ability due to brain damage also cause misunderstandings.

The reaction of the relatives and friends

This may be at least as important as that of the patient. Usually acceptance of reality is easier if there is a clear cause-and-effect, paraplegia due to trauma being easier for people to understand than that due to a virus causing transverse myelitis. Where the patient or a relative is not entirely satisfied with the explanation of cause of the illness, anger, frustration and even complaints may persist. The patient and family may only listen attentively and remember those things that they wish to hear, rather than all the information that is given. Honest discussion, where all the staff say the same thing, is vital; this takes time and several separate appointments with ample time for discussion and questions, on what can and what cannot be achieved. Truth is important but must be imparted gradually; it is unhelpful to say more than the person can understand or tolerate at any one time. Partial truths may be needed early on, but untruths must be avoided or the essential trust will not be built up. One must concentrate on function that remains, and what can be achieved with rehabilitation, and encourage optimistic honesty between patient, relatives and staff. All must be aiming for the same goals, the family need to continue treatment at home, whether this be stretching of a spastic limb or encouraging maximum function and everyday activities at home. They need to be given the motivation to continue these activities for months or years.

THE AIM OF THE ASSESSMENT

(1) To provide a data base — to estabish the diagnosis; to record disabilities, their nature and their character (static, fluctuant, deteriorating).
(2) To produce a problem list.
(3) To draw up treatment plans.
(4) To treat.
(5) To review (3) and (4) as frequently as necessary to ensure treatment remains appropriate as needs change.

Suggested framework for taking a rehabilitation history

Presenting functional problems (date).
Other problems (numbered).
History of above (numbered).
Paediatric history of above (where relevant) including details of birth, milestones.
Past history of illness or operations.
Other health problems.
Dental care.
Vision.
Hearing.
Speech and communication.
Breathlessness.
Fatigue.
Personal history — schooling and education (with attainments).
Family history.
Work history.
Leisure history (including clubs and day centres attended) whether for normal population or for disabled.

Direct questioning may supplement the above. The following areas should be explored: the level of functioning, of dependence; the use of aids or of helpers; the exact nature of the difficulties.

Main upper limb functions — feeding, dressing and grooming, washing and bathing (activities of daily living, ADL).
Bodily functions — bladder and bowel function, menstruation, sexual function.

Mobility

Mobility is crucial for independence and can be divided into:
(a) Mobility on foot

How far does the patient walk?
Does he require a helper?
What mobility aids are needed?
What are the problems?
Discuss walking inside the house, emerging and outside, at work, at leisure and at school.

(b) Mobility by wheelchair
What wheelchair(s) has the patient?
Do these satisfy his needs? If not, why not?
Are they in good repair?

(c) Mobility by private transport
What transport is used?
Is the patient passenger or driver?
What aids or help are necessary to get in/out of the vehicle; what modifications are needed?
What are the problems?

(d) Public transport

(e) Travel, work and finance

(f) Family and social relationships

Some adults require only to be able to care for themselves. Others may have to do their own food preparation and domestic chores. Many (mostly women) run households for dependent children, elderly parents and spouses. These activities require both dexterity and mobility. The doctor should enquire into shopping and food preparation, washing of clothes, etc., householding, household maintenance (DIY), including gardening.

Vision

Acuity can be judged by the patient's behaviour in the consulting room, the ability to read a paper, or by formal testing with a test chart. Checking visual fields to confrontation is usually adequate, but if there is brain damage a target must be presented in both fields simultaneously to determine whether there is visual inattention on one side (shown by the patient ignoring the target on one side although noticing it if presented alone). This has obvious implications for driving and some occupations (Chapter 16).

Hearing

Bilateral loss of hearing is usually obvious, but it is quite possible to miss a complete unilateral loss, e.g. after head injury (Chapter 17).

Speech and communication

In everyday life communication is through speech, hearing and vision; non-verbal communication is important to all of us. If one or other sense is reduced the sensitivity of the remaining senses is heightened and the patient may have to learn to communicate in new ways. Detailed speech assessment is left to the speech therapist, but the doctor can certainly judge if there is any obvious receptive or expressive dysphasia (this is a very simplified classification), or if a speech defect is only dysarthria, in which the patient understands and formulates the correct words but articulation is impaired. Comprehension of advice will be normal in the latter, whereas dysphasia often makes it difficult to obtain the history, test sensation or to give advice. The patient may understand more by visual than aural communication, so gesture is important. If the patient does not speak English a translator is essential. A member of staff may be more helpful than the patient's family, who will often not ask the questions as given, or will give their own reply rather than that of the patient. This can be very misleading. The translator should not modify question or answer (Chapter 15).

Breathlessness and fatigue

These may coexist due to cardiac or respiratory disease, which is relatively easily assessed, but fatigue occurring with neurological conditions such as MS or stroke or due to rheumatoid arthritis may be an underestimated problem requiring adequate rest periods during treatment. Fatigue is a subjective phenomenon, difficult to quantify but worsened by depression, treatment of which will help. The characteristic symptoms of depression may be masked by the obvious symptoms and limitation due to the disability; some depression is inevitable (Chapters 13 and 14).

Activities of daily living (ADL)

Personal care, i.e. dressing, washing, bath and toilet needs, as well as cooking, eating and drinking will be considered by the occupational therapist (OT), together with other activities round the home that we all take for granted. If necessary with the aid of a home visit the OT will be able to advise on simple or more complex modifications at home; she will assess the ability to use the telephone, and control everyday items such as the front door, radio, television, lights and heating that able-bodied people take for granted. For home modifications the OT will liaise with the social worker in the Social Services Department, especially as provision varies widely from one area to another.

Bowels and micturition

Loss of independent control of these functions is socially unacceptable, whereas a wheelchair or visual handicap need not deny a patient integration in normal social life. Patients with urinary problems require careful urological assessment to decide on the cause. The patient may be asked to keep a daily micturition chart to determine when and how often it occurs. Too many, particularly of our older patients, may consider that some of their problems are due to their age and nothing can be done about them.

The professionals treating that patient must not make the same mistake. The problems may be mild in a patient with good mobility and easy access to toilet facilities, but when considering the bladder and bowel one also needs to know how far and fast the patient can move on the flat and on the stairs. Even if specific treatment cannot be given to improve sphincter control, improvement in mobility or the provision of easily accessible toilet facilities may solve the functional problem. More help may be provided by a builder than a urologist (see Chapter 29)!

Sexual problems

These may be physical due to spasticity, muscle weakness, pain or joint limitation, or due to psychological causes, often associated with anxiety or depression, or they may be due to drugs used for the illness. Lack of understanding of the condition with its consequent disability will compound the problem; concentration on residual abilities will help. Some patients have a poor self-image, seeing themselves as incomplete and damaged, which impairs their psychological and sexual function as well as every other aspect of their life (Chapter 30).

Mobility and independence

Limitation may be due to a number of different problems in any one disease. The amount of difficulty due to each must be assessed to allow treatment of these specific problems. In rheumatoid arthritis it may be pain requiring systemic drug treatment, limitation of joint movement requiring splintage and physiotherapy, or so much pain or instability of one or more joints that surgery or an orthosis is required. Alternatively weakness may be due to neurological complications of neuropathy or myelopathy, the latter requiring evaluation of the cervical spine. With neurological conditions such as stroke or MS there may be *muscle weakness* requiring exercise; *spasticity or contracture* requiring physiotherapy, drugs or even surgery; or it may be that *incoordination or sensory loss* pose far greater problems, and are relatively more resistant to treatment. It is no good treating the patient's gait disturbance as though it is due to muscle weakness when one of the other factors is the predominant problem. Frequently there is a combination of problems, so that treatment needs to be directed at each, depending upon their relative importance. For instance, sensory loss or astereognosis, often with body-image problems on the same side, cause much greater difficulty in everyday life than a moderate degree of muscle weakness. More severe weakness with resulting leg joint instability on walking may require an orthosis and/or shoe modification, which must be assessed and prescribed by the doctor, in discussion with the physiotherapist and the patient (Chapter 45).

The details of mobility aids may be left with the physiotherapist and the OT, both of whom must have a clear idea of aims and methods. The physiotherapist will aim to increase muscle strength and joint movement, improve coordination and produce improved motor function. She may provide walking aids, and will choose from a great variety of sticks, crutches, walking frames or trolleys, the choice is important for optimum individual function (Chapter 46). Wheelchairs (Chapter 43) will be assessed by the OT, but the doctor should know that a wide variety of pushchairs, self-propelled chairs and electric wheelchairs for indoor use is available under the Health Service. If the patient cannot manage one it is probably wrong. Providing a wheelchair without paying attention to the seating is a recipe for disaster and pressure sores. Outdoor powered wheelchairs may also be discussed, although here the patient will be obliged to buy it himself (Chapter 43).

Travel, work and finance

Independent travel on public transport is difficult if the patient has more than moderate disability, so it is important for the doctor to assess *outdoor mobility*, which may be a reflection of where the patient lives as much as of his medical condition. Advice on driving or other means of personal mobility is a vital part of the assessment, for without this, work will probably be impossible. If driving is being considered one must give a firm opinion as to whether the patient is or is not fit to drive, but only when one has a full assessment, which may need to include psychometric testing. If tuition is required one may advise the patient of the best place to go for this, and for advice on car modifications. If he is unfit to drive alternative means of outdoor mobility should be discussed (Chapter 47).

Work will involve consideration of return to the previous work, possibly modified, placement in an alternative occupation, or training for a new job. For a very few patients their disability is a positive advantage, opening opportunities which they had not previously considered. It is the doctor's job to make sure that this is done, by discussion with the patient and other professional staff including the OT and disablement resettlement officer (Chapter 41).

Finance is a bigger problem for disabled people than for the able-bodied, as disability often results in additional costs in transport, clothing, food and heating. The doctor will not know of all the allowances or other benefits available, so the patient must be directed to the social worker or welfare rights worker who can offer up-to-date advice as benefits change frequently. While money does not solve disability, lack of it certainly compounds the problem. Mobility allowance, constant attendance allowance, disability and other benefits are often available, but patients may not receive them without prompting and advice (Chapter 37).

Family and social relationships

It is right to concentrate first on the more obvious problems like mobility and everyday activities as noted by the patient and the professional staff, but once management of these is under way one must then help the patient to engage in social activities, in work, sports and leisure; he may need considerable help and encouragement to do so. A disabled person disables the whole family, to some degree *limiting their choice in life.* Explanation to the family jointly with the patient about the remaining ability and the treatment programme is vital from the beginning. Whilst the family must consider the needs of the disabled person these must not be so dominant that the rights and wishes of others are neglected. *The disabled person has duties as well as rights,* the same as any other member of the community. He must be encouraged to take up as much of previous life as possible and to develop new interests, not avoiding contact with others, many of whom will be misinformed about disabled people. The patient may wish to join a society of others with a similar condition. For spinal injuries this is useful, but for some other progressive conditions it may be unwise for the mildly handicapped patient to see the later possibilities. Others more disabled will receive support from these groups, and receive information on aids, benefits or other possibilities which should have been suggested by the rehabilitation staff. As the whole family is affected by the disability *the carers* need not only explanation and sympathy, but practical help and relief. A breakdown of the carer may necessitate a heavily disabled person being admitted to hospital or institution.

CONCLUSION

Rehabilitation is an enabling process to allow the disabled person to gain maximum independence and enjoyment of his life. The disabled person will frequently underestimate his ability and his acceptance by others, which will lead to social isolation and a rapid worsening of medical and social functioning. Adequate medical and social assessment of the disabilities arising due to the illness or injury will lead to better management, and go far to solve the problems. Even if these remain, the patient will benefit greatly from knowing that someone cares enough to spend time and trouble finding out what the problems really are, and explaining to the patient and family which problems can be overcome and which are insoluble. We aim for active realistic adult acceptance of the true situation and *restoration of choice* in life as far as possible.

6

The Rehabilitation Team and Functional Assessment

Anne Chamberlain

A team approach is vital in rehabilitation. However, to tie up a large number of busy professionals in a case conference for several hours is costly and must be seen to be an effective use of time. 'The team' is not a fixed entity: its composition varies according to need, but will usually include a doctor, a physiotherapist, occupational therapist and nurse. *It is the team's function to ameliorate the mismatch that exists between the patient and his environment by whatever mediating factors they can command (therapy, aids, equipment, etc.).*

GENERAL PRACTICE AND PRIMARY CARE/REHABILITATION AT HOME

Traditionally the general practitioner is the first point of a patient's contact with medical services. Increasingly, access to physiotherapy departments, and possibly occupational therapy departments, is open to GPs, and some practices have available the services of community (domiciliary) physiotherapists. To provide home treatment for all patients would be extremely expensive in physiotherapy time (the skilled professional's time is not necessarily best used in travelling). Nevertheless, there are patients who need home treatment (such as those with severe rheumatoid arthritis) who are so exhausted by long ambulance journeys that they derive no benefit from physiotherapy in an outpatient setting. There are others who are chair- or bedfast.

Some patients' families need *advice* rather than treatment (e.g. a patient with a new stroke who is not admitted to hospital). Relatives caring for the patient require instruction in handling and lifting him, and require this help as soon as possible after (say) the stroke has occurred. We also find patients with remarkably severe disability managed at home (except possibly for intermittent care in a Younger Disabled Unit) and they need the services of many people, principally the community nurse.

Community occupational therapists assess patients at home for aids, equipment and adaptations, and less commonly, provide treatment there. Speech therapists and others such as dieticians are rarely available to health centres and patients at home. Where a Disabled Living Centre exists in the locality it may be a useful point of contact for the GP who will require a variety of services, for his patients with vastly different problems.

The care of the patients with chronic disease takes place largely at home: furthermore, most disabled people dislike living in institutions, so that there are now considerable pressures which will result in more severely disabled people remaining for longer at home, hopefully with more support being available to them there. General practitioners are the key figures in the care of these patients: an average GP will have some 300 people on his list with disability and 100 of these will have substantial problems. It is important that he considers himself a member of the disability team, and draws on the expertise of those professionals mentioned in this chapter who can best assess and help his patient, particularly by meeting in the patient's home.

OUTPATIENT REHABILITATION

Much work is done in separate physiotherapy, occupational therapy and speech therapy departments of many hospitals and where the patients' problem is simple, therapy in one department only is acceptable. But frequently severe disability brings with it problems which are complex and cross departmental boundaries. To make most effective use of the skills of the members of these individual departments it is vital that communication between them is good. The team is smallest in the outpatient clinic where it is helpful for the doctor conducting the clinic to have with him a physiotherapist and occupational therapist. In this way, all may observe (say) the patient's walking, and the physiotherapist (who may have been a member of the original treating team) may need only a few minutes to remind the patient and carer of simple exercises which continue to be necessary. Indeed the most vital participant in any exchange of information is *the patient*, frequently excluded from the discussion of aims and goals, with predictable results. The second most important person is the carer. The writer remembers well a useless outpatient appointment kept by an aphasic, hemiplegic Chinese elder who, although he had a large and caring family, arrived at outpatients on a trolley, totally alone.

The occupational therapist will be alerted to the domestic problems the patient is experiencing and may decide to do a domiciliary visit; or may liaise with social services to speed up delivery of ramps and rails, or may assess for, and expedite the acquisition of, other aids and adaptations (e.g. stairlift). She may provide advice on return to work and may have visited employers, having assessed the patient when working in the occupational therapy department. She may have set tasks of increasing complexity for the patient to do at home so that each week progress is made and recorded. A disablement resettlement officer (DRO) may rarely be available to come into the clinic, but more usually the occupational therapist at the clinic plans the patient's therapy in the workshops of the occupational therapy department, so that his performance increasingly approaches that necessary for return to work or entry to the Employment Rehabilitation Centre (ERC), and she will liaise with the DRO and ERC. She may also be available to go into schools and further education colleges to encourage good rehabilitation practice there, helping to integrate patients into normal education, work and leisure.

CORE TEAM FOR INPATIENT REHABILITATION

Patients must not be scattered throughout different wards, but must be brought together so that the benefits of the consistent policy of a rehabilitation ward may be available to the patient. The team at this stage usually consists of doctor(s), nursing staff, physiotherapist, occupational therapist, speech therapist, medical social worker and (possibly) health visitor and clinical psychologist. All should see the patient in the physiotherapy or occupational therapy department so that they have an accurate picture of the patient as he is currently functioning. All will then have the opportunity to give a thumbnail sketch of the patient as each sees him (at the ensuing case conference) giving as much relevant, factual information as is necessary to build up a picture of the patient 'in the round'. Each professional has a slightly different framework against which she assesses the patient, and may initially set goals different from those aimed at by others. It is essential that these different aims are articulated and common short- and long-term aims agreed. Thus it might be that the doctor assumes a patient will return to work and believes the patient could achieve this, albeit with difficulty. The social worker may know, however, that the patient has been made redundant, therefore independence in the home, adapting hobbies so that the patient can continue them despite disability, may be a more suitable aim. In some cases the spouse may need or wish to continue work. Where this leads to leaving the disabled patient at home for prolonged periods, rehabilitation must aim to make the patient independent or safe in the necessary basic tasks such as use of a toilet. He may need to be able to get himself a snack, or at least eat and drink food left for him. The minimum support to be provided will have to be ascertained. Day care at a day centre is usually insufficient in this situation as transport arrives for the patient at unpredictable times, often long after the working spouse should have left for work.

Sometimes it will be apparent that the patient works well in the physiotherapy department but considers it the nurse's duty to do everything for him when in the ward — a reflection perhaps of institutionalisation, or even of his attitude to his wife! Rehabilitation is a learning situation and most relearning is done outside the therapy department. The therapists' good work can be undone by incorrect management on the ward or at home, and the importance of the ward staff and the patient's helpers sharing common aims and methods with therapists is obvious. The patient will also be motivated by perceived success; on a general ward he may merely feel that he remains, week after week, unable to walk or unable to go home. In the rehabilitation department, walking will be broken up into many small, achievable stages. The aim is to replace feelings of failure and inadequacy by a sense of achievement. Even so, in a deteriorating situation such as multiple sclerosis it may be difficult for patients and carers to see any progress. It may be wise, therefore, for the team to anticipate deterioration and put in sufficient adaptations, aids and support so that persistent decline in function is not highlighted. This particularly applies to motor neurone disease, where the prescriber may lag behind the disease throughout the whole of its course, the patient never receiving help appropriate to his needs at any one point in time.

ASSESSMENT BY TEAM

Some patients always succeed in gaining a large, and sometimes disproportionate, amount of attention. Others need much and get little. Regular, systematic review ensures that none get forgotten. We review all inpatients two-weekly, with the proviso that where great changes have occurred we can discuss them more frequently. Thus a standard assessment is made of all patients within a week of admission, again during the week before discharge and at the first post-discharge outpatient visit. Similarly, if it transpires that a patient has been inappropriately referred (usually all referrals are screened before acceptance) rehabilitation can be terminated and the patient returned to the referring doctor. Therapists should not be asked to continue treatment which is placebo only, or where gains are agreed to be too small in proportion to the effort expended by staff and patient.

Discharge is *planned*, the date often being given a week or more in advance, when the patient has undertaken several successful visits to relatives or home and has stayed overnight there. These increasingly lengthy visits are necessary to reveal the areas of difficulty which must be tackled before discharge, and to demonstrate to relatives the need for them to learn effective ways of mobilising the patient (for instance, transferring from bed in the morning, or getting in and out of a car). The family and the patient gain confidence as home stays are repeated. Frequently the occupational therapist and physiotherapist will do a *domiciliary visit* well before the discharge date, to allow time for access rails to be installed, ramps to be ordered, a commode delivered, etc., and for the patient to use these when on weekend leave.

Patients coming from a distance are less easy to help: the range of facilities available to them through the local social services department and health services may not be known; it can then be helpful to invite the local community nurse or social worker to attend the case conference before details of discharge and support at home are finalised. So, too, when another member of the family who may either require the patient's help, or may assist him, is looked after by another service (e.g. by the community psychiatric nurse). (We recently had a patient who had to be fit enough to return to look after her apathetic and dementing husband: his discharge from the psychiatric hospital was tailored to his wife's recovery.) Those patients who live in rural areas may not have available the range of day care services found in large cities: on the other hand small communities can be very caring.

Patients with *multiple disabilities* are particularly difficult to help, and sometimes extraordinarily difficult to place (e.g. the older adult confined to a wheelchair who also has a recent decline in mental function).

Nature of assessment during treatment

The type of assessment is functional: it refers to the activities the patient needs to return home or to progress to a Part III institution (i.e. local authority 'home' where he must usually be able to wash, dress and feed himself and get himself to the dining room) or private or voluntary home. These end-points are related closely to immediate goals set. A standard assessment form provides a quick global checklist of relevant skills and levels of attainment. It complements full therapy assessments. No distinction is necessary between the performance of tasks with or without an aid, but it will usually be crucial to know whether another person is required to supervise or physically assist with a basic task. One should also consider the *critical interval*, the length of time a patient can safely be left unattended. One needs to know why a patient needs such intermittent help and how it is proposed that this should be provided — or whether there are other ways of dealing with the problem. For instance, a hemiplegic patient living alone may not be able to get up and walk to the toilet at night unless wearing his calliper. The problem might be solved by getting a night sitter (expensive and rarely available), or perhaps by giving further physiotherapy and antispastic agents to improve walking ability, or by altering the design of the calliper or, finally, by the use of a urinal (perhaps with a one-way valve) kept in or beside the bed. Urinary problems in the day are a frequent cause for calling for help; crutchless knickers in females, or a commode wheelchair or a slipper urinal, are possible solutions, but a severely disabled arthritic might be quite unable to use any of these.

Patient activities in a rehabilitation unit

Each patient in an inpatient unit has a structured day's programme written up on a ward wall-chart, usually consisting principally of half-hour sessions of physiotherapy, occupational therapy, keep-fit activities, attendance at the workshop, and speech therapy if required. Gradual changes to this programme will be made as the patient gets fitter and more mobile. Wherever possible the patient should be responsible for getting himself dressed, groomed and to therapy sessions on time, and should gradually assume responsibility for the care of his clothes. Day clothes (preferably simple ones such as a track suit) that allow active games, are preferred. Slippers are banned and replaced by comfortable, functional shoes (perhaps trainers with velcro fastenings). Visitors are welcomed: they often help with the feeding of patients or join in games and other activities that take place when the day's formal activities are ended. They are encouraged to handle the patient correctly, to become competent in taking him out and accompanying him in a variety of normal activities.

Individual responsibilities of the team members

A brief word is necessary about the various members of the team. A *consultant physician* or surgeon is in charge of most rehabilitation units and clinical responsibility still ultimately results with him or her. It will often be necessary to *allow the patient some risks*, for life is never free of them and is for living, as much by disabled as by able-bodied people; however, the consultant has to satisfy himself that any risks (e.g. of return to home) are reasonable. It is important that such a consultant has junior staff, at SHO level they gain valuable experience which they will use in whatever discipline they eventually find themselves; a considerable expansion of rehabilitation services is required in the UK and provision must be made for this in Senior Registrar appointments, probably rotating with related disciplines (Report of Royal College of Physicians, 1986).

A *rehabilitation officer*, recruited from any of the disciplines, is found in bigger units and may organise day-to-day management of the unit and patient timetables.

A *clinical psychologist* is of great assistance to a unit, particularly where that unit is dealing with brain-injured patients, or when patients make heavy emotional demands on staff who themselves may need support and advice. The clinical psychologist has a basic degree in psychology, followed by training within the health service.

Nurses constitute the biggest group within the health service, and are vital for the rehabilitation process. The morale and ethos of the rehabilitation ward will be much more influenced by the ward sister than by doctors. Unless she understands the need for continuous and considerable cross-professional communications the patient will not have the chance of using his time in a rehabilitation unit (or indeed in any ward) most profitably. If she allows junior nurses, say, to walk a patient in a manner different from the method he has practised in *physiotherapy,* the patient becomes confused about how he should be performing. If the toilet facilities on her ward are cold, uninviting, and inaccessible to a wheelchair, the patient will not learn wheelchair independence. (If there is no mirror at seated height the female patient won't be able to practise making-up, for instance.) If there are no rails in the ward toilet, a patient who has been independent at home with these will quickly lose his independence. If the nurse bundles the patient into his clothes to be ready for his treatment session, which is perhaps labelled 'dressing practice' and performed twice a week, it will be perceived by the patient as an artificial process unrelated to life at home. However, if the *occupational therapist* comes onto the ward after breakfast when everyone is preparing for the day, the nurses, occupational therapists and patients can work in harmony, gradually getting the patient to do more for himself.

Nursing the disabled patient in hospital is a highly skilled 'hands-off' process, the nurse having to encourage independence without initially, at least, asking too much of the patient. Her first task is to welcome patient and helper, to allay fears, to explain and inform. The rehabilitation ward goes at a slower pace than the acute medical wards, and the surroundings are geared to encouraging the patient to take up responsibility for his own feeding, dressing, toilet and treatment. The nurse needs to know exactly how to position and handle the hemiplegic or paraplegic patient, how to restore self-confidence and confidence in the relatives. She needs to have time to spend with the patient, listening, reinforcing appropriate behaviour, encouraging new skills, perhaps playing games which are therapy in disguise. The rewards of such an approach are often highly gratifying, although the job will rarely be complete when the patient leaves the ward and the nurse hands on to the *health visitor* or community nurse.

Many patients have been subject to the imposed discipline of a large district general hospital where they are amongst patients with a variety of acute illnesses, whose treatment takes precedence. They need to be encouraged to take on decision-making again, and many have to be encouraged to look good again in their own clothes. This frequently involves the nurses in sorting out practicalities: where the dentures are that the patient should have brought with him, that spectacles need renewing, that a hearing aid is necessary. Patients have to be helped in the restoration of continence and in toileting themselves. Nurses need instruction in lifting and handling techniques, and in the use of wheelchairs. Staff will need to give much encouragement and support, as many patients have to make major adjustments and deal with grief at the loss sustained. Nurses will need to encourage socially acceptable feeding; all patients should join others in the dining room and can help set and clear tables; junior nurses may not be aware that in helping patients with social skills they may be ensuring the sustained success of independent living. Those who are highly dependent on others for their physical well-being need to nurture relationships with carers.

Relatives, too, are finding this time a great strain; after the life-and-death crisis of an acute admission they are confronted by unpleasant realities. They will have many anxieties and may have to be helped gently, and firmly, to take over the care of their relatives, at first for a few hours, later a day, or overnight or for a weekend. They may begin to realise that the job ahead is difficult, restricting and perhaps unrewarding.

A great number of persons converge on the ward, and it will be one of the nurses' tasks to liaise. There will also be a variety of highly skilled practicalities to attend to — the acquisition of bladder and bowel control, prevention or healing of pressure sores, helping the patient use aids (say for feeding or hygiene). Pain may be present in a phantom limb, and insomnia may be an indication of anxieties. Frequently there will be at least one person in the ward with a difficult personality which will not make the nurse's task easy. The Royal College of Nursing has post-qualification training courses in rehabilitation nursing.

Siting of the rehabilitation ward in a District Hospital

The patient admitted to a rehabilitation ward has usually had his medical condition investigated and made stable as far as possible (e.g. polycythaemia, hypertension, amputation of a limb). He may still feel tired but should not be so unwell that he cannot take part in the programme of activities arranged for him. The rehabilitation ward needs to be adjacent to the rehabilitation facilities, to permit the interchange of ideas and free mixing of staff, and allow patients to get to therapy with minimal help. This reinforces the patient's idea of himself as independent, able to determine and direct his own activities.

The liaison health visitor

Traditionally, the prime function of a health visitor in Britain has been to provide advice and support for mothers of under-five-year-olds, to prevent illness and disability in this group and to direct them towards help. There are other groups in the population who are equally at risk, including the adult disabled and elderly, and these groups greatly benefit from the help of a health visitor. Patients appreciate that the health visitor is primarily a nurse, who has practical skills and has undergone a further year's training in health visiting.

In Leeds we have been fortunate in having health visitors as part of our team for many years: the supportive and preventive work they do is of considerable importance, particularly as patients feel most vulnerable in the early weeks after discharge, when there are no longer numerous professionals to help. At home, if a transfer to the toilet is done incorrectly the patient may fall to the floor. Or the carer's back may be hurt if she was lifting or helping the patient using incorrect methods. The health visitor has known the patient in hospital and has seen how he performed; she has details of his exercise and drug regimes, knows of his attendances at outpatients and can sort out these and many other matters. After a shorter or longer period this specialist health visitor hands on the patient to the local health visitor.

The health visitor usually visits the home before the patient's return there, and interviews the main carer there. The carer is frequently under great stress and appreciates the health visitor's attention to the carer's needs.

A second visit is made shortly after the patient's discharge, when an assessment is made of the patient's function in the same manner as in hospital. Home exercises are checked, goals agreed and a record card given. This is brought by the patient to the doctor at outpatients. the health visitor sees her work under three headings:

(1) the search for health needs,
(2) the stimulation of awareness of these, and
(3) the facilitation of health-enhancing activities.

The health visitor must assess, plan, implement and evaluate so that the patient is encouraged to maximise his potential and participate as much as possible in life around him.

Home nursing services

Other nursing and care services are developing for patients at home, but their availability and nature are highly variable. District nurses (community nurses) undertake many nursing procedures at home, such as the giving of injections and dressing of pressure sores. Some will bathe patients, dress and undress them, procedures which can be handed over quite satisfactorily to less highly qualified personnel such as bath attendants and care attendants. The Cross Roads Scheme is a widely used method of delivering such care.

Occupational therapy

An occupational therapist undergoes a three-year training, leading to a diploma or degree. Thereafter most occupational therapists tend to specialise, either in physical or psychiatric rehabilitation, and after some rotation into various subspecialist areas will usually remain for several years in specialist work (such as a head injury workshop, with paediatrics, in a prison, or doing community work) (Chapter 34).

Physiotherapy

Physiotherapists also undergo a three-year training, either to a diploma or degree standard (Chapter 35). After qualification they often rotate through various specialties (e.g. cardiac, neurology, paediatric) and usually eventually settle in one subspecialty in which they develop considerable expertise.

Speech therapy

The speech therapist will also have completed a three-year degree course. She is responsible for assessment and treatment of the patient's communication problems, including the prescription of communication aids, and can offer further assistance to patient, carers and staff as outlined in Chapter 15.

Social worker

Social workers have usually obtained a degree and postgraduate qualifications, and are employed by the local authority's department of Social Services, being seconded to hospital work. As our system of benefits is complex they may spend much time helping a patient with financial matters, but have considerable skills in counselling (sometimes in sexual counselling). All applications for social service care (in the form of day centres, residental care) are made through them (Chapter 37).

Support of the team and of carers

Some patients can be very hard to help; while some characters make those working with them feel appreciated, others nag incessantly and yet others, such as those with motor neurone disease, or with very adverse social situations which are insoluble, cause the staff considerable emotional 'wear and tear'. It must be recognised that the team itself, and individual members, from time to time need support and help: some staff and carers without support may, after years, 'burn out'. Usually, however, if the case conferences are well-conducted, enjoyable and productive, this will be sufficient support for most staff.

Carers are rarely so fortunate. They are unprotected by terms of employment; they are of all ages, in all situations, some with and some without mental, financial and physical strengths. They often have multiple responsibilities.

The patient's illness affects the carer from the outset. The carer who is a relative is often expected, by the dependant, to provide an extraordinary level of care. As time goes on the carer, too, may become isolated and may need emotional recharging more than the patient. She may need practical help and guidance in sorting out priorities. She may sometimes feel that the patient's needs are recognised, whereas hers are not.

It is important then to recognise that the demands on carers are high, and that their lives have become more difficult and more restricted. They should have ready access to professionals, the opportunity for some relief, and some support (perhaps from a carers' association). They should be allowed some control of plans made for the patient. Finally, it should be appreciated that the caring situation is never static and needs changing help and support.

FUNCTIONAL ASSESSMENT

It is important that all professionals in rehabilitation evaluate the work they do, for they are a scarce resource to be used effectively. Appropriate measurements are essential tools of evaluation. Many clinicians are exercised by the difficulty of defining the activity of a disease — is an inflammatory arthritis inactive when any vestige of morning stiffness remains, or only when the ESR is normal? That is, do we accept a clinical or a laboratory definition? In reality it is of greater importance, particularly to the patient, to assess function. Function is the final common pathway through which disease is expressed. In what way is the illness interfering with his life? Is it disease activity or residual damage which is giving rise to the patient's problems? This is an important question in vocational rehabilitation, for until disease activity is suppressed (if possible) and the patient's condition has become static, it is difficult to make an assessment of residual skills which will be helpful in a long-term work placement or for vocational training. The interaction of disease, patient and environment will be constantly changing, and handicap will thus fluctuate.

There are as many measures of disease activity (almost) as there are diseases. Perhaps a few examples in the field of rheumatology will help to clarify the situation. *Clinically*, the disease may be measured by asking about individual features of the illness, enquiring whether the patient is well, how many painkillers he uses daily, what is the duration of morning stiffness. It may also be useful to ask the patient to keep a diary in which he records what symptoms are occurring, with what frequency, and in what quantity. These features may be given a numerical value. A joint count may also be performed in infalmmatory polyarthritis. *The Ritchie Articular Index* (RAI) (Ritchie *et al.*, 1968) is such a measure. Unlike many other indices it has been validated: when one observer records, measurements are accurate on the three-point grading scale which may be used on different occasions, i.e. *intra*-observer error is small. However, *inter*-observer variability using the same three-point scale is unacceptably high; only the presence or absence of tenderness is reliable (Hart *et al.*, 1985). The RAI is time-consuming but it is a useful measure, particularly in research, in evaluating drug therapy.

Counting the number of inflamed joints may be helpful in determining whether an antirheumatic agent is becoming effective, but it gives no insight into how a patient is managing his day-to-day existence. Laboratory tests and radiological results give even less information, although they will indicate the damage which has resulted from disease. To determine how a disease is interfering with the patient's functioning one must measure function in a variety of spheres relating to normal activities. Desirable features in a questionnaire for patients are shown in Table 6.1.

MEASURING FUNCTIONS

Over the past 40 years or so many attempts have been made to measure function. One of the earliest gradings was again in rheumatology: Steinbrocker's functional Grades (1949) (see Chapter 10). This had four grades (from normal activity through diminished vocational or domestic work to bed- or chair-bound) which were quick to score in the outpatient situation. Nevertheless the grading has many problems and the distance between grades is inconsistent. Some statements about patients' ability, such as inability to do their normal work, depend very much on the nature of this and the availability of the help of others and of labour-saving equipment. Loss of a job also depends, at least partly, on the prevailing economic climate. The scale is thus measuring handicap rather than disability since it

Table 6.1: Desirable features in a questionnaire for patients

It should have been piloted.

It should be:

- short;
- written in clear, correct, simple, unambiguous language in easily read print;
- well laid out, to lead the eye from one question to the next and to prevent sections from remaining unfilled;

and should:

- ask only appropriate and relevant questions;
- use linking phrases from question to question which make the exercise feel personal, not remote, and which do not allow the interviewer to introduce bias;
- always allow the participant to contribute something (an open question to conclude, is helpful);
- thank the person interviewed;
- be analysable (preferably with boxes lined up for ease of transfer to computer for analysis)

depends at least partly on environmental factors. Further, the scale has never been validated, a finding common to many of the earlier functional activity scales (see Liang *et al.*, 1985). It also suffers from the problems of most scales used in clinical practice, where it may be impossible to have an interval scale, (see below) in contradistinction to muscle power measured with a dynamometer.

Scales may be nominal, ordinal, interval or ratio scales. A scale will be *nominal* where, for identification purposes, the data are labelled, e.g. male/female, married/divorced/single. It may be *ordinal* where data are ranked in order, e.g. 1st, 2nd, 3rd. The Barthel Index (Mahoney and Barthel, 1965) (Table 6.2) is an example of an ordinal scale of measurement. Where the data are ranked on a standard scale and the difference (say) between points 1 and 2 on the scale is the same as (say) between points 3 and 4 the scale is an *interval* scale (e.g. temperature). Finally, when that scale has a true zero the scale may be said to be a *ratio* scale, e.g. the time taken to complete a test.

The sophistication of measurement dictates the range of statistical techniques which may be employed in the analysis of data derived from the test.

Other *clinical* tests are frequently used, such as walking time for a fixed distance, the time to climb stairs and the time to rise from a seat. These all depend very much on local conditions and may not be reproducible (which chair? which stairs?) and thus have limited use. Stride length is said to have much general applicability in predicting recovery after stroke. In the clinical situation (and particularly with inpatients who need to be assessed by occupational therapists before discharge) an activities of daily living (ADL) assessment is frequently undertaken. Testing and charting these assess-

Table 6.2: The Barthel Scale (from Mahoney and Barthel, 1965)

Item		Code
Dressing	_____	10 = Independent: ties shoes, copes with zips, etc. 5 = Needs help but does half in reasonable time 0 = Dependent
Feeding	_____	10 = Independent: reasonable speed 5 = Needs help; e.g. cutting 0 = Unable
Grooming	_____	5 = Face/hair/teeth/shaves all alone 0 = Dependent
Toilet	_____	10 = Independent 5 = Needs help 0 = Unable
Bathing	_____	5 = Independent 0 = Dependent
Bed/chair transfer	_____	15 = Totally independent 10 = Minimal help needed 5 = Able to sit, but needs major help 0 = Unable
Ambulation	_____	15 = Independent for 50 m—may use aid 10 = 50 m, but with help of person 5 = Wheelchair, but independent—50 m 0 = Immobile
Stairs	_____	10 = Independent 5 = Needs help 0 = Unable
Bladder	_____	10 = No accidents, manages catheter alone, if used 5 = Occasional accidents, or needs help with catheter 0 = Incontinent
Bowels	_____	10 = No accidents 5 = Occasional accidents/needs help with enemas, etc. 0 = Incontinent
Total	_____	

ments varies greatly from hospital to hospital, from OT to OT. ADL forms have rarely been validated, but each probably has considerable local value. Nevertheless, some are lengthy, and it could be asked whether several tests within each assessment are really measuring the same dysfunction. The ADL section of the Stanford Health Assessment Questionnaire (Fries *et al.*, 1980) originally included some 30 such items. With little loss of sensitivity, questions have been reduced to eight key areas. Similar findings have been reported by Smith *et al.* (1977) in stroke. It is not helpful to use a new, or a non-validated, series of tests of self-care activities. Comparisons can best be made between different treatments or styles of management when these are compared using well-established indices such as the

Barthel Index or Katz index of independence in ADL (Brorsson and Asberg, 1984) (Table 6.3). However, these give no indication of the patient's way of life, as they record only ability or inability in basic functions, and a better index of the patients' ability to use his time constructively or happily may be the Frenchay Activities Index (Holbrook and Skilbeck, 1983) (Table 6.4).

In many instances apathy or depression will be suggested by low scores in this test, and by scores declining since the onset of illness, and it may be worthwhile progressing to tests of affect such as the Wakefield Inventory (Snaith *et al.*, 1971) and the more recent Hospital Anxiety and Depression Scale (Zigmond and Snaith, 1983) (Tables 6.5a and 6.5b). Other tests of well-being are referred to later. Some tests are better administered as self-reported questionnaires (Spiegel *et al.*, 1985). When intellectual function is impaired it may be useful to administer a test of orientation such as that developed by Quersti and Hodkinson (1972) and quoted in Wade *et al.*, (1985). These authors also mention the Mini-mental state (devised by DePaulo *et al.*, 1980 modified by Dick *et al.*, 1984) as helpful (Table 6.6). Of course, if deficits are complex and important the help of a psychologist is invaluable. Two valuable new test batteries for perceptual and other skills are now available — the Rivermead Perceptual Assessment Battery (Bhavani *et al.*, 1983) and the Chessington OT Neurological Assessment Battery (Tyerman *et al.*, 1987). Both have been validated.

One should consider the needs of the household: simple recording of the time the patient may be left comfortably and safely is useful (perhaps recording the exact need which requires intervention). This is the Interval Measurement referred to by Isaacs and Neville (1976).

In the clinical situation, as in a case conference, the details of inter- and intra-observer variability are of little importance. The central purpose of the functional chart is to make staff aware of the patient's past and present performance in a variety of self-care and domestic areas. Progress has to be monitored, lack of progress has to be investigated and variation in performance from department to department has to be explained and dealt with. In this situation it is acceptable to use any charting system which fulfils local needs and is reasonably reproducible.

Measuring individual functions (Tables 6.7 and 6.8)

It may be worth separating out those functions which need to be improved, and observing the effect of therapy. The purpose for which one measures needs thought: a simple goniometer for joint movement is often adequate for clinical use, but in a clinical trial of therapy would be better replaced by a light or telemetry goniometer, or perhaps one that records the maximum range reached. Similarly, the Davis bag used for measuring grip strength

Table 6.3: The Katz Index of Independence in ADL (Katz *et al.,* 1963)

The Index of Independence in Activities of Daily Living is based on an evaluation of the functional independence or dependence of patients in bathing, dressing, going to toilet, transferring, continence, and feeding. Specific definitions of functional independence and dependence appear below the index.

(A) Independent in feeding, continence, transferring, going to toilet, dressing and bathing.
(B) Independent in all but one of these functions.
(C) Independent in all but bathing and one additional function.
(D) Independent in all but bathing, dressing and one additional function.
(E) Independent in all but bathing, dressing, going to toilet and one additional function.
(F) Independent in all but bathing, dressing, going to toilet, transferring and one additional function.
(G) Dependent in all six functions.
Other: Dependent in at least two functions but not classifiable as C, D, E or F.

Independence means without supervision, direction, or active personal assistance, except as specifically noted below. This is based on actual status and not on ability. A patient who refuses to perform a function is considered as not performing the function even though he is deemed able.

Bathing (sponge, shower or tub)
Independent: assistance only in bathing a single part as back, or disabled extremity or bathes self completely.
Dependent: assistance in bathing more than one part of body: assistance in getting in or out of tub, or does not bathe self.

Dressing
Independent: gets clothes from closets and drawers puts on clothes, outer garments, braces, manages fasteners, act of tying shoes is excluded.
Dependent: does not dress self or remains partly undressed.

Going to toilet
Independent: gets to toilet: gets on and off toilet: arranges clothes: cleans organs of excretion: (may manage own bedpan used at night only, and may or may not be using mechanical supports).
Dependent: uses bedpan or commode or receives assistance in getting to and using toilet.

Transfer
Independent: moves in and out of bed independently and in and out of chair independently (may or may not be using mechanical supports).
Dependent: assistance in moving in or out of bed and/or chair, does not perform one or more transfers.

Continence
Independent: urination and defaecation entirely self-controlled.
Dependent: partial or total incontinence in urination or defaecation, partial or total control by enemas, catheters, or regulated use of urinals and or bedpans.

Feeding
Independent: gets food from plate or its equivalent into mouth (precutting of meat and preparation of food, as buttering bread, are excluded from evaluation).
Dependent: assistance in act of feeding (see above): does not eat at all, or parenteral feeding.

Table 6.4: The Frenchay Activities Index (modified from Holbrook and Skilbeck, 1983)

Activity	Score
In the past 3 months:	
Preparing main meals Washing up	0 = Never 1 = Under once weekly 2 = 1–2 times a week 3 = Most days
Washing clothes Light housework Heavy housework Local shopping Social occasions Walking outside > 15 mins Actively pursuing hobby Driving car/going on bus	0 = Never 1 = 1–2 times in 3 months 2 = 3–12 times in 3 months 3 = At least weekly
In the past 6 months:	
Travel outings/car rides	0 = Never 1 = 1–2 times in 6 months 2 = 3–12 times in 6 months 3 = At least twice-weekly
Gardening Household/car maintenance	0 = Never 1 = Light 2 = Moderate 3 = All necessary
Reading books	0 = None 1 = 1 in 6 months 2 = Less than 1 a fortnight 3 = Over 1 a fortnight
Gainful work	0 = None 1 = Up to 10 hours/week 2 = 10–30 hours/week 3 = Over 30 hours/week
Total (maximum possible score = 45)	

can be held in several different ways, and is an accurate instrument. The pinch grip meter will almost certainly prove more reliable. It gives much more information such as the time to reach (and descend from) the maximum, fatigue rate, work done (Helliwell *et al.*, 1987).

The use of questionnaires

It is sometimes believed of questionnaires that 'the longer the better', that *something* will come out of the lengthy questionnaire that wasn't thought of at its inception. Only weariness, on the part of the patient and the investigator, ensues.

Table 6.5a: HAD Scale (Hospital Anxiety and Depression Scale, Zigmond and Snaith, 1983)

Name: Date:

Doctors are aware that emotions play an important part in most illnesses. If your doctor knows about these feelings he will be able to help you more.
This questionnaire is designed to help your doctor to know how you feel. Read each item and place a firm tick in the box opposite the reply which comes closest to how you have been feeling in the past week.
Don't take too long over your replies: your immediate reaction to each item will probably be more accurate than a long thought-out response.

Tick only one box in each section

I feel tense or 'wound up':
- Most of the time
- A lot of the time
- Time to time, Occasionally
- Not at all

I still enjoy the things I used to enjoy:
- Definitely as much
- Not quite so much
- Only a little
- Hardly at all

I get a sort of frightened feeling as if something awful is about to happen:
- Very definitely and quite badly
- Yes, but not too badly
- A little, but it doesn't worry me
- Not at all

I can laugh and see the funny side of things:
- As much as I always could
- Not quite so much now
- Definitely not so much now
- Not at all

Worrying thoughts go through my mind:
- A great deal of the time
- A lot of the time
- From time to time but not too often
- Only occasionally

I feel cheerful:
- Not at all
- Not often
- Sometimes
- Most of the time

I can sit at ease and feel relaxed:
- Definitely
- Usually
- Not often
- Not at all

I feel as if I am slowed down:
- Nearly all the time
- Very often
- Sometimes
- Not at all

I get a sort of frightened feeling like 'butterflies' in the stomach:
- Not at all
- Occasionally
- Quite often
- Very often

I have lost interest in my appearance:
- Definitely
- I don't take so much care as I should
- I may not take quite as much care
- I take just as much care as ever

I feel restless as if I have to be on the move:
- Very much indeed
- Quite a lot
- Not very much
- Not at all

I look forward with enjoyment to things:
- As much as ever I did
- Rather less than I used to
- Definitely less than I used to
- Hardly at all

I get sudden feelings of panic:
- Very often indeed
- Quite often
- Not very often
- Not at all

I can enjoy a good book or radio or TV programme:
- Often
- Sometimes
- Not often
- Very seldom

Table 6.5b: HAD Scale (contd.)

Name: Date:

	A
	3
	2
	1
	0

D	
0	
1	
2	
3	

	A
	3
	2
	1
	0

D	
0	
1	
2	
3	

	A
	3
	2
	1
	0

D	
3	
2	
1	
0	

	A
	0
	1
	2
	3

D	
3	
2	
1	
0	

	A
	0
	1
	2
	3

D	
3	
2	
1	
0	

	A
	3
	2
	1
	0

D	
0	
1	
2	
3	

	A
	3
	2
	1
	0

D	
0	
1	
2	
3	

FOR HOSPITAL USE Patients Name/No:

D(8-10)__________

A(8-10)__________

Table 6.6: The mini-mental state (after Dick *et al.*, 1984; DePaulo *et al.*, 1980)

Test	Score
Orientation (one for each correct answer)	
Year, month, day, date, time	0–5
Country, town, district, hospital, ward	0–5
(in USA: state, county, town, hospital, floor)	
Registration	
Examiner names three objects. Patient asked to repeat three names.	
One for each correct:	0–3
Then to learn three names for later.	
Attention and calculation	
Subtract 7 from 100, then from result, etc.	
Stop after 5 (100, 93, 86, 79, 72, 65)	0–5
(Alternative: spell 'world' backwards)	
Recall	
Ask for three objects learnt earlier	0–3
Language	
Name a pencil and watch	0–2
Repeat 'No ifs, ands or buts'	0–1
Give a three-stage command. Score one for each stage	0–3
(e.g. 'place index finger of right hand on your nose and then on your left ear)	
Ask patient to read and obey a written command on a piece of paper stating: 'Close your eyes'	0–1
Ask patient to write a sentence. Score if it is sensible, has a subject and a verb	0–1
Copying	
Ask patient to copy a pair of intersecting pentagons	0–1
Total score	0–30

Table 6.7: Criteria for designing or choosing equipment to assess function

1. Know what function you want to study
2. Know relevant features of that function, i.e. background data
3. Isolate that function

Table 6.8: Equipment to be used in clinical situations

This should be:

1. Simple to *use* (and repair) (even if complicated under the wraps)
2. Reliable and sturdy (some equipment spends most of its time being modified)
3. Cheap
4. Transportable
5. Data analysable and storable
6. Checked for validity, reproducibility, random error

The good questionnaire fulfils a specific need and answers precise problems, whether these relate to a currently unsatisfactory situation which needs to be defined, or whether it aims to document the results of intervention. One frequently has to compromise between obtaining all the information one would wish and the practicability of doing this.

Measures of health and well-being

The Stanford ADL form is only a small part of a five-part Health Assessment Questionnaire (Fries *et al.*, 1980), other sections attempting to cover the personal and health service costs of illness. The Nottingham Health Profile (Hunt *et al.*, 1980) is frequently used in the UK. The Arthritis Impact Measurement Scales (AIMS) (Meenan, 1982) also gives a more complete picture. The Index of Wellbeing, covering mobility, physical activity and social function, was the basis of AIMS with the Rand Health Insurance study being grafted onto this. It is notable that many of these tests consider the wider effects of disability, as they look at personal, social and sexual function. Some may be concerned also with the emotional impact of the disease, and some with its economic impact on the patient and on society.

There are very many tests in existence: the reader is urged not to invent new ones, but, if possible, to ensure that, for research purposes at least, he uses validated tests.

REFERENCES

Bhavani, G., Cockburn, J., Whiting, S. and Lincoln, N. (1983) The reliability of the Rivermead Perceptual Assessment Battery and implications for some commonly used assessments of perception. *Br. J. Occup. Ther.*, *46*, 17–19

Brorsson, B. and Asberg, K. H. (1984) Katz Index of Independence in ADL. *Scand. J. Rehabil. Med.*, *16*, 125–32

DePaulo, G. R., Folstein, M. F. and Gordon, B. (1980) Psychiatric screening on a neurological ward. *Psychol. Med.*, *10*, 125–32

Dick, J. P. R., Guiloff, R. J., Stewart, A. *et al.* (1984) Mini-mental state examination in neurological patients. *J. Neurol. Neurosurg. Psychiatry*, *47*, 496–9

Fries, J. F., Spitz, P., Kraines, R. G. and Holman, H. R. (1980) Measurement of patient outcome in arthritis. *Arth. Rheum*, *23*, 137–45

Hart, L. E., Tugwell, P., Watson Buchanan, W., Norman, G. R., Grace, E. M. and Southwell, D. (1985) Grading of tenderness as a source of interrater error in the Ritchie Articular Index, *J. Rheumatol.*, *12* (4), 716–17

Helliwell, P., Howe, A. and Wright, V. (1987) Functional assessment of the hand: reproducibility, acceptability and utility of a new system of measuring strength. *Ann. Rheum. Dis.* *46*, 237–43

Hodkinson, H. M. (1972) Evaluation of a mental test score for assessment of mental impairment in the elderly. *Age Ageing*, *1*, 233–8

Holbrook, M. and Skilbeck, C. E. (1983) An activities index for use with stroke patients. *Age Ageing, 12,* 166–70

Hunt, S. M., McKenna, S.P., McEwen, J., Baackett, E.M., Williams, J. and Papp, E. (1980) A quantitative approach to perceived health status: a validation study. *J. Epidemiol. Comm. Health, 34,* 281–6

Isaacs, B. and Neville, Y. (1976) The needs of old people. The 'interval' as a method of measurement. *Br. J. Prev. Soc. Med., 30,* 79–85

Katz, S., Ford, A. B., Moskowitz, R. W., Jackson, B. and Jaffe, M. W. (1963) Studies of illness in the aged. The Index of ADL: a standardised measure of biological and psychological function, *J. Am. Med. Assoc., 185,* 914–19

Liang, M. H., Larson, M. G., Cullen, K. E. and Schwartz, J. A. (1985) Comparative measurement efficiency and sensitivity of five health status instruments for arthritis research. *Arth. Rheum., 28,* 542–7

Mahoney, F. I. and Barthel, D. W. (1965) Functional evaluation: the Barthel Index, *Maryland State Med. J., 14,* 61–5

Meenan, R. F. (1982) The AIMS approach to health status measurements: conceptual background and measurement properties. *J. Rheumatol., 9,* 785–8

Ritchie, D. M., Boyle, J. A., McInnes, J. M., Jasani, M. K., Dalakos, T. G., Grievson, P. and Watson Buchanan, W. (1968) Clinical studies with an articular index for the assessment of joint tenderness in patients with rheumatoid arthritis. *Q. J. Med., 37,* 393–406

Smith, M. E., Geraway, W. M., Akhtar, A. J. and Andrews, C. J. A. (1977) An assessment unit for measuring the outcome of stroke rehabilitation. *J. Occup. Ther., 40,* 46

Snaith, R. P., Ahmed, S. N., Mehta, S. and Hamilton, M. (1971) Assessment of the severity of primary depressive illness. *Psychol. Med., 1,* 143–9

Spiegel, J. S., Hirschfield, M. S. and Spiegel T. M. (1985) Evaluating self-care activities: comparison of self-reported questionnaire with an occupational therapist interview. *Br. J. Rheum., 24,* 357–61

Steinbrocker, O., Traeger, C. H. and Batterman, R. C. (1949) Therapeutic criteria in rheumatoid arthritis, *J. Am. Med. Assoc., 140,* 659–62

Tyerman, R., Tyerman, A., Howard, P. and Hadfield, C. (1987) *The Chessington O.T. Neurological Assessment Battery,* Nottingham Rehab., 17 Ludlow Hill Road, West Bridgford, Nottingham NG2 6HD

Wade, D. T., Langton Hewer, R., Skilbeck, C. E. and David, R. M. (1985) *Stroke: a critical approach to diagnosis, treatment and management,* Chapman & Hall, London

Zigmond, A. S. and Snaith, R. P. (1983) The Hospital Anxiety and Depression Scale, *Acta Psychiat. Scand., 67,* 361–70

FURTHER READING

Functional Assessment in Rehabilitation Medicine, ed. Carl Granger and Glen E. Gresham, Williams and Wilkins, 1984, Baltimore/London

Physical Disability in 1986 and Beyond: A report of the Royal College of Physicians, London

Part 2

Musculoskeletal Disorders

7

Management of Chronic Pain

Magdi Hanna

Pain is a unique and highly subjective experience, dependent upon a complex interplay of an individual's cognitions, emotions, interpersonal relationships and culture. Attempts to define pain have been hampered by this intrinsic complexity. Aristotle concluded that 'pain is an agony of the mind or a feeling of state', but excluded it from the classification of the five senses. Sherrington defined it as the 'physical adjunct of a protective reflex, playing a part in the survival of mankind'. Mountcastle's definition includes both physical and psychological elements in stating that 'pain is that sensory experience evoked by stimuli that injure or threaten to destroy tissue, defined introspectively by every man as that which hurts', while Merskey defines pain as 'unpleasant sensory and emotional experience associated with actual or potential tissue damage'. Even these more recent definitions seem inadequate and incomplete in the context of chronic pain, which is now recognised as a distinct medical entity in which pain persists after all possible healing has occurred, or it is at least no longer simply a symptom of injury or disease. It becomes a pain syndrome quite distinct in its composition from that of acute pain (Table 7.1).

Table 7.1: Pain syndrome

	Acute	Chronic
Aetiology	Known, detectable	Unclear, very difficult to detect
Duration	One month or less	Weeks–years
Psychological	Anxiety	Depression, behaviour and personality changes
Treatment	Relatively simple, logical–objective, usually effective	Complex, may require multiple methods
Result	Complete cure	Incomplete cure

PAIN RELIEF UNITS

The aims of pain relief units are:

(1) to deal with all types of pain (including cancer pain) from an early stage;

(2) to provide an advisory and treatment service at home and in hospital;

(3) to provide time (and patience) for patients to express their pain problems and for the doctor to create good rapport;

(4) to provide a wide spectrum of modern techniques of pain treatment;

(5) to work closely with family physicians, specialists and paramedical staff;

(6) to teach physicians and other medical staff, e.g. nurses, physiotherapists and pharmacists about pain;

(7) to conduct research.

MANAGEMENT OF CHRONIC PAIN

(a) The treatments available for chronic pain are diverse, and rarely specific owing to the varied pathology and psychological responses of those affected.

(b) Treatment may take a long time, and may be unsuccessful.

(c) Careful counselling to achieve proper evaluation, diagnosis and sympathetic understanding is essential.

(d) The understanding of patients and relatives of the treatment itself, its effects and/or side-effects, are important in gaining trust and continuous cooperation.

(e) It may be necessary to combine several therapeutic methods for the best results, e.g. drugs and transcutaneous nerve stimulation, nerve block and antidepressant.

(f) Many chronic pain syndromes are difficult to treat and require *specialist* management.

(g) The analgesic effect of drugs also depends on the brand of tablet employed because of bioavailability variations and differences in placebo response from one patient to another.

Table 7.2: Methods available for chronic pain therapy

1. Drugs
   A. Analgesics–antipyretic analysis (mild), narcotic analysis
   B. Adjuvant–tranquillisers, e.g. diazepam, chlorpromazine
   C. Antidepressant
   D. Others
2. Nerve blocks
3. Cryoanalysis, radiofrequency
   Surgery and radiotherapy
   Surface methods — cold spray, electrical transcutaneous nerve stimulation (TCNS)
4. Acupuncture
5. Physiotherapy and hypnosis

Drugs

Analgesics are the backbone of chronic pain therapy. To achieve the best results follow these principles:

(1) there should be a clear plan of action using a range of drugs from mild to strong;

(2) drugs should be given orally if possible;

(3) knowledge of the duration of action and half-life of commonly used drugs is essential to prevent erratic analgesia;

(4) with analgesia there is a ceiling effect, beyond which a higher dose does not produce more analgesia, only more side-effects;

(5) opioid addiction/dependence is rare provided drugs are used correctly.

Analgesics may be classified into two groups;

(a) Mild analgesics

Examples:

paracetamol, codeine, dextropropoxyphene, mefenamic acid, diflunisal, indomethacin, naproxen, other non-steroidal anti-inflammatory (NSAID)

This group is used for mild to moderate pain, i.e. headache, myalgia, arthralgia, mild neuralgia, widespread bone pain and other pain arising from integumental structures (rather than deep visceral pain). All NSAID (i.e. aspirin-like drugs) cause some gastric irritation including mild to severe bleeding. The addition of codeine or other opioid to an NSAID increases analgesic efficacy. Constipation is inevitable with codeine unless laxatives are added.

(b) Strong analgesics

'Narcotic agonists' (examples):

morphine, methadone, diamorphine (heroin), meperidine, methadone, dextromoramide.

'Narcotic agonists/antagonists' (examples):

buprenorphine, nalbuphine, pentazocine.

These drugs act on the opiate receptors in the central nervous system (CNS) and spinal cord. Morphine is the most commonly used of the strong analgesics and the standard by which others are judged. It has a combination of depressant and excitatory effects on the CNS. The depressant effects promote analgesia, hypnosis, tranquillisation and suppression of cough. Excitatory effects cause vomiting but rarely cause anxiety or restlessness. Constipation is common. Morphine has traditionally been given by injection 10–20 mg i.m. (Table 7.3) but modern practice favours alternative methods of administration, usually oral. Despite its poor efficacy (10 mg i.m. morphine=55–60 mg orally), morphine is now available in a slow-release formula.

Narcotic agonists/antagonists

Buprenorphine is the most widely used of this class of narcotics. It is 20–30 times as potent as morphine 0.3 mg i.m. = morphine 10 mg i.m. It is as effective as morphine and pethidine. Its duration of action is around 8 hours. It is available for parenteral or sublingual routes of administration. Tolerance does not appear to develop in chronic pain patients, and it has a low abuse potential.

Its major drawbacks are nausea, vomiting and the difficulty in reversing its effects with naloxone. Other side-effects are drowsiness, constipation respiratory depression, bradycardia and lowering blood pressure. Buprenorphine should not be given in combination with narcotic agonists, e.g. morphine.

Tranquillisers

Phenothiazines and benzodiazepine are used in chronic pain, for their anti-anxiety effects, hypnotic effects as well as muscle relaxant. They may be of use in combination with mild analgesics:

Table 7.3: Alternatives to morphine solution (all these drugs are given orally)

Name	Duration of action	Tablet	Morphine equivalent	Comment
Diamorphine (heroin)	4 hours	Used in mixture	Diamorphine : morphine = 1 : 1.5	Identical in use to morphine
Morphine sulphate continus (MST)	12 hours	10 mg	Morphine 5 mg 4-hourly	Useful new preparation; 30 mg, 60 mg and 100 mg tablets available
Phenazocine (Narphen)	6–8 hours	5 mg	25 mg	Useful strong analgesic in tablet form; usually start with ½ tablet 6 hourly
Dextromoramide (Palfium)	2 hours	5 mg	15 mg (peak effect)	Too short-acting for regular use, good for occasional 'breakthrough pain'
Dipipanone Co. (Diconal)	4 hours	10 mg (with cyclizine 50 mg)	5 mg	Addition of cyclizine causes marked sedation, especially if two or three tablets required
Levorphanol (Dromoran)	6–8 hours	1.5 mg	8 mg	Useful strong analgesic
Methadone (Physeptone)	Very long	5 mg	7.5 mg (for single dose)	Accumulation occurs with regular administration
Nepenthe (undiluted)	4 hours	1 ml	12 mg	Normally used in solution with aspirin
Oxycodone pectinate (Proladone) suppository	8 hours	30 mg suppository	15 mg 4-hourly	Excellent analgesic suppositories

(a) when further use of mild analgesics seems ineffective;

(b) when severe side-effects are associated with the use of a mild analgesic;

(c) in order to delay the use of narcotics.

Anti-depressants

Antidepressants work in two ways: firstly by causing mild elevation of mood and allaying anxiety, and secondly by promoting night sedation. Amitriptyline and prothiaden may have a direct analgesic action, due to interference with serotonin transport in the CNS. The combination of tricyclic antidepressant with phenothiazine is helpful in post-herpetic neuralgia and phantom limb pain.

Anticonvulsants

Anticonvulsants such as carbamazepine, phenytoin and sodium valproate work in trigeminal neuralgia, atypical facial neuralgia, pain in diabetic neuropathy and central pain.

Nerve blocks

Nerve blocks give worthwhile pain relief in up to 60 per cent of patients, e.g. visceral cancer pain; ischaemic pain, acute herpes zoster, minor causalgia and low back pain. Their purposes are diagnostic, prognostic and therapeutic by interruption of sensory pathways.

(1) *Diagnostic* blocks use local anaesthetic to identify the exact nerve radiating to the painful area (bupivacaine 0.5 per cent or lignocaine 1–2 per cent).
(2) *Prognostic* blocks assess the degree of pain relief resulting from a block; if the result is encouraging, definitive treatment can then be done by repeating the block with neurolytic agents (cryoprobe or radiofrequency).
(3) *Therapeutic* block
    (a) *Topical* infiltration of local anaesthetic is used for tender spots and trigger areas (painful scars).
    (b) *Somatic* (local anaesthetic or neurolytic, e.g. phenol, alcohol)
        (i) peripheral nerve
        (ii) brachial plexus
        (iii) epidural
        (iv) intrathecal
    (c) *Sympathic* (using local anaesthetic or neurolytic)
        (i) stellate ganglia plexus block

(ii) cardiac plexus block
(iii) lumbar sympathetic
(iv) coeliac plexus block
(v) *or* i.v. guanethidine

(d) *Cryoanalgesia* This technique freezes a peripheral nerve at −70°C and interrupts pain impulses, but does not alter it morphologically. It is helpful in many pain problems, especially intercostal neuralgia, atypical facial neuralgia, coccydynia and persistent trigger points.
(e) *Radiofrequency.* Radiofrequency causes destruction of pain fibres by high-frequency (50–100 Hz) electrical current. Its effect is more precise and lasts longer than neurolytic agent or cryoanalgesia, and is very useful in trigeminal neuralgia, mechanical back pain and for percutaneous cordotomy in unilateral cancer pain.

Physical methods

(a) Local anaesthetic spray/massage/heat or cold

Simple methods such as these should be tried first. They are helpful in:

(i) mild post-herpetic neuralgia
(ii) facial pain
(iii) joint pains

(b) Electrical stimulation

The aim of transcutaneous nerve stimulation (TCNS) is to stimulate large myelinated afferent nerve fibres and thus activate local inhibitory circuits within the spinal cord to reduce or diminish pain transmission.

For practical purposes, the aim of TCNS is to activate the large fibres without producing muscle contraction or dysthesia. One of the most important points is the positioning of the electrodes. The optimum site should:

(a) be very near to the area of maximum pain;
(b) preferably be in the distribution of the affected nerves (this is not essential).

The nature of the electrical stimulation should:

(a) produce some paraesthesiae felt by the patient in order to have a good effect;
(b) have higher frequency boosts which seem to offer better results than low frequency;

(c) have pulse width and amplitude adjustments for the patient to achieve comfortable paraesthesia.

The duration of using a TCNS machine varies considerably from patient to patient: some have very good relief lasting hours or days following 20 minutes of stimulation, and some only have relief when stimulated for 2–4 hours or even 24 hours, and may require either to have the machine constantly or maybe have implanted electrodes. TCNS is almost free of complications; the only side-effect commonly reported by patients has been allergic dermatitis from the jelly.

Acupuncture

Probably one of the oldest methods of pain treatment, requiring intact peripheral nerve pathways from the site of stimulation. Although its mechanism of action is still unclear, it could be through B-endorphin release and the opioid systems in the CNS. There is no doubt that acupuncture is effective in some patients with chronic pain states, e.g. neck pain, back pain, trigger points, arthralgia and headaches.

Psychotherapy and hypnosis

Patients suffering from intractable pain undergo severe personality, emotional and psychological changes. These will magnify the frustrations and disappointment of failure to recover from the pain and result in a vicious circle of depression and anxiety, leading to more pain and depression, etc. The use of ventilation therapy, behavioural therapy, group therapy, deep relaxation, positive reinforcement and continuous encouragement, should be an integral part of the whole strategy of managing chronic pain patients.

SOME COMMON CHRONIC PAIN SYNDROMES REFERRED TO PAIN RELIEF UNITS (Table 7.4)

1. Neuralgia

Neuralgia could be defined as pain in the distribution of a peripheral nerve, often accompanied by signs of nerve dysfunction. Neuralgic pain presents as paroxysmal, spontaneous and hyperpathetic.

It may be aching, burning or lancinating with superimposed attacks of severe pain, like stabbing. Neuralgia could be the product of mechanical

Table 7.4: Chronic pain syndromes referred to a pain clinic

Post-herpetic neuralgia
Trigeminal neuralgia and atypical facial neuralgias
Nerve entrapment
Migraine
Phantom pain, e.g. limb, breast
Causalgia
Ischaemic legs
Sympathetic dystrophy syndrome (Sudeck atrophy)
Raynaud's disease
Spinal mechanical pain
Spinal cord injury
Pain in advanced cancer
Central pain

(entrapment, trigeminal neuralgia), toxic, metabolic (diabetes, alcoholism), inflammatory (post-herpetic) or idiopathic. Analgesics (mild to strong), although widely used, are extremely disappointing and ineffective. Anticonvulsants, e.g. carbamazepine 200–600 mg t.d.s. have been found to be effective in trigeminal neuralgia and occasionally in post-herpetic neuralgia. Surgery has been used in selected cases of trigeminal neuralgic with good results, but in general peripheral neurectomy or rhizotomy are not beneficial. Nerve blocks with LA with or without steroids are helpful in nerve entrapment neuralgia, and cryoanalgesia may prolong the effect. Sympathetic blocks are useful, particularly in acute herpes zoster and early post-herpetic neuralgia. TCNS was found to be helpful in 30–34 per cent of neuralgias, especially in combination with central medication. Finally physical, emotional and psychological support to these patients is essential to achieve lasting rehabilitation.

2. Phantom pain syndrome

Phantom pain following amputation of limbs is now a well-recognised syndrome. Its incidence could be as high as 70 per cent. It seems that the incidence is much higher in patients with a severely painful limb prior to surgery compared with those with painless limbs.

Phantom limb pain can be differentiated from stump pain as the latter is usually caused by a local neuroma, whereas the former is likely to be centrally mediated.

Phantom pain can also follow other organ surgery, e.g. mastectomy, orchidectomy and following AP resection of rectum.

Surgical approaches to this syndrome are fruitless. Non-surgical approaches offer better results in the form of centrally acting drugs, especially antidepressants, in combination with phenothiazines or anticonvulsant and TCNS.

3. Causalgia and post-traumatic dystrophy syndrome

These syndromes have the following factors in common:

pain which is usually burning in character,
sympathetic dysfunction,
delayed functional recovery and trophic changes.

These symptoms could occur after any kind of trauma (fractures, laceration, strain and surgical incision). They usually occur in the extremities. In causalgia there is partial or total nerve injury. All these syndromes, if ingored, result in intractable pain with trophic changes and loss of function. The best line of treatment is to identify these syndromes early and intercept the pathological reflex activity by means of sympathetic nerve blocks, e.g. stellate ganglion block using i.v. guanethidine or by using i.v. ketamine (5-HT antagonists) in modified Beir's block. Active physiotherapy should be accompanied by the above treatment.

With intractable pain TCNS and antidepressants may be of some help.

4. Low back pain

Low back pain (LBP) is probably one of the most common syndromes referred to pain clinics all over the world. In many instances patients have undergone multiple examinations, numerous investigations and vast arrays of procedures and still suffer from LBP. The result may be a progressive deterioration in the physical and psychological status of the patient, added to the economic effects related to possible loss of income.

The management of chronic LBP

(a) Full and detailed history, which includes a detailed drug history.
(b) Full physical assessment and reappraisal of all investigations.
(c) Full psychological evaluation with special emphasis on social factors, secondary gain, familial interaction and personality inventory (depression and hysteria mainly).
(d) The emphasis should be conservative and not surgical, unless there is a clear indication of nerve root compression or spinal instability.
(e) Epidural injection with LA (bupivacaine) or with depomedrone 80 mg in selected cases of LBP due to root irritation or minor disc

herniation, can be of great help. The epidural should be as near as possible to the segment causing pain.

(f) Facet joint injections under X-ray screening in patients with postural defects can be extremely rewarding exercises. Diagnostic block can be followed by cryotherapy or radiofrequency of the affected joint if prolonged relief is not achieved by the LA injection.

(g) TCNS may be effective in some cases, especially those with predominant muscle spasm and the postoperative pain.

(h) Antidepressants, e.g. prothiaden and amitriptyline, are important for secondary depression and insomnia, especially in the intractable LBP associated with possible root damage, e.g. arachnoiditis.

(i) Long-term physical and psychological rehabilitation may be the only way to avoid a totally disabled patient.

5. Spinal cord injury

Pain following spinal cord injury can either manifest itself early following the injury or it may be quite delayed (possibly years after). The mechanism is usually multifactorial, including:

(a) musculoskeletal (e.g. spasm),

(b) phantom pain,

(c) autonomic disturbance as in causalgia,

(d) psychological aspects of the injury.

Treatment should aim at all the above factors, i.e. combination therapy of psychological and physical, e.g. sympathetic, blocks where applicable, control by drugs, e.g. antidepressants, and possibly TCNS.

6. Pain in advanced cancer

Pain in cancer can offer a unique challenge to the physician, even though it may accompany a dynamic, progressive and ultimately fatal pathology. With the proper uses of analgesics and nerve block techniques, pain control could be totally achieved, and this may be extremely rewarding for the medical and nursing staff concerned. The strategy of treatment is as follows:

(a) Select NSAID and mild analgesic in mild pain and specifically in pain associated with bony metastasis.

(b) Consider adjuvant drugs if pain is not totally controlled by mild analgesics, e.g. phenothiazines, benzodiazepines or psychotropic drugs.

(c) Nerve blocks should be considered early rather than later, e.g. coeliac plexus block in upper abdominal cancer pain, intrathecal injection for perineal pain.

(d) If pain is severe and generalised narcotic drugs should be given. The dose should be titrated to the need of the individual patient.

(e) Analgesic drugs should be given as regular medication and not only on demand.

(f) Side-effects of strong narcotics should be anticipated and prevented from the start; e.g. constipation — use regular laxatives, and for nausea use regular antiemetics.

FURTHER READING

Advances in Pain Research and Therapy, Vol. 7, Beneditti, C., Chapman, C.R. and Moricca, G. (eds), Raven Press, New York, 1984

Proceedings of the 4th World Congress on Pain, Raven Press, New York, 1985

Textbook of Pain, Wall, P.D. and Melzack, R. Churchill Livingstone, Edinburgh

Persistent Pain, Lipton, S. (ed.): Vol. 1, Academic Press, London, 1980; Vol. 2, Academic Press, London, 1981; Vol. 3, Academic Press, London, 1985

Psychology of Pain, Sternbach, R. (ed.), Raven Press, New York, 1986

The Challenge of Pain, Melzack, R. and Wall, P. D. (eds) Penguin, Harmondsworth, Middlesex, 1982

Neural Blockade and Pain Management, Cousins, M. J. and Bridenbaugh, P. D. (eds), Lippincott, Philadelphia, 1980

Goodman & Gilman's The Pharmacological Basis of Therapeutics, 7th edition, Gilman, A.G., Goodman, L.S., Rall, T.W. and Murad, F. (eds), Macmillan, London, 1985

Pain Terms; a list with definitions and notes on usage. Recommended by the IASP Subcommittee on Taxonomy. *Pain*, 1979, *6*, 249–50

Wall, P. D. Causes of intractable pain. *Hospital Update*, *12*(12), 969–74 (December 1986)

8

Locomotion: Analysis of Gait, Normal and Abnormal

John Goodwill

Walking is an activity that we all take for granted. It is basically a means of moving a multi-jointed body forwards from one point to another. While maintaining balance the body weight is taken on one leg, the stance side hip extends as the opposite leg swings forwards to gain distance and take the body weight in its turn. Movement depends upon intact nerves and coordinated control of muscle contraction and relaxation, the muscles acting on levers (bones) moving about the axes of the joints to produce movement or to control joint position. Energy is used usefully to propel the body forwards but it is also expended by the 3–5 cm sinusoidal movement of the centre of gravity both in the vertical and horizontal planes, by the acceleration of the leg in early swing phase, and by shock absorption and deceleration late in swing phase (Inman, 1967). Whether the gait is normal or abnormal the gait pattern used is that which is most energy-efficient, unless pain or the need to maintain joint stability is dominant. The more that the body is moved up and down the less efficient walking becomes as a means of propulsion, and in running even more energy is wasted in this manner. In walking part of at least one foot is in contact with the ground all the time, whereas in running there are periods during the gait cycle when both feet are off the ground.

WALKING IS DIVIDED INTO SWING AND STANCE PHASES

For each leg *stance phase* is that part of the gait cycle when any part of the foot is in contact with the ground, and *swing phase* is when the foot is clear of the ground. As the body weight is transferred from one leg to the other there is a *period of double support* when some part of each foot is on the ground. For each leg the proportion of time in stance to swing is about 60 : 40 in average walking (Figure 8.1).

The swing phase commences as the toe leaves the ground, the body weight transferring to the other leg by contraction of the opposite hip

Figure 8.1: Distance and time dimensions of walking cycle: *step length* is the distance between *contralateral* heel-strikes; *stride length* is the distance between *ipsilateral* heel-strikes; *cadence* is step frequency (steps per unit of time). (From *Human walking*, by V.T. Inmann, H.J. Ralson and F. Todd; reproduced by kind permission of the publishers, Williams & Wilkins, Baltimore and London, 1981)

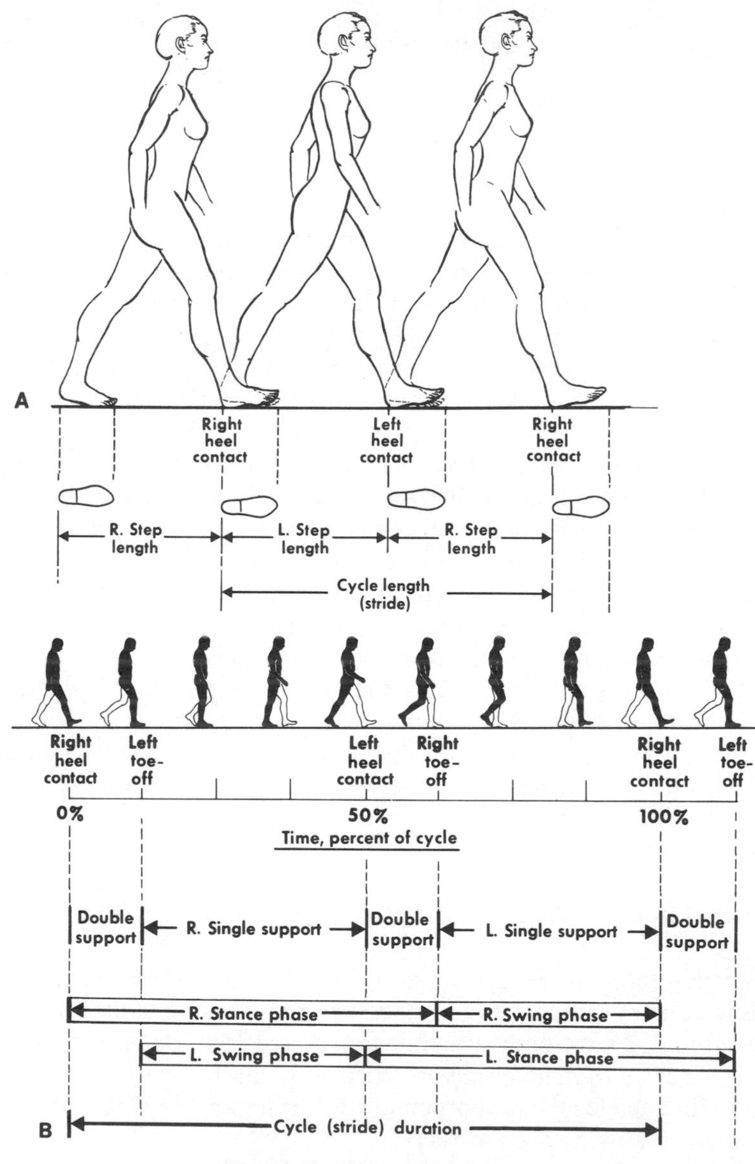

abductors and extensor muscles, with contraction of quadriceps and hamstrings to control the knee. *The swinging leg* flexes and abducts at the hip and dorsiflexes at the ankle to clear the ground, the pelvis dropping down (up to 5°) on that side as the foot leaves the ground.

The leg accelerates early in swing and decelerates late in swing phase. As swing phase continues the hip progressively flexes, the knee extends and dorsiflexion of the foot enables the leg to swing through to *heel-strike, the first part of stance phase.* At this time the ankle is controlled by contraction of dorsi and plantar flexor muscles; as the ankle plantar flexes into *foot flat* the body weight is transferred on to that foot. The lateral border of the foot hits the ground slightly before the medial side, the foot then pronating so that the foot is flat on the ground. The pronation/supination (eversion/inversion) movement at the subtalar joint is needed to maintain normal balance. *While the opposite leg swings through* the pull of the calf muscles stabilises the foot and then lifts the heel on the stance side (*heel-off*). The supporting knee flexes in late stance phase and while the opposite leg swings through the body weight moves forward over the foot. The metatarsophalangeal joints dorsiflex as the toes are on the ground while the remainder of the foot is rising. Stance ends with *toe-off.*

Rotation: in the last 25 per cent of stance phase the knee flexes further and the *tibia externally rotates 8–9°*. The tibia rotates internally during late swing and early stance phase. The *pelvis and femur externally and internally rotate* by about 4° and 6° respectively at the same time and in the same direction as the tibia rotates.

As walking speed increases the knee flexion increases in swing and in late stance phases, and the whole gait cycle takes place more quickly; stride length increases, and there is a reduction in stance phase and double-support time as a percentage of the gait cycle. When walking is very fast the stance phase shortens even more until the period of double-support is lost and the person is running (Kirtley *et al.*, 1985; Antonsson and Mann, 1985). In a slow shuffling gait there is a prolonged double-support time, so that stance phase may be 90 per cent of the total gait cycle and the speed is slow. Faster forward progress cannot be achieved by maintaining the same cadence (steps/minute) and increasing the stride length only, because energy consumption is then increased; the cadence as well as the stride length must be increased (Saunders *et al.*, 1953).

GAIT ANALYSIS

Murray *et al.* (1964) used a photographic method of gait analysis in 60 normal men walking at a cadence of 112 steps per minute and did not find any difference in stride *width* (mean 8.0 cm) or in the duration of the gait cycle (mean 1.03 seconds) in relation to age, height or weight, although taller men took longer steps and men over 60 years of age had shorter step and stride lengths. Similar results were found by Kirtley *et al.* (1985).

When comparing two groups of women, aged 20–35 and 60–84 years, Payne and Blanke (1985) found no difference between the two groups in vertical or lateral movement of the centre of gravity, pelvic or tibial rotation, or stride *width*, although the younger women took longer steps and had a greater range of ankle movement than the older women. Murray *et al.* (1970) examined the gait of 30 normal women in five decades from 20 to 70 years, comparing this with the gait of the men who they had studied previously (Murray *et al.*, 1964). They found that the women had greater lateral pelvic shift, smaller excursion of the arms, and less knee flexion in stance and in swing.

They then compared the same subjects walking in high-heeled (6 cm) or flat-heeled (2 cm) shoes; wearing the former the stride length was shorter (133 cm as against 152 cm) but the walking cadence (steps/minute), stride width, stance and swing duration were the same in high- or low-heeled shoes. The walking speed was slower, mean 163 cm/s compared with 188 cm/s. Methods of gait analysis are discussed in Chapter 36.

ENERGY COST OF WALKING

Walking is most efficient at about 80 m/min requiring about 0.8 cal/m per kg of body weight. The fit person in a hurry uses more energy per unit distance. The disabled person walking slower also uses excess energy and fatigues more easily, but will adjust his pace to maintain a level of oxygen consumption that does not make him feel breathless. Energy cost of walking is well reviewed by Fisher and Gullickson (1978).

RANGE OF JOINT MOVEMENT IN WALKING

A full range of joint movements at all weight-bearing joints is not needed for normal gait, but some movements are more important than others. In normal walking *the hip* has extended 15° by the end of the stance phase and flexes up to 30° in late swing. *The knee* needs to extend in late swing phase but is slightly flexed at heel-strike; to hit the ground with the knee straight would increase the shock of impact through the leg, whereas a slightly flexed knee going on to increased flexion during stance phase with eccentric quadriceps action is more shock-absorbing. The knee flexes about 40° in late stance, flexing further to 60° in early swing. *The ankle* dorsiflexes 15° at heel-off and then plantarflexes 20° at toe-off and in early swing phase. It is evident that limitation of movement at these joints which still allows the required range for walking may have little effect on normal gait. The angles may increase as walking speed increases (Figure 8.2).

Figure 8.2: Position of leg joints: (a) in swing phase; (b) in stance phase

(a)

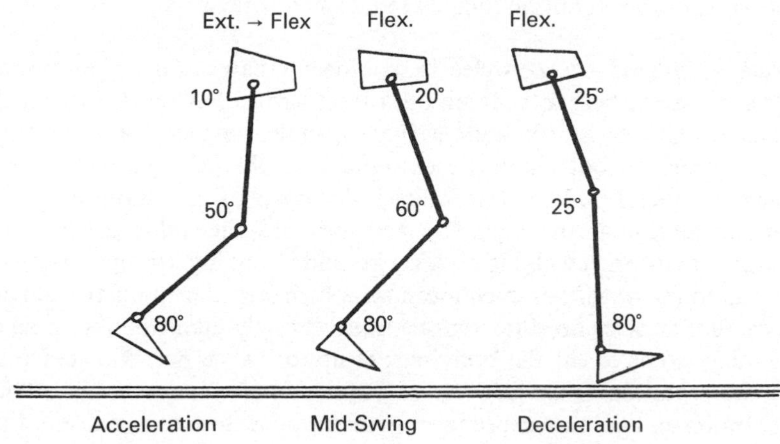

(b)

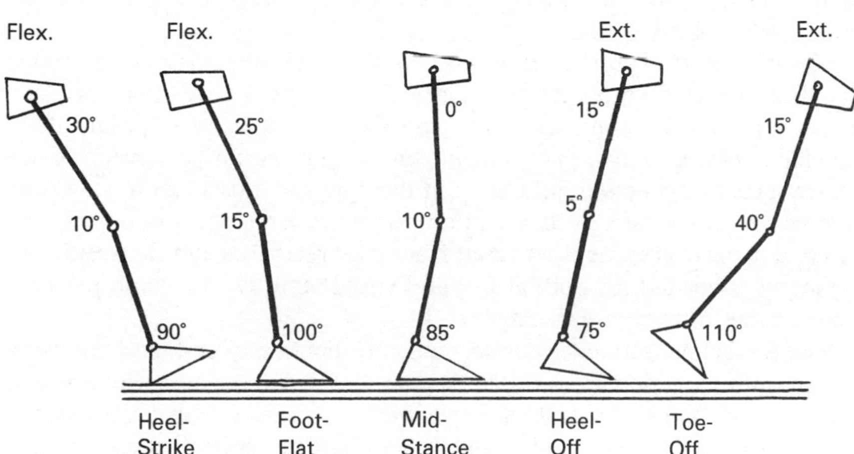

MUSCLES USED IN WALKING

Anterior tibial muscles are used throughout swing phase to dorsiflex the ankle, and in early stance until foot-flat.

Calf muscles act mainly in mid-stance to provide heel-off.

Quadriceps contract in early stance to stabilise the knee, and in late stance and early swing to bring the flexed knee forward to gain step length, whilst the *hamstring* muscles are used particularly in late swing and early stance to help stabilise the knee.

Hip abductors and extensors contract mainly in early stance to support the body weight; *hip flexors* in swing phase to bring the leg forward, while the *hip adductors* contract mainly in late stance phase.

Walking up or down steps clearly requires a greater range of movement and muscle strength than walking on a level surface. When going up, the calf muscles have to lift the body weight on to the next step, and the ankle of the supporting foot plantarflexes more than the 20° required in level walking; conversely when descending, the ankle of the supporting foot dorsiflexes more than the usual 15°. The hips and knees flex less on going *downstairs* than when walking on level ground but going *upstairs* may have to flex up to 80° or 90°, or even more for a high step. On stairs the quadriceps and hip muscles need to contract more strongly than when walking on flat ground, so as to lift the body weight up, or to support the stance leg while the other leg is lowered on to the next step. The latter is often a bigger problem, and may cause more pain in the arthritic knee or hip than going upstairs. In the same way weakness of hip or knee muscles from neurological or other diseases can make it more difficult to go downstairs than upstairs. Also when going up the body is leaning forwards, and the patient is less likely to fall.

The neurological control of gait is complex and only partly understood, but there are rhythm-generating centres in the spinal cord, one for each limb, coordinated by interneurones and fixed at an early stage in infant development (leg flexion occurs mainly in swing phase and extension in the stances phase of gait, with inhibition of the opposite muscle groups). These centres are controlled by descending pathways from the brainstem and cerebral hemispheres. Sensory input from joint receptors and the vestibular apparatus is needed for normal gait and visual input is important, particularly if either of these are damaged.

The cerebellum influences timing and coordination of gait, and the basal ganglia influence posture so that disease of the latter causes immobility (Martin, 1967). The physiological reasons for reciprocal arm movements are not clear, but they aid walking and reduce energy consumption. Jackson *et al.* (1983) found that walking was difficult if the ipsilateral arm moved forward with the leg or if the arms were strapped to the trunk. The neurological control of gait is well reviewed by Joseph (1985).

ABNORMAL GAIT

A leg that is short by 4–5 cm or more causes obvious dipping of the pelvis towards that side during stance phase, the patient leaning towards that side, while excessive flexion of the opposite knee and hip is used to clear the ground with the contralateral foot.

Pain in the hip or knee will be worse in stance than swing phase, the proportion of the former being decreased causing asymmetry of gait. In walking joint movement and step length are reduced (Tesio *et al.*, 1985). Also during stance on the painful side the hip may not be able to support the body weight adequately, giving rise to excess dipping of the pelvis towards the swinging leg, i.e. waddling.

Pain in the ankle or tarsal joints is felt mainly during early stance phase as the force of the body weight is taken on the hindfoot, the pain may ease as the heel leaves the ground. It is at this time, later in stance phase, that the *metatarsophalangeal joints* are passively dorsiflexed as the body weight moves forward over them. Because of this movement and the extra force through the forefoot, pain at these joints is worse late in stance phase, although it can be reduced by an outside rocker bar on the shoe (Chapter 45).

Limitation of joint movement

Fixed flexion at the hip will require increased lumbar lordosis to maintain erect posture when the knee is straight and weight-bearing. If the hip is so much flexed that the knee cannot be fully extended normally in the first part of stance phase, the flexed knee can only be stabilised by stronger contraction of the quadriceps or by the patient leaning forward on a stick, resulting in reduced step length on the normal side (Figure 8.3). *Fixed hip adduction* causes inability to abduct the hip during *swing phase*, the patient tilting the pelvis to the opposite side to compensate. Fixed flexion or adduction of the hip causes apparent shortening of the leg, which may require a shoe raise. In *stance phase* severe fixed adduction may make the patient unstable; falling to the affected side is prevented by use of a stick on that side.

Limitation of hip flexion is not a problem for walking because the joint only needs to flex 25–30°, and by the time this severity of limitation occurs the associated hip pain is usually the bigger problem. However, going up steps or sitting down requires up to 90° hip flexion, and will be difficult for many patients.

Fixed flexion of the knee over 25° causes the ground reactive force (line of body weight) to lie well behind the knee axis during stance phase, requiring stronger quadriceps contraction to support the body weight. In addition the heel stays clear of the ground so that the stance phase starts with the toe hitting the ground rather than with the normal heel-strike. In swing phase the leg cannot reach out as far as normal to gain a normal step length (Figure 8.3).

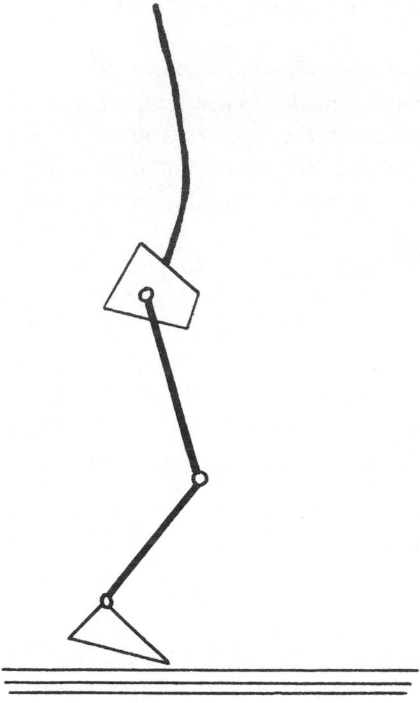

Figure 8.3: Fixed flexion of the knee and hip causes an increased lumbar lordosis and in stance phase the heel may not reach the ground

Limited flexion of the knee, or pain on flexion, limits the normal joint movement in late stance and early swing phase of gait, causing reduction of step length on both sides and an inefficient gait pattern. With a *fixed straight knee* the ipsilateral pelvis has to rise excessively. It is easier with a knee fixed in 15° flexion; however, there is still greater movement of the centre of gravity than is normal.

Ankle joint limitation on its own causes little problem until the movement is reduced to 10° up or down, when the foot tends to be put down and taken up in one piece, with loss of the normal heel–toe gait. There is a small increase in knee and hip flexion to compensate (Saunders *et al.*, 1953). However, there is often limitation of tarsal joint movement as well, which limits the normal pronation–supination of the foot.

Flaccid muscle weakness

Flaccid foot drop, as in common peroneal nerve paralysis, poliomyelitis, or muscular dystrophy, requires excessive lifting of the foot during swing phase in order to clear the ground, which is done by lifting the pelvis on the ipsilateral side with excessive flexion of the hip and knee. Stance may start with a toe- rather than a heel-strike, unless there is only moderate dorsiflexion weakness, when the whole foot meets the ground at one time, causing a slapping sound.

Calf muscle weakness limits the force available to lift the body weight up during attempted heel-off. Heel-off is delayed until heel-strike occurs on the opposite side, and the ground reactive force passing through the foot (line of body weight) is kept further back for longer than is usual. There is an increased flexor moment about the knee, requiring increased quadriceps contraction to counteract it. Excessive ankle dorsiflexion may result, which can be controlled by an orthosis limiting dorsiflexion (Lehmann *et al.*, 1985).

Quadriceps weakness: the knee axis passes through the femoral condyles 2–4 cm above the joint line, being forward in extension and moving back as the knee flexes. *Knee stability* during stance phase is normally maintained by quadriceps power, although weakness may be partly or wholly compensated by strong hip extensor muscles. During stance phase these can force the femur back to over-extend the knee, moving the knee joint axis back behind the line of body weight as the centre of gravity moves forward rapidly. This will then prevent knee flexion while the cruciate ligaments prevent excessive extension. During late swing phase normal knee extension is achieved by the inertia of the forward-moving leg; strong hip extensors decelerate the thigh, allowing the lower leg to swing forward to a good heel contact.

Weakness of hip and knee flexor muscles: this causes reduced hip flexion in early swing phase and reduced knee control in later swing and early stance phases, resulting in excessive lifting and forward rotation of the ipsilateral pelvis with a forward 'flip' of the leg, including some circumduction.

Hip girdle muscle weakness causes a waddling gait because the hip is not supported normally in stance phase, allowing excessive dipping of the opposite side of the pelvis. This is seen in muscular dystrophies and in other myopathies such as osteomalacia and hypothyroidism. Often the quadriceps muscles are also weak, causing additional problems with knee stability. When standing still any attempt to stand on one leg causes dropping down of the unsupported side of the pelvis, because the hip on the stance side is not supported normally by the hip abductors and extensors (Trendelenberg sign).

Paraplegia

If the patient has complete leg weakness he may walk using elbow or Canadian crutches and knee–ankle–foot orthoses with the knees locked in extension; the ankles are supported to prevent plantar flexion. This stiff-legged gait works because the pelvis is lifted for each step by the latissimus dorsi, and the remaining abdominal and spinal muscles, the point of fixation being the shoulders which are supported by strong downward thrust on the arms through straight elbows to the crutches. *The higher the lesion the more energy is required for walking* and above T 11–12 it usually becomes a wasteful activity for most adults, although there are a few exceptions (see Orthotics, Chapter 45). Even normal subjects use twice normal energy walking with either under-arm or elbow crutches, no difference being found between these two types of crutches (Fisher and Patterson, 1981); however, Dounis *et al.* (1980) found that in five normal subjects the Canadian crutch (with a rigid complete circular top) was more energy-efficient than the elbow crutch, the distance walked per litre of oxygen used being an average of 61.3 m compared with 53.3 m. Children can walk efficiently with higher lesions than adults, as is seen in many children with spina bifida who walk when young but stop doing so when they reach their teens. These children may use plastic or metal above-knee orthoses (KAFO), a hip guidance orthosis or a swivel walker (Rose, 1986).

Cauda equina lesions produce a wide variety of patterns of leg weakness; although they have flaccid paralysis, contractures can be a major problem if these are not prevented. If the quadriceps are spared, ankle–foot orthoses will provide foot and ankle support, and the normal knee control will allow a near-normal gait pattern using a walking aid. If quadriceps are weak, then knee–ankle–foot orthoses are needed, and the patient will walk with a stiff-legged gait as described above.

Gait in upper motor neurone lesions

Spastic drop foot causes the foot to catch during swing phase, and the spasticity of the calf muscles has an inversion moment about the subtalar joint causing the foot to go into equinovarus. At the start of stance phase the toe rather than the heel reaches the ground first, and the outer border of the foot may reach the ground markedly before the inner border, the foot then being forced flat by the body weight. If there is severe varus the body weight pushes the foot into more inversion. The patient may bear all or most of his weight on the outer border of the foot throughout stance phase. The axis of the subtalar joint passes about 45° downward and 12° outwards from the navicular, backwards, out and down to the outer posterior aspect of the calcaneum, so that the tendo achilles has a medial (inversion) moment about this axis (Hall, 1959). Although the vertical distance from the line of pull of the tendo achilles to the joint axis is small, the strength of the muscles is so much greater than that of the other invertors, that this vector of force provides the main mechanical force inverting the subtalar joint (Lapidus, 1955), at the same time as it plantarflexes the foot at the ankle joint (Alexander *et al.*, 1982) (Chapter 45) (Figure 8.4).

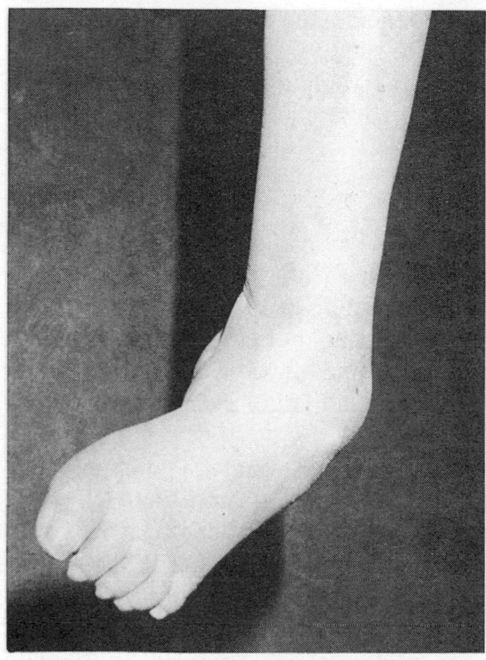

Figure 8.4: Spastic equinovarus foot showing the position to be prevented (stroke with spastic hemiplegia)

Most commonly spastic equinus is part of *hemiplegia due to stroke*, in which there is not only spastic weakness of the arm and leg but also impairment of superficial sensation, possibly also of joint position sense and often of body image, all of which affect gait. The stance phase is shortened on the affected side, but the duration of single leg support does not correlate with the degree of motor recovery (Brandstater *et al.*, 1983). If there is some remaining power in the quadriceps and hip muscles, the patient learns to keep the knee locked to enable him to take weight through the affected leg in stance phase; however this makes it difficult for him to initiate swing phase. The ipsilateral side of the pelvis is also rotated backwards, thus aggravating the problem (Wall and Ashburn, 1979). Slow movement of the paretic leg during swing phase prolongs stance on the opposite leg; the latter is also prolonged due to the slower than normal weight transference from the weak to the good leg during the period of double support (Eke–Okoro and Larsson, 1984). Step length on the weak side is shortened to 67–92 per cent of normal (Tesio *et al.*, 1985). There are thus many abnormalities of gait with which patient and therapist have to contend, and clearly the ability to maintain single leg support while the good leg swings through is the main determinant of gait.

The combination of *stroke and leg amputation* is not uncommon (Varghese *et al.*, 1978) and presents a considerable challenge to rehabilitation. Nevertheless in that series of 30 patients, ten achieved useful walking in their home, although only three were able to walk outside the house, all of the latter having the hemiplegia and the amputation on the same side.

Effects of contracture

Fixed plantarflexion due to contracture of the calf muscles, as may occur with prolonged spasticity due to stroke or head injury, causes the tibia to be angled back when the foot is flat on the ground. This helps to lock the knee in extension in early stance and weight-bearing, but later in stance phase it precipitates early heel-off and can prevent knee flexion. This either effectively increases leg length and increases rise and fall of the centre of gravity, or greatly limits step length in the other leg.

Fixed flexion of the knee and/or hip can occur even with good physiotherapy, more often due to head injury than stroke; more than 25° fixed flexion of either will cause gait problems. The knee is bent in stance phase in either case, and even if fixed equinus is absent the heel is off the ground in order to keep the line of body weight over the supporting foot. Step length is shortened because the knee cannot extend in the latter part of swing phase, and walking aids are often needed to maintain stability (Figure 8.3).

Parkinson's disease

This condition causes bradykinesia, the rigidity resulting in difficulty in initiating movement and a slow shuffling flat-footed gait. Knuttson (1972) found the reduced walking speed and prolonged gait cycle were due to diminished stride length, with an increased period of double support and reduction of associated trunk and arm movements. In normal gait right and left steps are usually equal but he found only four of his 21 subjects had a symmetrical gait pattern. Ankle plantarflexion was reduced at the end of stance phase, causing difficulty in initiating swing, and there was also reduction of hip flexion, and of knee flexion and extension. These combine to reduce the speed and amplitude of leg movement, and the gait problems are aggravated by the variability of the whole disease.

Cerebellar ataxia

This condition presents considerable problems. The patient walks on a wide base, the incoordination affecting all parts of the gait cycle and encouraging a prolonged stance phase to prevent falling. If a stick is used, the support base can be kept wide while the feet are brought into a more normal position. This gait problem is largely unresponsive to physiotherapy, even using biofeedback with the patient viewing his gait pattern in a mirror placed in front of him. The difficulties may be aggravated by ataxia of the arms and/or trunk, or by muscle weakness or position sense loss, all of which often occur in the diseases that cause cerebellar ataxia.

ACKNOWLEDGEMENT

I am grateful to my in-house artists Miss Anne-Marie Goodwill and Mr Mark Goodwill for the line diagrams, and to Gordon Rose, FRCS, and Robin Luff, FRCS for helpful comments on the script.

REFERENCES

Alexander, M.C., Battye, C.K., Goodwill, C.J. and Walshe, J.B. (1982) The ankle and subtalar joints. In *Measurement of joint movement. Clinics in Rheumatic Diseases*, 8, no. 3

Antonsson, E.K. and Mann, R.W. (1985) The frequency content of gait. *J. Biomech.*, *18*, 39–47

Brandstater, M.E., de Bruin, H., Gowland, C. and Clark B.M. (1983) Hemiplegic gait: analysis of temporal variables. *Arch. Phys. Med. Rehabil.*, *64*, 583–7

Dounis, E., Steventon, R.D. and Wilson R.S.E. (1980) The use of a portable oxygen consumption meter (Oxylog) for assessing the efficiency of crutch walking *J. Med. Eng. Tech.*, *4*, 296–8

Eke-Okoro, S.T. and Larsson, L.E. (1984) A comparison of the gaits of paretic patients with the gaits of control subjects carrying a load. *Scand. J. Rehabil. Med.*, *16*, 151–8

Fisher, S.V. and Gullickson, G. (1978) Energy cost of ambulation in health and disability, a literature review. *Arch. Phys. Med. Rehabil.*, *59*, 124–33

Fisher, S.V. and Patterson, R.P. (1981) Energy cost of ambulation *Arch. Phys. Med. Rehabil.*, *62*, 250–6

Hall, M.C. (1959) The normal movement at the subtalar joint. *Canad. J. Surg.*, *2*, 287–90

Inman, V.T. (1967) Conservation of energy in ambulation. *Arch. Phys. Med. Rehabil.*, *47*, 484–8

Jackson, K.M., Joseph, J. and Wyard, S.J. (1983) The upper limbs during human walking. Part 2: Functional. *Electroencephalog. Clin. Neurophysiol.*, *23*, 435–46

Joseph, J. (1985) Neurological control of locomotion. *Dev. Med. Child Neurol.*, *27*, 822–9

Kirtley, C., Whittle, M.W. and Jefferson, R.J. (1985) Influence of walking speed on gait parameters. *J. Biomed. Eng.*, *7*, 282–8

Klepsteg, P.E. and Wilson, P.D. (eds) (1954) *Human limbs and their substitutes*, McGraw-Hill, New York

Knuttson, E. (1972) An analysis of Parkinsonian gait. *Brain*, *95*, 475–86

Lapidus, T.W. (1955) Subtalar joint, its anatomy and mechanics. *Bull. Hosp. Joint Dis.*, *16*, 179–95

Lehmann, J.F., Condon, S.M., de Lateur, B.J. and Smith, J.C. (1985) Gait abnormalities in tibial nerve paralysis: a biomechanical study. *Arch. Phys. Med. Rehabil.*, *66*, 80–5

Martin, J.P. (1967) *The basal ganglia and posture*, Pitman, London

Murray, M.P., Drought, A.B. and Kory, R.C. (1964) Walking patterns of normal men. *J. Bone Joint Surg.*, *46A*, 335–60

Murray, M.P., Kory, R.C. and Sepic, S.B. (1970) Walking patterns of normal women. *Arch. Phys. Med. Rehabil.*, *51*, 637–50

Payne, P. and Blanke, D. (1985) Comparison of gait parameters of young and elderly women (Abstr). *Phys. Ther.*, *65*, 686

Perry, J. (1969) Mechanics of walking in hemiplegia. *Clin. Orthop.*, *63*, 23–31

Rose, G.K. (1986) *Orthotics: principles and practice*, Heinemann, London

Saunders, J.B. deC., Saunders, M., Inman, V.T. and Eberhart, H.D. (1953) The major determinants in normal and pathological gait. *J. Bone Joint Surg.*, *35A*, 543–58

Tesio, L., Civaschi, P. and Tessari, L. (1985) Motion of the centre of gravity of the body in clinical evaluation of gait. *Am. J. Phys. Med.*, *64*, 57–70

Turnbull, G.I. and Wall, J.C. (1985) The development of a system for the clinical assessment of gait following a stroke. *Physiotherapy*, *71*, 294–8

Varghese, G., Hinterbuchner, C., Mondall, P. and Sakuma, J. (1978) Rehabilitation outcome of patients with dual disability of hemiplegia and amputation. *Arch. Phys. Med. Rehabil.*, *59*, 121–3

Wall, J.C. and Ashburn, A. (1979) Assessment of gait disability in hemiplegics. *Scand. J. Rehabil. Med.*, *11*, 95–103

FURTHER READING

Inman, V.T., Ralston, H.J. and Todd, F. (1981) *Human walking*. Williams & Wilkins, Baltimore

Ohlsson, E. (1986) Gait analysis in hip and knee surgery. *Scand. J. Rehabil. Med.*, Suppl. 15

9

Osteoarthritis and Spinal Pain

Anne Chamberlain

INTRODUCTION

Degenerative joint disease (DJD) is common. Defined radiologically it is present in a large proportion of the population, its frequency increasing with age. Such findings apply equally to the axial skeleton as to peripheral joints. However, radiological signs are frequently present without symptoms so that indicators of the effects of the disease, in functional terms, are more meaningful.

Pathogenesis

The pathological changes, which start in the cartilage where fibrillation occurs, include an attempt at repair with osteophytosis. Radiologically loss of joint space is seen with sclerosis of underlying bone with cysts and osteophytes. These pathological changes have for many years been assumed to be due to 'wear and tear'. There is increasing evidence that, whilst such an explanation may be reassuring to a patient, it really says little about aetiology and pathogenesis, which is certainly multifactorial (Table 9.1). We should distinguish primary osteoarthritis, where causes are unknown, from

Table 9.1: Causes of osteoarthritis

Trauma, mechanical damage, instability, hypermobility, obesity
Genetic factors
Age-related
Hormonal (e.g. acromegaly) and biochemical factors
Old inflammatory joint disease
Other joint disease
Avascular necrosis (including sickle cell disease)

secondary disease, where previous damage to the joint is documented. Primary disease may be further subdivided: there is a group, mainly composed of younger females with a positive female family history who develop Heberden's nodes and degenerative joint disease from their 40s onwards. The distribution of joint involvement is shown in Figure 9.1.

Predisposing causes for osteoarthritis relate not only to articular cartilage but to the underlying bones, to the ligaments of the joint, and to the synovium. It is important to elucidate them as they have a bearing on prognosis, prevention and treatment.

Although lack of lubrication in a joint is of some significance, and the viscosity of synovial fluid is lower than in healthy joints, there is considerable evidence that factors related to joint loading are of importance. Further, in some sports osteoarthritis is not a common sequel (e.g. football) although in others such as parachuting, where meniscus tears are not infrequent, osteoarthritis may result. It seems that areas of cartilage within a joint may become conditioned by regular use to withstand considerable stresses without damage, but unaccustomed stress in an 'untrained' area may result in joint damage (Seedhom and Swann, 1987). Where a joint is subjected to usage for which it is not designed, osteoarthritis may also result (e.g. in the shoulder in subjects who propel their wheelchair manually for years). Joint laxity, incongruity and abnormal lines of weight-bearing all appear relevant.

Cartilage abnormalities and cartilage loss due to previous inflammatory arthritis also lead to osteoarthritis.

Natural history

Surprisingly little has been written on the natural history of untreated osteoarthritis but clinicians appreciate that few if any patients show reversal of radiological changes even though there may be prolonged periods of clinical remission or symptoms may remain static. Often, modification to lifestyle can assure that moderate disease has a 'nuisance' value only.

Clinical features of peripheral joint osteoarthritis (Table 9.2)

The main complaints of patients are: (1) pain, (2) loss of range and function, (3) stiffness.

1. Pain

This arises from a variety of causes and structures within and around the joint. It usually lasts for many hours and is aching in character, relieved by rest and exacerbated by usage of the joint (such as by weight-bearing). In

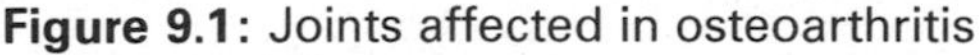

Figure 9.1: Joints affected in osteoarthritis

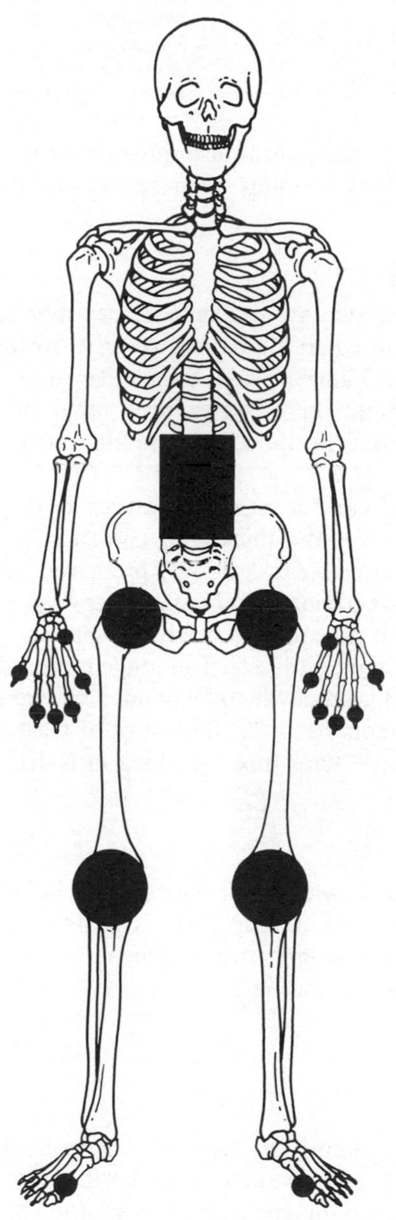

Table 9.2: Clinical features of osteoarthritis

Symptoms	Signs
Gelling on inactivity	Local tenderness
Absent/mild early morning stiffness	Little or no synovial swelling
Pain on use/weight-bearing	Soft tissue swelling
Loss of function	Bony swelling
	Joint crepitus
	Loss of joint range

the later stages, or when the joint is also inflamed or traumatised, pain may prevent the patient from sleeping. Its severity may be an indication for operation.

2. Loss of range and function

The muscles across the joint are weakened. They then atrophy and are less able to protect the joint when the patient is active so that the joint is more easily traumatised and liable to subsequent 'flare-ups'. The joint capsule may shorten and thicken; there is a reduced range of movement and the joint adopts an abnormal position, e.g. the hip and knee will show fixed flexion.

Loss of range arises early from muscle spasm in response to pain, later from loss of muscle power and thickening and shortening of joint capsule. The central range of movement is usually preserved. Loss of full range of movement is not always of functional importance (e.g. loss of a few degrees of elbow extension is of no consequence but inability to straighten the knee makes movement on stairs difficult). The range required for common tasks related to the involved joint needs to be defined so that the aims of therapy are clear (e.g. all patients need 90° flexion of at least one knee to mount stairs, but only a few, perhaps those working in restricted areas, need full flexion).

3. Stiffness

There may also be joint swelling and even mild inflammation with early morning stiffness. More frequently there is gelling; i.e. after a period of inactivity the joint is resistant to movement. After a few minutes of movement the discomfort vanishes.

Systemic effects

Osteoarthritis has no systemic effects, so that the patient feels well, albeit in pain; *laboratory investigations* such as the erythrocyte sedimentation rate (ESR) and full blood count are normal, tests for rheumatoid factor are negative.

MANAGEMENT

The aims are: (a) relief of pain and stiffness, (b) restoration of function.

Relief of pain and stiffness

This is fully dealt with in Chapter 10 but a few points may be made.

(1) *Analgesia.* Although some patients' pain may be adequately controlled by occasional, or even regular, analgesics, a significant number benefit from the regular use of nonsteroidal anti-inflammatory drugs. Twice-daily dosage interferes less with work than more frequent dosage. In the elderly, simplification of medication regimes is important. It should also be remembered that older people metabolise drugs less completely and more slowly than younger persons. They may also have trouble in opening tablet containers.

(2) *Local steroids* often give good relief of localised joint pain and may allow the physiotherapist to begin building up muscle power across the joint. The frequency of joint injection is the subject of much argument, as is the type of corticosteroid used: in the elderly, immediate relief of pain and preservation of function will be more important than any possible delayed joint destruction arising from steroid use.

(3) *Other factors.* Attempts must be made to reduce the load on the affected joint, principally by weight reduction, by the use of walking aids, and by high seating (in lower limb osteoarthritis). The patient who is active, interested and engaged in life and physical activities is less vulnerable to pain and depression than the housebound, apathetic subject.

Restoration of function

Rehabilitation in osteoarthritis is less complex than in many neurological diseases where cognitive and other functions are impaired. It is often an easier task than in inflammatory disease as relatively few joints are involved, and the course of the disease is more predictable. Nevertheless, some patients learn only with difficulty, or are unwell with a variety of other diseases. In addition, loss of activity is usually insidious, so that numerous small restrictions of activity have been accepted.

Physiotherapy

The general aims and methods used in physiotherapy are detailed in Chapter 35. The general purposes for which physiotherapy is prescribed in osteoarthritis are:

> to relieve pain, mobilise stiff joints, prevent and diminish contracture, encourage correct function (e.g. gait), strengthen weak muscles related to the arthritic joint and to restore and maintain function.

For some patients the time and energy required to attend a hospital outpatient department for repeated, regular treatments may be quite disproportionate to the benefit gained. The patient may be better helped by being *taught* exercises, then doing these at home. However it is difficult for an unsupervised patient to remain enthusiastic about time-consuming, often boring exercises. Patients frequently default unless a scheme of regular recording with regular supervision is devised (Chamberlain *et al.*, 1982).

Local physical methods of treatment

Local methods (heat, cold, short wave diathermy, transcutaneous nerve stimulation) relieve discomfort temporarily, and allow the patient to undergo active exercise, but do not alter the course of the disease. The choice of physical modality is a matter of therapist's or patient's preference. The patient should be encouraged to improvise as necessary at home, and must understand that such measures will not influence the course of osteoarthritis; however, he should be informed that regular exercise in osteoarthritis has been shown to decrease pain, will stabilise the joint in its functional range and may protect somewhat against repeated trauma.

Exercises

Exercises may be assisted, against gravity or resisted. Two principal groups can be distinguished: those to improve maximal strength and those to increase endurance (lower weights, more repetitions). In osteoarthritis the latter is more often required, together with exercise to increase range of movement.

Recreational exercise

Sport is useful, being a natural progression from individual exercises, and more enjoyable. There is evidence (Ekblom *et al.*, 1975) that even those with inflammatory arthritis benefit from a greater level of physical fitness. It may also have a preventive value, preserving the integrity of cartilage. Inappropriate sport, such as fell-walking or mountaineering, may have to be given up, and activities such as swimming and cycling, which are non-weight-bearing, substituted. Exercise may have to be alternated with rest, or at least reduction of load on the involved joints.

Walking aids

These take a significant proportion of the load off a diseased weight-bearing joint (Chapter 46).

Occupational Therapy

Problems should be tackled according to the joints involved and the perceived priorities of the patient. The occupational therapist is responsible for environmental modifications, such as rails on stairs, and in the toilet and bathroom; for kitchen alterations if necessary, for obtaining ramps and for seating changes such as high seats, high lavatory seats and wheelchairs (Chapters 39, 42 and 43). On occasion, a supporting splint (e.g. in osteoarthritic thumb) will be helpful to the patient and can be made by orthotist or occupational therapist. The occupational therapist should consider the interaction between the patient's osteoarthritis, his work and his method of transport.

Patient and family education

Many patients will have been subjected to outdated advice from friends and acquaintances, and even their doctors have been known to tell them 'You'll just have to live with arthritis'. This is only partly true: there is no *cure*, but there are numerous things which can be done to make life pleasurable again and to relieve the adverse effects of osteoarthritis to a great extent. The enthusiastic and educated cooperation of the patient is required, and one should dispel his fears that he will be helpless. Coordinated management usually ensures a relatively independent patient. The natural history of the condition is explained: patients with osteoarthritis have a normal lifespan and remain otherwise well. Certain drugs, physical measures and even changes in lifestyle may be used to relieve pain and reduce stresses to affected joints.

The patient will probably not remember much of what is said in the anxious situation of a clinic. It is a good policy to provide the patient with a booklet on osteoarthritis (e.g. from the Arthritis and Rheumatism Council). Booklets on specific problem areas, such as the neck or lumbar spine, and the effect of arthritis on marriage, e.g. due to hip involvement, are also available from the ARC and are discussed in detail in the appendix to Chapter 10. It is useful for other members of the family to read these and be a party to decisions on any necessary changes in lifestyle.

Surgery in Osteoarthritis

If pain remains uncontrolled and disability increases despite intensive treatment, surgery should also be considered. It should be considered for those whose condition is less severe, but whose livelihood is threatened, or who have a dependent family and perhaps handicapped spouse. Those who do not understand the purpose of surgery, who wish to remain dependent, or who are unprepared to work to achieve good results are less good candidates either for surgery or for other rehabilitation techniques. Results tend to be better than in inflammatory arthritis: the hips and knees afflicted in osteoarthritis respond better to prosthetic surgery than the smaller joints involved in rheumatoid arthritis; 'bone quality' and the integrity of surrounding structures are more likely to be preserved.

OSTEOARTHRITIS IN SPECIFIC JOINTS

(This section deals only briefly with specific disabilities, with the aim of providing the reader with a model for considering arthritis of lower limb joints. Preservation of function in upper limb joints is dealt with in the subsequent chapter on inflammatory arthritis.)

Osteoarthritis of the hip

The patient with osteoarthritis of the hip may have had an antecedent abnormality such as congenital dislocation of the hip, a slipped epiphysis or perhaps inflammatory arthritis. However, most patients give no such history of previous hip problems.

His (or her) main complaint will be *pain*, at first localised to the groin or radiating to the knee, but later perhaps accompanied by backache due to fixed flexion with increased lumbar lordosis. Pain is associated with limp and shortening of the affected leg, and is worse on weight-bearing.

The patient will experience many restrictions, associated with loss of joint range, and weak musculature, and with the fixed flexed and adducted posture; he has difficulty on mounting stairs, and on rising from the seated position (as from an easy chair or lavatory). Kerbs and high bus steps, and getting into the bath, are difficult; putting on shoes, socks and tights, and cutting the toenails present problems.

Examination reveals hip deformity with the hip in the adducted, externally rotated and flexed position. The ranges of flexion, extention, rotation and abduction are limited to a variable degree and shortening is present. If both hips are involved the intermalleolar separation is restricted: when reduced to 20 cm or less one can anticipate inability to mount high steps and kerbs and, in females, pain and difficulty with intercourse. Progressive restriction of intermalleolar separation is an indication of the need for surgery. *Weakness* of the muscles surrounding the hip may be marked, gluteus medius being commonly affected.

Management

The patient's *pain* is brought under control as discussed previously. Rest is interspersed with activity and there should be daily periods of prone lying to counteract the tendency towards flexion deformity.

Exercise aims to increase the power of gluteus medius, and to improve abduction and extension. Muscles are frequently so weak that exercises are done initially in sling suspension; hydrotherapy is invaluable though frequently unavailable; home exercises on a regular daily basis are necessary to maintain function. Where surgery is imminent it is worthwhile recalling the patient for exercises preoperatively so that he may more easily do these postoperatively.

The use of a *walking stick* is encouraged as the stick transmits half the body weight and relieves the joint load. Obese patients should be encouraged to reduce their weight — often a difficult task since with decreasing mobility calorie requirements may be reduced.

Shoes. A heel raise and, later, whole shoe raise to (almost) compensate for a short leg is required on the affected side to keep the pelvis level and reduce the incidence of subsequent back pain.

Preservation of mobility

Chair seats need to be high, with arms to assist in rising and decrease the load on the joint. Lavatory seats should be raised. Osteoarthritis subjects are big consumers of wheelchairs, accounting for some 15 per cent of prescriptions. A folding wheelchair, used in conjunction with a car, is helpful to many. Some require a wheelchair outside the house or even in it, but before this stage is reached, urgent consideration should be given to the possibility of surgery. It is much easier to mobilise postoperatively the patient who has been active on a frame or crutch than one who has been in a wheelchair for a long period.

A car is the single most useful aid to the patient with mobility problems, enabling him to participate in a wide variety of normal social activities. Automatic transmission on the car may be helpful.

Pedestrian mobility is considerably enhanced by good repair and planning of paths and roadways: arthritics find it hard to negotiate slippery, unswept flagstones, uneven surfaces, undropped kerbs and numerous steps, and are greatly helped by sensitive town planning which locates shopping and community facilities within range.

Preservation of normal activities

Many patients cannot perform tasks in the kitchen if required to stand for a long time, but can work well when sitting at a table or on a high stool working at higher surfaces. Those who need to use a walking appliance will find difficulty in carrying (say) a cup of tea or tray whilst using it, and will appreciate a trolley.

Numerous aids to help pick up objects from the floor, put on tights, etc, are available.

Shopping and householding will need to be modified in the light of the disability; energy can be conserved by the use of easy-care fabrics, by washing machines and tumble-driers, food can be bought in bulk, carried by a helper and stored in fridge and freezer. All these adaptations are helpful but many are too expensive for arthritis subjects whose earning ability is compromised. (Occupational therapy, Chapter 34).

Environmental modifications such as access rails and the installation of a shower, a downstairs toilet or stairlift are helpful in preserving the patient's independence (Chapter 39).

Osteoarthritic knee

The patient with osteoarthritis of the knee may have degenerative changes in any one or all of three compartments of the knee, medial, lateral or patellofemoral, with symptoms which are slightly different initially. Pain in the former two are mainly along the joint line on the affected side. Patellofemoral osteoarthritis is associated with pain in the front of the joint, early atrophy of the quadriceps muscle, loss of *sideways* mobility of the patella and loss of the last few degrees of extension. Pain is again associated with activity, with weight-bearing and with a reducing flexion and extension range; it is relieved by rest. Patellofemoral osteoarthritis often presents early with pain on descending stairs.

Functional difficulties are experienced with kneeling, climbing stairs and kerbs and uneven surfaces, and in rising (as from bed, chair, lavatory, car seat). Climbing stairs becomes impossible if there is less than 90° of flexion at both knees. There is a tendency for the patient to spend increasing periods inactive in a chair, where the knee takes up the same, comfortable position, the quadriceps wastes further, and a fixed flexion contracture results. The patient cannot walk on flexed knees for more than the shortest of distances and becomes chair- (or wheelchair)-bound. Rarely the situation is compounded by *instability*, by varus or valgus deformity that worsens on weight-bearing.

Examination confirms the pain as arising from the knee with localised tenderness related to the compartment involved. The knee is rarely hot, but there is often an effusion, with or without other deformity (e.g. valgus or varus perhaps only evident on weight-bearing), quadriceps wasting and weakness are always present. Standing and walking are observed: less time is spent with weight on the affected knee than on the good side, there is a limp and there may be instability.

Management

Management is similar to that in the other major weight-bearing joint, the hip. That is, pain is managed and function improved as much as possible. Changes in lifestyle may be necessary, as may environmental modifications at home and at work.

Rest with the knee extended as far as possible (by using a stool when sitting and *splinting* and the use of reversed dynamic slings (Dickson) are helpful, particularly when the latter are carried out for prolonged periods such as overnight. Accompanying pain can be relieved by anti-inflammatory agents and occasionally by injection of steroids into the joint when there is acute pain and effusion.

Exercise to strengthen principally the quadriceps muscles (but also the hamstrings) must be done regularly and frequently. In severe flexion deformity we ask the patients to record that they have exercised for five minutes each hour, or for a corresponding amount of time whilst watching television or doing other congenial, sedentary activities.

Relief of the load through the joint can again be achieved by treating obesity, and by using walking sticks and other mobility aids. Ellis *et al.* (1979) showed that up to seven times body weight is transmitted through the knee on rising from a low chair. High seating with armrests is much more suitable. Restriction of mobility is combated by the use of mobility aids, wheelchairs, trolleys and cars. Access rails and bath aids are usually necessary. Householding and self-care adaptations, and environmental modifications are needed. The unstable knee is difficult to splint. The telescopic valgus-varus (TVS) orthosis may help, as may a Cinch splint (see Chapter 45). Surgery should be considered before the patient retreats to a wheelchair existence.

Osteoarthritis of the first metatarsophalangeal (MTP) joint

This is common, and causes a surprising amount of disability, probably because body weight is normally transmitted through the joint at the end of the stance phase of gait, at push-off.

The patient complains of local pain and limps, bearing less weight for a shorter time on that side. A soft tissue bursa may develop over the first metatarsal head; the second toe may sublux or dislocate, and both the second and third MTP joints may become painful if there is an associated hallux valgus. Many patients complain more of the cosmetic deformity and have difficulty in wearing fashionable shoes.

Management

Surgery may eventually be required, but before this, obesity should be controlled and the patient should obtain appropriate footwear, i.e. shoes of sufficient width and depth — particularly around the MTP joint. An outside rocker also reduces pain.

Osteoarthritis of the hand

Osteoarthritis of the hands is frequent; Lawrence *et al.* (1966) quote the incidence of grades 2–4 of osteoarthritis of the distal interphalangeal joints as 22 per cent in males and 29 per cent in females. It causes relatively mild symptoms compared with the numerous serious and complex changes seen in rheumatoid arthritis. There is local *pain*, particularly on repetitive movement, associated with swelling of the joint (and squaring of the heel of the hand). This is relieved by rest for the first carpometacarpal joint only, use of a splint for work and for rest, by local steroid injection, by pain-relieving drugs, and occasionally by surgery.

Functional difficulties of fine movement and thumb stabilisation can be analysed by the occupational therapist. They result in numerous minor but frustrating difficulties of grip. Sometimes the patient's job may become impossible (e.g. the seamstress, or a craft worker).

BACK PAIN

Introduction

The total cost of treating backache is huge. Most of the adult population can expect occasional short periods of pain but there is a considerable amount of chronic backache also. The definition of chronicity is debatable: perhaps backache has attained a chronic phase after several weeks or months. Alternatively it could be said to have occurred when (a) sickness absence has reached six weeks or (b) hospital admission has taken place, and certainly (c) when continuous pain has been present for over a year.

Epidemiology

There are many useful indicators of the frequency of backache. Thus in the UK more than one million adults seek the advice of their GP each year, and more than half a million hospital consultations ensue. Fifty thousand subjects are admitted to hospital and 7,000 undergo surgery. Seven hundred and forty-seven days per 1,000 employed males are lost yearly (Benn and Wood, 1975).

Backache is associated with sciatica in approximately one-sixth of subjects; slightly more men than women suffer, and of those affected some three-quarters are under 65 years, and half are 45–60 years.

Anatomy

The vertebrae are supported by paraspinal muscles, by the inter- and supraspinous ligaments between the vertebral spines and by the anterior and posterior longitudinal ligaments which are attached to the discs and to the margins of vertebral bodies. Pain may arise from any of these ligamentous structures, from periosteum, from the posterior apophyseal synovial joints, from nerve endings near the blood vessels of the muscles and from pressure on the nerve roots of the cauda equina. Nociceptors are thus present in all the structures of the spinal segment under consideration, and the exact origin of pain in any patient may be obscure. Much interest has centred around the intervertebral disc and the structures nearby.

Diagnosis

The exact anatomical and functional diagnosis in a case of backache is notoriously difficult to determine, and is characterised by symptoms rather than signs which can be more effectively measured: hence the uncertainties concerning the efficacy of various treatments. A short list of the main causes of chronic backache is given in Table 9.3.

History

Back *pain* is the *sine qua non* of these conditions. Its site should be pointed out by the patient, as should its radiation. Some patients interpret words differently from doctors: they may complain of back pain but point to the groin, with pain radiating from here to the buttock or greater trochanter. Such pain is suspicious of hip pathology. Pain is commonest in the L4/L5/S1 region with radiation to the lateral or posterior aspects of the leg. Such pain may arise commonly from disc pathology or soft tissue lesions. It may be exacerbated by coughing when the nerve root in the leg is irritated, (Table 9.4).

Paraesthesiae may be associated (again the complaint of numbness has

Table 9.3: Causes of low back pain

1. *Mechanical or soft tissue causes*
   (a) Limited movement
      (i) Disc lesion
      (ii) Osteochondritis (Scheuermann's disease)
      (iii) Localised limitation (no evidence of (i) or (ii))
   (b) Mobile lumbar spine—ligamentous
   (c) Spondylolisthesis, spondylolysis

2. *Arthritis*
   (a) Osteoarthritis
   (b) Ankylosing spondylitis

3. *Bone disease*
   (a) Tumour:
      primary
      secondary deposit
      myeloma, lymphoma
   (b) Infection:
      tuberculous
      pyogenic
   (c) Vertebral softening/collapse:
      osteoporosis
      osteomalacia and hyperparathyroidism
   (d) Paget's disease

4. *Visceral causes*
   (a) Gastric or duodenal ulcer
   (b) Pancreatic carcinoma
   (c) Renal causes
   (d) Gynaecological
   (e) Aortic aneurysm
   (f) Arterial obstruction

to be analysed with care) and arise from neural tissue, usually nerve root pressure from a disc lesion.

Aggravating factors

Pain from the spine and associated ligaments (so-called mechanical pain) is usually worsened by prolonged standing and by particular movements or positions of the spine, but may be relieved by walking. Viscerogenic back pain does not have these associations.

Pain in the calf on walking suggests arterial insufficiency if it eases on resting. Such claudication must be differentiated from that of the cauda equina due to spinal stenosis. The latter is frequently found down the whole leg on exercise, sometimes with neurological signs developing, and may take 30 minutes or so to resolve.

Table 9.4: Features of lumbar root lesions

Root	Motor weakness (main)	Reflex diminished or absent	Sensory signs/symptoms
L2	Hip flexors and adductors	—	Usually none/thigh
L3	Hip flexors Knee extensors	Knee	Usually none/front of thigh
L4	Knee extensors Foot invertors	Knee	Medial aspect of calf and ankle
L5	Knee flexors Ankle/hallux dorsiflexors	—	Lateral aspect of calf Medial half of dorsum of foot
S1	Knee flexors Evertors of foot Plantar flexors of ankle and toes	Ankle	Plantar surface of foot

Pain at night is of serious import and may be of neoplastic origin, associated with dull, persistent pain throughout the day.

Early morning stiffness is characteristic of inflammatory joint disease and found in the back in ankylosing spondylitis and related spondarthritides.

Disturbance of bowels or micturition suggests serious pathology, as does any systemic disturbance, such as weight loss, anaemia or ill health. A past history of neoplasia is suspicious.

Handicaps and disabilities are rarely respecters of aetiology, and are not useful diagnostically. Personal care, domestic function, mobility on foot and by public transport, within and outside the house, are affected, as spinal movements obviously occur in numerous activities, in employment, domestic, sexual and social spheres.

Examination

A full examination (frequently including a rectal examination) is necessary. It may reveal associated signs of disease (such as café-au-lait spots). The spine should be observed with the subject standing, lying and moving.

(a) *Standing*: the patient is palpated for tender spots and the movements of the spine observed and measured. Commonly a segment may be seen to be rigid. The Trendelenburg test, in which the patient stands on each leg in turn, checks the muscle power of the hip on which the patient is standing.
(b) *Supine*: the abdomen is examined, straight leg raising (SLR) is ascertained and a full neurological examination undertaken.
(c) *Prone*: the examiner presses on each vertebral spine in turn and

tests for sacroiliac pain. The femoral stretch test can be usefully performed.

Laboratory tests

It is unnecessary to investigate most patients with pain of three months' duration or less. Later a full blood picture and ESR provide preliminary useful screens, with further tests as appropriate.

Radiology

Radiology rarely helps in the diagnosis of early or acute back pain. Spondylolisthesis, Scheuermann's disease, osteoarthrosis, ankylosing spondylitis, septic lesions, osteoporosis, and narrowing of disc spaces indicative of disc degeneration, may all be visible on routine radiology. Myelography with water-soluble contrast is of value in investigating nerve root pain if surgery is to be considered. Ultrasound scanning, as developed by Porter (1980), may be of epidemiological use, and computerised tomography (CT) has value in the demonstration of disc herniation, spinal stenosis and facet arthritis (for instance) but inter-observer agreement has been reported as small. Magnetic resonance imaging (MRI) probably also has a role.

Biomechanics

The mechanical integrity of the disc influences all surrounding structures: when the disc degenerates greater loads are imposed on the facet joints. There is also altered stress distribution on the end plates and subchondral bone of the vertebrae and encroachment on the nerve root canal.

The disc is the largest avascular structure in the body. Deficient nutrition first affects the boundary zone between the nucleus annulus where fissuring begins. Motion has been found to increase the flow of nutrients into the disc (in dogs) and smoking and vibration to decrease it. Hansson and Roos (1981) demonstrated the frequent presence of healing microfracture of the trabeculae of subchondral bone near the endplates.

Disc pressure measurement

Much work has been done by Nachemson since 1960 to define the intra-disc pressure in a variety of situations. Most studies were done at the level of L3 where the disc transmits some three times body weight. Intradisc pressure is lowest during supine lying: it is higher in unsupported sitting than in standing. The pressure in the disc increases 30 per cent during rising to standing. Flexion and rotation induce high loads on the lower spine.

There is little difference in the transient loads on the disc during the two types of lifting (back lift and leg lift) when the distance of the weight lifted from the trunk is standardised. Indeed the major factor governing intradisc pressure during lifting is lever arm length: the object to be lifted should be as near the body as possible to minimise load on the back.

Corsets and braces diminish the load through the lumbar spine by some 30 per cent irrespective of the type of corset.

Intra-abdominal and intrathoracic pressures are related inversely to disc pressure. Many authors have indicated the pain-relieving effects of increased intra-abdominal and intrathoracic muscle pressure, and the value of strong abdominal muscles in lifting.

The above basic data have consequences in back care and rehabilitation which will be detailed later. Other factors connected with load on the spine, such as sheer, are also likely to be of importance.

It is impossible to survey exhaustively all causes of backache. Mention will be made of only a few commoner conditions.

Lumbar spondylosis. Radiologically proven degenerative changes may occur in symptomatic and in symptom-free patients; the changes of lumbar spondylosis consist of disc degeneration, disc space narrowing, osteophytosis and sclerosis of lumbar vertebrae. Osteophytes are found at the margins of the vertebral bodies and may be associated with the osteoarthritic changes which usually coexist in and around the apophyseal interfacetal joints.

Non-specific backache of mechanical origin may occur in the presence or absence of radiological signs of lumbar spondylosis. There is chronic or persistent pain, often with acute exacerbations, with or without limitation of spinal movement, not associated with other disease or with abnormal laboratory findings. The hypermobility syndrome occasionally needs to be considered as a cause of backache. Spinal instability can result in pain, as shown by the relief of pain accompanying surgical stabilisation in spondylolisthesis.

Prolapsed intervertebral disc (PIVD) is less common than the above, but may occur at any time in adult life. The signs and symptoms are those related usually to posterolateral herniation of the disc, often after trivial stress. They consist, therefore, of pain, local and referred, and of paraesthesia and numbness related to the nerve root affected. In recent years it has come to be appreciated that the smaller is the lateral recess the greater the severity of the consequences of prolapse.

Spondylolisthesis is the forward movement of one vertebra on a lower one, usually L5 on S1 or L4 on L5. The usual cause is a break or elongation in the pars interarticularis. It results in severe back pain and may arise secondarily from degenerative spondylosis. If severe or increasing it may require surgical treatment. However, it may be a coincidental finding on X-ray.

Spondylolysis is a stress fracture through the pars articularis, usually at L5 or L4 without forward displacement of the vertebra. The spine is lordotic, pain is localised and worse on extension.

Osteoporosis causes persistent dull ache in the back, worse with activity, without neurological features and evident radiologically. Crush fractures may later cause severe local pain. Treatment is controversial, and includes calcium, fluoride, or oestrogens.

Ankylosing spondylitis results in a rigid (bamboo) spine with associated sacroiliitis, neck involvement, peripheral arthritis and occasionally uveitis. Chest movement may also be diminished and radiology is characteristic.

Backache must not be considered to be of psychological origin unless there are positive features of depression, or other psychiatric disorder, and investigations are normal.

Treatment of back pain

This is difficult and often unsatisfactory, and assessment of the value of the numerous treatment regimes is notoriously difficult: unsubstantiated claims of success abound. The major problems are (a) poor diagnostic criteria, (b) confused terminology, (c) few objective markers of success and (d) many trials have been designed by advocates of a particular treatment and lack the necessary objectivity about response to treatment.

Back care

(a) Prevention

Prevention of repeated attacks of pain is of considerable importance. Some occupations and sporting activities predispose to backache and even to spondylolisthesis. The lifting of heavy weights by an untrained lifter should be avoided: lifting techniques should be taught and loads should be placed as near the body as possible. Physiotherapists and occupational therapists are both available to give advice, and where necessary should also advise on the ergonomics of the home and the workplace, liaising with the DRO, personnel officer or health and safety officer at the place of work. Literature on back care needs to be freely available. Various back schools have had considerable success, and the work of some of these has been evaluated (Moffet *et al.*, 1986). It is worth surveying the patient's history for avoidable precipitating factors, but screening of job applicants is more controversial as those without radiological abnormalities of the lumbar spine may develop occupation-related backache whilst some of those with such defects may not. Nevertheless where backache threatens work, the help of DRO, or occupational psychologist, or assessment at an ERC may be useful (Chapter 41).

Posture is important. Patients are more comfortable lying flat on a firm mattress, perhaps with a board underneath. Nachemson's work also indicates the importance of *good seating* with a small incline to the back of the seat, with lumbar support, and armrests to spread the load. Long periods of driving in vehicles with poor seating or poor suspension may be unhelpful.

Shoes are rarely discussed. However, since the spine acts as a shock-absorber it is reasonable to increase the efficiency of shock absorption from the ground to the less resilient older spine by ensuring that the heels of shoes are of a resilient material or contain an energy-absorbing insole such as Sorbothane.

(b) Treatment of low back pain

Most patients with backache will recover quickly whatever treatment is given (or even without it). Certification data indicate that in those incapacitated for work the mean period off work was almost 26 working days (Social Security Statistics, 1976). Choler *et al.* (1985) demonstrated that of 7,504 patients who were off work for backache (but not hospitalised) nearly 90 per cent were back at work in six weeks, and 60 per cent had returned in one week.

Work itself is of importance in the management of back pain. Chaffin (1979) and Keyserling (1982) demonstrated that a mismatch between the patient's physical ability and the requirements of the job increases the frequency of low back pain injury at work. On the other hand, inactivity is unhelpful, for activity helps the injured segment heal quicker. Further, when back exercises are taught, supervised activity and gradual return to work seems to have therapeutic value. The whole question of the epidemiology and classification of backache and resultant disabilities is complex and is well reviewed by Wood (see Jayson, 1980). Similarly, the relationship of backache to occupation is not easy to analyse, and the reader is referred to the writings of Anderson (see also Jayson).

It is notoriously difficult to establish the effectiveness of a huge variety of treatments in backache. Many methods, such as flexion and extension exercises, short-wave diathermy, ultrasound, muscle relaxants, non-steroidal anti-inflammatory drugs, biofeedback programmes and local injections have no significant effect on the natural history as judged by return to work.

Obesity should be controlled. The spine should not be subjected to more load than necessary. Obese individuals tend to assume a lordotic posture and have poor abdominal musculature.

It is valuable to relieve pain as fast as possible using all available methods. Bed rest in the acute phase is of value. Non-steroidal anti-inflammatory drugs or analgesics should be available in adequate dosage. A lumbar *corset* is frequently prescribed and often brings relief: the mechanism of this is obscure. It may be that the back is kept warm, that forward flexion is prevented or that intra-abdominal pressure is raised. It is possible that *corsets should be used in acute episodes of pain only*, thereafter the patient should be weaned to exercise. Heat may be used to relax muscles as a preliminary to exercise.

It is difficult to know the value of spinal exercises since weakness of the muscles around the spine is rarely evaluated. Nevertheless, it is reasonable to train the quadriceps to take the required load of body weight, the arm muscles to increase the power of the lever, the abdominal and paraspinal muscles to withstand loads. Clinical trials of exercise therapy have yielded variable estimates of their use, but indicate that isometric exercises to strengthen the muscles of the back and abdomen are useful. Back extension exercises are advocated by some, but may produce undesired increase in back pain. Hydrotherapy appears valuable and it is helpful to encourage regular swimming thereafter.

Traction

'Continuous traction in a hospital bed serves no other purpose than as an effective means of keeping the patient in bed.' This may be an extreme statement: many find relief is useful but only temporary. Intermittent outpatient therapy is capable of producing demonstrable temporary improvement in epidurographic appearances as well as improvement in pain and straight leg raising.

The value of *chymopapein injection into a disc* prolapse is debatable but may relieve sciatica and backache. The risk of allergy probably precludes a second injection.

Passive manipulation has its advocates and may be helpful, but not in the presence of clear disc pathology.

Severe persistent low back pain may be helped by the various pain-relieving techniques detailed in Chapter 7.

Surgery for a lumbar disc lesion

This is indicated for:

(1) sacral root pressure causing bladder symptoms,

(2) (probably) gross muscle weakness in one nerve root distribution,

(3) (probably) moderate muscle weakness in two nerve root distributions,

(4) persistent pain radiating down the leg (not usually for back pain itself).

In each case the diagnosis must be proven by special X-rays (radiculogram, CT or MRI). Surgery for spinal instability is not considered here.

CHRONIC NECK PAIN

Cervical spondylosis

Radiologically degenerative changes are seen which are similar to those in the lumbar spine, and indeed often coexist. There is a similar cluster of symptomatology and signs, viz. local pain and tenderness (usually C6/7 with diminishing frequency upwards), referred pain and referred paraesthesiae from the affected roots (see Table 9.5). Cord compression is rare but requires urgent relief: its management is outside the scope of this chapter.

Symptoms last several weeks and are frequently recurrent; they occur in the absence of laboratory findings. They cannot be directly related to the radiology and it is probably more honest to consider their treatment as the management of chronic neck pain. The differentiation of pain of serious import from that of spondylosis or soft tissue abnormality follows the diagnostic lines discussed under lumbar pain.

Table 9.5: Features of cervical root lesions

Root	Motor weakness (main)	Reflex diminished or absent	Sensory signs/symptoms
C5	Shoulder abduction, elevation, external rotation	Biceps	Deltoid region
C6	Elbow flexion and adduction of humerus	Biceps (?) supinator	Thumb and forefinger
C7	Extension of elbow of wrist of fingers of thumb	Triceps	Middle finger
C8	Finger flexors, some wrist flexors, sometimes thenar muscles	—	Little and ring fingers
T1	Intrinsic muscles of hand	—	Medial surface of forearm

The principles of management are similar to those in low back pain, allowing for the fact that less weight is transmitted through the cervical spine.

Prevention

(1) The avoidance of trauma to the neck is desirable, e.g. by the use of correct seating and a headrest in the car.

(2) Activities and positions known to precipitate pain (such as hanging clothes on a washing line, carrying heavy loads or moving heavy equipment) are to be avoided.

Treatment

Pain has to be relieved by non-steroidal anti-inflammatory drugs or analgesics; anxiolytic agents (such as diazepam) have their uses, as do physical methods and relaxation techniques which relieve or prevent spasm in the paraspinal muscles. *Rest* is often prescribed in a collar. The collar does not have to be large, rigid or uncomfortable to provide a measure of relief, and its manner of doing this is a matter of conjecture. A soft collar, often of polythene, or foam, perhaps covered with cotton, is satisfactory. In an emergency, rolled-up newspaper inside a scarf is helpful. The collar is often worn all day, later perhaps at night only, or during exacerbations, or during activities known to cause pain (such as washing the hair). It is probable that, like the lumbar corset, the collar should be gradually replaced by active exercise. The head is supported by a pillow at night with a second pillow under the neck (Chapter 45, Orthotics).

The physiotherapeutic methods for dealing with neckache are various, and parallel those in lumbar pain; heat, cold, massage, manipulation techniques, transcutaneous nerve stimulation, relaxation regimes, are all used. All bring relief to individuals, but the relative value of the various methods is unproven. Since pain usually subsides within a few weeks it is reasonable for the physician to use any one or more methods as available and appropriate.

Most physiotherapists limit their techniques in the presence of objective neurological findings; where these are progressing or are of cord compression the above measures are inappropriate, and the help of a neurologist (and usually of a neurosurgeon) is sought.

REFERENCES

Benn, R.T. and Wood, P.H.N. (1975). Pain in the back: an attempt to estimate the size of the problem. *Rheumatol. Rehabil.*, *14*, 121–8

Chamberlain, M.A., Care, G. and Harfield, B. (1982) Physiotherapy in osteoarthrosis of the knees: a controlled trial of hospital versus home exercises. *Int. Rehabl. Med.*, *4*, 101-6.

Chaffin, D.B. (1979) Manual materials handling. *J. Envir. Pathol. Toxicol.*, *2*, 31–66
Choler, U., Larsson, R., Nachemson, A. and Peterson, L.E. (1985) *Ont i ryggen-Forsok med vardprogram for patienter med lumbala smarttillstand.* SPRI Rapport 188/85. Stockholm, Socialstyrelsens Planerings och Rationaliserings Institut
DHSS (1978) *Social security statistics 1976*, HMSO, London
Dickson, R.A. and Wright, V. (1984) *Integrated clinical science: musculo-skeletal disease*, Heinemann, London
Ekbolm, B., Lovgren, O., Alderin, M. *et al.* (1975) Effect of short-term physical training on patients with rheumatoid arthritis. *Scand. J. Rheumatol.*, *4*, 80-6
Ellis, M.I., Seedhom, B.B., Amis, A.A., Dowson, D. and Wright, V. (1979) Forces in the knee joint whilst rising from normal and motorised chairs. *Eng. Med.*, *8*, 573-80
Hansson, T. and Roos, B. (1981) Microcalluses of the trabeculae in lumbar vertebrae and their relation to the bone mineral content. *Spine*, *6*, 375–80
Jayson, M. (1980) *The lumbar spine and back pain*, 2nd ed, Pitman, London
Keyserling, W.M. (1982) Strength testing as a method of evaluating ability to perform strenuous work. In M. Stanton-Hicks and R. Boas, (eds), *Chronic back pain*, Raven Press, New York, p. 149
Lawrence, J.S., Bremner, J.M. and Bier, F. (1966) Osteo-arthrosis. Prevalence in the population and relationship between symptoms and X-ray changes. *Ann. Rheum.* Dis., *25*, 1-24
Moffett, J., Kleber, A., Chase, S.M., Portek, B.S. and Ennis, J.R. (1986) A controlled, prospective study to evaluate the effectiveness of a back school in the relief of chronic low back pain. *Spine*, *11*(2), 120-2
Nachemson, A. (1981) Disc pressure measurements. *Spine*, *6*, 93–7
Porter, W. (1980) Measurement of the spinal canal by diagnostic ultrasound. *Lumbar Spine Back Pain 2*, 231
Seedhom, B.B. and Swann, A. (1987) The relationship between the stiffness of normal articular cartilage and the predominant levels of applied stress. Implications for osteoarthrosis. (In preparation)

FURTHER READING

Copeman's Textbook of the Rheumatic Diseases (1986), J.T. Scott (ed.), 6th edn, Churchill Livingstone, London
Dickson, R.A. and Wright, V. (1984) *Integrated clinical science: musculo-skeletal disease*, Heinemann, London
Nachemson, A.L. (1975) Advances in low back pain. *Clin. Orthop. Related Res.*, *200*, 266-78
Jayson, M. (1980) *The lumbar spine and back pain*, 2nd edn, Pitman, London

ADVICE TO PATIENTS

Osteoarthritis Explained, A Handbook for Patients, Arthritis and Rheumatism Council
Backache and disc ('slipped disc') disorders, A Handbook for Patients, Arthritis and Rheumatism Council

10

Rheumatoid Arthritis and Other Inflammatory Arthropathies

Vera Neumann and Verna Wright

INTRODUCTION

Three to six per cent of the population of developed countries suffer from severe disability. In approximately a third of these patients arthritis is the cause. Thus arthritis has both a large social impact and far-reaching economic consequences. In 1981 Chamberlain and Wright estimated that 37 million working days were lost annually because of arthritis in the UK.

Although osteoarthritis is commoner than the inflammatory polyarthritides it causes less disability; it affects few joints at a time, and damage is slower to develop and usually less severe. Numerically the most important *inflammatory* joint disease is rheumatoid arthritis (RA) which affects 3 per cent of women and 1 per cent of men in Britain today. The other inflammatory arthropathies include the seronegative spondarthritides (psoriatic arthritis, ankylosing spondylitis, Reiter's disease, enteropathic arthritis), crystal synovitis (gout and calcium pyrophosphate deposition disease), connective tissue disorders such as systemic lupus erythematosus and joint sepsis. Crystal synovitis and joint sepsis are readily treated with drugs provided these conditions are recognised early enough. The connective tissue disorders (other than RA) are seldom associated with destructive arthropathy and these diseases will not be considered further here. Among the seronegative arthritides, enteropathic arthritis, Reiter's disease and ankylosing spondylitis seldom present long-term rehabilitation problems. Early diagnosis with appropriate advice about back care, exercise and posture will prevent problems in most patients with ankylosing spondylitis. (see Chapter 9). In one survey (Wordsworth and Mowat, 1986) of ankylosing spondylitis only 16 per cent of patients were obliged to stop work as a direct result of their disease. Psoriatic arthritis is also usually mild. In one study two-thirds of patients never required time off work despite suffering from the disease for more than ten years (Roberts *et al.*, 1976). Where severe problems do arise, the principles of rehabilitation are much the same as in RA. For this reason, and because of RA's numerical importance, this chapter will concentrate on management of RA.

RHEUMATOID ARTHRITIS

The joints most commonly affected by RA are the proximal interphalangeal and metacarpophalangeal joints of the hands, the metatarsophalangeal joints of the feet, and the knees. Slightly less commonly affected are the elbows, shoulders and tarsus (Figure 10.1). Hips and neck involvement also occur later in the course of the disease. The disease usually presents as symmetrical joint pain, stiffness and swelling, most commonly before the age of 45. As the disease progresses the joints develop erosions and lose cartilage. Muscle weakness and wasting, and laxity or even rupture of tendons and ligaments, may also make joints unstable. As a result joint subluxation and dislocation can occur, impairing the joint's function and accelerating damage to articular cartilage. This can have severe consequences, for instance joint instability in the neck may result in spinal cord damage. Involvement of tendons and synovial sheaths can result in 'trigger' fingers, or tendon rupture with inability to extend or flex the finger.

Extra-articular manifestations

The commonest systemic feature of RA is anaemia. This may occur as a feature of chronic inflammation, or secondary to treatment with anti-inflammatory or second-line drugs. Tiredness is one consequence of anaemia, so unless it is treated attempts at rehabilitation will be hampered. The underlying cause should be identified and treated appropriately.

Sjögren's syndrome, in which the lacrimal and salivary glands fail to secrete normally, is common. The lungs may be involved (pleural effusions, alveolitis, nodules). The heart may be diseased (pericarditis, aortic incompetence, myocarditis). Vasculitis is also seen, and may cause skin lesions (rash, ulcers). Occasionally vasculitis affects the vasa nervorum leading to mononeuritis multiplex. Three other neurological complications are recognised: entrapment neuropathy, the commonest example of which is carpal tunnel syndrome; myelopathy as a consequence of cervical spine instability; and rarely a symmetrical sensorimotor neuropathy.

Aetiology

The cause of RA is unknown. Our understanding so far is that the disease develops when a patient with a genetic predisposition encounters an

Figure 10.1: Joints affected in rheumatoid arthritis. Dark circles are joints most frequently involved

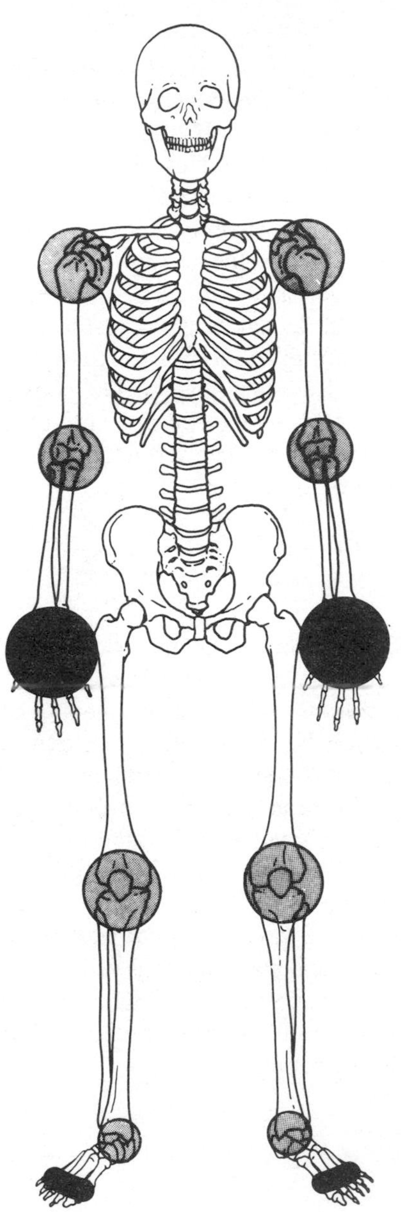

environmental trigger (possibly a silent infection in the bowel). This stimulates autoantibody production, one example of which is the production of IgM rheumatoid factor against the patient's own IgG. The immune complexes thus formed are deposited, complement activated and an inflammatory process ensues. Although we do not yet know what the postulated environmental trigger is, and know of no treatments which 'cure' RA, several drugs are available which retard the disease progression.

Prognosis

Certain features are associated with more severe disease. These include seropositivity, the presence of anaemia or other systemic features at onset, presence of nodules and possession of the HLA type DR3 antigen. Even so prognosis is difficult to predict, not least because the patient's ability to cope with medical, surgical and physical treatment can have a huge influence on his or her ultimate disability. Some 87 per cent of patients manage a more or less normal life, albeit with pain (Figure 10.2). However, the 4 per cent quoted in Functional Class 1 (Brattstrom, 1973) may well be an underestimate. The only large household survey of RA prevalence in the population, carried out in Wensleydale (Lawrence, 1965), revealed a significant proportion of RA sufferers who had never even consulted their GP, let alone a specialist.

Function Class	%	Capability
I	4	Manage the demands of daily living without impediments.
II	83	Manage, despite pain, stiffness and curtailed mobility in joints the essential demands of daily life. Generally partake in productive work.
III	11	Have considerable problems with or cannot manage dressing, hygiene, food, work or home. Are generally non-productive.
IV	2	Totally disabled (confined to bed or a wheel-chair). Tie up another person in their every-day life.

Figure 10.2: Disability in RA (after Brattstrom, 1973)

ASSESSMENT OF THE ARTHRITIC

Fortunately confusion about diagnosis no longer presents major problems. The American Rheumatism Association diagnostic criteria for RA are now widely accepted and applied. However, assessment of disease activity in RA causes considerable problems.

One reason for this confusion is that 'active' RA is generally taken to mean symptoms and signs of active joint inflammation (pain and morning stiffness accompanied by swelling and tenderness of affected joints). These clinical features correlate well with the ESR and elevation of acute phase proteins such as C-reactive proteins (CRP). Whilst it is almost invariably true that patients with persistently 'active' disease ultimately have greater joint damage than those with less 'active' RA it does not follow that such patients also develop the most severe functional disability or deformity. Indeed, functional disability and deformity may fail to correlate. For these reasons it is probably best to assess disease activity and disability separately, and consider management for these two areas independently.

Disease activity can be assessed by clinical examination and scoring for joint inflammation, e.g. the Ritchie Articular Index (see Chapter 6) supplemented by the ESR or plasma viscosity. Measuring acute phase proteins such as CRP will help, particularly where accurate objective measures of disease activity are needed such as in clinical trials.

Functional activity can be assessed by one of several schemes. The oldest of these is the Steinbrocker Classification. In 1949 Steinbrocker and colleagues proposed that functional disability be classified into four categories:

Class 1: Complete functional capacity with ability to carry on all usual duties without handicap.
Class 2: Functional capacity adequate to conduct normal activities despite handicap of discomfort or limited mobility of one or more joint.
Class 3: Functional capacity adequate to perform only little or none of the duties of usual occupation or of self-care.
Class 4: Largely or wholly incapacitated with patient bedridden or confined to wheelchair, permitting little or no self-care.

These functional classes are useful when assessing the response of groups of patients to a new therapy. In order to plan rehabilitation of an individual with RA more detailed assessment of his or her particular disabilities is required: the patient may be asked to complete a Health Assessment Questionnaire (Table 10.1).

TREATMENT OF RHEUMATOID ARTHRITIS

The long-term aims of treatment must be to reduce pain, to minimise joint destruction and to improve the function of the patient. Treatment falls into three broad categories: medical/drug therapy, physical therapy and surgery. Not all patients require surgery but for successful management, all three aspects must be considered.

Medical/drug treatments

Non-steroidal anti-inflammatory drugs (NSAID) are used to control pain and stiffness, and are often supplemented by simple analgesics. Local injection of steroids into joints may also provide considerable, though usually short-lived, relief from joint inflammation. Neither of these treatments will alter the course of the arthritis. The drugs which are thought capable of modifying RA include gold, penicillamine, hydroxychloroquine and sulphasalazine. Treatment with one of these 'second-line agents' should be commenced in patients with features of acute inflammation such as morning stiffness, painful tender joints, elevated ESR and acute phase proteins. Patients usually begin to respond within three months. If they fail to do so, or develop an adverse reaction, an alternative second-line drug is used. With many of these therapies, such as gold and pencillamine, regular monitoring, including monthly blood and urine tests, is essential to avoid potentially lethal toxic reactions. These therapies should not be given to patients unwilling or unable to cooperate with regular monitoring. This is even more important in those few patients who fail to respond to the usual second-line drugs and require more toxic drugs such as azathioprine,

Table 10.1: Health assessment questionnaire (modified from Fries *et al.*, 1980)

Name ____________ Date ________

We are interested in learning how your illness affects your daily life. Please feel free to add any comments on the back of this page.

PLEASE *TICK* THE *ONE* RESPONSE WHICH BEST DESCRIBES YOUR USUAL ABILITIES *OVER THE PAST WEEK:*

	Without *any* difficulty	With *some* difficulty	With *much* difficulty	Unable to do
1. *Dressing and grooming*				
— dress yourself, including tying shoelaces and doing buttons?	☐	☐	☐	☐
— shampoo your hair	☐	☐	☐	☐
2. *Rising*				
— stand up from an armless straight chair?	☐	☐	☐	☐
— get in and out of bed?	☐	☐	☐	☐
3. *Eating*				
— cut your meat?	☐	☐	☐	☐
— lift a full cup or glass to mouth?	☐	☐	☐	☐
— open a new carton of milk (or soap powder)?	☐	☐	☐	☐
4. *Walking*				
— walk outdoors on flat ground?	☐	☐	☐	☐
— climb up five steps?	☐	☐	☐	☐
5. *Hygiene*				
— wash and dry your entire body?	☐	☐	☐	☐
— take a bath?	☐	☐	☐	☐
— get on/off the toilet?	☐	☐	☐	☐
6. *Reach*				
— reach and get down a 5 lb object (e.g. bag of potatoes) from just above your head?	☐	☐	☐	☐
— bend down to pick up clothing from the floor?	☐	☐	☐	☐
7. *Grip*				
— open car doors?	☐	☐	☐	☐
— open jars which have been previously opened?	☐	☐	☐	☐
— turn taps on/off?	☐	☐	☐	☐
8. *Activities*				
— Run errands and shop?	☐	☐	☐	☐
— get in/out of a car?	☐	☐	☐	☐
— do chores; e.g. vacuuming, housework or light gardening	☐	☐	☐	☐

methotrexate, cholorambucil or cyclophosphamide.

Systemic steroids are not 'disease-modifying', but are useful in two categories of patients. Oral steroids are used in the elderly, who can often be maintained for several years on a small dose of prednisolone (7.5 mg per day or less). Pulsed intravenous methylprednisolone is used in acutely ill patients where a two to three-month delay before responding to long-term therapy is unacceptable; for instance where a patient's job is in jeopardy, pulsed steroids can be used to bridge the gap until a second-line drug starts to work and thus enable the patient to return to his employment (Neumann *et al.*, 1985).

Whenever drugs are administered this must be done in suitable packaging. Child-resistant bottles for tablets are often also 'rheumatoid-proof'. The patient should be aware of what toxic reactions can occur with their drug treatment, and which of these reactions are potentially serious, and should be reported immediately to the doctor. It is good policy to supply patients with record cards noting their current drug therapy, and with information leaflets concerning any potentially toxic treatment such as gold and steroids.

Rehabilitation

The aim is to enable a patient to minimise disability and dependence. The patient will expect and need therapy to relieve pain in inflamed joints, but those treating the patient must also consider change in the patient's behaviour and lifestyle, and modifications of the patient's environment.

When a patient first presents with RA, therapy to relieve pain and stiffness will involve a combination of drugs, resting the most inflamed joints and using simple physical modalities such as heat, or ice. The patient should immediately be encouraged to take an active role in his own treatment — for example by applying his own heat or ice packs at home. The patient should also learn about 'joint protection'. In some centres courses are available for patients; elsewhere, early referral to occupational therapy and physiotherapy should be arranged.

Joint protection

Deformity occurs in rheumatoid joints for at least three reasons: the joint itself becomes mis-shapen; the ligaments and capsule around the joint become lax; and associated muscles become weak. The relative importance of these factors varies from one joint to another and from patient to patient.

'Joint protection' is based on the hypothesis that if a joint is used in a way which minimises strains on the ligaments and the capsule, and if muscle power is maintained, the risk of long-term damage and deformity is reduced. If this hypothesis is correct, teaching a patient techniques to minimise load or strain on inflamed joints, encouraging the use of appropriate aids and teaching exercises to maintain range of movement and muscle strength should reduce long-term disability.

The following paragraphs describe application of joint protection principles to specific joints. Over the course of many years the joints bearing the brunt of the disease will vary, and thus the components of joint protection will be continuously varying. Regular assessment by the occupational therapist and physiotherapist is therefore necessary so that the patient can be taught the relevant aspects of joint protection.

Hands and wrist. The 'pinch' grip used when gripping small objects (e.g. turning keys and taps) increases the risk of subluxation of the metacarpophalangeal joints and derangement of the IP joint of the thumb, both common deformities in RA (Figure 10.3). Provision of such things as tap- or key-turners, which either use a lever principle to reduce the effort needed, or have a large grip, can reduce the strain on the metacarpophalangeal joints and hence the tendency for these to sublux. Scissors with a spring handle rather than a two-finger grip are also helpful.

Patients should avoid load-bearing with the involved hands, and should not use the knuckles when rising from a chair. This stresses the finger PIP and MCP joints and wrists. Whenever heavy objects are carried *both* hands

Figure 10.3: Hand deformity in RA — unstable thumb gripping

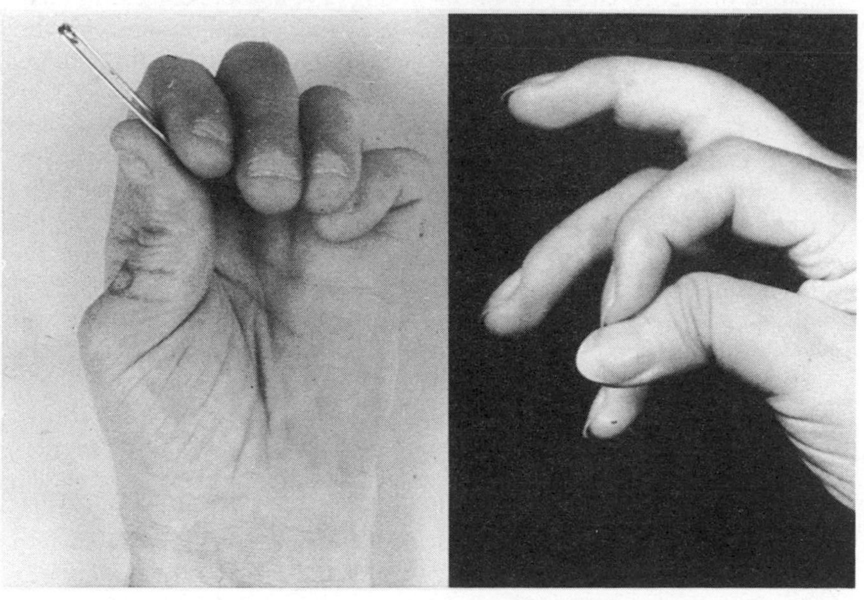

should be used, and where possible the weight should also be supported on the forearm. Provision of aids such as long-sleeved oven gloves, so that heavy pans can be carried on the forearm, will help this. A working wrist splint which holds the *wrist* in slight ulnar deviation (5°) will also reduce the strain and tendency to radial deviation at this joint. A rigid splint (usually made of a low-temperature thermoplastic) can also be supplied to maintain this position whilst the patient is resting at night.

The patient should be encouraged to practise ulnar deviation of the wrist with a slightly clenched fist, or maximal abduction of the thumb, which exercises extensor carpi-ulnaris. Weakness of this muscle is said to increase the likelihood of radial deviation at the wrist which occurs with ulnar deviation at the MCP joint.

Elbows. Maintenance of range of movement, and avoiding heavy loads on the joints are both important. Loss of extension can be tolerated in one elbow, and results in little functional disability but when both elbows have fixed flexion over 45° the patient will have several problems, including driving a car; during eating, drinking, dressing; and in particular in reaching the perineum and carrying out personal hygiene. The embarrassment that this causes can be avoided by providing appropriate aids, but if the problem can be prevented by regular exercises to maintain elbow movement, this is of course preferable.

Small losses of pronation and supination can cause significant disability. This movement is required for basic household tasks such as opening jars, turning keys, etc. Pronation is also vital for those whose work involves the operation of a keyboard. One of our young patients was obliged to reconsider a career in computing when she found operating the computer keyboard impossible because both elbows were fixed in a 'neutral' position.

Shoulders. These joints are particularly likely to lose range of movement, and the patient must be encouraged to put the shoulders through a full range each day. Patients often believe they should struggle on with a difficult task which they can just manage, such as carrying a heavy shopping bag, whereas it would be better to use a shopping trolley or a spouse! A trolley within the house for transporting heavy objects can also be invaluable. Where shoulder movement has already become restricted, provision of aids such as a long-handled comb can do much to preserve independence and self-respect.

Spine. Attention needs to be drawn to *sitting and resting positions*, particularly when doing close work such as sewing, other handiwork or reading. The patient may need to wear a collar to maintain a correct neck position and a head restraint is desirable in the car to prevent neck injury in an accident.

Hips and knees. The knees are usually involved early in the course of RA. Quadriceps weakness and wasting are a rapid, almost inevitable consequence, and destruction of cartilage may ensue later. This, together with damage to the joint capsule and associated ligaments, can lead to an unstable knee joint which usually adopts a valgus position. During weight-bearing on such an unstable joint some of the load may be transmitted to non-bony structures rather than along the long axes of the bones. Since ligaments are not designed to support body weight they may rupture. The instability and deformity is therefore increased and the destructive process is accelerated.

Fixed flexion is often seen in the badly damaged knee. Left untreated this leads to flexion deformity in the hip and may prevent the patient from standing. The other important consequence of hip involvement in RA is loss of abduction, which leads to difficulties in intercourse and childbirth in women.

To avoid these problems the principles of joint protection need to be applied by the patient. This means:

(a) Putting hip and knee joints through a full range of movement each day. Swimming (using breast-stroke) should be encouraged, since this uses a wide range of joint positions with reduced weight-bearing.

(b) A daily period of resting or sleeping prone, to encourage extension at the hip and knee. A pillow may be placed under the *chest* to make this more comfortable.

(c) Encouraging exercises to strengthen adjacent muscles. Quadriceps strengthening exercises are easy to perform and vital, since knee stability is lost if this muscle becomes weak.

(d) The treatment of obesity to reduce the load on weight-bearing joints. However, the position of the joints at the time of weight-bearing is also important. For example, rising from a chair where the seat is raised and the hip is in a semi-flexed rather than a fully flexed position is considerably easier than rising from a 'bucket seat'. The ARC booklet 'Are you sitting comfortably' is helpful when choosing chairs for arthritics (see Appendix) (see also Chapter 42).

Strategically placed supports such as grab-rails in bathrooms, toilets and on stairs serve the same purpose (Chapter 39). Unfortunately, similar features are seldom incorporated into car design. It is a common sight to see the arthritic patient struggling to pull himself out of his car by grabbing the edge of a swinging car door.

Resting positions for knees and hips should not be those which encourage deformity. Patients may choose to rest with a pillow under the knees, but this encourages flexion of hip and knees. It is preferable to provide resting splints for the knees which restrict the degree of flexion.

Treatment of established deformities has to be undertaken not infrequently even where patient and clinicians have been diligent in managing the disease. Where flexion deformity of the knee has developed serial splinting with progressively straighter plaster splints may reduce the deformity, but it usually returns rapidly unless the treatment is backed up by physiotherapy. Prosthetic surgery for the knees may eventually be required. Hip flexion may also require surgical intervention. Total hip replacement is usually the appropriate procedure in the adult with severe RA. 'Anterior release' of the hip is occasionally performed, but is more relevant to the treatment of juvenile chronic arthritis than RA. The latter operation will only produce lasting improvement if it is reinforced by persistent and intensive physiotherapy and adequate relief of pain. Reversed dynamic slings to maintain extension can be useful prior to, and after, surgery.

Where lateral instability in the knee is a problem an orthosis with steel struts hinged at the knee such as the Cinch, Can-Am, etc, can be used; this may help to relieve weight-bearing pain (see Chapter 45, Orthotics). The more active patient probably requires intensive active physiotherapy coupled with prosthetic surgical treatment.

Walking aids may be used to increase stability and reduce the load borne by the legs, but the patient and therapist must remember that the increased loads borne by the arms when sticks or crutches are used can accelerate damage to these joints. Axillary or elbow crutches are seldom suitable for the rheumatoid patient. When walking sticks are used, the handle should be broad or be moulded to conform to the patient's hand, as does the handle of the Fischer stick. Sometimes supplementing this with a wrist splint is helpful. Where crutches or a walking frame are necessary the 'gutter' type should be chosen for their more even distribution of load (see Chapter 46).

In more severely affected patients, where walking or standing requires considerable effort, it is often helpful to provide a wheelchair at least for outdoor use. This avoids the situation where the patient expends all his or her energy getting from 'A' to 'B' and is then unable to carry out any useful activity at 'B' (see Chapter 43).

Modification of the environment can do much to ease the strain on damaged hips and knees. For example, the kitchen layout should take account of the fact that the sink is the most-used equipment; it should be central and have adjacent work surfaces at a convenient height. Some work may be done seated, and storage should be carefully planned to minimise difficulties of reaching and carrying, and to conserve energy. These principles can be applied to all tasks by those who understand the principles of joint protection.

Ground floor accommodation with easy access is ideal, but other factors such as helpful neighbours or family nearby should be taken into consideration before moving patients away from 'unsuitable accommodation'. Even for the severely disabled, major housing modifications such as stairlift installations (Chapter 44) and provision of ramps may be cheaper and more convenient than moving house (Chapter 39).

Ankle and foot. Ankle stability depends on the integrity of ligaments holding the tibia and fibula together and connecting these two bones to the talus and calcaneum. If these ligaments become stretched or eroded by the rheumatoid process, pronation and eversion of the foot tends to develop. Rarely Achilles tendon rupture may occur, particularly at the site of nodules within the tendon. These features only occur in more severe disease. Subtalar joint involvement with valgus deformity occurs more frequently, and leads to loss of inversion and eversion. This causes difficulty and pain when walking on uneven ground.

Involvement of metatarsophalangeal joints occurs in the majority of RA patients, and pain arising from these joints is often a presenting feature of the disease. The common deformities which occur are separation and downwards subluxation of the metatarsal heads, with associated 'claw-toe' deformities, hallux valgus and bunion formation. As a consequence the metatarsal heads no longer rest on protective fat pads and ulcers can develop at pressure points under the metatarsal heads.

Protection of the ankles and feet in RA inevitably depends on weight reduction and load reduction. In addition the patient usually needs altered footwear and must recognise this as an ongoing problem. Initially all that most patients need is a broader shoe with thicker soles and lower heels. Full-length metatarsal supports can be fitted into the patient's shoes. Wedges or heel cups should be tried for hindfoot symptoms. Unfortunately patients often have difficulty finding footwear broad or deep enough to accommodate these orthoses. These patients, and those with more severe deformities, will need made-to-measure shoes. These are in a variety of available styles and colours. Ready-made 'comfort' shoes and training shoes designed to take orthoses are also now available. Where ankle problems exist a boot will give additional support. Whatever footwear is used, fastenings must be straightforward (e.g. velcro) so that patients can manage despite hand involvement. Ankle–foot orthoses are available for those with ankle or subtalar instability causing pain on weight-bearing, but many patients prefer to use foot supports only (Chapter 45).

As stressed earlier, both doctor and patient must recognise not only that adequate footwear will prevent calluses and pressure ulcers developing, but also that the foot shape is likely to alter from year to year and footwear will need regular adjustment. This is particularly important in those few patients who also have a sensory neuropathy.

Some 50 per cent of patients with RA have difficulty with cutting toenails, and referral to a chiropodist is useful, particularly when the patient lives alone and grip is poor.

Surgery

This may be required early in RA to repair existing structures such as ruptured tendons (most often finger extensors) or to relieve pressure on trapped nerves (e.g. carpal tunnel syndrome). Synovectomy may be useful in early disease and in monoarthritis, but is not practical where many joints are inflamed simultaneously and seldom provides long-lasting relief.

Great advances have been made in the field of *prosthetic surgery* — prostheses for total hip and knee joint replacement have been improved in reliability and durability. Other prosthetic joints are less well-tried but should be considered where involvement of a particular joint is causing significant disability. Tendon prostheses are available, but are only rarely used in RA.

When prosthetic surgery is contemplated, the damage to the particular joint, the disability caused by this damage and the availability of a suitable prosthesis are among the factors to be assessed. The patient's fitness for an anaesthetic also needs consideration; advice should be given on smoking, obesity and dental hygiene (Chapter 32). The patient should also be fit enough to make use of the prosthesis afterwards, and sufficiently well-motivated to carry out appropriate exercises regularly both before and after surgery. For this reason a physiotherapist's assessment prior to surgery is invaluable. Age alone is not a bar to prosthetic surgery, though since the life span of prostheses is limited it is best to postpone surgery of this type in children or young adults as long as possible. Severe involvement of the atlanto-axial joint or other cervical joints should be brought to the anaesthetist's attention.

Prostheses are available for *finger and MCP joints.* Arthrodesis is usually preferred for severe wrist involvement. Arthrodesis of the thumb IP joint accompanied by prosthetic surgery to the MCP joints is a common procedure used to restore a 'pinch grip' where this has been lost.

The surgical procedures most frequently performed, and of proven value, are the release of trapped tendons or a trapped median nerve in the carpal tunnel or repair of ruptured tendons. *Wrist* synovectomy and excision of the lower end of the ulna may be used for less severe wrist involvement.

Excision of the upper end of the radius and synovectomy at *elbow or shoulder* are performed for pain relief with some success. Prostheses are available for both these joints but have variable results.

Prosthetic surgery for the hips and knees has been mentioned already, and can be very successful. Arthrodesis of the knee is fortunately now only rarely needed. Early synovectomies are occasionally of value in the knee.

Removal of the metatarsal heads and correction of hallux valgus are common and useful procedures for *forefoot* arthritis. Triple or talo-navicular arthrodesis is used where *hindfoot* symptoms fail to respond to physical therapy and orthoses. So far ankle prostheses have only a poor success rate, and arthrodesis is usually preferable for the treatment of severe painful involvement. Pain arising from the ankle and subtalar joints can be difficult to distinguish clinically, although the latter is more common. Obviously the source of pain needs to be clearly established before surgery is contemplated.

For a more detailed description of these procedures the reader is referred to a general rheumatology test. It is, however, important to note that surgery almost invariably requires intensive rehabilitation both before and after the procedure. In prosthetic surgery, above all, muscle strength needs to be preserved so that the prosthesis is adequately supported.

SOCIAL CONSEQUENCES OF ARTHRITIS

Severely handicapped patients may be entitled to mobility and attendance allowances and should be encouraged to claim these (see Chapter 37). Those who are working but have found travelling difficult, and are registered as disabled, may qualify for the 'fares to work' scheme. Some patients, particularly skilled women, are better continuing at work, thus gaining sufficient financial resources to pay for domestic help and a car. A home help can ease the burden of household tasks and sometimes the shopping. 'Meals-on-wheels' may also be appropriate. If the patient's job is inappropriate for his disability, or if the patient has no work, the Disablement Resettlement Officer may be able to help (see Chapter 41).

Chronic disability in any member of a family puts a strain on the family. Social workers and psychotherapists may be of help where marital disharmony occurs. Curiously, in RA, if the arthritis is already apparent at the time of marriage, the marriage tends to be stable, but where the arthritis develops later, discord and divorce are more common. Perhaps this occurs because partners find it difficult to accept and adapt to altered abilities in their spouse, but can accept disabilities if prepared for these initially (Wright and Owen, 1976). Sexual counselling may be helpful (see Chapter 30). Patient support groups such as Arthritis Care and the NASS (National Ankylosing Spondylitis Society) can also help. These organisations provide social contact, thus easing the social isolation which severe arthritis can bring to patients and their relatives. Informal discussions and formal talks arranged by the societies can increase understanding and hence ability to cope with the arthritis. They also provide other services such as advice about suitable holiday accommodation. The addresses of these organisations are in the Appendix.

SUMMARY

The patient with RA has a variety of problems which may change repeatedly over the years. Though drug therapy of RA differs from that of other arthropathies, many of the functional problems are similar and the disease serves well as a model of rehabilitation in inflammatory arthropathies. In all these disorders a close liaison between the doctor and other health professionals (physiotherapist, occupational therapist, orthotist, social workers) is essential for successful treatment, and depends partly on assessment and modification of the patient's lifestyle and environment. Drug therapy alone is not enough.

APPENDIX: USEFUL ADDRESSES

The Arthritis and Rheumatism Council
41 Eagle Street, London WC1R 4AR.
This charitable organisation sponsors research into arthritis and produces booklets, leaflets and fact sheets to educate patients and medical staff about the rheumatic diseases. Currently booklets and leaflets available include:

Introducing Arthritis
Your Arthritis and Your Home
Rheumatoid Arthritis Explained
Osteoarthritis Explained
Ankylosing Spondylitis
Gout
Lupus: SLE
Marriage, Sex and Arthritis
A New Hip Joint
When your Child has Arthritis
Backache
Neckache
Polymyalgia Rheumatica (PMR)
Tennis Elbow
Are you Sitting comfortably?

The National Ankylosing Spondylitis Society (NASS)
6 Grosvenor Crescent, London SW1X 7ER

Arthritis Care
6 Grosvenor Crescent, London SW1X 7ER

REFERENCES

Brattstrom, M. (1987) *Joint protection and rehabilitation in chronic rheumatic disorders*, Wolfe Medical Publications, London

Chamberlain, M.A. and Wright, V. (1981) The arthritic patient. In S. Mattingley (ed.), *Rehabilitation Today in Great Britain*, Update Books, London, pp. 148-51

Fries, J.F., Spitz, P., Kraines, R.G. and Holman, H.R. (1980) Measurement of patient outcome in arthritis. *Arth. Rheum.*, *23*, 137-45

Lawence, J.S. (1965) Surveys of rheumatic complaints in the population. In A. St. J. Dixon (ed.), *Progress in clinical rheumatology*, Churchill, London, p. 1.

Neumann, V., Hopkins, R., Dixon, J., Watkins, A., Bird, H. and Wright, V. (1985) Combination therapy with pulsed methyl prednisolone in rheumatoid arthritis. *Ann. Rheum. Dis.*, *44*, 747-61

Roberts, M.E.T., Wright, V., Hill, A.G.S. and Mehra, A.C. (1976) Psoriatic arthritis — follow-up study. *Ann Rheum. Dis.*, *35*, 206-12

Steinbrocker, O., Traeger, C.H. and Batterman, R.C. (1949) Therapeutic criteria in rheumatoid arthritis. *J. Am. med. Assoc.*, *140*, 659

Wordsworth, B.P. and Mowat, A.G. (1986) A review of 100 patients with ankylosing spondylitis with particular reference to socio-economic effects. *Br. J. Rheum.*, *25*, 175-80

Wright, V. and Owen, S. (1976) The effect of rheumatoid arthritis on the social situation of housewives. *Rheum Rehabil.*, *15*, 156-60

11

Amputations

Robin Luff

INTRODUCTION

Limb ablation is often life-saving, may relieve great suffering and can sometimes allow for greater function, yet this involves stressful surgery resulting in bodily mutilation, distortion of the body image and usually a degree of loss of function. To the surgeon, amputation may represent failure of attempted limb salvage and thus a personal defeat, whilst to relatives and carers limb loss may appear as the final evidence of total dependence. However, a planned — and perhaps primary — amputation may be looked upon positively as the first stage of a scheme of rehabilitation permitting a pain-free independent existence.

The purpose of this chapter is to recommend practices of amputee management which can greatly improve the lot of the patient. Whilst based on the practices of the English Artificial Limb Service, the general principles can be applied to other forms of organisations dealing with amputees.

INCIDENCE

The annual incidence of new amputations is similar throughout the developed countries. The actual figures discussed below relate to England and are shown in Table 11.1; the gross totals have decreased by 4 per cent in the past five years. The great majority of patients lose a lower limb, and much of the following relates to the management of such amputees. Approximately equal numbers of above- and below-knee amputations are performed (Table 11.2) but for a number of reasons, particularly energy requirement (Waters *et al.*, 1976) and ease of rehabilitation, amputation conserving the knee joint is of immense value. *With this in mind and using a team approach, at least twice as many amputations can be performed below the knee as above* (Ham *et al.*, 1987). Most amputees are elderly — 78 per cent were aged over 60 — and the majority of these have coincident

Table 11.1: Number of new amputees presenting for prosthetic treatment in England in 1985

One leg	4,540	(87%)
Both legs	494	(9%)
One arm	164	(3%)
Both arms	5	
Others	11	
Total	5,214	

The total for bilateral leg amputees includes those who have become bilateral having previously been seen as unilateral amputees (Department of Health and Social Security statistics)

Table 11.2: Number of lower limb amputations performed in England in 1985

Hindquarter	20	
Hip disarticulation	30	
Above-knee	2,670	(47%)
Knee disarticulation	229	
Below-knee	2,574	(45.5%)
Syme	67	
Partial foot	57	
Digital	2	
Total	5,649	

The above-knee total includes an unknown number of Gritti–Stokes procedures (Department of Health and Social Security statistics)

disabilities, especially respiratory and myocardial disease. The rehabilitation plan must take all disabilities and handicaps into consideration if the optimum result is anticipated. The numbers of upper limb loss at the various levels are shown in Table 11.3.

PREVALENCE

The amputee population in England is as follows:

All cases	63,000
Upper limb	11,000
Lower limb	52,000

The high prevalance of arm amputees in the population, combined with the very low incidence, results from the better prognosis of the underlying causes of arm ablation. *For lower limb amputees, the overall prognosis is*

Table 11.3: Numbers of upper limb amputations performed in England in 1985

Forequarter	7
Shoulder disarticulation	7
Above-elbow	60
Elbow disarticulation	4
Below-elbow	37
Wrist disarticulation	7
Partial hand	10
Digital	13
Total	145

(Department of Health and Social Security statistics)

poor (English and Gregory Dean, 1980); *nearly a third of unilateral leg amputees lose the other limb within three years and half of them will die within five years, mostly from progression of vascular disease.* The prevalance of limb deficiency in the UK is 132 per 100,000 of the total population, 4,500 amputees per health region, or approximately three such patients per family practitioner.

AETIOLOGY

The DHSS figures used as the basis of the above discussion result from cases of limb deficiency referred for prosthetic treatment, and must thus underestimate the true amputee population. Bearing this in mind there are nearly eleven times as many limbs lost from disease as are lost from trauma (Table 11.4). The great excess of amputation resulting from vascular disease is apparent, and such amputations are further classified in Table 11.5. The relationship between apparent level of vascular occlusion and level of limb loss is complex (O'Dwyer and Edwards, 1985). There is overlap between cases assigned to diabetic causes rather than vascular as these conditions not uncommonly are concurrent. Personal experience suggests that more cases are occurring as a result of endoprosthetic arthroplasty and internal fixation of fractures. Advances in chemotherapy and tumour resection with limb conservation appear to be reducing the number of amputations for malignancy. The predominant tumour types leading to amputation are osteosarcoma with considerably fewer fibrosarcomas and squamous cell tumours; other types of malignancy are relatively rare. Survivors of tumour surgery and congenitally limb-deficient patients are a small but important group with the prospect of many years of artificial limb use.

Table 11.4: Causes of upper and lower limb amputation in patients presenting for prosthetic treatment in England in 1985

Trauma	444	(8.5%)		
Disease	4,770	(91.5%)		
Vascular			3,332	(64%)
Diabetes			1,080	(21%)
Infection			104	(2%)
Malignancy			191	(4%)
Congenital			43	
Other			20	
Total			4,770	
Total	5,214	(100%)		

(Department of Health and Social Security statistics)

Table 11.5: Vascular causes of amputation in patients presenting for prosthetic treatment in England in 1985

Atherosclerosis	2,977	(89%)
Embolism	206	(6%)
Thromboangiitis	29	(1%)
Varicose ulceration	59	(2%)
Other	61	(2%)
Total	3,332	(100%)

(Department of Health and Social Security statistics)

MANAGEMENT OF AMPUTEES

Time-honoured procedures in amputee management aim for primary healing of the stump — and therefore often an unnecessarily proximal amputation level — with discharge from hospital and subsequent referral for assessment for prosthetic treatment. This practice can result in prolonged inpatient stay, repeated visits for outpatient physiotherapy and continued poor use of prostheses (Ham *et al.*, 1987). Alternatively, *all those concerned with amputee care can act together as a team actively working towards the optimum rehabilitation plan for each patient*; such teams are already at work in Dulwich (Ham *et al.*, 1987) and Roehampton (Engstrom and Van de Ven, 1986) in London and in Dundee (Scotland) and widely in the USA. A typical team will consist of: the amputating surgeon, physiotherapist, nurse, prosthetic clinician and prosthetist. Others such as the social worker, clinical psychologist and occupational therapist are involved as necessary, with roles related to the usual phases of management of any patient (Chapter 6): preoperative, surgical, postoperative and in this case prosthetic. After discharge from hospital when the patient attends a prosthetic clinic for continuing care, the team should still be active but will now include the family practitioner.

PREOPERATIVE PHASE

A full medical and social assessment (Chapter 5) should be made and all relevant social benefits discussed (Chapter 37). Where time permits, general health and fitness should be improved, body weight reduced when necessary and tobacco consumption reduced or eliminated. Nurses, who have the greatest amount of time in contact with the patient, can make valuable contributions to assessment. It is helpful for the patient's family to be included at this early stage.

The physiotherapist plays a vital role at this point in management; the patient must be prepared for surgery and for the subsequent rehabilitation, but in addition the activities of the team must be coordinated. The preparation of a patient for general anaesthesia is assumed, and in addition a careful assessment of disabilities and resulting handicaps is necessary (Chapter 5). In particular, auditory, sensory and visual handicaps must be evaluated and corrected where possible. Balance and coordination should be assessed and improved as needed, and muscle group power and joint movement ranges determined for upper and lower limbs; joint contracture is best reduced at this time and it is thus essential that the therapist has time with the patient preoperatively. The more proximal amputation levels usually require a degree of wheelchair dependence and an assessment for this purpose should be made, taking into account likely handicaps, home environment and intended use (Chapter 43). A stump support board should be fitted to wheelchairs supplied for below-knee amputees and a suitable pattern is shown in Figure 11.1. An alternative design is described by Ham and Whittaker (1984).

There are specific aspects of medical input to the team assessment, particularly related to evaluation of the peripheral circulation and condition of what will be the remaining limb; foot care by a chiropodist should start as an inpatient and continue after discharge. Adequate pain relief must be established as soon as possible, and maintained. There is understandable concern about pain, phantom limb sensation and phantom pain; reassurance about analgesia, the common occurrence of phantom limb sensation and the transient nature of phantom pain is invaluable. It is rare (0.02 per cent after one year, DHSS Statistics, 1986) for phantom pain to remain troublesome after one year. At this time the patient must be encouraged in the attitude that amputation is a positive decision to improve general health and regain mobility.

The level of amputation should be decided preoperatively, based on

Figure 11.1: Simple stump board design to support a below-knee stump which has a minimal dressing; stump bandaging is unnecessary and interferes with inspection of the stump during early mobilisation

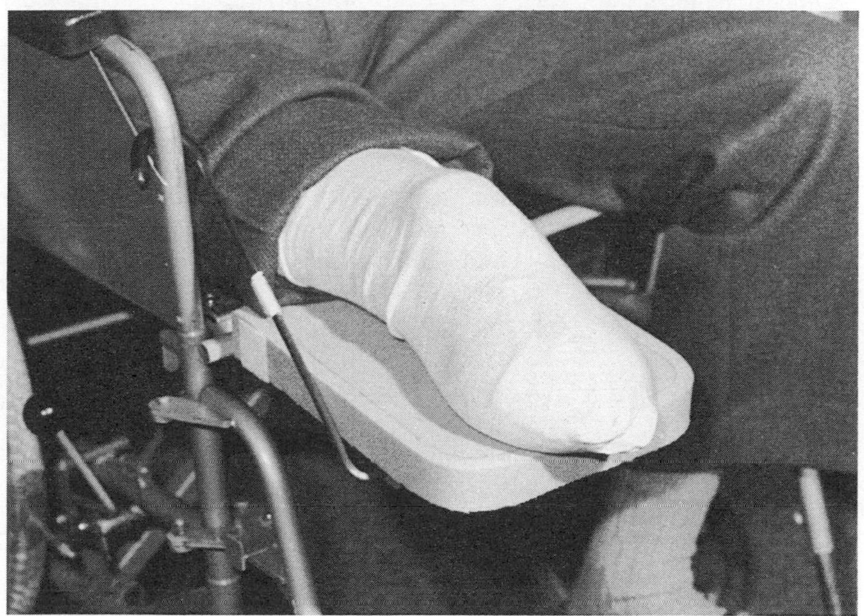

information obtained from: clinical assessment, investigation, and the anticipated result of rehabilitation. Many surgeons rely solely on clinical assessment to determine amputation level, but this leads to an excess of proximal amputations; thus 30 per cent of amputations in one series healed below the knee even when no femoral pulse was palpable (O'Dwyer and Edwards, 1985). Unfortunately, no single technique gives sufficient accuracy to be used in isolation, but the following have been found to be useful guides in level assessment:

transcutaneous oxygen pressure measurement,
isotope clearance techniques,
Doppler indices,
thermography.

Arteriography and digital subtraction angiography are of value in planning vascular reconstruction rather than amputation.

Rapid, uncomplicated healing of a stump fashioned at the most distal level possible represents the ideal in amputee management, and the importance of preserving the knee joint whenever possible has been mentioned.

The relevance of making a realistic plan for rehabilitation becomes apparent in the case of a patient who will never use a prosthesis; in this situation a below-knee stump will go into fixed flexion and be a considerable additional handicap. In such a case the preoperative decision on level should be for a knee disarticulation or Gritti–Stokes amputation (Campbell and Morris, 1986).

Whenever possible, and particularly in difficult cases, the prosthetic clinician and prosthetist should take part in the preoperative assessment to assist in planning rehabilitation with regard to the level of amputation. The team decision should be discussed with the patient, whose opinion should be taken into account. A visit from an established amputee may be of benefit and suitable individuals may be identified by prosthetic clinics or through the National Association for the Limbless Disabled.

SURGICAL PHASE

The following section is given for guidance only; a general review of surgical techniques is given by Vitali *et al.* (1986) and the lower limb procedures described by Malt (1978). Not all texts of general surgery are in line with current attitudes to amputation surgery, and the reader should exercise caution in their use.

Skin. Scars should not be formed across load-bearing areas of the stump, and flaps must not be undermined during construction; the amputating surgeon must thus understand modern prosthetic practices. Skin closure is best performed using adhesive strips, e.g. Steristrip.

Muscle. Three aspects of the surgical handling of muscle must be considered: length, volume and reattachment.

Muscle groups must be divided so that reattachment can be performed maintaining physiological tensions; otherwise the imbalance in muscle forces will predispose to contracture. Bulk in myocutaneous flaps must be reduced by adequate muscle trimming, otherwise a bulky stump results which will considerably delay prosthetic treatment and give rise to continuing problems. Inadequate trimming is one of the common errors leading to an unsatisfactory stump (McColl, 1986). The topic is amplified by Dederich (1967).

Nerve. Neuroma formation after amputation is inevitable, and is best managed by ensuring that these are allowed to form deep to fascia and protected within soft tissues. Attendant vessels should be dissected free, ligated separately if necessary, and the nerve placed on gentle traction and cleanly divided.

Blood vessels. Arteries and veins should be ligated separately to avoid fistula formation. Diathermy should be avoided in the residual limb but frequently there is little bleeding; *the absence of bleeding is not an indication for amputation at a higher level, as wound healing depends on the microcirculation.*

Bone. For any level of amputation, bone must be divided at the correct length and *cut edges must be rounded and, in the below-knee stump, bevelled.* This avoids high tissue loading over bone surfaces having small radii of curvature; the skin in the above-knee stump in Figure 11.2 is obviously at risk.

Drainage. Haematoma formation following inadequate haemostasis causes stump oedema which will delay prosthetic treatment. Careful haemostasis and the use of a fine-bore suction drain, e.g. Redivac, for the first 48 hours is essential. Bulky, passive drains can cause adherent scars.

Dressing. A standard postoperative dressing should be applied and left for 48 hours when, if all is well, the drain should be removed and the dress-

Figure 11.2: An above-knee stump where the myoplasty has retracted from the end of the femur which is prominent beneath the skin. The high pressures which result commonly cause ulceration. A similar result is seen after mid-thigh amputation performed without myoplasty construction

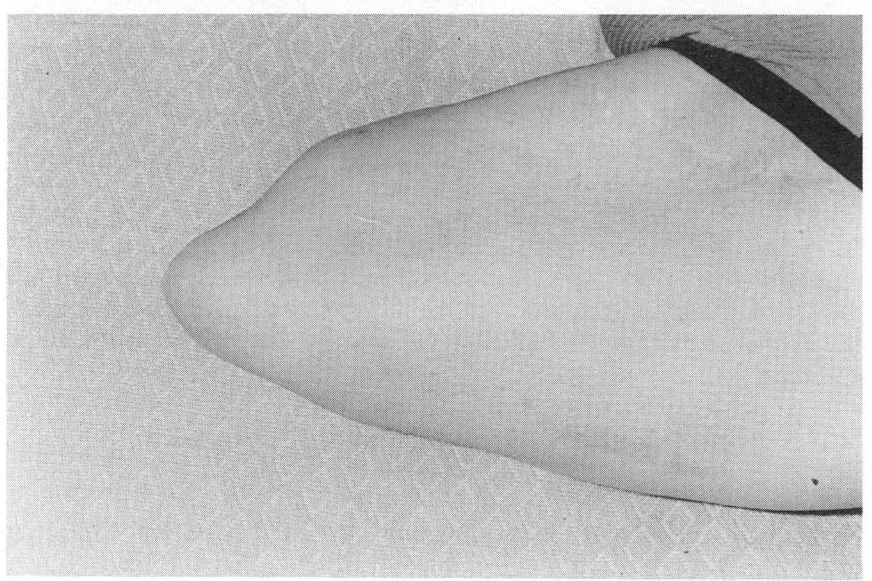

ing reduced to the minimal thickness of absorbent dry material. The supportive nature of Tubifast is helpful. *Conventional stump bandaging and the use of elasticated dressings such as Tubigrip must be avoided*; there is no evidence of benefit in modern practice and considerable risk of harm. The circulation in a dysvascular stump is already sufficiently at risk. Postoperative plaster dressings can control stump oedema but require great attention to detail and have no advantages over minimal dressings and early walking aid use. A rigid post operative dressing will not control flexion contracture but, if applied for this reason, may cause secondary stump injury.

Analgesia. Pain relief must be adequate both before and after surgery. Ward staff should cooperate in arranging doses of analgesia to precede physiotherapy by a suitable interval.

Amputation levels

Digital and ray amputations

Descriptions of the many techniques can be obtained from orthopaedic surgery texts; no prosthetic treatment is necessary. Forces acting on the foot should be distributed using shoe fillers made from, e.g., Plastazote or by custom-made — 'surgical' — footwear.

Transmetatarsal amputation

This useful level is indicated where disease, vascular or mechanical, is confined to the distal part of the foot and when *a viable flap based on the sole can be constructed.* The distal forefoot is amputated through a dorsal incision with division of the metatarsal necks. The wound is closed with a flap based on the distal sole of the foot. A shoe filler is required which allows the continued use of existing footwear, usually with an excellent gait.

Partial foot amputation

Amputation at this level may be considered in the traumatised foot and exceptionally in distal vascular disease; the common techniques used are the tarsometatarsal operation — Lisfranc's amputation — and the mid-tarsal — Chopart's amputation. All techniques produce a stump with inherent muscle imbalance which is worse at the more proximal levels; better long-term results are obtained if muscle-balancing procedures are employed (Marquardt, 1973). Prosthetic treatment is necessary.

Syme's Amputation

This modified disarticulation of the ankle joint is indicated, when the heel has adequate blood supply and protective sensation, in: chronic infection (especially diabetes), trauma, congenital deformity and vascular disease (only if the heel is viable). Syme's original technique is still applicable; the talo-tibial joint is opened from the front and the os calcis freed from the heel pad by subperiosteal dissection. The foot is discarded and the malleoli excised with rounding of the resulting bone edges. The heel pad is brought over the end of the stump, sutured in place and carefully strapped to stabilise its position. (In children particularly, stabilisation can be ensured by Kirschner wires.)

The well-healed stump is durable and should be fully end-bearing but is bulky. Prosthetic treatment is necessary although limited mobility indoors is possible without a prosthesis. Stump shape dictates the design of limb, which is often unsightly but functionally excellent.

Below-knee amputation

This level can combine excellent appearance and an efficient gait, and is applicable for any of the causes of limb ablation already described. It is the next level of choice after the transmetatarsal amputation in dysvascular limbs. (Bone overgrowth can occur following this trans-diaphyseal amputation in children and special techniques are necessary to overcome this (Marquardt, 1981).) Below-knee amputation is best performed as a one-stage procedure including a formal myoplasty. For optimum results the stump at this level should be the correct length for the patient. A short stump causes prosthetic difficulties but is manageable, whereas a long stump (Figure 11.3) usually causes repeated stump difficulties and leads to surgical revision. Two approaches are recommended in deciding stump length: bone may be divided either at the level of maximum calf bulge or at a length equivalent to 8 cm per metre of the patient's height (or one inch per foot!). The long, posterior-based myocutaneous flap described by Kendrick (1956) and elaborated and brought into standard use by Burgess *et al.* (1971) remains the most frequently used technique. There are a number of advantages, both surgical and prosthetic, in the skew flap procedure described by Robinson *et al.* (1982) but it must be recognised that these have not been demonstrated in a formal trial.

Prosthetic treatment is necessary, and if the stump is correctly fashioned after accurate selection of level, even very elderly patients can regain independent mobility. Cosmetic and functional results are excellent and a normal walking gait is possible.

Through-knee disarticulation

As neither major muscle handling nor bone section is involved, this level of amputation can be performed quickly and under minimal anaesthesia. It is thus the ideal operation for a patient who could have a successful below-knee operation but is assessed as highly unlikely to benefit from prosthetic treatment. It is contraindicated, if prosthetic treatment is contemplated, in:

Figure 11.3: A very long below-knee stump — 23 cm from knee joint line to the end of the soft tissues of the stump. Prosthetic problems will occur frequently and stump revision will probably be necessary

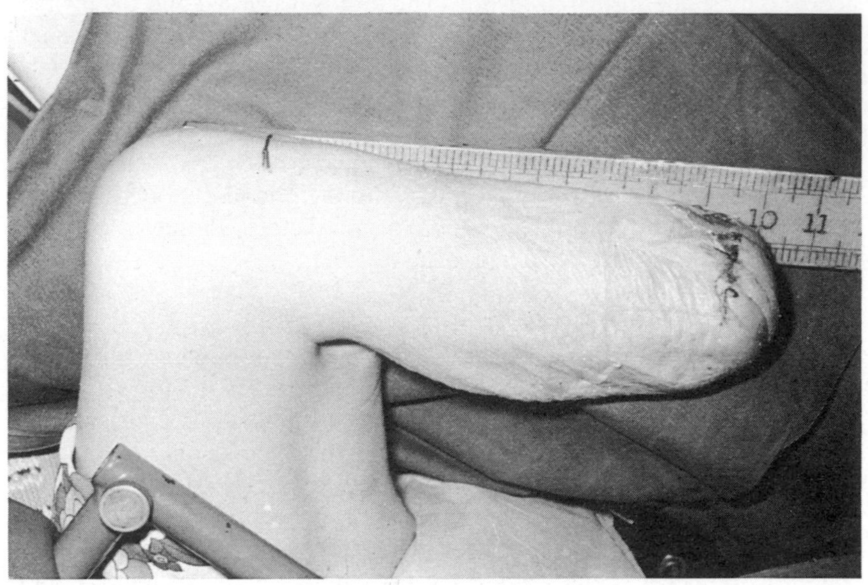

an osteoarthritic knee, the presence of fixed flexion at the hip (>20 degrees) and in young adults (especially female).

Lateral skin flaps produce the best scar, and retention of the patella, stabilised by tenodesis in front of the femoral condyles, controls rotation of a prosthesis. The heads of the gastrocnemius should be preserved to maintain blood supply to the flaps. The stump is capable of full end-bearing and will mature rapidly; early definitive prosthetic fitting is often possible.

Gritti–Stokes amputation

This modified disarticulation of the knee, described separately by Gritti (1857) and Stokes (1870) is much favoured by some surgeons and generally disliked by those involved in prosthetic treatment. Indications and contraindications are as for the true disarticulation but with the additional benefits of using shorter flaps and faster initial healing (Campbell and Morris, 1986).

The disarticulation is followed by excision of the articular surfaces of the patella and femoral condyles; the raw bone surfaces are then opposed and stabilised together. This amounts to the construction of an extensive open fracture in a dysvascular limb, and although skin healing readily occurs, there is considerable doubt about the success of bony union.

The stump is at best partially end-bearing and gives rise to a number of prosthetic difficulties.

Mid-thigh amputation

This, the most commonly performed of the proximal amputation levels, is indicated when removal of pathology and tissue viability require amputation above the knee. When prosthetic treatment is not contemplated, a long stump — ideally through knee or Gritti–Stokes — is valuable, but is an additional handicap if prosthetic use is likely. Similarly, a very short stump has inbuilt muscle imbalance and will cause prosthetic difficulties; when amputation around the lesser trochanter of the femur is required, a hip disarticulation should be performed. *Ideally, 12 cm clearance from the end of the soft tissues of the stump to the knee joint line should be achieved.*

The femur should be divided in the middle third to give the required clearance and the bone edges then adequately rounded. A formal myoplasty (Murdoch, 1984) is necessary as simple flaps often result in protrusion of the femur through the myoplasty with consequent discomfort.

Prosthetic treatment is necessary; the stump is incapable of end-bearing and a proximal bearing socket is required. The energy cost of amputation above the knee must be appreciated; for a given walking velocity, Peizer and Wright (1970) report an energy need twice that of a non-amputee.

Hip disarticulation

Indications at this level are tumours, trauma and occasionally very severe aortoiliac obliterative atherosclerosis. Because of the importance of certain areas in force transmission, scars should not be formed over the ipsilateral ischium or the iliac crests.

Hindquarter amputation

Malignancy, when surgical treatment offers a reasonable prognosis, is almost the only indication for this very extensive amputation. Scars over the remaining ischium and iliac crest should be avoided.

Upper limb amputations

These are almost always performed for either trauma or malignancy, and length of the remaining limb should be preserved, using plastic surgery as necessary. In general, disarticulation should be avoided, as should a very short stump except when a very short humeral stump can be fashioned to improve the shoulder contour. Adherent scars and superficial neuromas should be avoided as described above, and formal myoplasties constructed when possible, as this will help preserve muscle function which may be of value in establishing control of externally-powered prostheses.

Congenital limb absence

Digital vestiges — so-called nubbins — should be left intact unless the adult patient insists on removal, as the nubbin may be of some value either as a source of sensory information or as a possible control mechanism for an upper limb prosthesis. The value of limb vestiges can be seen in the phocomelic adult driving an adapted car (Chapter 47).

POSTOPERATIVE PHASE

Medical and surgical input

Individual responsibilities of the amputation team members should be coordinated by the physiotherapist. In particular, dressings and analgesia should be managed as suggested previously. Diabetic control must be achieved and a simple regime established. Proper care of the remaining foot is essential for dysvascular and diabetic amputees; such care must be provided for diabetic patients who may have visual and sensory deficits. The foot should be kept clean and dry, and toenails must be kept short and tidy; in particular they should be trimmed squarely across and not cut down into the lateral nail fold. Any sign of infection, bacterial or fungal, should be treated vigorously. If the prescription of special footwear changes during prosthetic treatment, the prosthesis may also need alteration. Diabetic foot care and relevant orthotic aspects are further considered in Chapter 45.

Therapist input

A recent publication (Engstrom and Van de Ven, 1986) has described the role of the physiotherapist in amputee management in some detail. Early walking aid use should be started according to an established routine; this term has a specific meaning in amputee treatment over and above the provision of walking frames, crutches and sticks. The most commonly used aid is the pneumatic post-amputation mobility aid whose acronym 'PAM aid' (more properly PPAM aid) has confused many a doctor in hospital training. *In an otherwise satisfactory stump this may be applied in almost complete safety five days post-operatively to a stump with normal blood supply (Figure 11.4) or after seven days in a dysvacular stump with great benefit to both early gait re-education and ease of early prosthetic treatment* (Redhead *et al.*, 1978). This aid, or an alternative, the 'Tulip' limb, have maximum ease of use in the below-knee amputee, although the PPAM aid can be used for above-knee limb loss if a shoulder diagonal strap is also used. The 'Femuret' aid is a further possibility for the above-knee amputee and has advantages in its functional resemblance to a temporary prosthesis.

Such aids accelerate healing and speed the resolution of oedema; in

Figure 11.4: A young amputee using the pneumatic post-amputation mobility aid (PPAM aid). Note the simple rocker end; more recent designs of early walking aid use an ankle articulation and foot

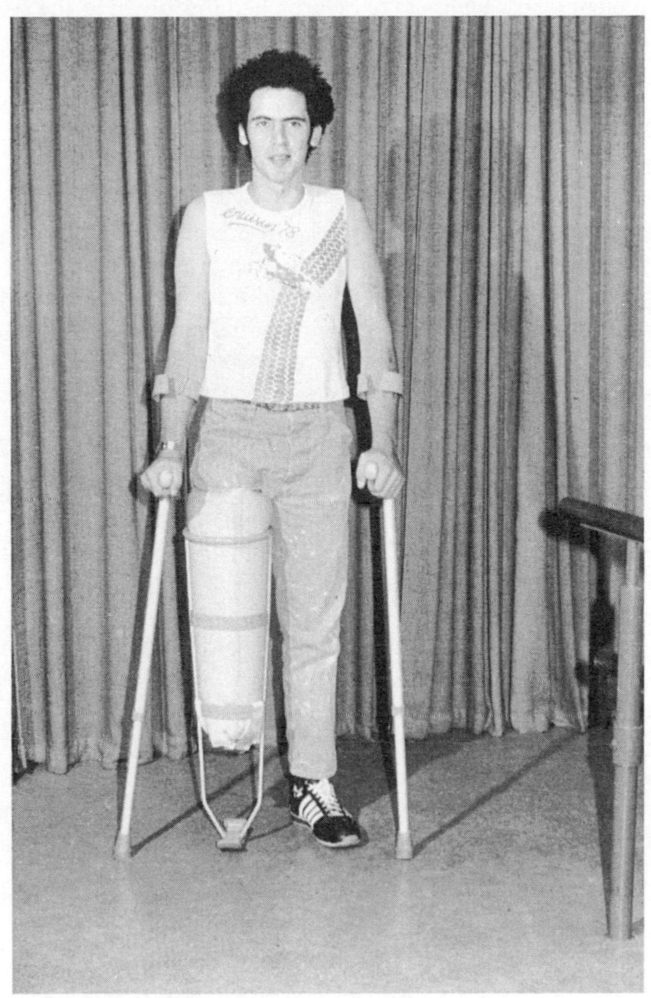

addition, valuable information is obtained about the likelihood of successful prosthetic treatment. Care should be exercised in their use in the presence of infection, but early walking aids can otherwise be used at the above postoperative intervals even if the wound is incompletely healed, provided that it is stable.

As mentioned above, a suitable wheelchair must be available from a well-maintained hospital stock. A double amputee, particularly bilaterally above the knee, is dangerously unstable in a standard-wheelbase wheelchair and should use a chair with the wheelbase extended backwards by three inches to maintain stability. Alternatively, a backrest kit may be used which displaces the body weight forward in the chair. In the absence of the above, sufficient lead weights may be attached low down at the front of the wheelchair as an emergency and temporary measure. All such patients should use a waist belt (Chapter 43).

PROSTHETIC PHASE

The prosthetic clinician, prosthetist and therapist should reassess the amputee between one and three weeks after limb ablation. Much more frequently the patient will have been discharged from hospital and will be attending for intermittent therapy as an outpatient. *Such patients must be referred to a prosthetic clinic before discharge from hospital.* If doubt regarding prosthetic treatment persists at the time of discharge, referral should still be made; this avoids delay which otherwise would prejudice successful prosthetic treatment (Jamieson and Hill, 1976).

The rehabilitation plan, modified as necessary (see also Chapter 8) has the following outline:

early fitting of a temporary prosthesis,
early gait retraining,
initial prescription of a definitive prosthesis,
further gait training,
modification of the definitive prescription.

Similar concepts apply to the upper limb amputee but retraining for function replaces gait in the above description, and temporary prostheses are rarely used.

Prostheses

A prosthesis is a part supplied to correct a deficiency; a prosthetist (not a 'fitter'!) is a professional who practises prosthetics. An artificial limb, which is an exoprosthesis, consists of the following components: a socket, articulation(s), overall structure, means of suspension, alignment devices, cosmetic cover, and power source. Such limbs may be temporary or definitive in nature and will differ in terms of construction, sophistication of function and cosmesis. Essentially, the temporary prosthesis is supplied quickly to allow very early rehabilitation when considerable changes in stump volume are anticipated. Volume change is one component of the process termed *stump maturation,* which includes scar tissue resolution, a degree of muscle atrophy, limited changes in the bone end and the development of load-bearing tolerance; volume changes occur in the first few weeks but the other changes take many months. Knee locks for stance phase stability, additional suspension and simple cosmesis are usually incorporated. In contrast, a definitive prosthesis will often have a self-suspending socket, sophisticated control of swing and stance phase and detailed cosmesis, but may take some weeks to fabricate, align and finish. An example of a fully finished definitive prosthesis is shown in Figure 11.5.

Figure 11.5: Blatchford's above-knee Endolite prosthesis. The polypropylene suction socket and carbon fibre endoskeleton are clearly seen. The single-axis knee has a built-in stabiliser and the rod for the shin-mounted pneumatic swing phase control is visible behind the knee. The prosthesis, draped in its shaped foam cosmesis and covered with a stocking, is shown in the right of the picture

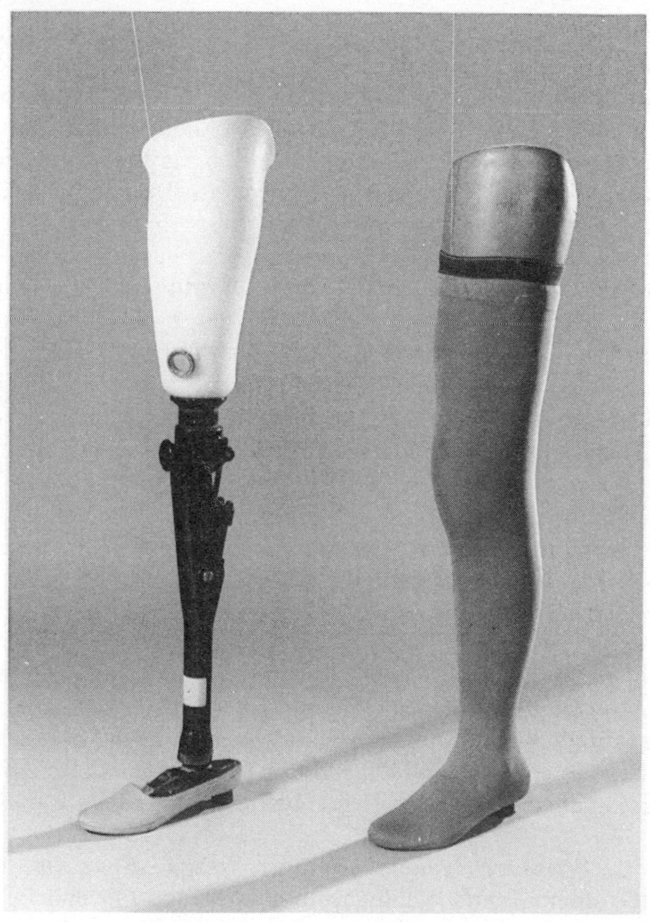

Socket. This, the principal interface between the patient and the prosthesis, is the single most important component in any prosthesis, and may be:

Proximal-bearing, e.g. ischial; patellar tendon-bearing (PTB), many upper limb prostheses.
End-bearing, e.g. knee disarticulation; Syme.
Total surface bearing, e.g. some mid-thigh sockets.

Total surface contact should be achieved whenever possible to prevent distal stump congestion. The traditional materials, wood, leather and metal, are still in common use but are being superseded by glassfibre laminates, rigid (polypropylene) and flexible polymers. In some sockets, liners are an integral part of the socket system; these are made from resilient polymers or leather and are formed together with the hard shell of the socket. *Liners must not be interchanged between sockets.*

Articulation(s). These are required to replace ablated joints and must thus afford an acceptable range of movement together with control of movement in swing and stance phases of gait. An artificial knee joint is uniaxial or polyaxial, and can be controlled either by alignment and the user's muscle power only — e.g. a free knee — or have control mechanisms built in. The structures which can be incorporated to control swing phase are: *elastic return, friction devices, return spring, pneumatic piston, hydraulic piston.* Stability of the knee in stance phase depends on: *alignment, stabilisers, locks.* The locks may be semi-automatic, in which case the amputee locks the knee by extension and has a stiff knee gait, or an optional lock which may be used for stiff-knee walking or simply for stability when standing. Ankle joints may be uniaxial or polyaxial as in Figure 11.6. Modern prostheses, in which hip joint function must be replaced, incorporate an adjustable stride length limiter and polyaxial hip joint.

Structure. Prostheses are either endoskeletal or exoskeletal in structure, the former being the more modern modular system based on an axial tube (e.g. Figure 11.7) and the latter the traditional limb types in which the load-bearing structure also forms the cosmetic cover.

Alignment devices. These must allow for translational and rotational adjustment in all three planes (longitudinal translation is equivalent to length alteration). Such devices may be deleted from the limb after alignment has been established, and this reduces the final mass of the prosthesis, but further alignment changes will then be difficult.

Suspension. Prostheses require support during the swing phase to maintain the stump interface and ensure control, and this may be achieved

Figure 11.6: Patellar tendon-bearing (PTB) prostheses. Left to right: Blatchford's PTB Endolite with carbon fibre skeleton, polypropylene supracondylar socket and Multiflex ankle; Otto Bock modular PTB limb with lightweight metal skeleton and polypropylene socket within which the liner can be clearly seen; PTB modular assembly prosthesis, now obsolete but still in widespread use in the United Kingdom

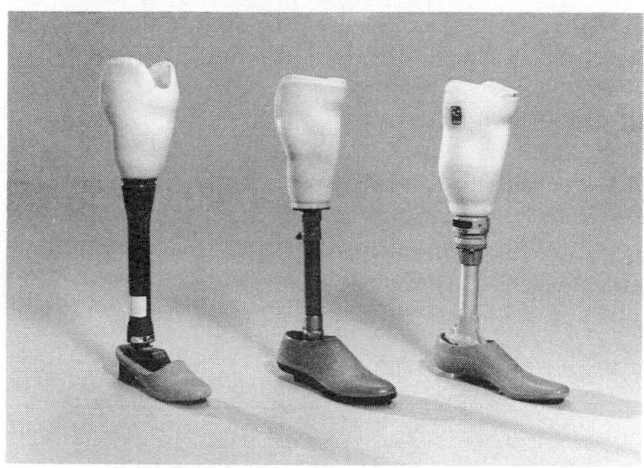

by additional suspension or by using a self-suspending socket design. Additional suspensions vary with the type of prosthesis:

Cuffs, straps, braces, belts — for all levels.
Pelvic band and external hip joint — for mid-thigh stumps and occasionally more distal levels (Figure 11.8).
Soft suspensions, e.g. the Silesian belt.

Cosmesis. In exoskeletal limbs the shaping of the limb, in wood, metal or glassfibre laminate, is both structural and cosmetic, whereas the endoskeletal limb has a modular central structure over which is draped a soft cosmesis of shaped foam which is then covered by a plastic skin or stocking. There are as yet unsolved problems regarding the shaping of the knee cosmesis in such limbs.

Power sources. Almost all prostheses use the amputee's body power in combination with gravity to produce useful movement and function, but some upper limb devices, because a useful power/weight ratio can be achieved, employ external power sources.

All lower limb prostheses from Syme's level proximally require a complete prosthetic foot, and this is a component for which there have

Figure 11.7: Hanger's UltraRoelite prosthesis for the above-knee level shown in skeletal form to display the structure. The long four-bar link knee mechanism (Extraflex knee) is clearly seen. The socket is a modified quadrilateral brim total surface bearing socket design; the suction valve aperture is seen medially towards the end of the socket

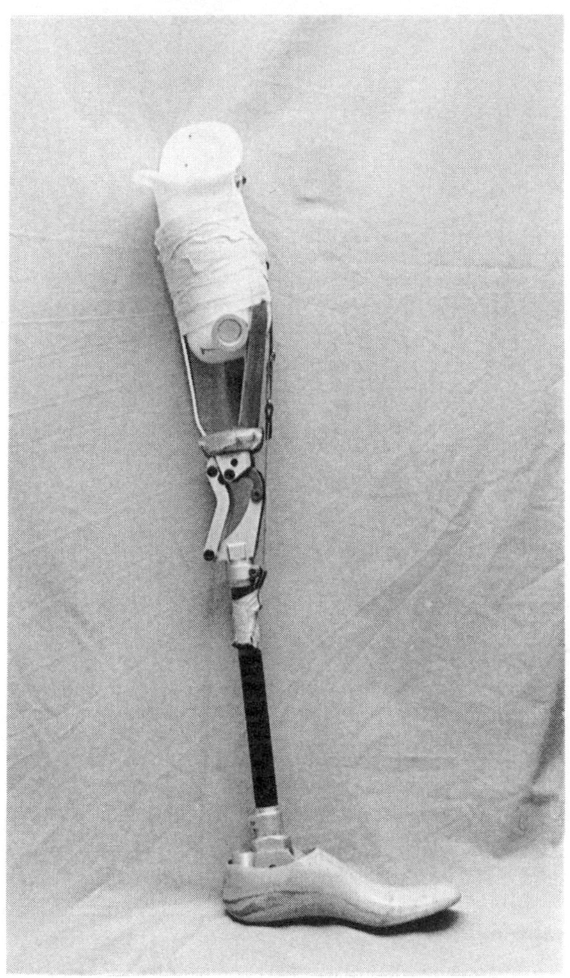

been many recent advances. Most feet are fashioned from wood or moulded from polymers and then attached to the rest of the prosthesis by a mounting bolt and ankle articulation. The Endolite foot has a carbon fibre keel incorporated into a moulded foot and a polyaxial (Multiflex) ankle joint. The solid-ankle–cushion-heel (SACH) foot eliminates the need for an ankle joint as the cushion properties of the

Figure 11.8: AK/BK temporary (or bypass) prosthesis. The rigid pelvic band, shoulder suspension strap and external hip joint can be seen. The leather thigh corset is closed by lacing and/or straps; the felt socket is made large enough to support any necessary dressings

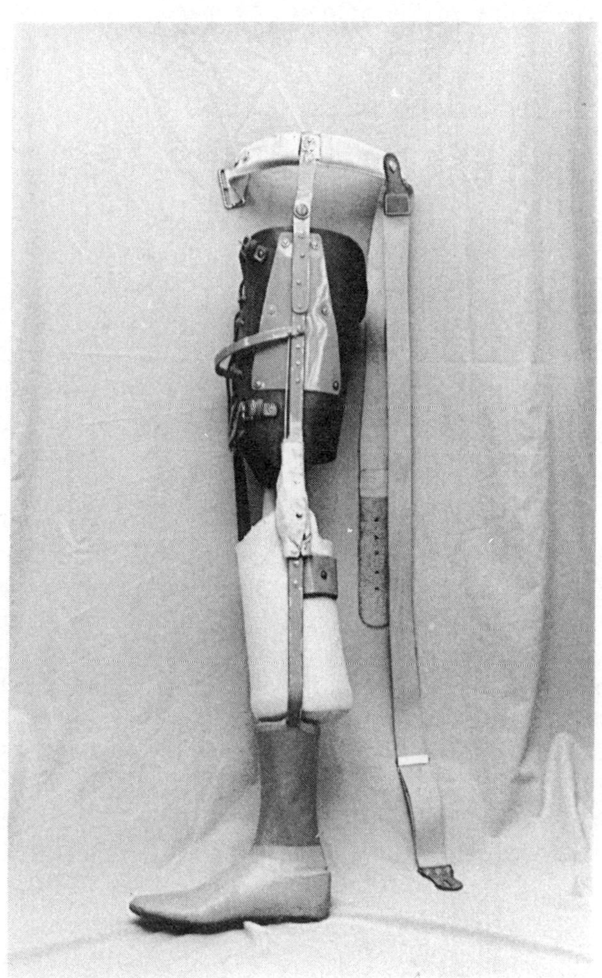

heel provide a polyaxial range of movement.

The interval between postoperative assessment and temporary limb delivery will vary from 1 to 14 days depending on amputation level, type of prosthesis prescribed and the time available for contact between prosthetist and patient. During this interval the patient should continue intensive physiotherapy. *The temporary nature of the first prosthesis should be emphasized, and responsibility for donning, doffing and adjustment of fit by number of socks by the amputee, encouraged.*

The prosthetist, and prosthetic clinician where required, should assess the prosthesis at delivery to confirm socket fit, limb configuration and alignment. The details of the checkout are beyond the scope of this chapter. The ability of the amputee to manage the technology of a prosthesis is a significant factor in determining temporary and definitive prosthesis prescription. Gait re-education using the temporary prosthesis then continues in the following sequence:

full weight-bearing and weight transfer;
walking within parallel bars, turning by stepping;
walking with sticks within parallel bars;
walking with one stick and one parallel bar;
free walking with two sticks or walking frame;
optimum gait with minimal walking aids.

Crutches — elbow, Canadian and axillary — are best avoided in elderly amputees; although the younger patient may prefer elbow crutches their use should be carefully monitored as dependence on such walking aids may delay rehabilitation.

The correction of socket fit by sock adjustment is core knowledge for any carer who has dealings with amputees. Socket fit may of course be effected in a number of ways in a suitably equipped prosthetic workshop — grinding, filling, lining, padding — but these are necessary only when the basic adjustment of fit has failed to maintain comfort, or results in loss of socket definition. In the individual, the adjusted fit at the start of a period of walking may not necessarily be correct at the end, and further socks may need to be added. Three types of stump sock are in common use:

(a) Nylon sheaths: these have insignificant thickness and are used to provide a free sliding surface to allow easy ingress and egress of the stump.

(b) Wool socks: almost all non-suction sockets are constructed to fit correctly when one wool sock is applied to the stump. Extra socks may be worn to compensate for stump shrinkage.

(c) Cotton socks: each of these has one-third the thickness of a wool sock, and cotton socks may thus be used to achieve fine adjustment of fit.

Sensible adjustment of fit will allow continued walking training whilst maintaining amputee comfort. As the amputee becomes confident in managing socket adjustment self-esteem increases, and as dependence decreases so walking improves. The reasonable limits of adjustment of fit by sock changes is dealt with in the more detailed discussion of the prostheses applicable to the various levels of amputation, which follows.

Prosthetics and amputation level

Partial foot

In the muscle-balanced, plantigrade foot a bootee or backsplint in polypropylene or ortholene with sole plate and toe filler is usually satisfactory. The equinus stump often seen after Chopart's amputation presents major prosthetic problems, particularly when attempting to distribute the forces of walking; a prosthesis immobilising the hindfoot and ankle and extending up the calf is necessary. All advantages of preserving the hindfoot and ankle are then lost.

Syme's amputation

The stump is bulbous and end-bearing. Modern designs have better appearance than the traditional kind but are still not very satisfactory except in congenital cases. A self-suspending socket, ankle articulation and foot must be provided. The three socket designs commonly encountered are:

(a) laced-up leather supported on side-steels;

(b) glassfibre laminate with a medial or posterior window which is opened to allow the stump to pass through the narrowed, suspending part of the socket and closed in use;

(c) glassfibre laminate containing a built-up Pelite liner.

Ankle and foot function are best replaced by a SACH unit.

Below-knee level

This is the first level which frequently requires a temporary prosthesis. Forces are taken through the patellar tendon with other pressure-tolerant areas of the stump used to support the stump at the correct position in the socket. An ankle articulation, foot and suspension must be provided. The socket contains a liner usually made from Delite, although Kemblo may be employed for heavy active users. The ankle can be uniaxal or polyaxial. Various suspensions are available and the following are frequently met: leather supracondylar cuff, elastic stocking and suspender belt or a self-suspending socket design. Sockets are designed to be a comfortable fit with one wool stump sock; if more than two wool socks are needed for comfort the amputee should attend a prosthetic clinic for adjustment.

Two types of *temporary limb* are used, of which the simpler is a basic PTB socket containing a Pelite liner, and uses cuff suspension, a uniaxial ankle and a simple cosmetic cover. Regrettably, some stumps are unsuited for early PTB fitting, when the above-knee-for-below-knee (AKBK) or bypass prosthesis (Figure 11.8) may be used. This consists of a leather thigh corset which transmits most of the forces and a felt socket with side steels and semi-automatic knee locks. With stump maturation the amputee progresses to a PTB. Indications for AKBK use are:

for very early fitting;
stable but incompletely healed surgical wound;
adjacent, unhealed surgical wounds interfering with PTB use;
poorly fashioned stump.

There are almost no contraindications for PTB prescription; even very short stumps can be satisfactorily treated with the addition of a short, stabilising thigh corset. The indications for *definitive thigh corset limb use* are:

instability of the knee, arising from mechanical derangement or gross muscle weakness;
specific activities related to employment or sport.

Such a prosthesis normally has side steels and unlocked external knee joints with a simple socket shape.

Knee disarticulation. This is a bulbous, end-bearing stump and in common with the Syme's stump can use a self-suspending socket with a built-up liner. Glassfibre laminate is normally used with Delite for the liner; no additional suspension is required. Sockets have also been fabricated from leather and metal. Knee and ankle articulations, a shin and a foot must be provided. The shin structure is determined by the endo- or exoskeletal nature of the limb. The ankle and foot are as for the PTB.

The knee joint presents difficulties as the physiological axis of the joint should pass through the femoral condyles and this inevitably entails compromises in limb design. The possibilities are:

(a) External knee joints alongside the femoral condyles causing widening of the knee contour.

(b) Four-bar, polyaxial knee distal to the femoral condyles which combines good appearance when standing with excellent function (but the longer thigh segment is unattractive when sitting).

The two knee systems may be compared in the limbs shown in Figure 11.9.

Figure 11.9: Pairs of through-knee prostheses (constructed for a child) showing the conventional knee joint design in the left-hand pair and the four-bar link (Hanger Roelite) on the right

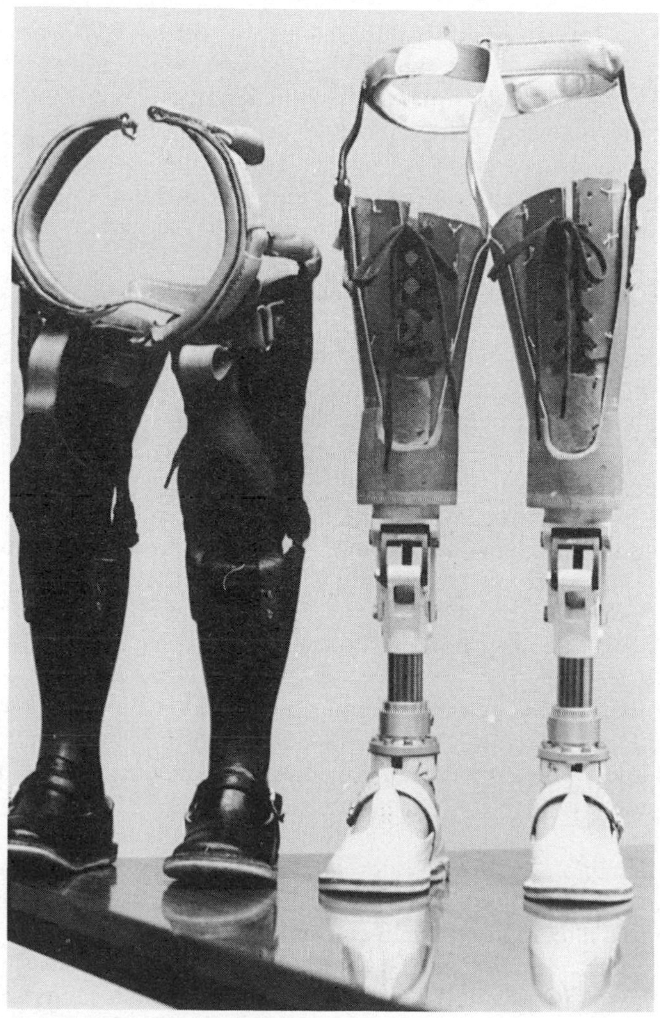

Similar prostheses may be used for stumps fashioned according to the technique described by Gritti and Stokes; the reduced ability to end-bear requires an ischial bearing socket. This slightly shorter, narrower stump which results gives a better appearance when combined with the four-bar link type of articulation. Temporary prostheses can be designed for these amputation levels but are rarely needed; they consist of a lace-up corset of leather which incorporates ischial bearing and has an end-bearing pad. As an alternative, a modified mid-thigh temporary limb may be used to which an end-bearing bar is added. Whatever approach is used, the end result is unattractive.

Mid-thigh. *This level requires that socket forces are taken proximally*; even in a properly constructed myoplastic stump, end-bearing is not possible without discomfort and damage to the stump. The prosthesis at this level has the following components: a proximally bearing socket, knee articulation allowing control of stance and swing phase, a shin piece connecting this to the ankle articulation and foot, any necessary suspension and the cosmetic covering. The possible variations are legion and only the major topics will be discussed.

There is no consensus regarding the optimum socket shape or material for this amputation level; recent work in the USA suggests that existing concepts may need complete revision since a new socket design (Sabolich, 1985) suggests that the ischium can be included within the socket whose surfaces allow a much more physiological alignment of the femur. In general terms there should be support to the end of the stump to avoid terminal engorgement; ideally all the tissues of the stump are adequately supported by a total surface bearing design (Redhead, 1979). The ischial area should be the major site of force transmission from the prosthesis and the stump must be correctly stabilised within the socket by proper design of the areas providing counterbalancing forces. Further description of this aspect of socket design is beyond the scope of this chapter.

Knee mechanisms. Both uniaxial and polyaxial knee joints may be used; the fit, active amputee will use a sophisticated swing phase control and a stabilised knee, whereas the elderly or unsteady amputee may use a locked knee for stability.

Ankle articulation. This may be either single-axis, allowing plantar and dorsiflexion only, or polyaxial. The single-axis ankle is relatively light and allows simple alteration of alignment and characteristics by change of the bumper rubbers. In addition, the extent of plantar flexion is easily altered to allow for variation in heel height. However, such ankle joints are limited when the amputee attempts to traverse a slope, as there is no lateral degree of freedom. A lateral articulation can be fitted, but this adds appreciably to the weight and reduces durability. A true polyaxial ankle unit, such as the Blatchford Multiflex, overcomes many of these difficulties but does not yet permit easy adjustment for change in heel height. The SACH ankle/foot unit is an alternative but is unable to deal with changes in heel height. This unit is ideal if the ankle is likely to be exposed to abrasive conditions.

Suspension. Prostheses for this level may be suspended or be self-suspending using a suction socket. The latter form, particularly in combination with a total surface bearing socket, gives an efficient interface between stump and prosthesis and enables excellent control, and therefore gait, with the added benefit of good appearance. Suction socket use (Figure 11.7) involves drawing the soft tissues of the stump into the socket in a controlled manner; this is by no means easy and is often the limiting factor in the application of suction designs to elderly amputees. The stump must be mature and not subject to fluctuation in volume, as such sockets are constructed to be a contact fit against the skin of the stump. All other designs of socket for this level incorporate sock use, and this will in turn allow for changes in volume. When, because of problems with either the patient's ability or with stump configuration, a non-suction design is used, a variety of forms of suspension may be considered. Traditionally the mid-thigh amputee used a rigid pelvic band attached to the thigh segment of the prosthesis by an external uniaxial or polyaxial articulation at the level of the hip (Figure 11.8). This affords excellent control of the prosthesis by acting as a hip guidance orthosis, but is probably unnecessary for many amputees. An alternative, offering good suspension and prosthesis control with better appearance, is to employ a version of the Silesian suspension in which diagonal straps descending from a waist belt provide vertical suspension and control of rotation. Other forms of soft suspension are encountered but are less satisfactory than the above.

Temporary forms of prostheses for the mid-thigh amputee are frequently encountered. These have metal or polypropylene proximal bearing sockets, a knee mechanism incorporating a semi-automatic lock for stance phase stability and a rigid or soft suspension. It is rarely possible to provide early fitting of a suction socket. Such limbs must have allowance within the socket for a degree of support to the end of the stump in order to reduce the formation of terminal oedema which is common in the unsupported stump. Recently, modern modular systems such as Hanger's Roelite have been used in their skeletal state as temporary limbs with subsequent upgrading to definitive designs.

The double mid-thigh amputee is not uncommonly encountered, and requires particular care in counselling as the energy cost of walking with bilateral prostheses is enormous. The established unilateral amputee who becomes bilaterally limb-deficient may well manage a pair of prostheses whose length is reduced to assist independent standing, improve balance and reduce the mass of the prostheses. Other bilateral mid-thigh amputees should be started, where this is indicated, using a pair of minimal length non-articulated temporary prostheses and then progress assessed; the majority (Van der Ven, 1981) reject prosthetic treatment. Occasionally, a double above-knee amputee may use a pair of ultra-lightweight, non-articulated limbs; these are purely cosmetic and are intended to improve appearance when seated, especially in a wheelchair.

Hip disarticulation, hindquarter. Prostheses for these levels are essentially similar in that they consist of a socket which embraces the pelvis, a hip articulation and thigh segment; the distal structures are as for the mid-thigh level. They differ in socket design, which for the disarticulation uses the ipsilateral ischium for force transmission whereas the hindquarter prosthesis must enclose and stabilise the abdominal wall and contents on the amputated side as well as make use of the contralateral ischium.

In the traditional forms of these limbs the hip joint is sited below the socket and is locked during walking. The Canadian design for this limb has advantages in terms of both function and appearance, which result from positioning of the hip joint somewhat anterior to the socket and allowing the hip to move during walking. Stride length, and therefore walking velocity, are altered using the hip limiter in contrast to the traditional design which, because of its locked hip, has a fixed comfortable walking speed. The gait pattern is acceptable for both levels of amputation but usually has a pronounced limp for the hindquarter amputee. Temporary limbs are rarely of any benefit at these levels.

Footwear

Virtually all prostheses are designed to accept normal footwear but amputees need careful instruction in selection of suitable items. Ideally, shoes should have full medial and lateral counters and reasonably wide, low heels. The contact surface to the ground should have good non-slip properties; leather soles and metal tips are to be avoided. Some studies of the biomechanics of amputee gait indicate that much energy is expended in accelerating and slowing moving segments. Energy consumption increases rapidly as mass is added to the distal part of the limb; *the amputee should use shoes of the lightest construction compatible with expected activities.* The alignment of any prosthesis is greatly affected by small alterations in heel height and *the importance of buying shoes of almost identical heel configuration must be appreciated.* Changes in heel height are easily accommodated by a prosthetist who will realign the ankle accordingly; some limbs can be fitted with an adjustable heel which the amputee can alter as necessary.

UPPER LIMB PROSTHESES

The unilateral upper limb amputee can cope with the activities of daily living remarkably well with little need for a prosthesis; the majority of such amputees will either not use a prosthesis at all, or will use one only occasionally. This may reflect the inadequacy of existing prosthetic systems

Figure 11.10: an externally powered below-elbow prosthesis (Hugh Steeper, Roehampton) showing the self-suspending socket, electrode for myoelectric control and cosmetic glove. Both power and span of this prosthesis are greatly improved compared to body-powered mechanical hands

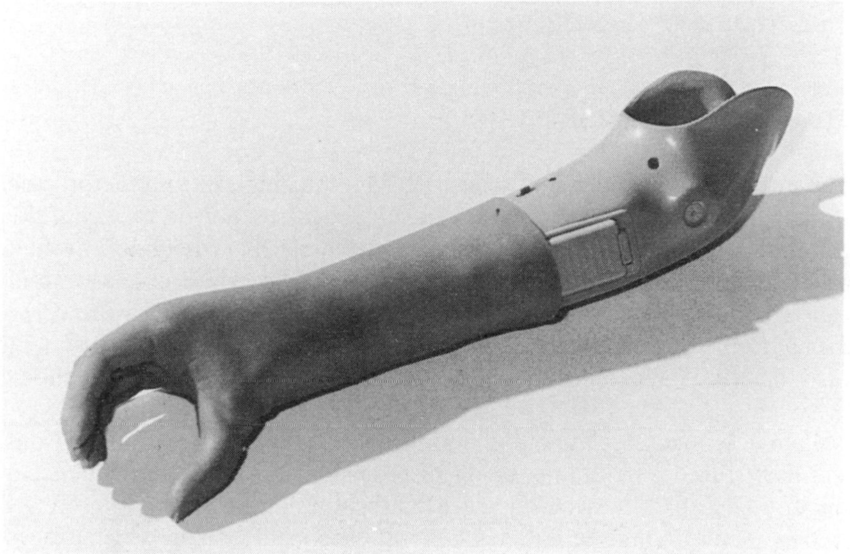

when compared to the ease of conversion to a one-armed existence. There are three principal groups of prostheses: *cosmetic*, *body-powered*, *externally powered*.

Purely cosmetic limbs are designed for appearance combined with comfort and minimal weight. Self-suspending sockets are used whenever possible and the non-functioning hand is covered with a high-definition glove. Passive elbow joints are fitted, sometimes with a forearm-mounted lock, for amputation levels above the elbow.

Body-powered prostheses use forces arising from movement of the residual and contralateral limbs to open and close some form of terminal device. Most of the prosthesis thus acts as an adjustable spacer between the stump and the terminal device (split hook, mechanical hand) to position the terminal device usefully in space. The mechanical efficiency of these systems decreases considerably in the more proximal levels of limb loss, and this is often the cause of rejection of any form of functional limb. The most useful of the terminal devices is some form of split hook, although this is aesthetically unattractive. The various types of mechanical hand offer much better appearance but function much less satisfactorily.

Externally powered prostheses offer reasonable power in a terminal device irrespective of the level of limb loss, usually with good cosmesis; the power sources used at present are almost always rechargeable batteries, although much work has been done in the past on systems powered by the expansion of compressed gas. Microswitch, servo and myoelectric control systems (Figure 11.10) are used and applied, sometimes in combination, to suit particular needs of the patient.

COMMON STUMP PROBLEMS

The integument forms the interface between the amputee and the prosthesis, and is subject to particular pathological processes; a wide variety of skin conditions may present on the stump and the excellent textbook by Levy (1983) puts the problem into perspective. Particular skin problems — folliculitis, sebaceous adenomas, abrasion, ulceration — *commonly arise from loss of fit, with or without suspension inadequacy.* If the basic adjustments of fit described above do not help, the advice of a prosthetic clinic should be sought.

Pain described in relation to a deficient limb may arise for many reasons, and this symptom should not be dismissed as the inevitable consequence of surgery. Such pain may be related to: a local lesion in the stump, referred pain or phantom limb sensation. A painful site in the stump which exacerbates the complaint needs careful investigation looking for a local lesion; neuromas, bone spikes and chronic osteomyelitis are the common problems and should be treated surgically. Referred pain merits assessment and treatment of the source. The management of pain associated with phantom limb sensation can be complex. The amputee must be reassured that the phantom experienced after amputation is common, and almost invariably settles with time. *Persistently troublesome phantom pain* requires careful assessment and then trial of treatments available. The management, including the psychological aspects, has recently been summarised by Moratoglou (1986), and the case that all non-invasive forms of treatment should be fully evaluated first is well made. Readily available treatment modalities include use of a vibrator, interferential treatment, transcutaneous nerve stimulation and a variety of drugs, of which tricyclic antidepressants and carbamazepine seem the most useful. In resistant cases, combined assessment with the prosthetic clinic, clinical psychologist and pain clinic consultant can be invaluable (Chapter 7); referral should not be delayed, since the longer pain has persisted, the more difficult is its treatment.

PROSTHETIC CARE IN THE UK

The UK is unusual in having a nationwide scheme for the provision of prosthetic care; the constituent countries, however, have developed individual approaches to amputee management. Prosthetic care in England is provided through the Disablement Services Authority of the Department of Health and Social Security, and will integrate in 1991 with the National Health Service. Medical care, funding and administration are supplied by the DHSS and prosthetic care and prostheses supplied by manufacturers contracted to the Department; care is provided within Artificial Limb and Appliance Centres (Disablement Services Centres). The rest of the UK has schemes which are integrated into the National Health Service, in which medical care is provided by health service consultant staff, and some prosthetists at least are similarly health service employees. Amputee care in Scotland is particularly well organised, with surgical care under the aegis of consultant orthopaedic staff and excellent teams cooperating in rehabilitation. Prosthetic care is available from prosthetists employed by the Scottish Home and Health Department, which also sponsors a highly regarded prosthetic training centre. Following the publication of the McColl report (1986) the movement to integrate the English service into the NHS has gained considerable momentum. Many countries worldwide have centres of excellence concerned with amputee care, but few offer the nationwide consistency of treatment which the UK provides.

THE FUTURE OF PROSTHETICS

The increasing use of early walking aids has led to the earlier fitting of the first prosthesis, and consequently has accelerated rehabilitation. Lightweight modular temporary limb systems will further reduce the delay in limb provision. Techniques for socket construction have outstripped the ability of prosthetists to produce consistently accurate information from which comfortable sockets may be made. The systems for computer-assisted design and manufacture of sockets hold tremendous promise in allowing controlled alteration in socket design and very rapid fabrication. New, transparent materials allow the stump to be seen during weight-bearing and walking, so that dynamic assessment of fit is becoming possible. Soft cosmetic coverings for endoskeletal limbs are improving, and may give a most satisfactory appearance and make a valuable contribution to swing phase control. Existing ankle and foot systems are almost entirely passive in function, but the recently described energy-storing and -releasing units offer considerable benefits to the active amputee. The endless search for greater comfort, better function and reduced weight can only produce the maximum rewards for the amputee when the quality of stump construction is uniformly excellent; amputation must be regarded not as an end in itself but as the construction of a new organ of locomotion.

Note. The views are those of the author and should not be taken as a statement of policies of the Department of Health and Social Security for the UK, although these are broadly in line with them.

REFERENCES

Burgess, E.M., Romano, R.L., Zettl, J.H. and Schrock, R.D. (1971) Amputations of the leg for peripheral vascular insufficiency. *J. Bone Joint Surg., 53A*, 874-89

Campbell, W.B. and Morris, P.J. (1986) A prospective randomized comparison of healing in Gritti–Stokes and through-knee amputations. *Ann. Roy. Coll. Surg., 68*, 1-4

Dederich, R. (1967) Technique of myoplastic amputations. *Ann. Roy. Coll. Surg., 40*, 222-7

Department of Health and Social Security (1986) *Amputation statistics for England, Wales and N. Ireland, 1985.* Statistics and Research Division, Norcross, Blackpool FY5 3TA

English, A.W.G. and Gregory Dean, A.A. (1980) The Artificial Limb Service. *Health Trends, 12*, 77-82

Engstrom, B., and Van de Ven, C.M.C. (1986) *Physiotherapy for amputees, the Roehampton approach.* Churchill Livingstone, Edinburgh

Gritti, R. (1857) Dell'amputazione de femore al terzo inferiore e della disarticolazione de ginocchio. *Ann. Univ. Med. (Milano), 161*, 5-32

Ham, R. and Whittaker, N. (1984) The King's Amputee Stump Board — a new design. *Physiotherapy, 70*(8), 300

Ham, R., Regan, J.R. and Roberts, V.C. (1987) Evaluation of introducing the team approach to the care of the amputee: the Dulwich study *Prosth. Orthot. Int. 11*, 25-30

Jamieson, C.W. and Hill, D. (1976) Amputation for vascular disease. *Brit. J. Surg., 63*, 683-90

Kendrick, R.R. (1956) Below knee amputation in arteriosclerotic gangrene. Brit. J. Surg., *44*, 13-17

Levy, W.S. (1983) *Skin problems of the amputee.* Warren H. Green Inc., St Louis

Malt, R.A. (ed.) (1978) *Amputations of the lower extremity.* Volume 3 of *Surgical Techniques Illustrated.* Little, Brown and Co., Boston

Marquardt, E. (1973) Die Chopart-exartikulation mit tenomyoplastik. *Z. Orthop., 111*, 584-6

Marquardt, E. (1981) Stump capping. In *The multiple limb deficient child. Atlas of Limb Prosthetics, Surgical and Prosthetic Principles*, American Academy of Orthopedic Surgeons, Mosby, St Louis, pp. 601-8

McColl, I. (1986) *Review of Artificial Limb and Appliance Centre Services*, Department of Health and Social Security

Mouratoglou, V.M. (1986) Amputees and phantom limb pain: a literature review. *Physiother. Pract., 2*, 177-85

Murdoch, G. (1984) Amputation revisited. *Prosth. Orthot. Int.*, 8-15

O'Dwyer, K.J. and Edwards, M.H. (1985) The association between lowest palpable pulse and wound healing in below knee amputation. *Ann. Roy. Coll. Surg., 67*, 232-4

Peizer, E. and Wright, D.W. (1970) Human locomotion. In G. Murdoch (ed.), *Prosthetic and orthotic practice*, Edward Arnold, London

Redhead, R.G. (1979) Total surface bearing sockets, *Prosth. Orthot. Int.*, *3*, 126-36

Redhead, R.G., Davis, B.C., Robinson, K.P. and Vitali, M. (1978) Post-amputation pneumatic walking aid. *Brit. J. Surg.*, *65*(9), 611-12

Robinson, K.P., Hoile, R. and Coddington, T. (1982) Skew flap myoplastic below knee amputation: a preliminary report. *Br. J. Surg.*, *69*, 554-7

Sabolich, J. (1985) Contoured, adducted–trochanteric, controlled alignment method (CAT–CAM): introduction and principles. *Clin. Prosthet. Orthot.*, *9*(4), 15-26

Southwell, M. (1983) *The history and design development of artificial limbs.* Thesis, Department of Industrial Design, Lanchester Polytechnic

Stokes, W. (1870) On supra-condyloid amputation of the thigh. *Med. Chir. Trans.*, *53*, 175-86

Van de Ven, C.M.C. (1981) An investigation into the management of bilateral leg amputees. *Br. Med. J.*, *283*, 707

Vitali, M., Robinson, K.P., Andrews, B.G., Harris, E.E. and Redhead, R.G. (1986) *Amputations and prostheses*, Baillière Tindall, London

Waters, R.L., Perry, J., Antonelli, O. and Hislop, H. (1976) Energy cost of walking of amputees. The influence of level of amputation. *J. Bone Joint Surg.*, *58A*, 42-6

12

Lower Limb Injuries

Fred Middleton

INTRODUCTION

Injuries to the lower limb are relatively common. Although overall the commonest single injury, certainly in the winter months, is fractured neck of femur in the elderly population, this chapter concentrates on injuries to young adults, a group who have particular problems currently in achieving full rehabilitation, and in particular in return to employment. Injuries to adolescents and young adults usually occur against a background of general good health and a high level of activity. Fortunately the majority of those who sustain lower limb injury recover fully — they suffer from temporary disability as opposed to chronic disability. During the past few years much of the thinking and action in regard to disability (Royal College of Physicians Report, 1986) refers to those people with chronic disability, and in particular to their management in the community. Insufficient emphasis is placed on the services which need to be provided for those with temporary disabilities — who will usually make a full recovery when adequate treatment and management are available — and therefore not swell the numbers of those with chronic disability. The importance of such services and their ability to return young injured back into employment, back to being providers and supporters in their community, is enormous, and assumes even more importance in today's situation of high unemployment. Those who are unable to return to work in their pre-accident employment are unlikely to be successful in obtaining alternative work. That those with temporary recoverable disability should be allowed to become chronically disabled in the community is a tragedy.

It is sometimes argued that those with recoverable disabilities should rehabilitate themselves, and yet there is no substantial evidence that the situation reported 20 and 30 years ago (Ferguson and MacPhail, 1954; McKenzie *et al.*, 1962) is inaccurate or invalid. It remains a fact that some 30 per cent of people with acute illness or injury, in whom the expectation would be a full recovery, are still significantly disabled a year after their injury, and have not returned to employment or taken up the running of their homes. The reason for this fact remains obscure, but the fact remains.

THE PATIENT

In an average health district, population 250,000, some 2,500 people are admitted annually with injuries (Royal College of Physicians Report, 1986). Of those some 1,000 are likely to have sustained lower limb injuries. In Bloomsbury Health Authority, London, in the years 1975 to 1985 some 200 patients were admitted annually with lower limb injuries to specialist rehabilitation facilities providing intensive therapy. The two largest groups comprised those with fractures of the tibia and fibula, and those following surgery for internal derangement of the knee. Those with fractures round the knee joint comprised almost as many as those with junction of lower and middle third fractures of tibia and fibula, reflecting the difficulty of achieving good results with this type of fracture. Fractured shaft of femur comprised a considerably smaller group. The most common site of fracture was supracondylar with consequent range of movement problems at the knee joint. This is not the place for discussion of early management of fracture. However, the underrepresentation of patients with closed injuries followed by internal fixation is likely to reflect the relatively good outcome from that situation. There is no doubt, however, that whatever the injury intensive rehabilitation can both shorten the recovery period and also result in an individual with significantly less disability (Nichols and Wynn Parry, 1966).

In complex injuries skilled surgical management is essential to good outcome, but must be complemented by adequate rehabilitation (Molloy and Wynn Parry, 1981).

Two smaller groups at the Medical Rehabilitation Centre, London, comprised 10–20 patients annually with major soft tissue injuries requiring specific ligamentous repairs mostly around the knee joint and those with extensive soft tissue injuries associated with fractures frequently involving nerve injury — most commonly to the common peroneal resulting in foot drop.

THE PROBLEMS

At any stage in the rehabilitation of those with lower limb injuries — from the moment of acute injury to total integration back into the community — there are five essential aspects directly relating to the lower limb which must constantly be considered (Nichols, 1976). These comprise (1) bone union, (2) soft tissue conservation, (3) joint mobility, (4) maintenance of muscle strength and coordination, (5) total patient care. If all these aspects are successfully managed then the patient is likely to return successfully to the community. Clearly this is not always the case, and frequently problems which prevent a successful outcome arise for entirely different reasons. It is therefore essential that the process of defining the patient's problems and needs should have adequate structure, ensuring that it takes place with as much comprehensiveness and accuracy as possible. Such a process will undoubtedly include:

(1) A review of the patient's general health.

(2) Assessment of his mobility.

(3) Assessment of specific deficit including muscle power, range of movement, tissue status, coordination and proprioception, balance, stamina, agonist–antagonist efficiency. Appropriate balance between these groups is essential for achieving good coordination of movement and maintaining stability of joints. The presence or absence of pain.

(4) Psychological status, mood, illness affect, learning ability. Education comprises a major component of any rehabilitation process. The ability to learn quickly and efficiently will greatly dictate the overall outcome. Frequently little attention is paid to whether components detrimental to this learning process exist — e.g. anxiety, depression, poor motivation.

(5) Social situation.

(6) Communication skills.

How this process of evaluation takes place differs greatly from one hospital to another, with very great variation in the amount of time and importance given to the process. Our practice at the Medical Rehabilitation Centre is initially to define problems in terms of impairment, disability and handicap as defined in the WHO Report (1980) (Chapter 2).

All patients referred to our Centre attend for one whole day, during which they are seen by each member of the interdisciplinary team. It is our experience that problems can only be defined if an appropriate range of skills are contained within the multidisciplinary team, e.g. it is unlikely that underlying anxiety, mood-related problems, or indeed significant personality traits or disorders, will be properly defined unless psychological skills are available to the team. The most frequent reason for referral to specialist rehabilitation facilities is for 'failure to progress' and the belief that the answer to this problem is 'further intensive physiotherapy'. In reality this means that effective rehabilitation has not been considered until far too late. To use specialist rehabilitation skills should be a positive decision taken at an appropriate time in the patient's management with clear reasons for referral and expectations of outcome. Requesting 'further intensive physiotherapy' is unlikely to contribute to the return to the community and to full employment, home management and full social life of young adults who are failing to cope with the complex problems of being temporarily physically disabled.

Skilled comprehensive evaluation of the patient carried out at an appropriate stage in the course of management following injury is perhaps the most crucial and most frequently neglected aspect of trauma patients' care.

THE SERVICE

Traditionally orthopaedic rehabilitation involves physiotherapy and occupational therapy. When one defines the problems of those entering rehabilitation services it is clear that their needs are as much for social and psychological support, counselling and education as for physical therapy. The rehabilitation team should therefore reflect the skills necessary to effectively resolve the patient's problems (Chapter 6).

The physical environment

A major advantage in most rehabilitation centres is the availability of space; in particular the availability of open areas where group activities can take place. Small private areas are also essential, but the individual should not be isolated from his peers. The rehabilitation unit should not be isolated from other medical services from which the patients have come, nor from the community which it serves. The concept of the converted country manor should become a matter for history.

The psychological environment

The objective should be to create active positive processes, with individuals restoring themselves to full ability — assuming responsibility for that process and for the outcome. In the 1950s and 1960s much emphasis was based on group dynamics. People with similar disabilities were placed in groups so that they would develop a competitive element. For some that was a successful strategy; perhaps more important is the realisation of individuals in the group that each is not unique in that they are setting out on a process to deal actively with common problems.

The process

It is frequently stated that rehabilitation is the management of disability in order to prevent handicap. Most management of those with lower limb injuries takes place within orthopaedic departments and physiotherapy departments of District General Hospitals. The majority of these patients recover fully, and there is no need for other special services. A major problem is the identification at an early stage of those individuals who are likely to become chronically disabled and therefore potentially handicapped. Where appropriate referral takes place achievement in terms of return to work, assumption of full domestic and social activities can be high, about 90 per cent of referrals returning to work (Sommerville, 1970).

On referral of the patient a full comprehensive multidisciplinary evaluation should take place. Out of this process should come clearly defined long-term objectives which in the case of the young injured adult are likely to comprise full mobility, both indoors and outdoors, use of public transport and driving, and also the assumption of full domestic, social and leisure activities.

In the context of the young injured adult expectation is one of minimal or nil long-term disability and therefore much of the management must be directed intensively towards correction of impairment. The rehabilitation team must be orientated towards strengthening of weak muscles, the achievement of joint range of movement while maintaining joint stability, the seeking of a high level of fitness and stamina and the reduction of detrimental psychological states, e.g. anxiety, depression, lack of confidence, inappropriate illness behaviour, etc. The patient must understand what is required of him, what results are to be expected and how these are to be achieved.

Muscle strengthening

In the small number of patients with nerve injuries, the most frequently damaged nerve is the common peroneal, either occurring at the time of injury or subsequently during immobilisation of the limb. With drop foot provision of an appropriate orthosis applied in neutral position should be carried out in order to prevent shortening of the Achilles tendon and also to maintain an appropriate gait (Chapters 8 and 45). Electromyographic analysis at an early stage will give a prognosis and indicate returning function. As soon as Grade 1 power returns appropriate biofeedback should be introduced.

In the early stages of recovery from lower limb fractures, while bone union is progressing and healing of soft tissues is occurring, maintenance of muscle bulk should be enthusiastically pursued. Persuasion of patients to carry out *isometric (constant-length)* quadriceps contractions on a regular and frequent basis is surprisingly difficult, and it may well be that in the early stages this is a good indication of which patients are going to require more intensive services. The carrying out of such exercises is ideally suited to group activities where introduction of more normal social interaction is also an advantage.

When bone union is established much greater emphasis can then be placed on the restoration of muscle power by the introduction of resisted *isotonic (constant-force)* exercises. These should be carried out specifically for the injured limb, but also for the patient as a whole. The use of predetermined circuits is an ideal way of carrying out this procedure in that it gives the patient confidence and feedback on his progress, and therapists can easily set short-term weekly objectives.

Use of *isokinetic (constant-velocity)* exercise is of particular use for those patients with injury around the knee joint where muscle function is of paramount importance in re-achieving stability across the joint. Exercise through the whole range of movement produces increase in muscle strength throughout that range. Because of the nature of isokinetic exercise equipment, input from the patient to the process can be accurately judged, and therefore gives clues to the patient's motivation, to the achievement of a positive attitude and to the return of confidence in the use of the injured limb.

Joint function

The achievement of a functional range of movement in a joint is a complex process, and one which is frequently poorly understood. During the process of immobilisation of fractures or soft tissue injuries, synovial adhesions occur. During the first two or three days following removal of plaster of Paris or traction the process of mobilisation involves breaking down these adhesions. This leads to inflammation of the synovium, pain, and occasionally an effusion in the joint. The patient should understand that this is a necessary process, that it is short-lived and that the symptoms can be controlled by analgesia, whether by drugs or by physical means in the physiotherapy department. The next phase of reachievement of range of movement will involve the breakdown of adhesions between the complex layers of extra-articular tissues. These adhesions are likely to be stronger, and the time scale involved therefore longer. In the early stages much of the achievement will be by passive stretching by the therapists, but this should gradually be taken over by active work by the patient using his own muscle strength across the joint and using his body weight. The use of occupational therapy workshops with static cycles (Figure 12.1) is particularly valuable in this regard, and sessions in OT which interchange between

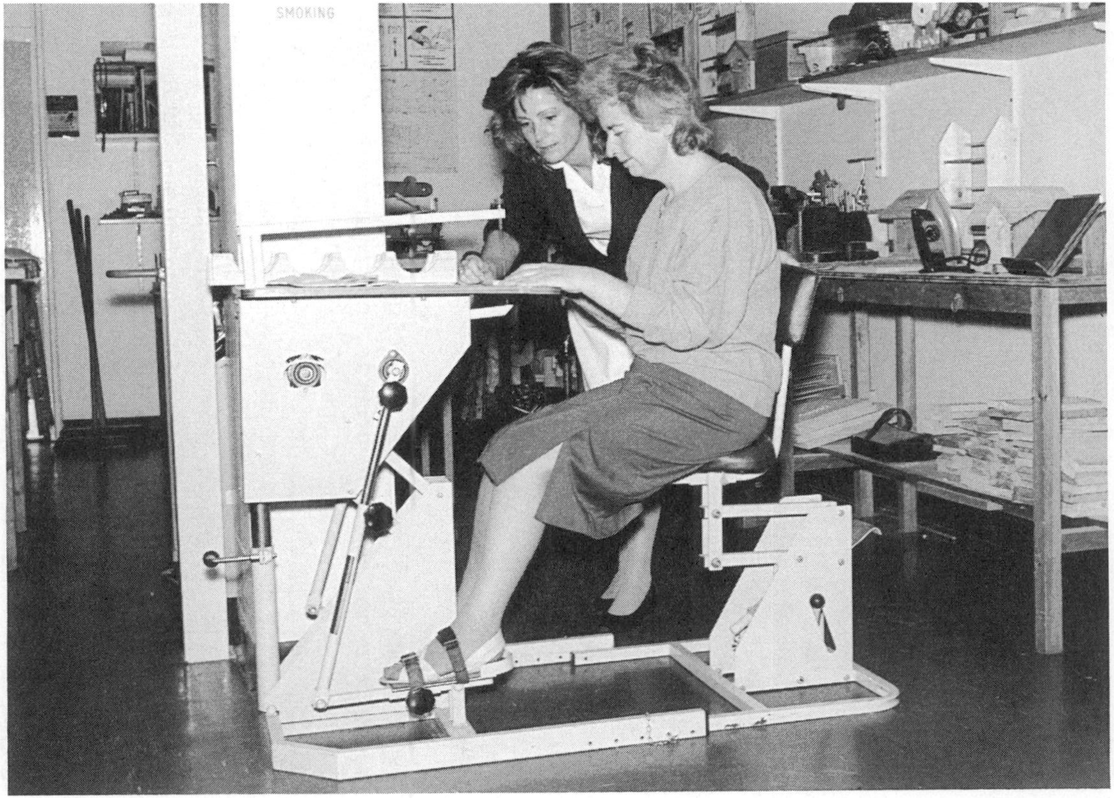

Figure 12.1: Patient using treadle fretsaw to regain range of movement at the ankle joint following Pott's fracture

the cycles and quads switches should form a significant part of the patient's programme at this time. Also at this stage discussions can commence with the OTs about the patient's work needs, so that an early decision can be taken as to what achievement the patient requires in order to return successfully to his employment. In this way, if a change of occupation becomes essential, this can be identified at the earliest possible opportunity and work towards training for a new occupation can be included positively in the overall programme, thus retaining the expectation of a return to full employment.

It is important that realistic goals, such as the achievement of full range of movement following ligament repair, should be entertained. The process must be one of progress towards functional achievement and understanding by the patient of the relationship between the range of movement and stability of the joint, particularly where this applies following reconstruction of ligaments around the knee joint. It is our experience that long-term disability is much more frequently related to instability of the joint rather than to loss of range of movement, and functionally a stable joint, even though lacking even 30–40° of range, is greatly to be preferred.

Walking function (Chapter 8)

During reachievement of mobility the important principle should be to maintain an adequate pattern of walking. This is not to say that aesthetics should be more important than function. However, the use of walking aids, elbow crutches and sticks in the early stages to achieve a balanced pattern of walking cannot be overemphasised, if the slow process of unlearning abnormal movements is not to significantly lengthen the process of rehabilitation.

Coordination and balance

The relearning of skills is an important aspect of the rehabilitation process. Proprioception plays an enormous part not only in our efficiency of movement but in the prevention of further injuries and degenerative wear in joints. The relearning of such skills is well suited to group activities involving functional goals. It is during this process that a return to a more normal social function and achievement of confidence is also acquired. It is for functions such as these that adequate space is essential within the rehabilitation facilities. The availability of hydrotherapy can add greatly to this process and shorten the overall period of rehabilitation requirements.

Stamina and fitness

During this process of rehabilitation regular medical monitoring of the patient's condition should be taking place, re-enforcing the concept that rehabilitation is a process involving the total individual. Patients at this stage should no longer consider themselves as being ill or sick. Good physical fitness should be sought by all, and to many will be important in relation to their employment and lifestyle. Return to physical fitness and stamina appropriate to the patient's previous way of life is an essential component within the overall programme. The achievement of such a state also contributes greatly to psychological well-being.

Social services

Full social evaluation at the beginning of the rehabilitation process will define social and domestic problems which may be major detriments to the recovery of the individual. For those patients with significant problems regular counselling sessions with the unit social worker should take place. These may be related to their entitlement to allowances but more long-term problems of family relationships, etc., may also become apparent. Physical illness frequently serves to bring to the fore pre-existing social and domestic stresses. Counselling and resolution of these issues should begin at an early stage of rehabilitation, but may well be more appropriately undertaken within the community resources of the patient and his family. Progress or lack of progress with these problems will have major implications for the patient's rehabilitation. Regular team conferences should take place during which achievements and failures are noted and new short-term goals defined (Chapters 3 and 37).

Time scale

It is a frequent criticism of rehabilitation units that patients spend too long in their programmes, and that the outcomes are indeterminate and vague. If appropriate long- and short-term goal-setting has been carried out during the rehabilitation process this should not occur. It is likely that the time of attendance in a particular unit will vary from extremely short (a few sessions), to a number of months where there are particularly complex problems of movement and stability of a joint. Whatever the time scale the process should be one of working towards clear objectives. Once the expected goals have been achieved the patient should be discharged, even if he is unable to function as well as before the accident. Subsequently there should be follow-up by the team at one month, three months and one year after discharge. As circumstances change new problems or difficulties may arise which may need further intervention by the rehabilitation team.

THE FUTURE

For some time it has been DHSS policy to concentrate resources at District General Hospital level and away from independent rehabilitation centres providing intensive facilities. Indeed by the end of 1986 virtually all such centres had closed or changed their role. The expectation is that therapy departments within the District General Hospital will extend their facilities and structural organisation to incorporate the provision of intensive rehabilitation for those with temporary disability; although there is little evidence of this occurring to any great extent and there is a persistent shortage of the required professionals to set up such a service. It is likely that considerable pressure will need to be brought to bear upon the DHSS if such an increase in role is to take place. The report of the Royal College of Physicians, 'Physical Disability in 1986 and beyond', concentrates its thinking and proposals on those individuals with chronic disability. If the numbers of chronically disabled are not to be swelled unnecessarily, then an equally intensive approach must be taken towards resolving the problems of those with temporary disability.

REFERENCES

Ferguson, T. and MacPhail, A.N. (1954) *Hospital and Community.* The Nuffield Provincial Hospitals Trust. Oxford University Press, Oxford, pp. 81-106

McKenzie, M., Weir, R.D., Richardson, I.M., Mair, A., Harnett, R.W.F., Curran, A.P., Ferguson, T. and MacPhail, A.N. (1962) *Further studies in hospital and community,* The Nuffield Provincial Hospitals Trust, Oxford University Press, Oxford, pp. 38-49

Molloy, M.G. and Wynn Parry, C.B. (1981) Helping the injured. In S. Matingley (ed.), *Rehabilitation today,* Update Books, London, pp. 152-60

Nichols, P.J.R. (1976) *Rehabilitation medicine,* Butterworths, London

Nichols, P.J.R. and Wynn Parry, C.B. (1966) Rehabilitation in fractures and dislocations. In C. Rob and R. Smith (eds), *Clinical Surgery,* vol. 12, Butterworths, London, pp. 236-264

Royal College of Physicians (1986) Physical disability in 1986 and beyond. *J. Roy. Coll. Phys. Lond., 20,* 160-94

Sommerville, J.G. (1970) Medical rehabilitation. *Ann. Phys. Med., 10,* 421-4

World Health Organization. (1980) *International classification of impairment, disability and handicaps,* World Health Organization, Geneva

Part 3

Energy-restricting Disorders

13

Cardiac Disability

Graham Jackson

CAUSES

Cardiovascular disease, mainly coronary artery disease, affects at some time over 50 per cent of the population. It may exert its effect clinically as angina pectoris, myocardial infarction or heart failure. Occasionally embolisation from an impaired left ventricle may have devastating consequences either in the cerebral or peripheral circulation. Less frequent now are the limitations imposed by valve disease with the declining incidence of rheumatic fever in western civilisation, but this still represents a major problem in the developing cultures. The one exception is elderly calcific aortic stenosis which can severely limit otherwise healthy people. Finally, specific heart muscle disease, whether secondary to a viral myocarditis or of unknown aetiology, can have a tragically sad effect on the younger population, whose lives are transformed from one extreme of physical and perhaps mental fitness to the other.

Patients have three forms of restriction — chest pain, breathlessness and/or fatigue and syncope. Peripheral arterial disease leading to claudication and cerebrovascular disease are associated but independent causes of restriction. The greatest problem involves coping with the consequences of coronary artery disease invariably involving rehabilitation following a myocardial infarct (WHO, 1985). In many ways, however, though demanding, this represents a relatively easy option in comparison to helping the heart failure patient adjust to his lifestyle changes.

A separate group in many ways are those who are recovering from coronary bypass surgery or valve replacement surgery. Here there are musculoskeletal problems imposed on the preoperative complaint and additional psychological and social factors caused by the operation and the high (sometimes unrealistically) hopes the patient and family may have of the result. The symptom-free operative result is usually fine, but those with residual restrictions are often very difficult to help because of the feeling that the intervention, with its pain, has 'failed'.

GENERAL OBSERVATIONS

Rehabilitation is about restoring disabled people as quickly and as sensibly as possible to a full physical, social and mental level of activity. This assumes a level of activity existed before the illness which the doctor or multidisciplinary team felt acceptable. This is not always the case; nor is it always the wish of an individual to do more, or live a different life after an illness compared to before. Health care teams involved in rehabilitation set ideal standards of activity which are conditioned in many ways by their own levels of activity, and by definition people actively involved in rehabilitation are most unlikely to be slothful. Yet many members of the community are quite happy leading a slothful existence, making the minimum effort and enjoying television and public houses. The problem we face in rehabilitation is restoring the person to where he was before the illness, and then we have to sell the idea that by various lifestyle changes a further illness may be prevented. The personality of each patient being so different, we must always adjust our objectives to the individual. Overzealousness in some will be met with a vigorous and positive response, but others will default and be lost to the efforts of secondary prevention (Bass, 1983).

THE HEART

The centre of our universe, the soul, the very reason we exist and so on; the heart is the most emotional aspect of our body and is in turn the most vulnerable to many of our emotions. When illness strikes the heart the emotional responses can exacerbate the problem, and no more so than in the situation of myocardial infarction.

MYOCARDIAL INFARCTION

Rehabilitation begins at the onset of the illness with as much communication as possible between the patient, spouse and family. The outcome will be related to personality (coping ability and comprehension of the illness), social background (work, housing, finances, responsibilities to family and their's to him), and family strengths and weaknesses (married, divorced, strength of spouse).

Normal reactions to an infarct are denial, anxiety and depression. The degree of the reactions is usually mild from 'why me', 'can't be' to a temporary bout of 'the blues'. Occasionally the reaction is pathological, invariably because of a preceding problem either recognised or not, and profound depression, or rarely a psychotic episode, may follow. Emotional disturbances can be expected in about 60 per cent of people admitted to a coronary care unit.

The onset of myocardial infarction is painful and frightening. In many ways how the patient copes depends on how he is dealt with initially. The immediate relief of pain with intravenous diamorphine with the antiemetic cyclizine helps the patients' and families' immediate fears which revolve around death. The family unit are relieved to be in a 'safe' environment (hospital) and the immediate alleviation of the major symptom reinforces in them the idea that whatever has or is happening the patient is 'in the right hands'.

CORONARY CARE UNIT

Initially the patient is anxious, tired and may still be in pain (Table 13.1). At this point the diagnosis should be explained in simple terms to both the patient and spouse at the same interview, so each knows what the other knows. I tell the patient the heart is bruised and sore and needs to rest, and the best thing he can do to help himself for the first day is rest in bed. I try to get the idea across even at this stage that the patient is helping himself also. I explain the monitors and gadgets as routine protection to try to give an impression of a team approach, with the patient the most important individual in the team.

Denial is a common problem, especially with professionals, particularly doctors.

> One eminent professor of cardiology developed chest pain during a lecture which he gave unusually poorly. He drove home (2 hours) and only on the insistence of his wife did he go to his own unit with his infarct.

Resorting to antacids, anything to avoid the obvious, leads to its own

Table 13.1: Patients' thoughts

What is wrong with me?
Am I going to die?
How can I stop this happening again?
Why can't my children visit?
I'm bored in hospital.
I'm lonely at night.
Why is my wife/husband so anxious?
What about my job?
Should I cancel my holiday?

problems, for in the first six hours the greatest mortality occurs.

Denial usually gives away to reality, but often in the Type A personality (aggressive, ambitious, impatient) it persists, and though this may be useful in the short term with regard to a positive approach to recovery, in the long-term it may be detrimental. It is estimated that 20 per cent of people two weeks after an infarct still doubt it happened. Men exhibit more denial than women, and it is invariably men who take their own discharge against advice.

Anxiety is universal — What is wrong with me? Am I going to die? The patient sees the deaths of others in the unit and then finds the severing of the umbilical cord unpleasant when he is transferred to a general ward. At this point more questions will arise, the opportunity to ask must be available and the questions should not be avoided. The doctor or nurse must sit on the bed and look at the patient, not talk down to him from the standing position. Patients with limited intelligence need more patience, not less time. Moving to the ward is accompanied by stating how pleased we are with the patient's progress and 'you don't need to be here any more'. At this point a plan for the patient should evolve now that the patient and family are more able to absorb the meaning of the illness and plan for the future. I outline the future as a series of two's:

two weeks — in hospital for healing and gradual mobilisation;
two weeks — at home very gradually increasing activity;
two weeks — at home accelerating back to normal with a positive approach to the future and a six-week medical assessment where we can either deal with problems or send the patient back to work.

Of course this is simple, but keeping it simple and straightforward is the key to recovery. Those who remain anxious may benefit from a short course of diazepam.

Depression may not be a problem but, if it is, it usually presents in the third day after leaving the coronary care unit. Concern over jobs in the current economic climate, especially for heavy goods vehicle or public service vehicle drivers; guilt, invariably because of heavy smoking, and helplessness are paramount. The male feels his 'manhood' is challenged — especially the younger male. With a positive approach to the future this is less of a problem. Pointing the patient at the future and planning the rehabilitation circumvents many of the problems without recourse to specific antidepressant therapy. If, however, depression persists psychiatric assessment is valuable before allowing drug prescriptions, because there may have been a preceding problem which needs specialist evaluation.

BOOKLETS

No matter how clearly the doctor or nurse feels they have expressed themselves, with the background of stress and anxiety the patient and family may misinterpret or become confused by the information given. Providing written information for the patient and spouse as soon as possible answers many of the asked and unasked questions which preoccupy all concerned. In a study I performed we found a far greater understanding of the illness, and a more satisfactory recovery, in those given written as well as oral information. They are not a substitute for talking, but complement and often enhance the interviews by prompting the patient to ask awkward and relevant questions. Sources include The British Heart Foundation and Stuart Pharmaceuticals (Jackson, 1979).

THE GENERAL WARD

Whilst this is a sign of progress it is also the time to begin the first aspects of physical rehabilitation. We have attempted to allay the anxieties of the patient and family and we now begin a positive move forward. Our own rehabilitation programme is run by specially trained physiotherapists. Where necessary patients with difficulties can be seen by a psychiatrist, who may enrol them in a group counselling session where concerns can be freely discussed and mutual reassurance given.

I must again emphasise the importance of education which will alleviate fear and anxiety. If the doctor really 'doesn't have time' to talk he should say so, but emphatically make the point that he is going to come back. Simple repetitive information is all that is needed. From the general ward and into convalescence recommendations on management and prevention must be given to the patient. Our inpatient programme is illustrated in Table 13.2.

AFTER DISCHARGE

The hospital environment is controlled and protective; naturally anxiety occurs when leaving. Feelings of fatigue usually follow the environmental change, but can also reflect too much physical activity. The patient should be told to anticipate this, and to be sure to rest and get a good night's sleep. If this proves difficult, night sedation should be ordered from the family doctor. Aches and pains previously discounted now assume greater importance, but they are invariably sharp and positional and not cardiac. The patient should be told the difference between cardiac and non-cardiac pain (Table 13.3).

Table 13.2: Inpatient exercise programme, coronary/CABG

Days 1 and 2 in ITU	(i) Routine breathing exercises (ii) Foot exercises and knee flexion
Days 3–4 to ward	*If patient is painfree for 24 hours,* then:
Day 3	(iii) Sit over side of bed (iv) Shoulder elevation (v) Shoulder shrugging
Day 4	(vi) Sit in chair
Day 5	(vii) Walk in ward
Day 6	(viii) Walk to toilet (ix) Straight leg raising in long sitting (x) Lifting technique
Days 7–8	(xi) Walk to stairs
Day 9 onwards	(xii) Stairs, gradually increasing amount (xiii) Introduce home exercise programme

Patients are usually discharged from Day 8 onwards and should be given a home exercise sheet and have the leaflet on coronary heart disease

Table 13.3: Chest pain characteristics

Cardiac	Non-cardiac
Tightness	Sharp (not severe)
Pressure	Knife-like
Weight	Stabbing
Constriction	'Like a stitch'
Ache	'Like a needle'
Dull	Pricking feeling
Squeezing feeling	Shooting
Soreness	Reproduced by pressure or position
Crushing	Can walk around with it
'Like a band'	Continuous: 'It's there all day, Doc'.
Breathlessness (tightness)	

GETTING BACK TO NORMAL

The days of prolonged rest and convalescence are over except for those who have sustained massive infarcts with substantial left ventricular damage. Early ambulation avoids physical problems such as deep venous thrombosis, as well as psychological problems such as anxiety and depression (Wenger, 1981).

PHYSICAL ACTIVITY

Physical activity programmes have not been shown to lengthen life or reduce subsequent cardiac events. They need to be tailored to the individual. If a satisfactory programme is adopted a subsequent increase in the sense of well-being and decreased anxiety follows. By taking part in a programme with others the group atmosphere is encouraged, opportunities for communication fostered and the sense of isolation and guilt diminished. Our initial home programme is shown in Table 13.4 and our gymnasium programme in Table 13.5. Following on from this our patients have continued exercises at home and formed a once-weekly coronary club. It is very rare for cardiac arrests to occur in a properly directed and supervised programme with individual prescriptions, but we have full resuscitation facilities on site (Cobb, 1986).

TREADMILL ECG

All our patients under 65 years of age who have sustained an uncomplicated myocardial infarct undergo routine treadmill exercise testing to their maximal ability within two to six weeks after their infarct. It has been shown that those with a positive test have an increased morbidity and mortality at one year (Figure 13.1) and that elective bypass surgery may be able to prevent subsequent infarction and death (Akhras *et al.*, 1984). In addition, by combining the treadmill test with the rehabilitation process we have been able to reinforce the recovery of the patient as well as to emphasise our continuing commitment to care and progress.

Table 13.4: Coronary home exercise programme to be followed during week after discharge

Name: ___________

	Day 1	Day 2	Day 3	Day 4	Day 5	Day 6	Day 7
Lying: straight leg lift							
Arms raise, and lower sideways							
Lying: knee bend and straighten							
Side bending in standing							
Squat for lifting practice							

Go for a short walk each day, gradually increasing the distance and keep up a fairly brisk pace.
For the first few days use the stairs only at night and in the morning; then gradually increase their use during the day.

ALWAYS REST if you feel any chest pain; or faint; or are short of breath.

Table 13.5: Rehabilitation programme — coronary outpatients

Name: __________ Age: _____ Date of coronary: _____

Pulse rate:
Before exercise
After
After 5 min rest

1. *Standing*
   Trunk side bending
2. *Standing*
   Trunk rotation
3. *Standing*
   Alternate knees to chest
4. *Standing*
   Arms circling with 4 lb.
5. *Lying*
   Straight lift alternate legs
6. *Prone lying*
   Straight lift alternate legs
7. *Lying with knees bent up*
   Raise bottom
8. *Lying*
   Lift medicine ball from chest
9. *Lying*
   Head and shoulders lift sitting
10. *Squats*
11. *Step-ups*
12. *Cycle*

SEXUAL ACTIVITY

Bartlett (1956) reported a marked increase in heart rate in both male and female at the time of orgasm, with increases of over 100 beats per minute. This was associated with respiratory rate increases of up to 60 per minute. Similar findings were reported by Masters and Johnson (1966). These vigorous responses may cause alarm in the mind of the physician advising the cardiac patient, so it is important to take into account the environment in which the studies were carried out, and the special circumstances of the volunteers.

Bartlett (1956) used married couples aged 22–30 years in a 'small experimental room fitted with a bed and other items conducive to a normal sexual response'. The bed was placed against a wall through which an opening had been made. The opening was covered with a thick sheet of

Figure 13.1: One-year mortality based on abnormal exercise test for ischaemia two to six weeks post infarct (+ve) compared to normal (−ve)

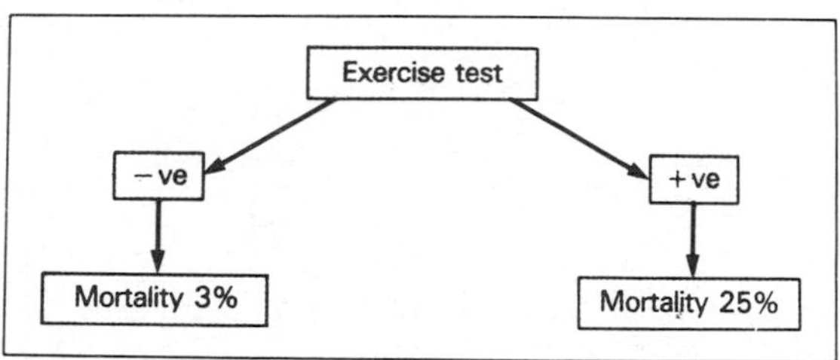

foam rubber through which ECG leads were passed and attached to the 'upper thighs and upper arms'. Respiratory responses were obtained by using a mouthpiece and the nose was 'lightly clamped'. The subjects pressed a button individually as intromission, orgasm and withdrawal occurred. This unnatural environment, and its formation, is similar to other volunteer studies which have included unmarried or divorced people, prostitutes and individuals with marital and sexual problems. It would be unwise to judge these physiological responses as representative of those achieved in the general population.

Fortunately, several studies are now available which look at a more representative sector of the population, and these can be used as a basis for initiating advice and guidelines to cardiac patients. Nemec *et al.* (1976) studied ten normal males aged 24–40 years, recording heart rate on a portable (Holter) ECG recorder and blood pressure on an automatic Doppler device. This study was conducted in the home environment with their wives.

The average resting heart rate was 60±8 beats per minute rising to 92±13 at intromission and achieving a maximal rate of 114±14 at orgasm. At 120 seconds of resolution the rate had already fallen to 69±12 beats per minute. Similar responses occurred whether the male was on top or underneath. Blood pressure rose from a mean of 112/66 mmHg at rest to 148/79 at intromission and a maximum of 163/81 at orgasm. Resting levels were achieved 120 seconds into resolution. Position again made no significant difference.

Hellerstein and Friedman (1970), evaluating middle-aged (47 years) patients with ischaemic heart disease reported an average maximal heart rate of 117 beats per minute (range 90–144) during sex, in comparison to 120 (range 107–130) during other activities. Similar findings were reported in patients with angina pectoris (Figure 13.2) who were studied in the UK, with heart rates during sex of 122±7.1 beats per minute and 124±7.2 during other activities (Jackson, 1978). Larson *et al.* (1980) compared the cardiovascular response to sex with stair climbing. The stair test involved

Figure 13.2: Twenty-four-hour ECG: top trace, heart rate; bottom trace, ST segment trend. During non-sexual activity (P) the heart rate response is similar to that during sexual activity (S)

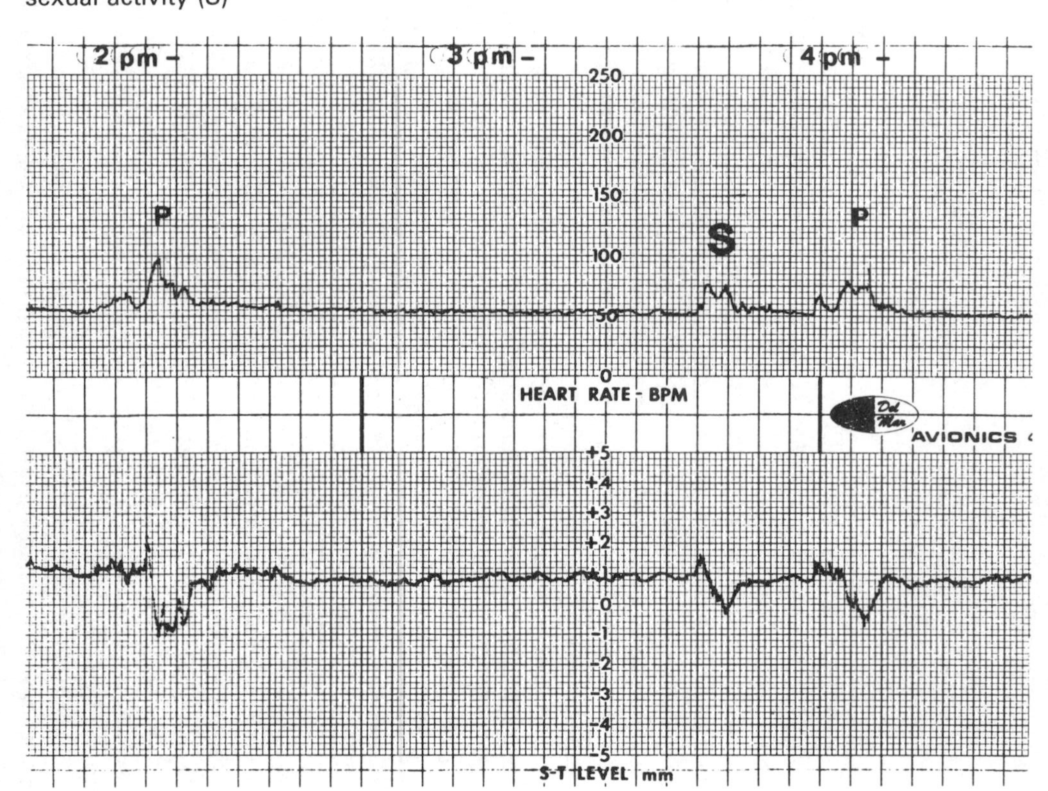

walking for 10 minutes then climbing 22 stairs in 10 seconds (the average English flight is 12–13 stairs). In the normals the mean maximal heart rate was 123±8 during sex and 122±5 on the stairs, whilst in the coronary patients it was 118±6 and 115±7 respectively. The systolic blood pressure rose modestly to 146±2 mmHg in the normals for both stresses, but in the coronary patients it was actually less during sex (144±6 mmHg) than on the stairs (164±7 mmHg) ($p < 0.01$).

A pattern of cardiovascular responses emerges. For the long-married or cohabiting couple (one assumes this can be so for homosexual as well as heterosexual relationships), the heart rate and blood pressure response is modest, achieving its maximum at orgasm. For middle-aged couples this occurs on average twice a week, with a maximal response representing only 15 seconds or so of the 16 minutes' average duration of sexual intercourse — representing less than 0.3 per cent of leisure time (Théroux *et al.*, 1979).

It is important to establish that sex is part of the normal lifestyle of an individual, whether he or she has coronary disease or not. As in any form of exercise, myocardial demand (heart rate and blood pressure) will increase. With appropriate background information the physician or nurse can place the demand in its appropriate context, reassure the needlessly concerned and by simple tests (for example, climbing two flights of stairs) enable individuals to lead full and satisfactory lives.

WORK

Up to 90 per cent of people can return to their previous occupation. Specific advice is needed for HGV and PSV licence holders who must lose their licence, and those doing heavy manual work. The disablement resettlement office may be able to help, but where possible, and providing finances are available in the current employment situation, early retirement may be the most sensible option. It must be made clear to the patient that this does not mean we are concerned about him medically. Interesting leisure activities may be suggested as a partial substitute.

TRAVEL

About four weeks after an infarct most patients are fit to drive, and certainly if they have had a satisfactory treadmill exercise ECG. They should avoid the stress of rush-hour traffic initially. Air travel is safe from six weeks, but may be undertaken earlier if essential (Chapter 47).

SECONDARY PREVENTION

Beta blockade

It is now clear that following myocardial infarction a treadmill ECG is essential to establish one-year risk (Chamberlain, 1983) (Figure 13.1). In addition, beta blockade has been shown to reduce one-year mortality by up to 20 per cent. However it is estimated that only one-third of patients will be able to tolerate beta blockade, and certainly the side-effects, if present, are not worth suffering for the benefit. I believe beta blockade should be introduced in all suitable cases postinfarct but discontinued if the treadmill ECG is normal, because the mortality is already less than 3 per cent, or when side-effects are rendering the individual tired, lethargic and depressed. No other class of drug has been shown to give the mortality benefit of beta blockade, though evidence in support of aspirin (300 mg) daily is accruing.

PREVENTION — GENERAL

Prevention must be the prime objective of all involved in any aspect of medicine. The major risk factors can be avoidable, e.g. smoking, or unavoidable, e.g. ageing. It is important to remember that risk factors are additive, and that individuals with one or more risk factors should be pursued vigorously (Figure 13.3). With the prospect of an additional 800 in 10,000 males reaching age 65 if primary prevention is successful, we can see the benefit both in the quality and quantity of life of the individual and cost to the community.

Results of the primary prevention trials have unfortunately been disappointing apart from a reduction in coronary mortality from stopping smoking. Certainly eliminating smoking, eating a prudent diet, increasing dynamic exercise and avoiding obesity sound sensible, but as a mass intervention there is little evidence to support a change in worldwide lifestyle. Selective screening, focusing on high-risk individuals and their relatives, concentrates efforts and resources on far fewer people with the chance of a greater impact on prevention. Here, in addition to smoking, there is a clear benefit from cholesterol lowering for those in the top quartile of serum cholesterol distribution. However, only one study supports this philosophy — The Lipid Research Clinics Coronary Primary Prevention Trial (LRC of cholestyramine 1984). Studying the top 5 per cent of cholesterol elevation those treated had a 19 per cent reduction in coronary deaths and non-fatal infarcts. Confidence limits, however, were poor, making it difficult to extend the intervention argument to lower-risk groups. Indeed it is overlooked in discussion that in the treated group there was an increase in

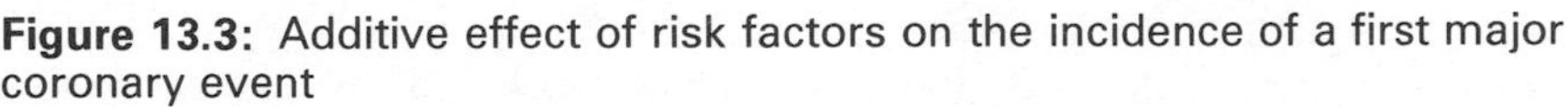

Figure 13.3: Additive effect of risk factors on the incidence of a first major coronary event

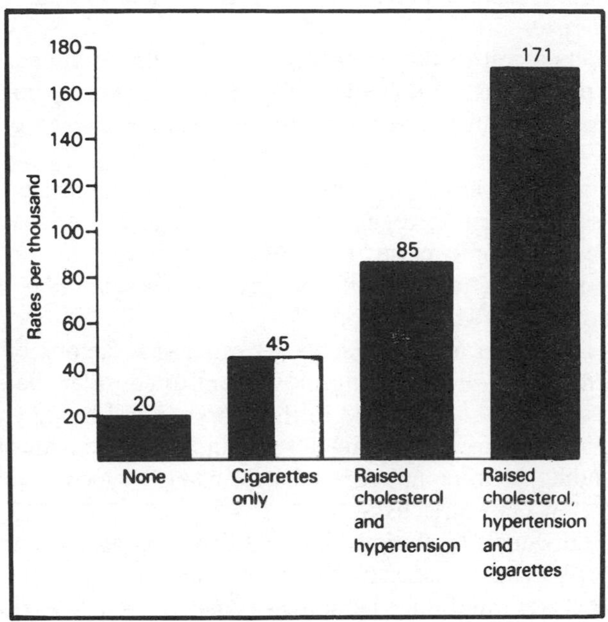

the incidence of oral gastrointestinal cancer.

Controlling hypertension benefits stroke incidence, but the data for mild to moderate hypertension and coronary heart disease are negative. The recent MRC trial of therapy in mild hypertension showed no benefit, but 20–25 per cent of healthy men were made unhealthy as a result of therapy (1985). Thus whilst those with elevated cholesterols and blood pressure are at risk, the risk is not that high so that in men of 40–55 years about two-thirds will be fit over the next 25 years without intervention. This means that major lifestyle changes, lipid-lowering agents and antihypertensives will in the majority have been unnecessary. However, the public are at the mercy of the marketing men, and no scientific argument will overcome the commercial interest in developing and profiting from low-cholesterol products.

PREVENTION — PRACTICAL

We must not punish our patients or instill them with guilt. We must concentrate on reducing smoking, which is responsible for 25 per cent of coronary deaths in those under 65 years and 80 per cent of men below 45 years. Cigarettes increase the myocardial workload by catecholamine stimulation, at the same time as reducing oxygen supply by carbon monoxide inhalation. This, combined with increased platelet adhesiveness, is a recipe for disaster.

All smokers are at risk, but especially those with additional risk factors such as hypertension or diabetes. The risk of a future infarct can be reduced by half within five years of stopping smoking (Figure 13.4) (Doll and Peto, 1976).

General practical advice should emphasise the importance of annual blood pressure screening, regular exercise if enjoyed, and avoidance of obesity, because people close to optimal weight feel better than when overweight. However, the slothful who hate exercise should be told to stop smoking and be otherwise left alone.

Stress is a problem in the presence of other risk factors, but not as an isolated entity. It is worth advising the patient to consider the emotionally demanding aspects of his lifestyle in the working and home environment. Regular holidays, non-stressful lunch time and home activities (gardening, walking, reading) help complete a lifestyle change which is easier for the patient to follow than expected.

Type A individuals (ambitious, competitive, aggressive, impatient) may be more at risk than the relaxed Type B counterparts. Here it is of interest that beta blockade can induce personality change from A to B, which may be useful in the appropriate patients with anginal pain.

Figure 13.4: Mortality from coronary disease is halved five years after stopping smoking

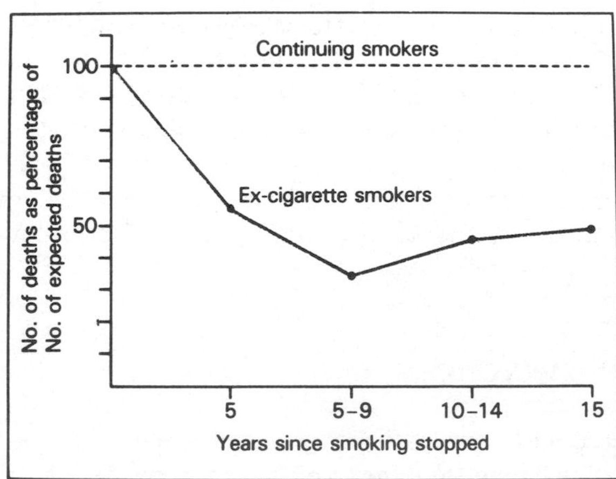

ANGINA

Angina is a chest pain brought on by effort or emotion and relieved by rest and sublingual glyceryl trinitrate. It is known that the extent of obstructive coronary artery disease that may induce anginal chest pain varies widely between individuals. The problem we have is in identifying those at risk of infarction and death whose prognosis may be substantially improved by coronary bypass surgery. Physical disability, in spite of optimal medical therapy, so that the individual cannot enjoy a satisfactory lifestyle demands further investigation to see if surgery can improve the quality of life. Too many people are confined to unacceptable limitations because of far too great an emphasis on conservative medical treatment. It is simply not good enough for a 50-year-old man to be unable to play with his children or enjoy sexual intercourse with his wife when symptom relief is possible with bypass surgery. Mild symptoms are easily accepted by patient and physician, but neither knows whether the anatomical problem is potentially dangerous. All patients under 65 years of age should undergo treadmill exercise testing to establish their risk status. If positive for ischaemia, angiography may identify a pattern of coronary lesions which, independent of symptoms, adversely affects prognosis, a prognosis which surgery will improve.

For the patient angina again means heart disease and the possibility of infarction and death. Counselling the patient on risk factor modification is essential, and weight reduction, blood pressure control and stopping smoking are essential beginnings in management. A frank discussion with patient and spouse is strongly advised. The patient must be encouraged to volunteer any difficulties he may have. It is easy to prescribe beta blocking drugs which are dramatically effective in reducing anginal attacks and increasing exercise performance. Particularly with everyday life they preserve the spontaneity of events, whereas nitrates sublingually can at the wrong time emphasise the underlying problem. Here one has the chance to benefit a sexual relationship — the enthusiasm must be tempered with the need to check for impotence which can be induced by beta blockade in up to 10 per cent, and which the British male rarely mentions.

Again there is no evidence that an exercise programme will lengthen life or protect the patient, but for the well-motivated a significant improvement in well-being is possible and, with training, exercise ability. Exercise, however, is to be enjoyed. It is no use jogging if it is hated; better to walk in the countryside, swim, dance or play tennis. Some prefer golf, others would sooner sit and fish. There has to be enjoyment or stress will be all that is achieved. Stress supplements other risk factors rather than acting as a powerful risk factor on its own. Certainly severe stress can cause a cardiac event providing there is an underlying problem, (Bass, 1983). It is recommended that those under stress try to effect lifestyle changes to reduce stress (see Myocardial infarction).

Booklets are available to help the patient and relatives, and should be used to supplement the advice given at consultation.

HEART FAILURE

This is one of the more difficult aspects of rehabilitation. If the failure reflects valvar damage, and medical therapy is unsuccessful, valve replacement can be dramatically beneficial. When the problem is heart muscle disease, from whatever cause, then controlling symptoms at the same time as maintaining activity requires the early use of vasodilator drugs (Fowler and Jackson, 1983).

Conventional therapy of heart failure involves diuretics and digoxin in appropriate cases. Diuretics are excellent in removing volume and relieving breathlessness, and certainly in mild heart failure this will be all that is necessary. However, as the need for diuretics increases so the volume decreases, until the critical balance between blood returning to the heart and blood leaving it is reduced too far. Breathlessness will be resolved, but cardiac output will not be increased and a dry-skinned, dehydrated, tired and lethargic individual will result.

Using vasodilator drugs early the blood returning to the heart (preload) can be reduced and the blood leaving the heart have the resistance reduced (afterload) thereby facilitating cardiac output. A 25–50 per cent improvement in performance can be achieved without the social inconvenience and debility of excessive diuresis. The quality of life improves for a substantial number of patients. We do not know yet if lengthening of life is possible, but the signs are hopeful.

Patients languishing on high-dose diuretics need a re-evaluation; they should be sought out.

CARDIAC SURGERY

The immediate problem is musculoskeletal pain from the thoracic spine and anterior chest wall, and pain from the leg scars as a result of vein dissection. The patients need to be aware this is going to happen, and again booklets supplement the advice given by doctors and nursing staff. The pain resolves slowly but in a small but significant number persists and interferes with mobilisation. Here a two- to four-week course of a non-steroidal anti-inflammatory drug is very helpful.

Surgical patients are in hospital an average of 10 days, and on discharge are mobile, climbing stairs, etc. It is important to emphasise to the patient and spouse that they have not had an illness but had one prevented or corrected. They cannot undo the good of the operation — it will not fall apart. Sexual relations can be resumed as so desired, but the sternal pain may be limiting. The side-to-side position or mutual masturbation will usually circumvent these problems.

Returning to driving, walking or swimming is done as early as possible, with the emphasis most positively on resuming normal life with a return to work at approximately eight to ten weeks. Occasional muscle pains should be warned about, particularly with front-wheel drive cars which do not have power-assisted steering. The myocardial infarct rehabilitation programme is helpful. If progress at six weeks is not as quick as expected, invariably the reason is lack of confidence, and enrolment in a rehabilitation programme is a great confidence booster.

CONGENITAL HEART DISEASE

With heroic surgery in childhood we now have a collection of severely limited adolescents whose demise has been postponed. The problems of heart failure, pulmonary hypertension and arrhythmias are compounded by the real problems of growing up. Their lives have been saved, only for them to die in adolescence or struggle vainly in the competitive atmosphere of the late teens and 20s. Heart transplantation perhaps offers an option, but again this is only palliative with a high chance of repeat in five to six years. Clearly if ever there was a need for the paediatric cardiologist to supervise into adulthood, and thereby maintain continuity of care and expertise, this is it. I would advise any family doctor faced with these problems to consult with the nearest paediatric centre for advice.

PROBLEMS ENCOUNTERED BY WOMEN

The problems of the woman with cardiac illness are sometimes forgotten. In many homes women still do much of the housework; they feel house-proud. Following a heart attack the patient comes home after eight to ten days and needs time to resume normal household activities. She needs help from husband, children or other relatives and friends; firm medical advice may help this to be forthcoming. Following heart surgery there can be additional concern about sexual activity with the woman lying underneath; this can give rise to fear of inducing damage or of causing pain. These fears need to be allayed and any pain treated.

There is a higher incidence of heart disease in men than women, the man still being the main breadwinner in most homes. The wife may need help coping while the husband is in hospital; help again may be encouraged by advice from the general practitioner or hospital staff.

SUMMARY

Cardiac illness is a family problem. All members need open simple advice about what is going on, what will happen and how everyone including the patient can contribute. Even without access to a formal rehabilitation programme most people will get through with education and common sense. It is the medical profession's responsibility to provide this basis for recovery.

REFERENCES

Akhras, F., Upward, J., Keates, J. and Jackson, G. (1984) Early exercise testing and elective coronary artery bypass surgery after uncomplicated myocardial infarction. *Br. Heart J.*, *52*, 413-17

Bartlett, R.G. Jr (1956) Physiologic responses during coitus. *J. App. Physiol.*, *15*, 469-72

Bass, C. (1983) Stress, personality and coronary heart disease. *Cardiol. Pract.*, *1*, 6-11 [Author's note: The most simple comprehensive review of stress and the heart]

Bruce, R.A., Fisher, L.D., Cooper, M.N. and Grey, G.O. (1974) Separation of effects of cardiovascular disease and age on ventricular function with maximal exercise. *Am. J. Cardiol.*, *34*, 757-83

Chamberlain, D.A. (1983) Beta adrenoceptor antagonists after myocardial infarction — where are we now? *Br. Heart J.*, *49*, 105-10

Cobb, L.A. (1986) Exercise: a risk for sudden death in patients with coronary heart disease. *J. Am. Coll. Cardiol.*, *7*, 215-19 [Author's note: This issue has an excellent symposium on the athletic heart]

Doll, R. and Peto, R. (1983) Mortality in relation to smoking: 20 years observations on male doctors. *Br. Med. J.*, *2*, 1525-36

Fowler, J. and Jackson, G. (1983) Cardiac failure: pathophysiology and therapy. *Update*, 197-204

Hellerstin, J.H. and Friedman, E.H. (1970) Sexual activity in the post coronary patient. *Arch. Int. Med.*, *125*, 987-99

Jackson, G. (1978) Sexual intercourse and angina pectoris *Br. Med. J.*, *2*, 16

Jackson, G. (1979) Sexual intercourse and post coronary patients. *Br. J. Sex Med.*, *6*, 44-8

Larson, J.L., McNaughton, M.W., Ward Kennedy, J. and Mansfield, L.W. (1980) Heart rate and blood pressure response to sexual activity and a stair-climbing test. *Heart Lung*, *9*, 1025-30

Lipid Research Clinic Coronary Prevention Trial (1984) *J. Am. Med. Assoc.*, *251*, 351-74

Masters, W.H. and Johnson, V.E. (1966) *Human sexual response*, Little, Brown & Co., Boston

MRC Trial of treatment of mild hypertension (1985) *Br. Med. J.*, *291*, 97-104

Nemec, E.D., Mansfield, L. and Ward Kennedy, J. (1976) Heart rate and blood pressure responses during sexual activity in normal males. *Am. Heart J.*, *92*, 274-7

Théroux, P., Walters, D.D., Halphen, C., Debaisieux, J.C. and Mizgala, H.F. (1979)

Prognostic value of exercise testing soon after myocardial infarction. *N. Engl. J. Med.*, *301*, 341-5

Wenger, N.K. (1981) Rehabilitation of the patient with myocardial infarction. Responsibility of the primary care physician. *Primary Care*, *8*, 491-507

World Health Organization (1985) *Rehabilitation after myocardial infarction.* WHO, Copenhagen [Author's note: an up-to-date comprehensive review]

14

Respiratory Disease

John Moxham

INTRODUCTION

Respiratory disorders are frequently chronic and disabling. Rehabilitation can seldom restore normal health, but much can be done to improve respiratory function and exercise capacity. Rehabilitation may halt the otherwise inevitable decline in pulmonary function and enable the patient to tolerate his symptoms of breathlessness and exercise limitation. Largely as a consequence of cigarette smoking disability is most commonly due to chronic bronchitis and emphysema.

CHRONIC BRONCHITIS AND EMPHYSEMA

The scale of the problem

Chronic bronchitis and emphysema is responsible for the personal disability and misery of tens of thousands of patients and imposes a huge social and economic burden on society. In the United Kingdom 10 per cent of absence from work and 10 per cent of the occupancy of medical hospital beds are the result of these diseases, and it is estimated that a quarter of males aged 50–59 have chronic bronchitis.

Therapy and rehabilitation

Since restoration of normal function is not possible in chronic bronchitis and emphysema, the aim of therapy is to reduce disability by tackling the interrelated problems of recurrent infections, airways obstruction, breathlessness, hypoxia and poor exercise tolerance. Factors aggravating chronic bronchitis, particularly cigarette smoking, must be withdrawn.

Infection

In acute exacerbations of chronic bronchitis an infective viral or bacterial pathogen is isolated in less than 50 per cent of cases. However, viral infections are frequently complicated by bacterial overgrowth and the majority of patients develop purulent sputum. Antibacterial therapy is therefore of the greatest importance. Whereas minor exacerbations are associated with increased airways obstruction and breathlessness, severe exacerbations are characterised by worsening hypercapnic ventilatory failure and up to 25 per cent mortality (Warren *et al.*, 1980). For most patients long-term chemoprophylaxis is not helpful, not reducing the number of exacerbations, but if intermittent treatment fails, a trial of continuous antibiotic therapy is justified. Prompt therapy of infection is important, and patients should always have available appropriate drugs to be taken when symptoms first develop. Immunisation against *H. influenzae, S. aureus* and *S. pneumoniae* has not been shown to be effective. Immunisation against the common cold virus is similarly ineffective but annual immunisation against influenza virus, using killed vaccine, may have some value and should be considered in the severely disabled patient with frequent infections.

Airways obstruction

In chronic bronchitis and emphysema airflow limitation is due to reduced elastic recoil of the lung, hypertrophy and oedema of the bronchial wall mucous membrane, excess mucus within the airways and contraction of bronchial wall smooth muscle. The increased resistance to gas flow within the bronchial tree increases the work of breathing and overall oxygen consumption. As a consequence of airways obstruction there is excess gas trapping in the lungs, hyperinflation, and disordered rib cage geometry, all of which shorten the respiratory muscles, make the diaphragm less curved and greatly reduce ventilatory capacity. Airways obstruction therefore increases ventilatory work at the same time as reducing ventilatory capacity. Sucessful treatment of airways obstruction reduces the work of breathing as well as improving the capacity of the thorax to achieve the ventilation required. This improvement reduces breathlessness, reverses ventilatory failure and improves exercise capacity.

Conventionally the airways obstruction of chronic bronchitis and emphysema is regarded as being irreversible. However, the majority of patients show a small improvement in lung function with therapy aimed at relaxing bronchial smooth muscle, and in the rehabilitation of severely disabled patients every effort must be made to provide optimum treatment for airways obstruction. The most important agents are selective beta-adrenergic agonists (salbutamol, terbutaline) best administered as an aerosol. Careful instruction in the use of metered dose inhalers is of critical importance, and a variety of modifications to basic inhaler design are available to help patients who have difficulty in mastering the correct inhaler technique. Drug in powder form administered by a rotahaler device may be an effective alternative to pressurised inhalers. For the few patients who find it impossible to successfully use a metered dose inhaler, beta-2 agonists can be administered from a nebuliser driven by an air compressor. Using a nebuliser the conventional dose of beta-2 agonists is large, i.e. 2.5 or 5.0 mg of salbutamol, and this therapy should not be initiated without specialist assessment. As a consequence of the large drug dosage, patients with chronic airflow limitation frequently report that nebuliser therapy is superior to that from metered dose inhalers. However, if metered dose inhaler therapy is increased to achieve maximum bronchodilatation, four to six 100 μg inhalations being taken rather than the standard dose of 200 μg, most patients are helped equally by the two methods of drug administration (Jenkins *et al.*, 1987).

Inhaled atropine analogues (ipratropium bromide) can be helpful instead of, or in addition to, beta-2 agonists and can be administered either by metered dose inhaler or nebuliser. It is important to establish optimum dosage.

Oral theophyllines available in slow-release formulation are of undoubted value in asthma, particularly when nocturnal symptoms are severe, but they are of marginal usefulness in chronic bronchitis and emphysema (Cochrane, 1984). They should not be prescribed long-term without critical review. Therapeutic and toxic drug levels are close, side-effects can be serious and it is frequently necessary to monitor blood theophylline levels. In addition to a bronchodilator action it is possible that theophyllines have a small beneficial action on the contractility of skeletal muscle, including the respiratory muscles, but the clinical importance of this remains uncertain (Moxham and Green, 1985).

All patients with severe airways obstruction should have a therapeutic trial of steroids, for example oral prednisolone 30 mg daily for a period of three weeks, providing there is no contraindication to this drug. If respiratory function unequivocally improves then inhaled steroids should be tried. Long-term oral steroids will not be indicated in most patients; such therapy requires regular assessment and long-term dosage should seldom exceed 7.5–10 mg daily, thereby avoiding drug complications. Careful clinical judgement is required in cases where there is subjective improvement in symptoms but no objective change in lung function or exercise capacity.

Mucolytic agents (e.g. bromhexine) reduce sputum viscosity but are of unproven value in chronic bronchitis. Occasional patients report substantial benefit from mucolytic agents, and when sputum retention is a major problem a therapeutic trial is justified.

Chronic hypoxia eventually causes secondary polycythaemia, possibly with increased risk of vascular thrombosis. Relief of hypoxia by treatment of the underlying primary pulmonary disease or by long-term oxygen therapy represents the most satisfactory way to reverse polycythaemia. Venesection is only effective in the short term, but alleviates the symptoms and avoids the complications of hyperviscosity (Harrison and Stokes, 1982). Most recently the clinical usefulness of erythropharesis is being evaluated.

Nutrition and body weight

With increasing disability many patients exercise less and gain weight, thereby increasing resting respiratory work. Severe obesity adversely affects chest wall mechanics. Many patients with chronic airways obstruction are depressed and some eat excessively as an expression of their psychiatric state. Appetite may be further stimulated if patients are successful in stopping smoking, or treated with oral steroids. Depression is positively correlated with the severity of breathlessness (Morgan *et al.*, 1983), and the treatment of depression as well as reduction in body weight may be helpful, although such therapy is frequently difficult. In contrast, with advanced respiratory disease, weight loss and muscle wasting is common, the respiratory muscles sharing in this atrophy. Inadequate nutrition, common in these patients, accelerates the wasting process and further diminishes respiratory reserve (Arora and Rochester, 1982). It is not yet clear whether supplementary high-calorie and high-protein diets can improve respiratory muscle bulk and pulmonary function. Diets high in carbohydrate increase carbon dioxide production, stimulate ventilation, exacerbate breathlessness and can intensify ventilatory failure: in some patients, therefore, dietary modification may be of value.

Oxygen therapy

During acute exacerbations of chronic bronchitis and emphysema oxygen therapy is necessary to avoid death from hypoxia, although in patients with hypercapnia oxygen must be given at low and controlled concentrations. From the rehabilitation point of view the more contentious question is the value of long-term domiciliary oxygen therapy. Studies suggest that long-term controlled oxygen therapy can benefit patients with severe chronic airways obstruction who have an FEV_1 of less than 1.2 litres, severe hypoxia ($P\text{O}_2$ 40–55 mmHg) and who do not smoke cigarettes. Not only is smoking and oxygen therapy dangerous, it also mitigates against the beneficial effect of treatment. An MRC study has looked at 87 patients with chronic bronchitis and associated hypoxia, hypercapnia, pulmonary hypertension and secondary polycythaemia. Half of the patients were treated with oxygen (2 l/min by nasal prongs) for 15 hours each day for five years, the other half did not receive oxygen. Those not treated with oxygen fared badly, with a five-year survival of 30 per cent, but those treated with oxygen did better, and their survival was almost doubled (Medical Research Council, 1981)). A similar American study compared oxygen therapy for 12 hours a day with oxygen for 19 hours each day, both groups having oxygen therapy throughout the night. Oxygen for 12 hours daily produced results similar to oxygen for 15 hours each day reported in the MRC study, but oxygen for 19 hours each day further prolonged survival and reduced the frequency and duration of hospital admissions (Nocturnal Oxygen Therapy Trial Group, 1980). The physiological evaluation of the patients in these studies suggested that oxygen therapy reversed secondary polycythaemia and prevented the progressive increase in pulmonary vascular resistance and pulmonary artery pressure that occur without oxygen therapy.

The administration of continuous oxygen presents formidable practical and financial difficulties. Until recently oxygen was supplied in cylinders in the UK and continuous therapy for up to 15 hours each day requires 15–20 1346 litre cylinders each week, at an annual cost of several thousand pounds. A more satisfactory alternative is the oxygen concentrator, routinely available in many countries, and recently introduced in the UK, which removes nitrogen from air and is a reliable and less expensive device. The oxygen concentrator has been extensively assessed in recent years, and the use of these devices is likely to become widespread in the near future. The present system of prescribing domiciliary oxygen is often unsatisfactory. Many patients receive oxygen without careful assessment and conversely patients who could benefit from oxygen therapy do not receive it. Oxygen is a difficult and expensive drug to administer, and in most cases should only be prescribed after careful clinical and physiological assessment by a thoracic physician.

Short-term and portable oxygen therapy

In practice most oxygen used by patients in their homes is for a few minutes, and often only on a few occasions each week. Patients report that they take oxygen in this way for relief of breathlessness. This may be correct because oxygen therapy reduces respiratory rate and therefore the work of breathing, but the effect of short bursts of oxygen therapy on the sensation of breathlessness has been little studied (Waterhouse and Howard, 1983).

The purpose of portable oxygen is to relieve hypoxia during exercise, and hopefully to increase exercise capacity. Small cylinders are available which weigh 2 kg and have sufficient oxygen to last approximately 30 min.

These cylinders require appropriate reducing valves to facilitate a flow rate of 2 l/min and they can be refilled from a larger oxygen cylinder in the patient's home. However, the process of refilling is rather difficult, and is frequently unsatisfactory. Currently several centres are evaluating the administration of oxygen at a low flow rate (½–1 l/min) directly into the trachea via indwelling fine catheters. This technique may be more acceptable to some patients and may also be more efficient, thereby prolonging the life of oxygen cylinders. Controlled trials of portable oxygen therapy have demonstrated a very small benefit in terms of exercise capacity, but some patients report a reduction in breathlessness even though they do not walk further. Further studies of portable oxygen therapy are urgently required, but it should not be forgotten that when patients claim benefit from portable oxygen they may well be correct, and the inability of physicians to document objective improvement may reflect the lack of precision of current techniques for evaluating exercise tolerance and breathlessness. The use of visual analogue scales to assess breathlessness has greatly improved the scientific study of this difficult symptom, and the effect of oxygen and drugs on dyspnoea can now be accurately assessed.

Hypoxia and oxygen therapy during sleep

Patients with chronic bronchitis and associated hypoxia, hypercapnia, secondary polycythaemia, pulmonary hypertension and cor pulmonale can have profound nocturnal hypoxaemia, particularly during rapid eye movement (REM) sleep (Flick and Block, 1977). Nocturnal hypoxaemia is much more severe in the 'blue bloater' than the 'pink puffer'; normal subjects and pink puffers do have nocturnal hypoxaemia but the level reached is much lower in the already hypoxic chronic bronchitic. Much of the hypoxia is caused by hypoventilation and irregular breathing patterns during REM sleep or increased ventilation–perfusion mismatch, and is not due to obstructive sleep apnoea. Oxygen therapy during the night (2 l/min by nasal prongs) can alleviate hypoxaemia and make hypoxic dips much less severe. Respiratory stimulants, particularly the new oral agent almitrine, may have a place in reducing nocturnal hypoxaemia, probably by improving ventilation–perfusion matching, but the clinical role of almitrine is still under evaluation (Howard, 1984).

Drug therapy for breathlessness

In patients with airways obstruction it is the 'pink puffers' with normal CO_2 values and mild hypoxia that are characteristically severely breathless. However, 'blue bloaters' may be equally incapacitated and dyspnoea can be particularly disabling in patients with pulmonary fibrosis. There is evidence that diazepam, promethazine and dihydrocodeine can reduce breathlessness in 'pink puffers', and the careful use of such therapy is justified in severe cases (Woodcock *et al.*, 1981). For the devastating dyspnoea frequently a feature of terminal respiratory failure diamorphine is helpful.

Obstructive sleep apnoea

Obstructive sleep apnoea may affect up to 1 per cent of the adult male population, particularly those who are middle-aged/elderly and obese, and those who snore. It is made worse by alcohol, sedatives and hypnotics (Saunders and Sullivan, 1984). When asleep the patients exhibit periodic breathing with episodes of apnoea during which strong inspiratory efforts are made against an occluded upper airway. Profound hypoxia occurs and patients develop polycythaemia, daytime somnolence, respiratory failure and cor pulmonale. Appropriate therapy can reverse these changes. Definite diagnosis requires a laboratory assessment of ventilation during nocturnal sleep. The site of airflow obstruction is within the pharynx and hypopharynx, but the exact site is variable between patients. The collapse of the pharynx is due to reduction in the activity of upper airway muscles acting on the soft palate, tongue and hyoid. Anatomical abnormalities frequently contribute; anatomical narrowing resulting in more negative intrapharyngeal pressures and a greater tendency to pharyngeal collapse. The greater the incoordination between inspiratory muscle and pharyngeal muscle activation the greater the pharyngeal collapse. Alcohol and sedatives depress brainstem activity, depress pharyngeal muscle activity and precipitate pharyngeal obstruction. Obstruction is relieved when the upper airway muscles are sufficiently activated, and this is frequently only possible by the recruitment of the higher nervous system and therefore the interruption of sleep. This mechanism is impaired by ethanol and sedatives and apnoeic episodes are prolonged, thereby intensifying hypoxia.

In the management of obstructive sleep apnoea, weight reduction is helpful but difficult to achieve. Tracheostomy is effective but presents management difficulties and many patients are reluctant to agree to this line of treatment. Nasal continuous positive airway pressure (CPAP) is uniformly effective (Sullivan *et al.*, 1984), but only recently have nasal masks individually fitted for each patient become available, and the technique remains rather cumbersome.

Palatopharyngoplasty (PPP), surgical reconstruction of the pharynx, can also be effective, but the site of obstruction may not be relieved in some patients and the long-term effects of surgery are not yet available. As yet surgery is little practised in the UK.

Drugs may also be helpful; particularly protriptyline (a non-sedative tricyclic antidepressant) which reduces the duration of rapid eye movement sleep, when obstruction is most severe as a consequence of the reduced activity of upper airway musculature (Brownell *et al.*, 1982). For many patients weight reduction and protriptyline should be tried before considering CPAP or PPP.

CHEST WALL DISORDERS – SCOLIOSIS AND MUSCLE WEAKNESS

Patients with severe scoliosis or rib cage deformity from thoracoplasty eventually develop hypercapnic ventilatory failure and cor pulmonale. These patients can be helped by ventilatory assistance using negative pressure tank, cuirass or jacket ventilation (Hoeppner *et al.*, 1984; Sawicka *et al.*, 1983). Patients with respiratory failure secondary to chronic respiratory muscle weakness can be treated in the same way, although some may be better managed with positive pressure ventilation via a tracheostomy. For many patients ventilatory support is necessary for short periods, and in practice nocturnal ventilation is frequently both convenient and effective. It is of note that such ventilatory support produces long-term improvement in ambulatory blood gas tensions, perhaps secondary to the intermittent rest of the hard-pressed respiratory muscles. For patients with scoliosis, and some cases of chronic stable or slowly progressive respiratory muscle weakness, the results of assisted ventilation treatment have been excellent, with enhanced quality of life for many years.

The value of intermittent assisted ventilation in patients with airways obstruction or pulmonary fibrosis is more doubtful. Although the breathing of alert normal subjects and patients with chest wall disorders can be 'captured' by mechanical ventilation this is seldom the case with patients with lung disease. In general, intermittent positive pressure breathing (IPPB) has not been helpful, although individual patients have reported benefit and further studies would be useful. Other techniques of reducing ventilation, and thereby respiratory muscle work, such as high-frequency ventilation and high-frequency oscillation, deserve further study.

SMOKING

Smoking is an important aetiological agent in chronic bronchitis, emphysema, lung cancer, and ischaemic heart disease, as well as causing cough, aggravating asthma and increasing susceptibility to pulmonary infection. All patients with chronic lung disease must stop smoking. If patients with chronic bronchitis and emphysema can stop smoking, particularly in the early stages of their disease, airways obstruction is improved. The problem for both patient and physician is how this is to be achieved (Higgenbottom and Chamberlain, 1984).

A powerful influence on successfully stopping smoking is whether a patient's spouse or cohabitant continues to smoke, and the physician needs to involve the patient's family in the task. It is as well to remember that up to 20 per cent of patients falsely claim to have stopped smoking. Nicotine is the most active pharmacological agent in cigarette smoke, exerting a powerful effect on the autonomic nervous system, and nicotine-containing compounds have been widely used as cigarette substitutes. The most extensively studied has been nicotine chewing gum, which has been shown to help those patients who ask for it and who are therefore highly motivated to stop smoking (Jarvis *et al.*, 1982). In patients with smoking-related diseases randomly allocated between nicotine gum, placebo, and advice only, long-term abstinence is less than 10 per cent, with no difference between the three treatment groups. Results from anti-smoking clinics offering advice and guidance show them to be relatively ineffective with less than 15 per cent long-term abstinence if biochemical verification of non-smoking is demanded. A physician's advice, particularly to the symptomatic patient, is more effective, as may be the advice of nurses and other health staff. The opportunity to advise patients to stop smoking should therefore never be let pass. Controlled studies suggest that hypnosis and acupuncture have little effect, and aversion therapy is seldom successful.

The majority of patients will continue to smoke despite all available measures to persuade them to stop. Can smoking be reduced? Smokers should be encouraged to smoke fewer cigarettes, switch to low-tar brands, not to oversmoke lower-tar cigarettes, take fewer puffs and inhale less. When cigarette smokers switch to cigars and pipes they continue to inhale, and can achieve increased tobacco smoke exposure.

REHABILITATION PROGRAMMES

Comprehensive rehabilitation programmes have concentrated on patient education, physiotherapy, breathing exercises and training schedules aimed at improving general fitness and specifically improving the performance of the respiratory muscles. Following rehabilitation programmes some investigators have reported improvement in overall performance, but controlled studies are few. Such programmes seldom improve lung function or gas exchange, but may enable patients to cope better with the limitations imposed by their disease. An evaluation of programmes should include assessment of exercise capability. In a five-year study of 252 male patients with chronic bronchitis and emphysema a programme of medical therapy, postural drainage, breathing and general exercises resulted in 25 per cent of patients returning to work compared to 3 per cent in a control group, and a reduced mortality of 22 per cent compared to 42 per cent in the control patients (Hass and Cardon, 1969). Studies have also demonstrated improved twelve-minute walking distance and increased work capacity on a bicycle ergometer. However, a recent double-blind study involving a large number of patients with chronic airflow limitation failed to show any improvement in exercise capacity, although patients reported subjective improvement (Booker, 1984). The available evidence suggests that any objective benefit from exercise programmes, in terms of spirometry or blood gases, is likely to be minor, but that patients' tolerance of their disability is improved. It is important to reassure patients with chronic airflow limitation and breathlessness that exercise, short of exhaustion, is not harmful.

CHEST PHYSIOTHERAPY

Studies of the long-term effects of chest physiotherapy, aimed at improving breathing patterns, have been few, and have been reviewed by Sutton *et al.* (1982). Slow purse-lipped breathing can improve blood gases. Abdominal (diaphragmatic) breathing leads to deeper and slower respiration but probably does not alter the distribution of ventilation. The aim of instruction in such breathing techniques is to produce a more relaxed breathing pattern and thereby reduce the work of ventilation and oxygen consumption of the respiratory muscles. This hypothesis remains untested.

Postural drainage is of undoubted benefit in patients with excessive bronchial secretions. It enhances mucociliary clearance, sputum volumes are increased and some studies have documented improved lung function (Cochrane *et al.*, 1977). The effectiveness of postural drainage is increased by coughing or forced expiratory manoeuvres. Postural drainage has little place in patients without sputum. Forced expiration 'huffs' increase the efficacy of postural drainage in cystic fibrosis. In patients with excessive secretions cough clears sputum from central and intermediate regions of the lungs but there is doubt about its efficacy in clearing peripheral airways. Most clinical studies have shown little immediate effect of physiotherapy on arterial blood gas tensions. In asthma vigorous physiotherapy, especially forced expiratory manoeuvres, can increase bronchospasm. During acute exacerbations of bronchitis, and in pneumonia, studies have shown no benefit from physiotherapy, and in the absence of excessive secretions it is difficult to justify physiotherapy for these patients.

Mucociliary clearance is decreased and basal collapse increased during general anaesthesia and surgery, particularly surgery to the upper abdomen. However, the case for routine physiotherapy in patients with chronic airflow limitation is not proven except for high-risk cases.

RESPIRATORY MUSCLE TRAINING

In patients with airways obstruction or pulmonary fibrosis the work of breathing is increased, and this excessive load is borne predominantly by the muscles of inspiration. With suitable training programmes limb muscle performance can be improved, and a large number of studies have been undertaken to assess the value of specific respiratory muscle training. In normal subjects Leith and Bradley (1976) documented substantial improvement in the strength and endurance of the respiratory muscles following training. Studies in patients with chronic airflow limitation, cystic fibrosis and quadriplegia have shown benefit in terms of respiratory muscle strength, endurance and exercise tolerance. However, other studies have shown little or no objective improvement, and as part of a general rehabilitation programme it remains doubtful whether specific training of the respiratory muscles is useful.

REFERENCES

Arora, N.S. and Rochester, D.F. (1982) Ventilatory muscle strength and maximum voluntary ventilation in undernourished patients. *Am. Rev. Respir. Dis., 126,* 5-8

Booker, H.A. (1984) Exercise training and breathing control in patients with chronic airflow limitation. *Physiotherapy, 70,* 258-60

Brownell, L.G., West, P., Sweatman, P., Acres, J.C. and Kryger, M.H. (1982) Protriptyline in obstructive sleep apnoea: a double blind trial. *N. Engl. J. Med., 307,* 1037-42

Cochrane, G.M. (1984) Editorial: Slow-release theophyllines and chronic bronchitis. *Brit. Med. J., 289,* 1643-4

Cochrane, G.M., Webber, B.A. and Clarke, S.W. (1977) Effects of sputum on pulmonary function. *Br. Med. J., 2,* 1181-3

Flick, M.R. and Block, A.J. (1977) Continuous in-vivo monitoring of arterial oxygenation in chronic obstructive lung disease. *Ann. Intern. Med., 86,* 725-30

Harrison, B.D.W. and Stokes, T.C. (1982) Secondary polycythaemia: its causes, effects and treatment. *Br. J. Dis. Chest, 76,* 313-40

Hass, A. and Cardon, H. (1969) Rehabilitation in chronic obstructive pulmonary disease. *Med. Clin. N. Am., 53,* 593-606

Higgenbottom, T. and Chamberlain, A. (1984) Editorial: Giving up smoking. *Thorax, 39,* 641-6

Hoeppner, V.A., Cockroft, D.W., Dosman, J.A. and Cotton, D.J. (1984) Night time ventilation improves respiratory failure in secondary kyphoscoliosis. *Am. Rev. Respir. Dis., 129,* 240-3

Howard, P. (1984) Editorial: Almitrine bismesylate (Vectarion). *Clin. Resp. Physiol., 20,* 99-103.

Jarvis, M.J., Raw, M., Russell, M.A.H. and Feyerbend, C. (1982) Randomised controlled trial of nicotine chewing gum. *Br. Med. J., 285,* 537-40

Jenkins, S.C., Heaton, R.W. and Fulton, T.J. and Moxham, J. (1987) Comparison of domiciliary nebulised salbutamol and salbutamol from a metered dose inhaler in stable chronic airflow limitation. *Chest, 91,* 804-7

Leith, D.E. and Bradley, M. (1976) Ventilatory muscle strength and endurance training. *J. Appl. Physiol.*, *41*, 508-16

Medical Research Council Working Party (1981) Long term domiciliary oxygen therapy in chronic hypoxic cor pulmonale complicating bronchitis and emphysema. *Lancet*, *1*, 681-6

Morgan, A.D., Peck, D.F., Buchanan, R. and McHardy, G.J.R. (1983) Effect of attitudes and beliefs on exercise tolerance in chronic bronchitis. *Br. Med. J.*, *286*, 171-3

Moxham, J. and Green, M. (1985) Editorial: Aminophylline and the respiratory muscles. *Clin. Resp. Physiol.*, *21*, 1-6

Nocturnal Oxygen Therapy Trial Group (1980) Continuous or nocturnal therapy in hypoxemic chronic obstructive lung disease. A clinical trial. *Ann. Intern. Med.*, *93*, 391-8

Saunders, N.A. and Sullivan, C.E. (1984) Sleep and breathing. In C. Lenfant (ed.), *Lung biology in health and disease*, Marcel Dekker, New York, vol. 21 pp. 299-363

Sawicka, E.H., Branthwaite, M.A. and Spencer, G.T. (1983) Respiratory failure after thoracoplasty: treatment by intermittent negative-pressure ventilation. *Thorax*, *38*, 433-5

Sullivan, C.E., Issa, F.G., Berthon-Jones, M., McAnley, V.B. and Costas, L.J.V. (1984) Home treatment of obstructive sleep apnoea with continuous positive airway pressure applied through a nose mask. *Clin. Resp. Physiol.*, *20*, 49-54

Sutton, P.P., Pavia, D., Bateman, J.R.M. and Clarke, S.W. (1982) Chest physiotherapy: a review. *Eur. J. Resp. Dis.*, *63*, 188-201

Warren, P.M., Flenley, D.C., Millar, J.S. and Avery, A. (1980) Respiratory failure revisited: acute exacerbations of chronic bronchitis between 1961–68 and 1970–76. *Lancet*, *1*, 467-71

Waterhouse, J.C. and Howard, P. (1983) Breathlessness and portable oxygen in chronic obstructive airways disease. *Thorax*, *38*, 302-6

Woodcock, A.A., Gross, E.R., Gellert, A., Shah, S., Johnson, M. and Geddes D.M. (1981) Effects of dihydrocodeine, alcohol, and caffeine on breathlessness and exercise tolerance in patients with chronic obstructive lung disease and normal blood gases. *N. Engl. J. Med.*, *305*, 1611-16

Part 4

Sensory and Communication Disorders

15

Speech and Communication

Pamela Enderby

> In the beginning was the word. The word itself, of which our works of art are fashioned, is the first art form, older than the roughest shaping of clay or stone. A word is the carving or colouring of a thought and gives to it, permanence. We do not yet know, if ever we are able to trace, how language first began, though we may deduce that words to express love were those first used, since love is the emotion, just as speech the instrument, that even in its lowest most primitive form, clearly distinguishes human beings from their humble cousins of the animal world.
>
> (Osbert Sitwell)

Speech and language are so much a part of ourselves that it is hard to distinguish one from the other. The way we relate to others, the way we express our thoughts and emotions, our angers and fears, are very much the way that we see ourselves and reflect our personalities to the world. Thus, it is possible to surmise that people with speech impairments or loss of speech not only have difficulty in asking for what they want, and other relatively mundane aspects of daily living, but also have difficulty in reflecting their being. Speech and language impairment may be looked upon as one of the most fundamental of handicaps, as it can strike at the very soul of the human being.

Speech therapy reflects the recognition that communication is an integral part of human nature not only by being involved in the surface structure of speech and articulation or of language and vocabulary, but by being committed to communication in its broadest sense. Frequently we see patients who will be unable to communicate in the conventional manner, but who will benefit from therapy by being able to be taught to reflect their expressions in alternative ways. Therapy extends beyond the sounds and words to their use and effectiveness. Thus, referral of such a handicapped person for assessment by the speech therapist is nearly always the most appropriate action, as it is difficult for somebody who is unfamiliar with speech therapy techniques and approaches to know who will, or who will not, benefit.

WHO SHOULD BE REFERRED FOR SPEECH THERAPY?

Any patient who has a congenital or acquired speech or language handicap, or who has a long-standing speech disability, but has not received attention for this disability for some time, should be referred. The therapist, following assessment, will be able to judge whether this patient would benefit from speech therapy. Many doctors are concerned that they are referring patients too early. This cannot be the case, and early referral is to be encouraged. If the patient is not in a position to benefit from direct therapy either because he is too ill, or the situation is unstable, the therapist will arrange for an appointment at a later time. Some patients benefit from the support, knowing that the symptom is not being ignored. Even though she is unable to work directly with the patient at that time, the therapist will be able to guide the family, relatives and staff at a time when they are greatly concerned and distressed, and do not know how to approach the patient because communication is compromised.

WHY SHOULD YOU REFER?

This question relates to the expectations of the speech therapist. It is important to remember that the term 'speech therapy' is, to a certain extent, a misnomer, as it gives the impression that we are involved only in articulation and elocution, rather than communication as a two-way process.

If we take this latter definition of speech therapy, it is not hard to see that the speech therapist is involved in the following activities:

(1) detailed speech and language assessment;

(2) specific speech and language remediation;

(3) improving communication skills in general, and introducing non-oral means of communication where appropriate;

(4) advice to nursing, medical, remedial and other staff on handling specific expressive and receptive difficulties;

(5) advice and support to patients and relatives.

It is clear that most speech-disabled people may benefit by contact with the speech therapist, despite the fact that a large number will be unable to be rehabilitated to normal communication. Coping with disability and functioning at the highest possible level may be realistic and satisfactory from both the patient's and relatives' point of view (Brown, 1981).

ASSESSMENT

It is absolutely essential that each speech-handicapped person is fully assessed. Assessment of the orofacial musculature, as well as deep and surface linguistic abilities including those of reading and writing, will assist the therapist to plan appropriate intervention. Objective assessments are important, as a number of patients will learn to hide their socially unacceptable disorder, and it is easy to assume or surmise inaccurate information, which will result in rehabilitation being based on sand rather than rock. Not only do assessments help to establish the degree of the defect, and the areas of retained ability, but also they can assist in the classification of the disorder, provide information required to plan treatment, and can quantify and qualify changes in abilities. This latter point is important, as subjective clinical judgement may well give a false impression with regard to progress. For example: a patient with impaired articulation may be thought to be improving as people become familiar with his attempts to speak, and therefore can interpret them more readily. We must ensure that improvement is in the patient and not limited to improvement in the therapist's interpretive skills!

There are over 15 detailed standardised assessments which are appropriate for the investigation of speech, language or voice disorders.

PHYSIOLOGY OF SPEECH AND LANGUAGE

Speech production

To produce normal-sounding speech it is essential that the organs involved in respiration, phonation, and articulation are of normal structure and coordinated effectively. Respiratory flow is the power source behind speech. The air is channelled through the larynx and either the vocal cords vibrate, creating the voiced sounds, e.g. *b, d, g*, and the vowels, or the vocal cords remain open, allowing the production of voiceless sounds, e.g. *p, t, k, sh*, etc. The quality of the voice, appropriate pitch, modulation and intonation require sophisticated coordination of activity and inactivity of the larynx. The sound is conveyed into the mouth via the pharynx. Air is allowed to resonate in the nasal cavities for two sounds in English — these are *m* and *n*. The voiced and voiceless air is modified by the articulators to produce the various consonants. The airstream may be stopped to produce the plosive sounds — *t, k, g, p, b*, or interrupted, causing the friction required for the fricatives or affricate sounds, e.g. *sh, ch*, etc. The movements required for speech have to be produced quickly in a well-sequenced, coordinated and precise fashion. The only difference between the two words 'pat' and 'bat' are that the vocal cords come into play at an earlier stage for the latter than for the former. Thus, any imprecision caused by neurological dysfunction, scarring, tumour, or obstruction, would alter the precision, quality, tone or speed of speech (Daniloff, 1973).

Lesions of the central or peripheral nervous system may interrupt the central control of speech production. For example, lesions in the brainstem may produce bulbar palsy where the speech will be thick, nasal and imprecise. In cerebellar disorders the speech may be explosive and intermittent, and normal flow of speech will be interrupted, showing hesitations and arrhythmia. In basal ganglia disorders speech will be quiet and monotonous. The articulation will be unclear due to underarticulation or restricted movement of the tongue and lips.

Language production

The production of language is less clearly understood, and recent research has shown that some of the simplistic ideas with regard to localisation of language may be erroneous. In most patients the localisation of language is within the dominant cerebral hemisphere. There is not the clear division between receptive and expressive language as was once thought. Furthermore, the role of the non-dominant hemisphere with regard to interpretation of subtleties of language, and involvement in intonation and initiation of speech, has recently attracted more attention (Brookshire, 1978).

SPEECH AND LANGUAGE DISORDERS

There are four main groups of speech and language disorders which we may encounter with the disabled adult.

1. Disorders of articulation

It is important to understand the difference between the term ‘speech’ and term ‘language’. Speech may be used to express audible utterances, whereas language refers to vocabulary and grammar, or the content of those utterances which may be expressed in gesture, writing or speech. Articulation disorders are a disruption of speech, and there may be many causes of these. Damage to the structures required for speech, i.e. the tongue, the lips, the palate, the vocal cords, the lungs, etc., may affect the tone and quality. A cleft in the roof of the mouth may result in speech sounding hypernasal. A tongue badly scarred following an accident may have difficulty in moving precisely to the right place to form the different interruptions to the airflow which result in sound. Therefore, damage to a certain part of the articulatory system would affect speech in a fairly predictable fashion.

Loss of neuromuscular control due to central or peripheral nerve involvement results in changes of tone, coordination or precision, resulting in speech we commonly term 'dysarthric'. The features of the dysarthrias are listed in Table 15.1.

The term 'anarthria' is used to describe a complete loss of speech due to impairment of neuromuscular control, and the term 'dysarthria' is used to describe abnormal speech as the result of disorders of neuromuscular control affecting articulation, respiration, phonation and intonation. The different types of dysarthria may assist in localising the neurological damage, as the speech symptoms are frequently characteristic (Darley *et al.*, 1975).

2. Language disorders

The most commonly acquired disorder of language is dysphasia, which is a disorder of processing and formulating language. The terms 'aphasia' and 'dysphasia' are commonly used interchangeably, although the former term strictly refers to a complete language loss. The most common cause of dysphasia is a stroke affecting the dominant hemisphere. Patients with this disorder may have difficulty in understanding what is said to them, understanding what they read, and using the vocabulary and grammatical structures required to formulate what they wish to express. These symptoms may also be reflected in writing. Although dysphasic patients frequently have receptive and expressive difficulties, there may well be a disparity between the modalities; i.e. the dysphasic may be able to understand more than he can express, or vice-versa (Darley, 1982). There are many different combinations of language symptoms, and some schools suggest these have diagnostic implications (see Table 15.2).

3. Disorders of fluency

The inability to express oneself fluently due to hesitations, repetitions or blocking of articulation may be termed stammering or stuttering, the latter term being more frequently used in America to describe the same condition. A number of stammerers will develop secondary problems associated with fear of speaking, causing muscular twitching, poor eye contact, or avoidance of words and situations. Stammering is remarkably variable, and a sufferer may go through periods when he has difficulty in speaking in most situations and then have periods when he can express himself with ease (Gregory, 1979).

Table 15.1: Hierarchy of speech and bulbar deficits associated with different dysarthria types

Spastic dysarthria

1. Poor movement of tongue in speech.
2. Slow rate of speech.
3. Poor phonation and intonation.
4. Poor intelligibility in conversation.
5. Reduced alternating movements of the tongue.
6. Poor lip movements in speech.
7. Reduced maintenance of palatal elevation.
8. Poor intelligibility of description.
9. Hypernasality.
10. Lack of control of volume

Mixed dysarthria

1. Reduced ability to elevate tongue
2. Reduced ability to produce lateral movements of tongue.
3. Restriction of pitch.
4. Poor phonation and intonation
5. Reduced alternation of lip movement.
6. Reduced phonation time.
7. Reduced intelligibility of conversation.
8. Reduced rate of speech.
9. Reduced intelligibility of description.
10. Reduced tongue movement in speech.

Extrapyramidal hypokinetic dysarthria

1. Reduced phonation and intonation.
2. Increased rate of speech.
3. Reduced intelligibility of conversation.
4. Reduced control over volume.
5. Reduced phonation time.
6. Reduced ability to elevate tongue.
7. Reduced intelligibility of description.
8. Inadequate tongue movements in speech.
9. Reduced alternating movements of tongue.
10. Dribbling.

Ataxic dysarthria

1. Poor intonation and phonation.
2. Poor tongue movement in speech.
3. Poor alternating movement of tongue in speech.
4. Reduced rate of speech.
5. Poor swallowing.
6. Reduced lateral movement of tongue.
7. Reduced elevation of tongue.
8. Reduced intelligibility of conversation.
9. Poor alternating movements of lips.
10. Poor lip movements in speech.

Flaccid dysarthria

1. Poor lip seal.
2. Abnormality of lips at rest.
3. Abnormality of spread of lips.
4. Dribbling.
5. Reduced elevation of tongue.
6. Abnormality of tongue at rest.
7. Poor alternating movements of tongue.
8. Reduced phonation time.
9. Poor intelligibility of repetition.
10. Poor intelligibility of description.

Table 15.2: Speech–language characteristics of various aphasic syndromes from the Boston Classification System

Aphasic syndrome	Conversational speech	Auditory comprehension	Auditory speech repetition	Confrontation naming	Reading aloud	Reading comprehension	Writing
Broca	Non-fluent	Good	Abnormal	Abnormal	Abnormal	Good or abnormal	Abnormal
Wernicke	Fluent, paraphasic	Abnormal	Abnormal	Abnormal	Abnormal	Abnormal	Abnormal
Conduction	Fluent, paraphasic	Good	Abnormal	Usually good	Abnormal	Good	Abnormal
Transcortical motor	Non-fluent	Good	Good	Abnormal	Abnormal	Often good	Abnormal
Transcortical sensory	Fluent, paraphasic, echolalic	Severely abnormal	Good	Abnormal	Abnormal	Abnormal	Abnormal
Mixed transcortical	Non-fluent with echolalia	Severely abnormal	Good	Severely abnormal	Abnormal	Abnormal	Abnormal

Adapted from: Benson, D. F. (1979) *Aphasia, alexia and agraphia,* Churchill Livingstone, New York. As published in SMCL Preprints, R. McNeil (1981)

4. Disorders of voice

Dysphonia (abnormal phonation) may be a symptom of neurological, organic or psychological disorder. Amongst the organic dysphonias are those resulting from polyps, nodules and oedema of the vocal cords. Stress and tension may also be an underlying cause of dysphonia without obvious organic involvement. Dysphonia is frequently looked upon as a cosmetic rather than an actual disability, but many patients will suffer personal and employment difficulties if this symptom is not treated. Aphonia results from laryngectomy, which may be required following irremediable cancer or trauma to the larynx (Greene, 1980).

MAIN SPEECH AND LANGUAGE DISORDERS ASSOCIATED WITH COMMON DISEASES OR CONDITIONS

1. Mental handicap

One of the largest group of people suffering speech and language handicap is those with mental handicap, the prevalence being 2,500 per 100,000. One of the main considerations is whether the speech and language is in line with mental ability, or are contributing substantially to lack of development. If speech and language are out of line with mental age, then remediation may substantially assist the person's functional improvement. Frequently the reduced demands, limited environment and associated disabilities can restrict the mentally handicapped person's language development, and treatment within realistic limits is possible. The mentally handicapped person may suffer from phonological disorders which may be a direct result of learning difficulties, requiring specific training to improve articulation, or he may have difficulty retaining vocabulary to express his needs and wants. In some cases simple signing systems, e.g. hand signs, Makaton, or Picture Signs — Blissymbolics — can extend communication, which helps the carer and the cared for.

2. Stuttering

The prevelance of this disorder is about 1 per cent. Frequently, children who have done poorly in therapy at school will have a different attitude to therapy when faced with motivating factors such as attracting and keeping girl/boyfriends or going for jobs.

The underlying causes of stuttering are much debated. There are schools of thought which dwell upon psychological aspects, and other schools which emphasise abnormal neurological transmission. It is likely that there is more than one cause which is exacerbated by the secondary problems associated with having a speech disorder for a long period of time, such as lack of confidence and situation-avoidance. Speech therapy can occasionally resolve somebody's fluency disorder, but in most cases aims to assist the person to control the stammer by using attitude and pacing techniques. Most approaches help the patient by teaching him techniques which control the speed and manner of expression. In conjunction with this it is important for the therapist to improve the person's attitude to speaking situations to increase his confidence, and assist the patient to overcome some of the habitual aspects of this disorder. Surprisingly it may be difficult for him to become accustomed to fluency if he has been used to being dysfluent for a long time. The speech therapist can assist the stutterer to have a realistic approach so that he can assert control over his speech.

3. Deafness

Approximately 200 persons per 100,000 population are severely deaf. Of these, 60 per cent have deafness to a level which impairs speech and language. If a person is born deaf, not only his speech but also his vocabulary will be limited, due to restricted learning opportunities. With acquired deafness, modulation of voice and the use of appropriate stress and pitch become involved at an early stage, whereas articulatory precision may deteriorate later. In addition to speech therapy, the hearing therapists and teachers of the deaf help in the management of this disability. This may include practical advice with regard to management of the hearing aid, teaching of lip-reading and speaking skills, and general advice on how to cope with such a hidden and isolating condition. A number of deaf persons will require intermittent assistance to ensure that their speech does not deteriorate to a level where it is difficult for others to understand (see Chapter 17).

4. Cerebral palsy

One hundred and seventy-five people per 100,000 suffer from cerebral palsy. This term is used to describe a heterogeneous group of disorders and disabilities with a variety of aetiologies that have the common elements of being developmental, neuromotor disorders that are the result of non-progressive abnormalities of the developing brain. Sixty per cent of persons with cerebral palsy will have a speech and/or language disorder. The majority will be dysarthric, but in addition there may be language disorders, due to specific problems such as dysphasia or developmental delay, memory problems or reduced intellectual function; these may be concomitant problems with the dysarthria (Hardy, 1983).

Cerebral palsied children are now attracting much more specialised educational assistance, but this has not always been the case, and there are many adults with cerebral palsy who have not had appropriate assessment and treatment. Frequently they do not get referred, as they have suffered their condition for so many years, everyone assuming that all has been done, but this is not necessarily so. Techniques and technology have developed rapidly, enabling us to help the more severely physically handicapped. Detailed assessment of the cerebral palsied person is essential to gauge the degree of mental, physical and speech disability, and thus appropriate therapy to maximise communication can be given. In some cases speech therapy can assist by helping the person to improve his articulation; in other cases alternative communication via communication aids or sign systems is more appropriate.

5. Stroke

The prevalence of speech or language disorder secondary to stroke is about 150 people per 100,000. The majority of these will have language disorder, i.e. dysphasia, which is commonly associated with a lesion in the temporal lobe of the dominant cerebral hemisphere. Inferior lesions are suggested to cause more impairment of comprehension, whereas posterior superior lesions cause non-fluent expressive dysphasia and frontal lesions cause fluent expressive dysphasia. Non-fluent dysphasia is demonstrated when the person grasps for words, repeats the same word frequently, and has a very restricted vocabulary. Fluent dysphasia is used to describe those patients who speak readily, but use jargon consisting mainly of nonsense words. Intonation may be preserved, assisting the listener to guess the speaker's intent (Lesser, 1978).

Bilateral cortical damage will result in spastic dysarthria, characterised by a strained, husky, weak voice, imprecise articulation and hypernasality. These patients will commonly have problems with swallowing and dribbling, particularly in the first two weeks post-stroke.

There is a common misconception that the main role of the speech therapist is to initiate and guide exercises which release, increase, develop or clarify the speech of the disabled person. It is important to emphasise in this chapter that this is only one element of the speech therapist's involvement with the post-stroke patient. As language is an integral part of human behaviour and relationships the approach to its remediation is necessarily eclectic. It is essential that the disorder is assessed so that all those caring for the patient are aware of the extent of his disabilities and the areas of retained ability. For example, a patient who has difficulty understanding the spoken words may have greater ability in understanding what he reads. This knowledge will help all those involved. The shock of losing one's speech is fundamental, and can be soul-destroying to all family members. The speech therapist is in a position to assist and support the family in their period of readjustment, which sometimes takes many months. A person's vocation, social life, self-esteem and personal hobbies can be destroyed by losing his power of communication; support and attention from a person with specialised knowledge may be of paramount importance (Enderby and Langton Hewer, 1985).

6. Other acquired neurological disease

Many people suffering from other acquired neurological diseases will have a speech disorder. The most common diseases which affect speech are: Parkinson's disease, multiple sclerosis, Friedreich's ataxia, muscular dystrophy, motor neurone disease, myasthenia gravis and Huntington's chorea. The prevalence for these acquired neurological diseases (excluding stroke) is 250 per 100,000. Of these, about half may develop a speech and language disorder. The majority of patients with these disorders will have dysarthria due to neuromuscular involvement. Additionally, many of them will have feeding and swallowing problems.

Many patients with Parkinson's disease will notice that their voice becomes quieter as the disease progresses. Others will find that they have difficulty in starting speech, or that their speaking rate increases and becomes festinant. The onset of this extapyramidal dysarthria is insiduous, and the patients themselves may not notice that they are having difficulty in making themselves understood until well after there is a major problem. There is some evidence that short intensive courses of speech therapy to improve self-monitoring, re-establish control over speaking rate and to improve breathing and phonation can assist the patient to re-attain some degree of clarity (Scott and Caird, 1981).

A few patients with multiple sclerosis develop dysphasia in addition to the more common dysarthria during the course of the disease. Occasionally both symptoms are temporary, and are related to an exacerbation in the condition. In other cases the symptoms persist and require attention. There may be some degree of intellectual involvement, which will affect the type of therapy appropriate. Many patients will benefit from learning compensatory methods which may assist the quality as well as the intelligibility of their speech, but a few will have difficulty retaining information; thus teaching a patient to improve the clarity of his articulation would be inappropriate, and using simple communication aids, or teaching the family prompting methods, may be more realistic. Medical textbooks often cite that the dysarthria associated with multiple sclerosis is cerebellar in origin, and describe 'scanning speech'. However, more recent studies show that the most common dysarthria is associated with upper motor neurone involvement, causing spasticity to the muscles of articulation.

Nearly all patients suffering from motor neurone disease will become dysarthric during the course of their disorder. A significant number will be anarthric (Newrick and Langton Hewer, 1984). Very few will have any intellectual impairment, and the frustrations and difficulties of coming to terms with a very distressing, progressive disease are heightened by the reduced ability to communicate effectively. The speech therapist's role is associated not only with ameliorating some of the bulbar symptoms, but also assisting with the management of adapting to non-vocal methods. Speech therapists can often understand disordered speech which others find difficult, and they frequently become the person who can most easily communicate with the patient, and have to take on the role of interpreter, as well as therapist. Again, we find the speech therapist's work goes beyond what is immediately apparent. She may frequently have to help the patient to understand, and come to terms with, other non-specific bulbar dysfunctions, e.g. emotional lability.

The majority of patients with dysarthria will have feeding and swallowing problems. Recently, speech therapists have become involved in the management of dysphagia. Certainly the techniques used to assist and improve muscular control and coordination for speech are not dissimilar to those which assist with swallowing, so this seems a natural development.

7. Laryngectomy

The prevalence of laryngectomy is approximately 3 per 100,000. Fortunately, the prevalence has reduced significantly in the past decade due to earlier detection and greater success with curative radiotherapy. The population now undergoing laryngectomy is older, with more additional handicaps. Furthermore, they tend to have either suffered larger lesions requiring more radical surgery, or have endured long courses of preoperative radiotherapy, which render healing more difficult. Thus the techniques the speech therapist used some ten years ago have had to be adapted, as the population has more associated difficulties.

Patients should be given the opportunity to learn oesophageal speech. This pseudo-voice is dependent on the patient injecting air into the upper oesophagus which is returned with some vibration, causing a sound which can be used for speech. Approximately one-third of patients will be able to learn oesophageal speech to a level which is sufficient for them to communicate in most situations and on the phone. Another one-third will be able to use oesophageal speech with their family and friends, but may not be skilled enough to use it elsewhere. Unfortunately, the remaining third of laryngectomy patients have a great deal of difficulty in learning this method of communication. It is likely that this is due to the type of surgery undertaken, which restricts the motility of the upper oesophagus. Oesophageal voice is limited in its range, and may require a great deal of concentration. It can be impeded by such things as chest infections and colds. It is now thought that all laryngectomy patients should have the back-up of an electrolarynx for augmentative use. Recently surgical vocal reconstruction techniques have attracted much attention. One of the more successful has been the 'tracheo-oesophageal shunt'. A small valve — many types have been tried — can be placed by the patient to maintain the patency of a surgically produced puncture between the trachea and oesophagus. By placing a finger on the stoma, the patient diverts air into the oesophagus and thus can produce 'oesophageal speech' with greater ease (Perry, 1984).

8. Head injury

The prevalence of patients disabled following head injury is hard to establish. However, it has been suggested that 160 persons per 100,000 have a severe speech and language disorder as the result of head trauma. A number of patients will have a combination of dysarthria, dysphasia and dyspraxia. Some may have a very specific isolated disorder, but many patients following head injury will have disorders arising from impaired concentration, cognition and memory. The speech therapists's role with the head-injured patient is very much as a member of the team and, as with many other disorders, her input may continue for many months as improvement of communication may be slow (Levin, 1981).

HELPING THE PATIENT WHO HAS DIFFICULTY IN UNDERSTANDING

These guidelines will assist communication with speech and language disabled, but should be modified according to severity of disorder.

A: Understanding the dysphasic patient

(1) When speaking to the dysphasic patient, keep in full view of him, so that your facial movement and facial expression can be observed — do not mouth or exaggerate your facial expression.
(2) Never underestimate a patient's comprehension
(3) Avoid long rambling conversations — they are almost always misunderstood.
(4) Do not demand too much of the patient when he is agitated.

Fatigue or emotional upset adversely affect comprehension and expression.

(5) Avoid noisy rooms. Some language-disabled patients are distractable and have difficulty in concentrating.

(6) Some limited gesture may help the person to understand, but it must not be exaggerated.

(7) Use repetition. If the patient has not understood a question or statement, repeat what you said but phrase it slightly differently.

(8) Speech should be a little slower than normal, and if hearing is good, the voice should be clear but not raised.

(9) Single words often convey less than a phrase or short sentence. Therefore it is best to talk to the patient using familiar words in short sentences with a slight pause.

(10) Do not change the subject too quickly.

(11) The patient will understand and express himself more easily when he is in familiar surroundings, talking about familiar things.

(12) Allow more time for a speech/language handicapped patient to start his response. Do not assume that he has not understood immediately. It takes more time for him to assimilate what has been said to him.

B: Helping the patient who has difficulty speaking

(1) Give the appearance that you have time to listen to the patient's attempt to speak. Do not guess at his utterance unless you are sure that he wishes you to do so.

(2) Communication in any way should be encouraged, e.g. if he can write or do a 'thumbs-up' sign, then these should be accepted.

(3) Encourage the person to use all the speech that is available to him, and give him opportunities to try and speak. Persons with speech difficulties often function at a lower level than they are capable of. They may well withdraw from speaking situations and inhibit their speech due to embarrassment and frustration.

(4) Try to avoid asking a question of a relative about the patient when he can answer for himself, e.g. 'Does he take sugar in his tea?'

(5) Talking to a speech-handicapped patient on his own will often reduce embarrassment on both sides.

(6) If a patient is learning to speak, he must 'want' to learn to speak; therefore encourage discussion which is motivating and stimulating.

(7) If the patient is having difficulty in expressing himself, allow him time. If he still fails, supply the words for him and encourage these to be repeated.

(8) If the patient uses one-word sentences, e.g. 'Out', encourage him, as this is meaningful, but expand the sentence for him by saying, 'I want to go out.'

(9) Sometimes it is easier for the staff and the patient to avoid speaking, due to the obvious effort on both parts. As far as possible these occasions should never arise.

(10) Dysphasic patients are at their best when the routine is familiar to them. Always promote some communication at regular times, e.g. always say, 'Good morning', 'How many sugars do you take?' etc. These questions will become familiar and he will be less tense, encouraging an improved response.

COMMUNICATION AIDS

Some patients who have difficulty in making themselves understood may benefit from a communication aid. These may assist existing speech to be more intelligible, e.g. an amplifier, or they may replace speech so that a person is able to communicate via the aid, e.g. a typewriter. However, all communication aids require a degree of language ability and therefore they are mainly used by people with speech disability with retained language, e.g. dysarthric patients. Thus the majority of those stroke patients who have dysphasia are unable to use a communication aid due to the inability to recall the words that they wish to express, making it impossible to express them through any mode, be it through speech, writing or communication aid. Therefore, unfortunately, there remain a greater number of speechless people who cannot benefit from the technology that is presently available.

There are more than 60 different communication aids available in Great Britain, and it is important that the patient is thoroughly assessed so that the correct equipment is given. The speech therapist has to assess the language abilities, the physical abilities, eyesight, hearing and psychological factors. She will work with the doctor, occupational therapist and physiotherapist, to assess these areas, and to determine the most suitable aid. Aids can be categorised according to the method of input. There are three groups of aids — direct select, scanning and encoding.

Direct select

Vanderheiden and Grilley (1976) explain that this is any technique in which the desired choice is directly indicated by the user. This can involve the use of any part of the body which may be able to directly make an indication of a symbol. Obviously, the easiest facility should be used, though the upper body is used in preference, when possible. This may be, for example, finger, elbow, chin, fist or eyeball. If these sites are ruled out, then the lower body, e.g. foot, may be chosen. Simple appliances which might aid this indication, such as head sticks, mouth sticks, hand sticks, may need to be considered. If direct selection is a possibility, then this method is preferred above the others. It is a recognised means of indicating wants and needs, requires low cognitive skills and becomes a rapid method with practice. However, it requires accuracy and a reasonable range of movement. The advantage of this method is its wide range of application. The moderately intelligible dysarthric person may use an alphabet board and point to the first letter of each word as he says it; or, aids using conventional keyboards such as electric typewriters and computers may be appropriate. Some aids which are specifically made for the handicapped, and which use the direct-select technique, are the Canon Communicator, which is a small, hand-held method of typing one's communication, or a Memowriter, which has not only a print-out facility, but also a light-emitting diode (LED) (Figures 15.1–15.3).

Scanning

This method of indication would be chosen for those severely speech-handicapped individuals who are also grossly physically handicapped. It is a relatively slow method and is cognitively more complex than direct selection. Methods of scanning are 'any technique in which the selections are offered to the user by a person or display'. Depending on the aid, the user may respond by signalling when he sees the correct choice presented (Vanderheiden and Grilley, 1976). The simplest scanning method is a run-through of yes–no questions. The individual uses a prepared signal to indicate the required item.

Linear scanning involves an item-by-item scan for the individual, indicating when his chosen subject is reached. Items may be displayed on a simple communication chart, or a clockface with an indicator. In group item scanning the letters, words or symbols are placed in rows or groups. The individual is encouraged to scan along a row, until he indicates when the appropriate column is reached. This column is then, in turn, scanned to reach the correct item (Figures 15.4 and 15.5).

Encoding

This technique is cognitively sophisticated, but is very useful for individuals who may wish to use a large vocabulary even though they may have limited movement. Encoding may be described as a method by which the individual makes his choice from a pattern or code of symbols which, when decoded, indicate his message. The code needs to be either memorised or set out on separate cards for reference. Morse code may be considered as such a method, where sequences of dots and dashes, when decoded, represent traditional orthography. Another simple encoding method may be to have on one card a list of commonly used phrases, with each of these being numbered. On another card there can be the numbers of the phrases. It is

Figure 15.1: Lightwriter with a larger keyboard, green dual display and memory facility

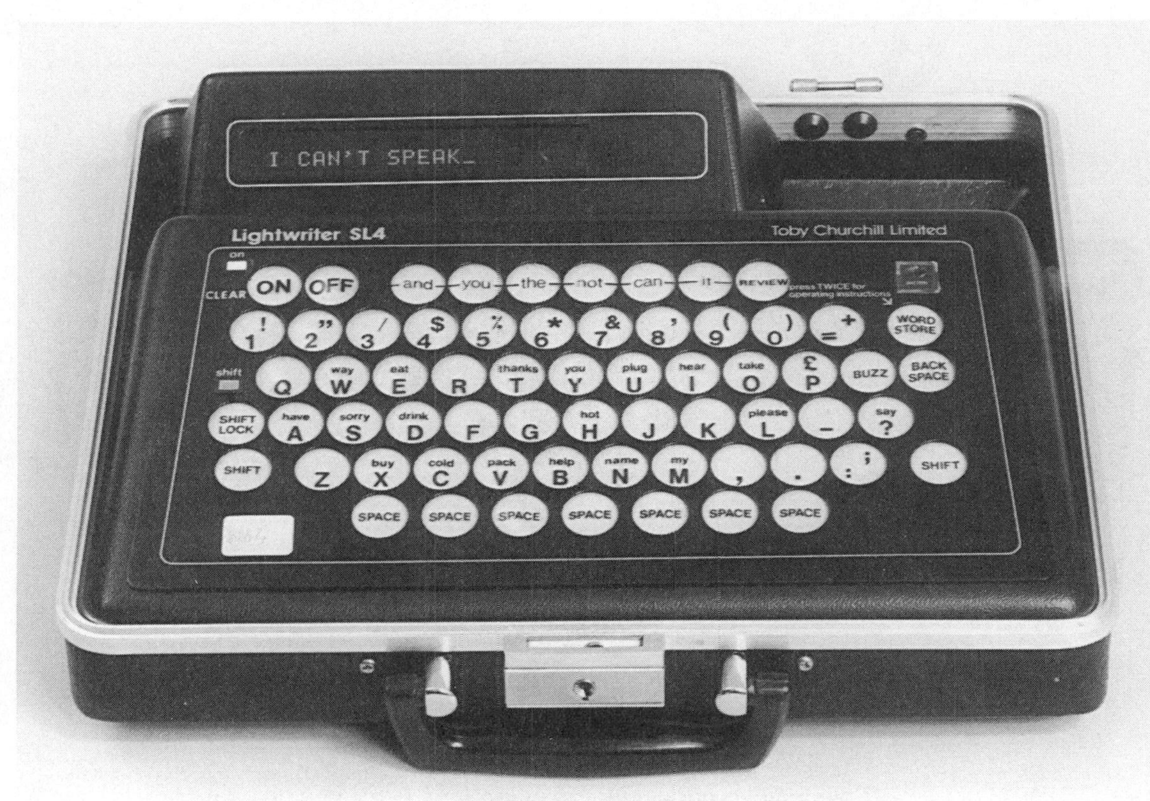

Figure 15.2: Canon communicator with print-out; simple message-taker

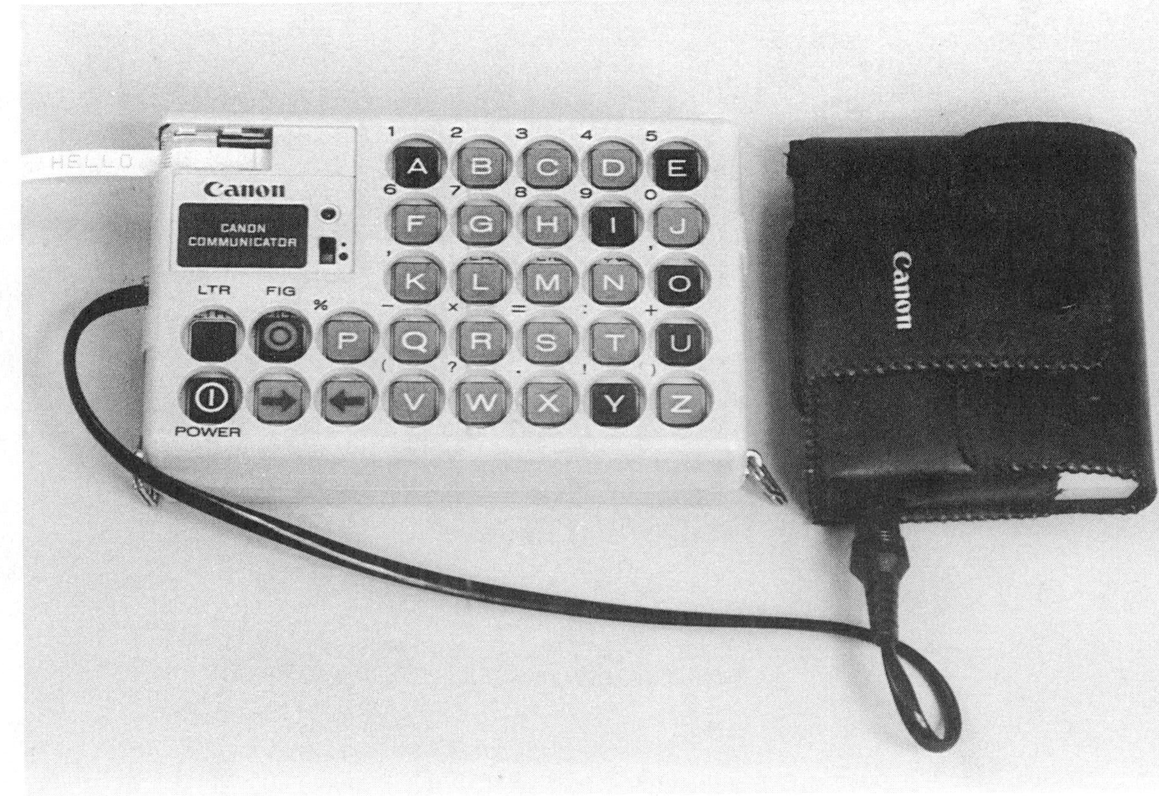

Figure 15.3: Microwriter, a flexible, portable electronic device which can be used with various terminal devices

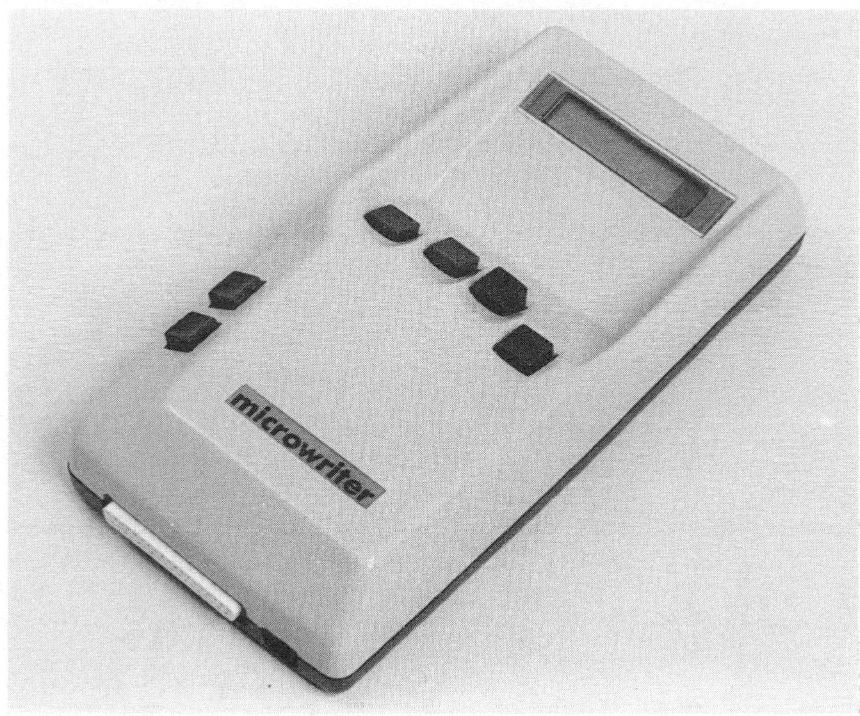

possible then for the individual to indicate a number by an arranged method, which will correspond to the appropriate phrase.

Encoding may be combined with direct-selection or with scanning, in order to indicate messages.

PROMOTING SUCCESSFUL USE OF COMMUNICATION AIDS

It is important that the therapist considers the environment in which the patient is going to communicate, as it is essential that communication is not seen as a one-way process. For example, if the main carer has hearing or eyesight problems this may directly affect the type of equipment that is most useful in that situation.

The patient should have a total communication system, and sometimes a sophisticated technical device has to be backed up with a simple picture board or sign system which can be available to the patient for longer periods, and can be used as back-up in the event of technical problems with

Figure 15.4: Possum 100 SP: light scanning communication aid, with numerous variations and with synthetic speech

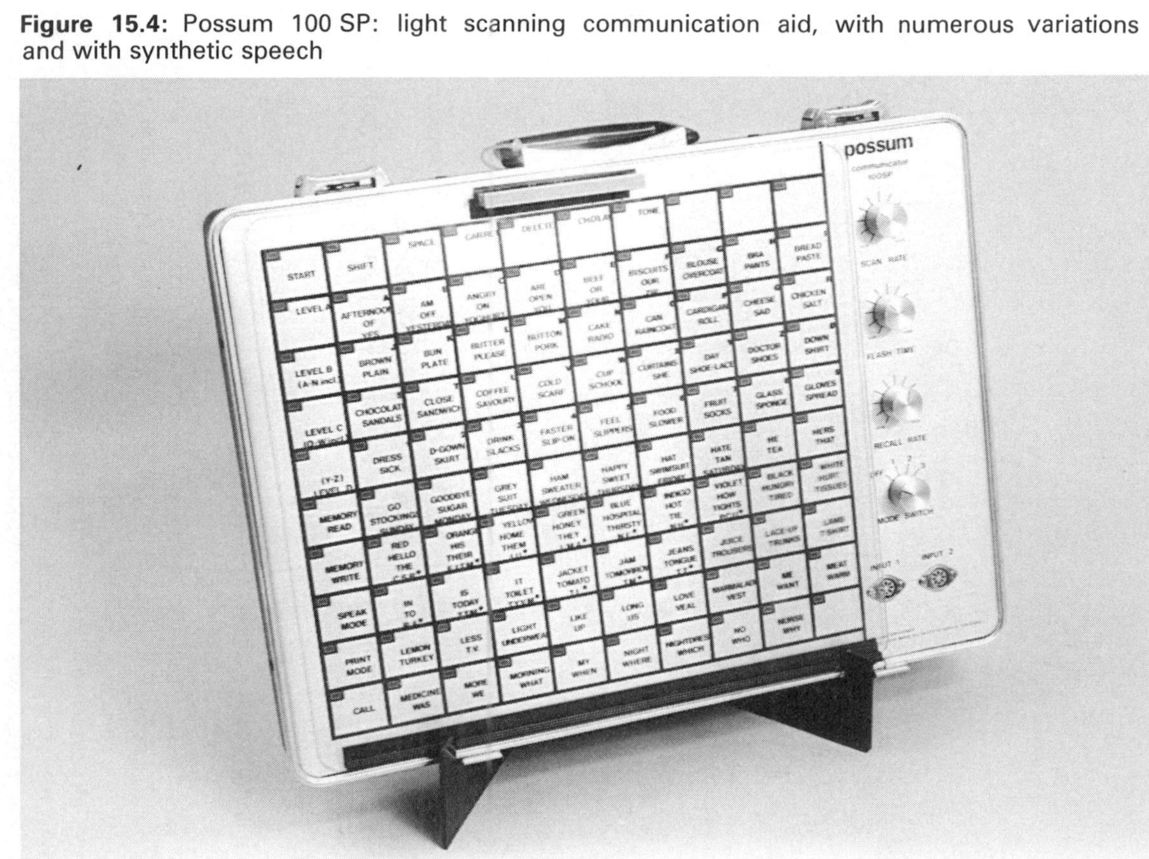

Figure 15.5: Toucan communicator: light scanning device which can be linked to computer, speech synthesiser; it has a dual display

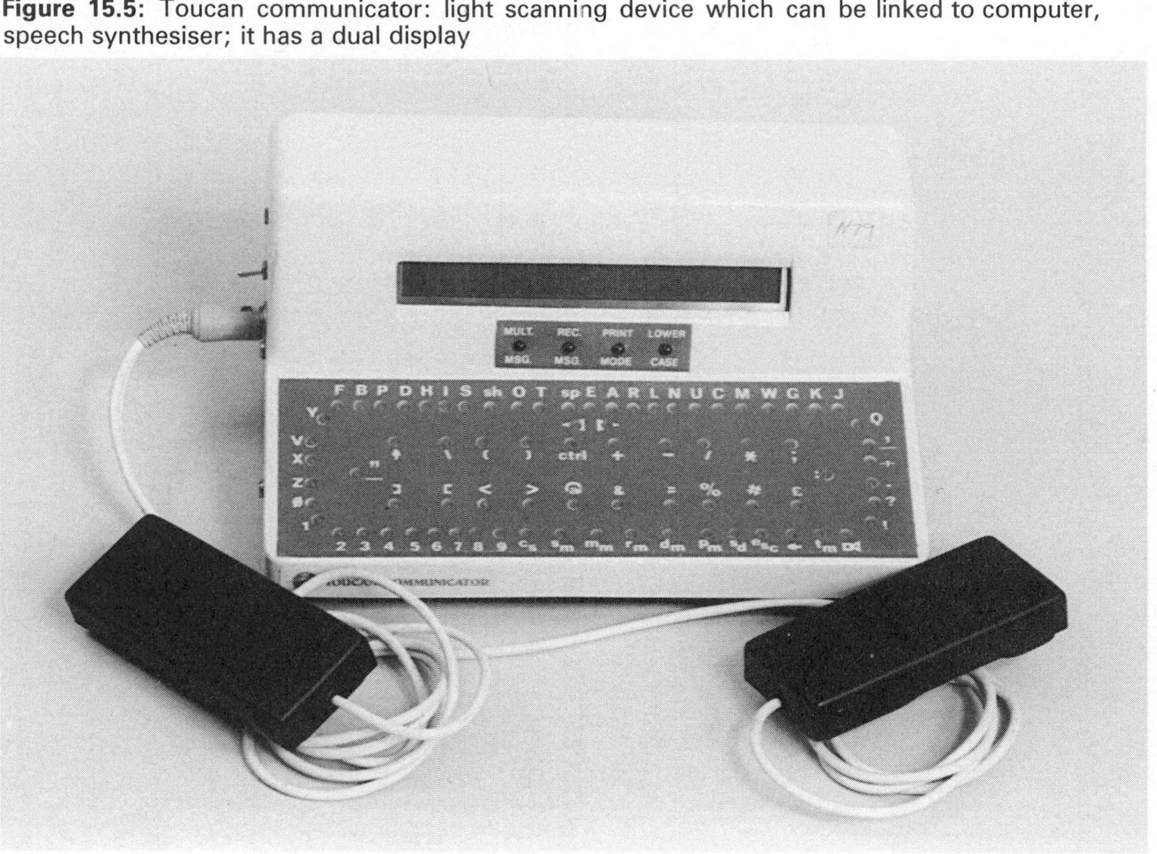

the aid. Continued access to the speech therapy department is required for any aid-user, as the interfaces may need to be adapted according to changes in the patient's condition, be it for better or worse, or if the patient's environmental needs change (Musselwhite and Louis, 1982).

Considerable help is available from communication aid centres; in addition many speech therapy departments carry a stock of aids for loan. In all cases patients who use communication aids can be helped by the following:

(1) Ensure that the aid is near and accessible to the patient.

(2) Encourage the patient to use the aid. No communication aid can replicate the speed of speech; patience on the part of both the listener and speaker is essential.

(3) Do not change the subject too quickly. The aid-user may be replying to one question, and if other questions are fired it is difficult for him to catch up.

(4) It is important that the communication aid is accepted and not looked upon as a toy or a joke. Some patients reject equipment that can be most useful because of the attitudes of other people around them.

(5) Many patients can communicate a little verbally or by facial expression. Encourage this, along with the rest of their communication, through their communication aid.

ASSISTING THE PATIENT WHO HAS SWALLOWING PROBLEMS

Many patients with neuromotor speech disorders may develop problems with swallowing, which are distressing not only to the patient, but also to the relatives. Frequently dysphagia can be secondary to stroke, motor neurone disease, multiple sclerosis, and in some patients with Parkinson's disease. To help the patient feed more comfortably and safely it is important to understand what is involved in the swallowing mechanism. There are three phases to swallowing: the *oral* phase, which takes place in the mouth and is under voluntary control; the *pharyngeal* phase, which takes place in the upper part of the throat; and the *oesophageal* phase, which carries the food from the back of the throat to the stomach. These last two phases are mostly under reflex control and thus we shall concern ourselves particularly with the oral phase, as it is the one over which we therapists have the most influence (Groher, 1984).

Symptoms corresponding to various neuromuscular swallowing difficulties

1. Disorders affecting preparation of the bolus

The patient may have difficulty in masticating, due to weakness of the buccal musculature or restriction of tongue movement which normally distributes food between the teeth for grinding, and then retrieves the food to form the bolus. Reduced labial closure may allow food or liquid to fall from the mouth while the bolus is being prepared. Some patients have reduced oral sensitivity which would affect this preparatory phase.

2. Disorders affecting propulsion of the bolus

The bolus, having been retrieved, has to be moved from the front to the back of the mouth, and this is usually done by elevation of the front of the tongue which squeezes the bolus backwards. Any restriction in the movement of the tongue will have an effect upon this propulsion. As the bolus moves posteriorly the palate is raised to seal the nose from the pharynx and prevent food regurgitation up into the naso-pharynx.

3. The swallow reflex

The swallow reflex is triggered by the sensory receptors in the anterior aspect of the faucial arch. Normally the timing of the reflex is such that the posterior movement of the bolus is not interrupted. Some patients do not trigger a reflex until the bolus has contacted the aryepiglotic fold, while others trigger the reflex only when the material has fallen into the pyriform sinuses. This delay in the reflex being triggered may result in slow eating or, more seriously, may give rise to aspiration.

4. Cricopharyngeal dysfunction

The cricopharyngeus muscle is in a state of tonic contraction during rest. During swallowing, respiration is halted and the cricopharyngeus must relax as the bolus approaches. If this does not happen the patient may feel that he is having to force food down his throat. He may complain of feeling a ridge or obstruction. The dysfunction of the cricopharyngeus muscle may be related to various upper motor neurone lesions, or due to fibrosis in this area.

There are many other swallowing problems which can cause distress and concern to the patient and his relatives. The speech therapist frequently works with the physiotherapist and dietician to analyse exactly the type of feeding problem that the patient is suffering, and to develop a feeding programme which will increase confidence and promote better integration of the retained facilities.

The following feeding programme may be adapted for individual patients, but gives the bases which may assist neurologically damaged patients.

Guidelines to help those with swallowing disorders

(1) *Posture.* Make sure that the patient is sitting comfortably, with head upright. Support the head if this is required.
(2) *Relax.* Ensure that the patient is in a calm frame of mind before eating or drinking. Stress and tension are often associated with exacerbating dysphagia.
(3) *Do not talk.* Avoid speaking during the meal. It may be helpful to be silent for a couple of minutes before eating or drinking.
(4) *Yawn.* Encourage the patient to yawn before eating if the throat feels tight. This may ease the constriction.
(5) *Feeding routine.* Encourage the patient to follow this purposeful routine:
  (a) place a small amount of food in the mouth;
  (b) close the lips tightly;
  (c) chew;
  (d) pause;
  (e) give purposeful swallows;
  (f) pause.
(6) *Food textures.* Avoid mixing fluids and solids, e.g. minestrone soup. Also avoid any foods which are crumbly. Frequently, smooth semi-solids are best for these patients. Food should neither be too liquid nor too solid.
(7) *Small meals.* It is advisable to have several small meals a day rather than two or three big meals.
(8) *Fatigue.* The patient should stop eating if feeling tired with the effort.
(9) *After the meal.* Drink a small amount of water to swill the mouth out, and cough to make sure that the throat and mouth are clear. Remain sitting for at least half an hour after eating or drinking.

CONCLUSION

Speech and language disorders are rarely restricted to the obvious defects which meet the ear. Frequently they cause misery to the patient and relatives, who may have difficulty in understanding a defect which is not visible, and which is frequently variable. The techniques available to the speech therapist have progressed over the past decade and our understanding, ability to analyse, and skills in remediation have grown. Therapists are now more aware of the realistic objectives which should be employed in active treatment of adult patients with acquired disorders. They are familiar with, and welcome being involved in, the caring aspects of the chronically disabled.

REFERENCES

Brown, B.B. (1981) *Speech therapy principles and practice*, Churchill Livingstone, Edinburgh

Brookshire, R.H. (1978) Auditory comprehension and aphasia. In D.F. Johns (ed.), *Management of neurogenic communicative disorders*, Little Brown & Co., Boston, pp. 103-29

Daniloff, R.G. (1973) Normal articulation processes. In F. Minifie, T. Hixon and F. Williams (eds), *Normal aspects of speech hearing and language*, Prentice Hall, Englewood-Cliffs, New Jersey, pp. 169-211

Darley, F. (1982) *Aphasia*, W.B. Saunders, Philadelphia

Darley, F., Aronson, A. and Brown, J. (1975) *Motor speech disorders*, W.B. Saunders, Philadelphia

Dickson, D. and Dickson, W. (1983) *Anatomical and physiological bases of speech*, Little Brown & Co., Boston

Enderby, P. (1986) Relationships between dysarthric groups. *Br. J. Dis. Commun.*, *21*, 189-97

Enderby, P. and Langton Hewer, R. (1985) The context and management of acquired speech and language. In B. Isaacs (ed.), *Recent advances in geriatric medicine*, Churchill Livingstone, Edinburgh

Gregory, H. (1979) *Controversies about stuttering therapy*. University Park Press, Baltimore

Greene M.C. (1980) *The voice and its disorders*, Pitman Medical, London

Groher, M. (1984) *Dysphagia*, Butterworths, Boston

Hardy, C.J. (1983) *Cerebral palsy*, Prentice-Hall, Englewood Cliffs, New Jersey, pp. 200-5

Lesser, R. (1978) *Linguistic investigations of aphasia*, Edward Arnold, London

Levin, H. (1981) *Linguistic recovery after closed head injury. Brain Lang.*, *12*, 360-74

Musselwhite, C.R. and Louis, K.W. (1982) *Communication programming for severely handicapped: vocal and non-vocal strategies*, College Hill Press, San Diego

Newrick, P. and Langton Hewer, R. (1984) *Motor neurone disease: can we do better?* A study of 42 patients. *Br. Med. J.*, *289*, 539-42

Perry, A. (1984) The speech therapist's role in surgical and prosthetic approaches to speech rehabilitation. In Y. Edels (ed.), *Laryngectomy: diagnosis to rehabilitation*, Croom Helm, London, pp. 271-89

Scott, S. and Caird, A. (1981) Speech therapy for patients with Parkinson's disease. *Br. med. J.*, *283*, 1088

Vanderheiden, G. and Grilley, K. (1976) *Non-vocal communication techniques and aids for severely physically handicapped*, University Park Press, Baltimore

READING FOR PATIENTS AND RELATIVES

Communication aids — a guide for people who have difficulty speaking, Research Institute for Consumer Affairs, 14 Buckingham Street, London WC2N 6DF

Help the Stroke Patient to Talk, Marie Crickmay. Charles C. Thomas, Springfield, Illinois, 1977

Communication in Parkinson's Disease, S. Scott, F. Caird and B. Williams. Croom Helm, London, 1985

Language remediation and expansion — workshops for parents and teachers, Catherine Bush. Communication Skill Builders, Tucson, Arizona, 1981

ADDRESSES OF COMMUNICATION AIDS CENTRES (CACs)

Speech Therapy Dept, Frenchay Hospital, Bristol BS16 1LE

Communication Aids Centre (Speech Therapy), Charing Cross Hospital, Fulham Palace Road, London W6 8RF

Communication Aids Centre, The Wolfson Centre, Mecklenburgh Square, London WC1N 2AP

Communication Aids Centre, The Dene Centre, Castles Farm Road, Newcastle-upon-Tyne NE3 1QH

Rehabilitation Engineering Dept, Rookwood Hospital, Llandaff, Cardiff, South Glamorgan CF5 2YN

Sandwell Health Authority CAC, Boulton Road, West Bromwich, West Midlands B70 6NN

FURTHER READING

Communication: equipment for the Disabled (ed. R.M. Wilshire). Oxford Health Authority

16

Visual Handicap

Roger Coakes

INTRODUCTION

The normally sighted adult who loses vision may face formidable social, economic and emotional problems. Help in overcoming these problems is available from a variety of agencies, but there is no clear-cut pathway for the rehabilitation of the visually handicapped. Indeed, it would be surprising if there were, for individual requirements vary considerably depending on the extent of the handicap, age, adaptability, emotional resilience and so on.

The aim of this chapter is to outline the causes of visual handicap, the practical steps that can be taken to maximise use of residual vision and the help that can be obtained from the various agencies concerned with the welfare of the blind and the partially sighted.

THE NATURE OF VISUAL HANDICAP

Visual handicap may result from loss of central vision, loss of peripheral vision or both. Less commonly it can be caused by a disorder of ocular motility and, very occasionally, there may be a psychogenic basis.

The macular area of the retina is responsible for the fine, discriminating vision necessary for reading and other detailed close work, and the visual acuity is a measure of this function of central vision. Colour vision is also predominantly a function of the central retina where the concentration of cone photoreceptors is greatest.

The outer part of the visual field is essential for full awareness of the immediate environment and, in particular, for navigation. The peripheral retina contains mainly rod photoreceptors which function more efficiently than the cone photoreceptors at low levels of illumination, and dark adaptation, essential for good night vision, is a function of the peripheral retina.

PARTIAL SIGHT AND BLINDNESS

Few people registered as blind are totally without sight; that is unable to differentiate between light and dark (Table 16.1). Generally speaking a person is eligible for blind registration if his visual acuity with both eyes together is less than 3/60, but a person with better, or even normal, visual acuity may be eligible if the field of vision is severely contracted. The definition of blindness is therefore deliberately vague, and for registration in the United Kingdom a person must be considered 'so blind as to be unable to perform any work for which eyesight is essential'.

There is no statutory definition of partial sight, but for registration purposes those with visual acuity between 3/60 and 6/60 are eligible, as are those with better visual acuity but whose visual fields are contracted. It should be noted that loss of vision in one eye, even if total, does not by itself constitute partial sight for registration purposes.

THE INCIDENCE AND PREVALENCE OF VISUAL DISABILITY

Approximately 12,000 individuals are registered as blind in England and Wales each year, of whom 72 per cent are over the age of 70 (Sorsby, 1972).

The prevalence of visual disability has been steadily rising as the population has aged, and approximately 340 per 100,000 of the population are now registered as blind or partially sighted. In 1980 there were officially 120,000 blind and 40,000 partially sighted individuals in England and Wales (DHSS, 1980).

These figures do not give a complete picture of the extent of visual disability in the community for many, especially the elderly, have vision that is poor but still too good for the purpose of registration. Cullinan (1977), in a community-based survey, found that 520 adults per 100,000 had a visual acuity of less than 6/18 when examined in their own homes, but less than one-third would have been eligible for blind or partial sighted

Table 16.1: The vision of those registered as blind

Level of vision	Percentage of total
Total blindness	3.4
Perception of light only	10.4
Hand movements to 3/60	58.8
Visual acuity better than 3/60	27.4

Source: Sorsby, A. (1966) *The incidence and causes of blindness in England and Wales, 1948–1962*, HMSO, London

registration on grounds of visual acuity alone. He also showed that visual acuity measured at home was considerably worse than when measured in a hospital clinic, and Silver and colleagues (1978), in a subsequent study, concluded that if hospital conditions of illumination existed at home the number of adults functioning as visually disabled would be substantially reduced.

THE CAUSES OF VISUAL DISABILITY

The leading causes of blindness in the UK are given by age in Table 16.2.

Senile macular degeneration

This is the commonest cause of blindness among persons over the age of 65. Distortion of central vision progresses to the development of a dense central scotoma and a fall in visual acuity to less than 6/60, but peripheral vision is retained. A small number of patients may benefit from laser photocoagulation but for the majority the condition is untreatable.

Diabetic retinopathy

This is now thc commonest cause of blindness in adults under the age of 65, affecting mainly diabetics who have been dependent on insulin for many years. Vision may be affected either through involvement of the macula with gradual loss of visual acuity, or from the development of new blood vessels on the surface of the optic disc and retina. Bleeding from these new vessels gives rise to repeated vitreous haemorrhage and leads eventually to retinal detachment and blindness. Laser photocoagulation of the retina and microsurgical techniques for repairing damaged retinae have greatly improved the visual prognosis of patients with diabetic eye disease.

Chronic glaucoma

The hallmark of this prevalent eye disease is gradual loss of the peripheral visual field with preservation of central vision, until the late stages of the disease, giving rise to 'tunnel vision'. Vision that has been lost cannot be regained, but lowering the intraocular pressure by drug, laser or surgical treatment can arrest or significantly slow the progress of the disease.

Table 16.2: Leading causes of blindness

20–44 years	Percentage	45–64 years	Percentage	65+ years	Percentage	All ages	Percentage
Diabetic retinopathy	20	Diabetic retinopathy	19	Macular degeneration	39	Macular degeneration	30
Myopic degeneration	20	Macular degeneration	14	Glaucoma	17	Glaucoma	15
Optic atrophy	20	Glaucoma	13	Cataract	13	Cataract	10
Uveitis	10	Myopic degeneration	9	Diabetic retinopathy	7	Diabetic retinopathy	9
Glaucoma	7	Optic atrophy	9	Myopic degeneration	5	Myopic degeneration	6
All others	23	All others	36	All others	19	All others	30
Total	100	*Total*	100	*Total*	100	*Total*	100

Source: Ghafour, I. M., Allan, D. and Foulds, W. S. (1983) Common causes of blindness and visual handicap in the west of Scotland. *Br. J. Ophthalmol., 67,* 209

Cataract

This is a very common cause of deteriorating vision in the elderly but, with few exceptions, it can be successfully treated, even in the very old and infirm. The modern practice of implanting an acrylic lens in the eye at the time of surgery has eliminated the optical distortion caused by thick post-cataract spectacles, and has encouraged the earlier treatment of cataract. Most patients with cataract who are registered as blind have coexisting untreatable ocular disease such as senile macular degeneration.

Degenerative myopia

The highly myopic eye is frequently unhealthy and prone to develop retinal detachment and chronic glaucoma. Atrophy of the choroid and retina, especially in the region of the macula, is the most common cause of disabling loss of vision in this condition, and is untreatable.

Other, less common, causes of visual disability include retinitis pigmentosa, an inheritable condition causing night blindness and 'tunnel vision', chronic ocular inflammation and neurological disease. Stroke may result in extensive visual field loss if the visual pathway or occipital cortex are involved, and repeated attacks of optic neuritis in multiple sclerosis lead to optic atrophy and progressive loss of visual acuity.

THE ROLE OF THE OPHTHALMOLOGIST

The majority of elderly patients with a visual handicap are referred by their general practitioner for specialist assessment, often after a sight test by an ophthalmic optician has revealed an abnormality that cannot be corrected by spectacles. Other sources of referral include social workers, geriatricians, diabetic physicians and physicians concerned with rehabilitation of the physically disabled.

The role of the ophthalmologist in the care of the visually handicapped is threefold. Firstly, where possible, to improve or restore sight and prevent further deterioration. Secondly, to ensure maximum use of the remaining vision by the provision of low vision aids and thirdly, where indicated, to initiate rehabilitation by clarifying the medical situation and registering the patient as blind or partially sighted.

LOW-VISION AIDS

A low-vision aid is any appliance which may be used to augment residual vision. The provision of one or more of these aids can dramatically improve the quality of life for the user and may allow a return to economic and social independence. A consultant ophthalmologist can prescribe an aid, refer the patient to a Low-vision Clinic within the Hospital Eye Service or send him to a private optician.

The simplest type of low-vision aid is the single-lens, hand-held magnifier which is readily available from opticians and a variety of retail outlets. These have the advance of being relatively cheap and easy to use but, being hand-held, they restrict manual tasks. Stand magnifiers may include an illumination system and variable focusing and are generally more satisfactory, especially for the elderly who often find it difficult to hold a magnifier steady in front of a book or newspaper.

Spectacle and head-borne magnifiers increase magnification by reducing the working distance between observer and object. The Keeler LVA 10 is a spectacle magnifier which can be prescribed in various powers giving magnification ranging from ×2 to ×8 and a field diameter of 100 mm to 33 mm.

If the observer to object distance is fixed a telescopic system, usually Galilean, can be employed. Telescopic aids may be hand-held or spectacle-mounted and designed for near or distance vision, but they tend to be heavy and rather difficult to use since they permit only a restricted field of view.

Closed circuit television (CCTV) systems allow a variable degree of distortion free magnification up to ×100 (Figure 16.1). A hand-held or mounted camera is used to scan a printed page, or other close work, and the field is displayed on the TV screen. The user is able to control contrast, which facilitates the reading of poor-quality print, and to reverse contrast to produce white print on a black background. Cost and lack of portability are disadvantages of CCTV systems but many visually handicapped individuals are able to work in a wide variety of desk jobs with their help. In Britain the prescription of CCTVs is limited to certain DHSS-approved Low-vision Aid centres but where they are required for work the Manpower Services Commission may pay for them.

The majority of patients referred to a Low-vision Aid clinic have macular disease, but this group has less success than those with diseases of the optic nerve or media, possibly because the average age of the patients is older, and the importance of adequate levels of illumination for the elderly with macular disease has been emphasised by Humphry and Thompson (1986).

Registration of the partially sighted and blind

In England and Wales this is carried out by a consultant ophthalmologist who completes the Form BD8. One part of this form, containing informa-

Figure 16.1: 'Magnalink' closed circuit television (photo courtesy of C. Davis Keeler Ltd)

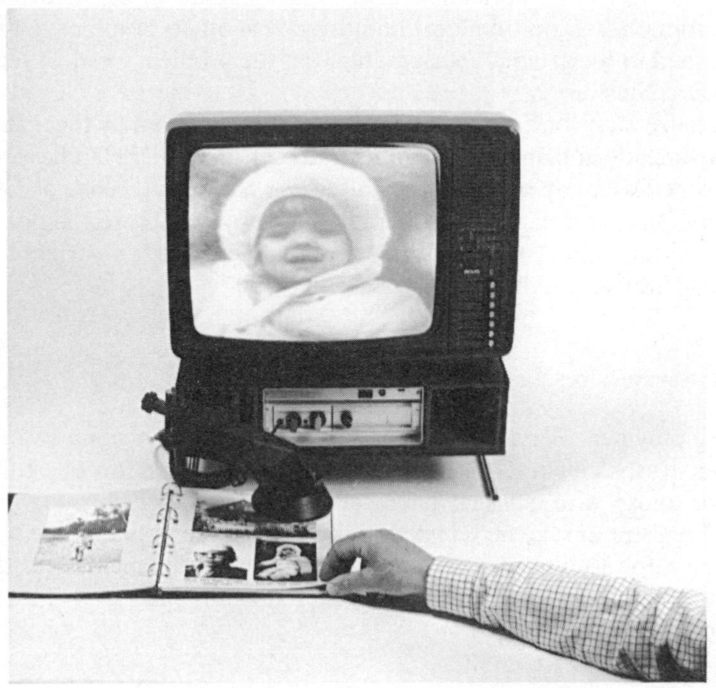

tion relating to the cause of blindness or partial sight, is used for the central collation of statistical data on visual disability; the other part is forwarded to the local authority whose statutory obligation it is to provide services for the visually handicapped.

AGENCIES PROVIDING HELP FOR THE VISUALLY HANDICAPPED

Local authority social services

Prior to the reorganisation of the social services in 1971 the blind and partially sighted were the responsibility of a specialist social worker, the Social Welfare Officer for the Blind (SWOB). Following the recommendations of the Seebohm Report (1968) social work specialisation fell into disfavour and the SWOB training course was abolished to be replaced by training for Technical Officers for the Blind to teach communications and daily living skills, and Mobility Officers for the Blind to teach orientation and mobility.

As a result of these changes much of the social work with the visually handicapped is now done by social workers with limited or no training in visual handicap, and both the quality and quantity of services provided vary enormously from one local authority to another. Some have retained or returned to social work specialisation but the problem exists of replacing SWOBs as they retire.

Specialist staff for the visually handicapped employed by local authorities may include at managerial level an Adviser on Visual Handicap and, at field work level, any or all of the following: SWOBs, Technical Officers, Mobility Officers, occupational therapists with special interest in non-visual or low-visual methods and sessional workers who teach a variety of skills including braille, cooking, typing, etc.

Manpower Services Commission (MSC)

The Employment Services Division of the MSC has a number of Blind Persons Resettlement Officers and Training Officers for the Blind. In addition those with a visual handicap who are not eligible for partially sighted registration can be referred to the MSC by an opthalmologist, social worker or Job Centre to receive help from the Disablement Resettlement Officer, though they must first be registered as disabled with the Department of Employment.

Voluntary agencies

The visually handicapped may be referred directly to the voluntary agencies by an ophthalmologist or social worker. In some areas the Social Services Departments have given the responsibility for social rehabilitation to these agencies. The largest and best-known is the Royal National Institute for the Blind, which provides a wide range of services. Other national agencies include the Partially Sighted Society, and St Dunstan's, which cares for those blinded during war service. In addition there are local voluntary societies and self-help groups in most areas.

British Broadcasting Corporation

The weekly BBC Radio 4 programme 'In Touch' has broadcast news and information for the visually handicapped since 1961. The BBC also publishes a quarterly bulletin summarising the information broadcast during the previous three months and a handbook *In Touch* (Ford and Heshel, 1977) which details aids and services for the blind and partially sighted. Both the bulletin and book are available in braille.

ASPECTS OF REHABILITATION OF THE VISUALLY HANDICAPPED

Psychological adjustment to visual loss

The emotional reaction to visual loss and its implications varies from one individual to another and depends to a large extent on the degree to which normal life has been disrupted. Resolution of the emotional problems is a necessary first step before the practical problems of visual handicap can be tackled.

The psychological reaction to loss is grief, and the gradual realisation of the fact and implications of loss has been termed the 'grief syndrome'. Its applicability to visual loss has been demonstrated by Fitzgerald (1970), and Hicks (1978) has outlined the phases of the syndrome which must be worked through to resolution. It is a gradually unfolding process in which there must be acceptance of the visual loss and its implications followed by rejection of unhelpful attitudes and emotions. Once these stages have been passed new patterns of behaviour and new relationships can be acquired.

At least one-third of patients registered blind under the age of 60 are in need of immediate counselling or psychotherapy (Todd, 1987). This applies particularly to those whose blindness is traumatic or genetic, where there is severe illness or multi-handicap and when the individual is mentally or socially unstable.

It is important that all patients are given a clear explanation of their visual impairment at an early stage, and this is the role of the ophthalmologist. The possibility or probability of blindness, if this has not already occurred, should be discussed and any false hope for a return of vision should be avoided as this may impair or retard successful rehabilitation.

The role of counsellor usually falls on the social worker, who is also responsible for assessing the patient's needs, planning a treatment programme and mobilising resources. There is unfortunately little or no specialist training in counselling related to visual loss, though generic social workers usually have skills in problem-oriented counselling.

Social implications of visual loss

For most newly registered blind and partially sighted persons there are also social implications of their visual handicap which are intertwined with the emotional and pscyhological reactions outlined above. Social isolation and loss of self-esteem, frequently compounded by stereotyped attitudes and increased dependence on others, are accentuated by restricted mobility and lack of information about rehabilitation and available benefits. Discussion and support groups set up by voluntary societies, adult education centres and some social services departments play a valuable part in restoring social confidence and facilitating the establishment of new relationships.

Communication — reading, writing and listening

Reading

Of all the limitations imposed by failing sight the one most often resented is the inability to read. If the loss of central vision is not too severe the individual may be able to read large-print books with the use of reading glasses and a good light, or a low-vision aid may be required. There are now over 1300 titles, both fiction and non-fiction, in the original Ulverscroft series which can be obtained from public libraries, but there are other large-print publishers and a list of these can be obtained from the Library Association.

For the blind, and those unable to use residual vision, there are two systems of embossed script read by the fingertips, the best known of which is braille. The English version consists of 63 symbols which are variations on the dots of a domino six. There are a great number of braille publications — between 500 and 800 per year — including the *Radio Times.* The other system is Moon, which consists of simplified Roman letters. It is easier for the elderly to learn but there is less literature available and, unlike braille, it cannot be written. Teaching of both systems is the responsibility of the local authority, but the service provided varies considerably from area to area.

Two different types of reading machine are available. The more widely used and cheaper is the Optacon, which converts the printed word to a tactile stimulus which is read by the user's forefinger. Training programmes for the use of these machines are run by the RNIB and Electronic Aids for the Blind.

The other reading machine, the Kurzweil, converts the printed word into synthetic speech, but the range of material it can cope with is limited and it is very expensive.

Writing

Many people with low visual acuity are able to write, and this is made easier if the contrast between ink and paper is improved by suitable choice of writing materials. For those able to type, large-print typewriters are available, though expensive, but typing is taught to newly blind persons in rehabilitation centres and at evening classes. Braille writing machines range from simple hand frames to sophisticated machines similar to typewriters, all of which can be obtained through the RNIB.

Listening

Registered blind people over the age of 16 are eligible for a radio set on free permanent loan from either the local Social Services Department or local voluntary society, and a sound-only television set which requires no licence can be purchased from the RNIB. Blind people who have an ordinary television set are entitled to a small reduction in the licence fee. Talking book machines are issued to the registered blind and to any visually handicapped person with defective reading vision (generally N12 or worse) whose application is supported by an ophthalmologist. There are several thousand titles recorded onto cassettes which can be played back only on these machines, which are available from the British Talking Book Service.

Mobility

To the newly blind loss of free movement is an additional handicap which saps self-confidence and increases the sense of isolation from the outside world. Mobility training is an essential early step in rehabilitation, and this is usually undertaken by the Mobility Officer employed by the local autority.

Moving about safely in the home is not usually a problem for the blind, with the exception of the very elderly, but lighting improvements may help the partially sighted. Outside the home the blind individual has to be taught ways of moving about safely and effectively using a variety of aids and techniques.

The white stick

There are several types of white stick, all available through the RNIB. The 'symbol cane', a collapsible stick made of sections of white tubing, can be used as a probe, but more useful in this respect is the long cane which has a special grip and is tailored to the user's height. It is swung in an arc roughly the width of the body to check the ground ahead. These sticks cannot be used for support, and the infirm may need a crook-handled white wooden walking stick that they can lean on.

Sonic aids

A variety of hand-held and spectacle-mounted devices are available which transmit a beam of high-frequency sound, some of which is reflected back by obstacles in the beam's path and converted into an audible or vibratory warning signal. These tend to be expensive but hand-held sonic aids may be borrowed for use under the supervision of a mobility officer.

Guide dogs

Registered blind persons over the age of 17 can apply to the Guide Dogs for the Blind Association for a guide dog. A doctor's certificate of fitness is required, as is the endorsement of the local blind welfare authority. If accepted by the Association the trainee attends one of its centres which are in Exeter, Leamington Spa, Bolton, Wokingham and Forfar.

Travel concessions

The mobile blind or partially sighted are entitled to a variety of local authority concessions, which may include free bus and underground passes, a taxi service and disabled person's railcard. Free escorts are available from the British Red Cross, and British Rail will arrange for blind persons to be accompanied to trains.

Daily living skills

Instruction in daily living skills, such as housekeeping, cooking and personal care, is normally given by Technical Officers for the Blind or Rehabilitation Officers who are qualified to teach both technical and mobility skills. Other important aspects of their work are adapatation of the home to provide the best possible environment for the visually handicapped person, and the provision of household aids. For the elderly and infirm a wider range of services is often required and the district nurse, health visitor, meals-on-wheels and home helps may be called upon to provide support.

Employment

Most people who are threatened with loss of vision are anxious about their future employment. Those in work are often best advised to hold on to their present job for, in many instances, visual disabilities can be overcome by the use of low-vision aids, changes in the pattern of work or even a change of job within a company, to one which is less visually demanding.

For the more severely visually handicapped employment services are provided by the Manpower Services Commission which works closely with the voluntary societies. Those registered as blind or partially sighted who are able to work may be registered with the Commission and obtain help in gaining employment through its two executive divisions.

Employment Services Division

Jobs are found for those registered blind, or as partially sighted and likely to become blind, by the Division's Blind Persons' Resettlement Officers (BPRO). Referral to the BPRO is normally done automatically by the local authority on receipt of a suitable BD8 registration form. The BPRO can arrange attendance, paid for by the MSC, at one of the RNIB's employment rehabilitation courses held at its centres in Torquay and Fife. These residential courses normally last between four and twelve weeks, and are designed to assess abilities and give realistic vocational guidance. A range of skills is taught from mobility and the use of low-vision aids to braille reading, typing, crafts and light engineering techniques. The Employment Services Division also employs Blind Persons' Training Officers, whose function is to help and advise both employee and employer at the place of work, and loan aids which are essential to employment, such as braille micrometers, typewriters and closed-circuit televisions.

Training Services Division

Most people completing an employment rehabilitation course are recommended for further training through courses run by the Division itself and by voluntary agencies. All these courses are free and a weekly allowance is given by the MSC. Courses are available in, among others, light engineering, shorthand and audiotyping, telephony, computer programming, piano tuning and physiotherapy. In the professional field, apart from physiotherapy, there are no special training schemes, but many visually handicapped people are able to follow the same courses as sighted students and qualify as teachers, solicitors, musicians and social workers. Financial assistance, where local authority grants are not given, is provided by the TSD's Professional Training Scheme.

Of those registered as blind and of employment age approximately one-third are in employment, one-third are unemployed (though the majority are not seeking employment) and one-third are considered unemployable, often by virtue of multi-handicap. Of those in employment a significant number, almost one-third, are in sheltered workshops or home-worker schemes run by local authorities and voluntary agencies.

Housing

The majority of the visually handicapped are elderly and many live alone or have a spouse who is infirm. For those who are unable to maintain an independent life, even with the help of support services, sheltered accommodation with a warden and some communal facilities are often a satisfactory alternative, but the pressure on local authority sheltered accommodation is great. The local authority is, however, obliged to provide accommodation for those 'in need of care and attention which is not otherwise available to them' and does so in the form of residential homes. Occasionally local authorities run residential homes specifically for the blind.

Housing for the blind and partially sighted is also provided by voluntary housing associations and private charities, and the RNIB publishes a list of homes for the adult blind.

Adult education and leisure

Participation in further education can play an important part in the rehabilitation of the visually handicapped person. Local education authorities often run special courses for the blind and partially sighted in subjects such as braille, tailoring, dressmaking, cookery, sports activities and dancing, which not only teach useful skills but increase confidence and self-esteem, and lead to social integration and further study. Many visually handicapped people join normal adult education classes, and some have graduated through the Open University, which offers special facilities including a weekend preparatory study course at which help and advice is given by counsellors and blind graduates.

The range of leisure activities in which the visually handicapped can participate is now large. Some, with the use of special equipment or techniques, such as braille playing cards and braille music, allow the blind to participate with the sighted, while other activities, particularly team sports, are of necessity so modified that they are more specifically for the visually handicapped. The popularity of sport is such that in cricket and five-a-side football national leagues have been formed.

The *In Touch* book lists the facilities available in the wide range of recreational activities for the visually handicapped, and the RNIB's Sport and Recreation Officer can supply information about the provision made for any particular sport or hobby.

ADDITIONAL HANDICAP

Sixty per cent of those persons registered as blind have at least one additional handicap (DHSS, 1976), and of these diabetes, deafness and physical disability pose particular problems.

Diabetes

Most visually handicapped diabetics are insulin-dependent and they experience increasing difficulty with self-injection as their sight deteriorates. Good illumination, and the use of a magnifier which leaves both hands free, help distinguish the calibrations on the syringe, but when magnification is no longer sufficient a pre-set syringe or, if mixed doses are used, a click-count syringe is needed. Inserting the needle into the insulin bottle is aided by the use of a funnel-shaped needle guide which fits over the cap of the bottle, or by a plastic location tray, manufactured by Hypoguard, which holds both syringe and bottle in correct alignment. The same firm also produce an audio urine meter which allows self-monitoring of the urine glucose level.

The British Diabetic Association publishes a bi-monthly newspaper which is also recorded on cassette for the visually handicapped.

Deafness

Most deaf–blind patients have acquired their disabilities in old age, and many can be helped by a combination of hearing and low-vision aids. The problems of the profoundly deaf–blind, usually younger people suffering from congenital rubella or Usher's or Norrey's syndrome, are of a different order of magnitude. Communication is the greatest problem and a number of different techniques are used to overcome it. Some employ the tracing of letters on the deaf–blind person's palm, but if braille or Moon can be read other methods can be more effective. The RNIB's communicator disc, which has a moving pointer and braille or Moon letters, and the more sophisticated Tellatouch, a 'typewriter' which forms braille letters one at a time on a touch cell, allow the sighted and deaf–blind to communicate.

Various aids employing tactile stimuli as warning signals are helpful to the deaf–blind, for example an alarm clock with an attached vibrator which is placed beneath the pillow, and the RNIB supplies a white stick with two red bands denoting deaf–blindness. Rehabilitation facilities are available through several blind associations and the Deaf–Blind Helpers League.

Physical disability

Loss of manual dexterity — from arthritis, stroke, multiple sclerosis or other neurological disorder — limits the use of touch and the ability to use many of the aids designed for the visually handicapped. Modified switches and controls on domestic and electrical appliances, which can be operated by the forearm, can be fitted, and the Talking Book can be modified to incorporate a semi-automatic cassette changer. Stand or spectacle-mounted low-vision aids are generally easier to manage than a hand-held magnifier, and at times an advantage can be obtained by the construction of a frame, incorporating the low-vision aid, that can be attached to the patient's chair or bed. For the recumbent, bedridden patient prismatic glasses can allow a book to be read, or television watched, at 90° from the direction of gaze. Unfortunately there is usually little that can be done to help the patient whose reading difficulties stem from grossly defective ocular motility or homonymous hemianopia following stroke.

Multi-handicap

This term is generally used to imply a combination of visual, physical and mental handicaps, and is applied to the young rather than the elderly. Most have spent their childhood in residential centres though a number of adults fall into this category following severe trauma or neurological disease. The range of disability is wide, from those who live at home and work in sheltered schemes to those who, through lack of suitable residential facilities, become long-term residents of hospitals for the mentally handicapped. There are a very small number of specialist residential homes for the blind and partially sighted, with additional severe handicaps, the largest of which is the Royal School for the Blind at Leatherhead.

ACKNOWLEDGEMENT

In preparing this chapter I am grateful for the advice of Mrs Mary Todd, adviser to the visually handicapped at King's College Hospital, London.

REFERENCES

Cullinan, T.R. (1977) *Visually disabled people in the community.* Health Services Research Unit Report No 28, University of Kent at Canterbury

DHSS (1976) *An investigation into some aspects of visual handicap.* Statistical and research report series No. 14, HMSO, London

DHSS (1980) *Registered blind and partially sighted persons. Year ending March 31st 1980*, HMSO, London

Fitzgerald, R. (1970) Reactions to blindness: an exploratory study of adults with recent loss of sight. *Arch. Gen. Psychiatry*, *22*, 370-9

Ford, M. and Heshel, T. (1977) *In touch: aids and social services for blind and partially sighted people*, BBC Publications, London

Hicks, S. (1978) Psycho-social and rehabilitation aspects of acquired visual handicap. *Trans. Ophthalmol. Soc. UK*, *98*, 252-61

Humphry, R.C. and Thompson, G.M. (1986) Low vision aids — evaluation in a general eye department. *Trans. Ophthalmol. Soc. UK*, *105*, 296-8

Seebohm Report (1968) *Report of the committee on local authority and allied personal social services.* Cmnd 3703, HMSO, London

Silver, J.H., Gould, E.S., Irvine, D. and Cullinan, T.R. (1978) Visual acuity at home and in eye clinics. *Trans. Ophthalmol. Soc. UK*, *98*, 262-6

Sorsby, A. (1972) *Incidence and causes of blindness in England and Wales, 1963-68*, HMSO, London

Todd, M. (1987) *Working with people with loss or threatened loss of vision.* King's Fund Publication (in press)

USEFUL ADDRESSES

British Diabetic Association
10 Queen Anne Street, London W1M 0BD

British Talking Book Service for the Blind
Mount Pleasant, Alperton, Wembley, Middlesex HA0 1RR

Guide Dogs for the Blind Association
Alexandra House, 9-11 Park Street, Windsor, Berkshire SL4 1JR

Hypoguard Ltd
Dock Lane, Melton, Woodbridge, Suffolk TP12 1PE

Library Association
7 Ridgmount, London WC1E 7AE

National Deaf/Blind Helpers League
18 Rainbow Court, Paston Ridings, Peterborough PE4 6UP

Partially Sighted Society
Secretariat Office: Breaston, Derby DE7 3UE. Publications and aids: 40 Wordsworth Street, Hove, East Sussex BN3 5BH

Royal National Institute for the Blind
224/6/8 Great Portland Street, London W1N 6AA

St Dunstan's Organisation for Men and Women Blinded on War Service
191 Old Marylebone Road, London NW1 5QN

Ulverscroft Large-Print Books
The Green, Bradgate Road, Anstey, Leicester LE7 7FU

A comprehensive list of organisations for the blind is contained in the *Directory of Agencies for the Blind*, published by the RNIB.

17

Auditory Disability and Handicap

Dafydd Stephens

INTRODUCTION

Hearing disability, reflected in difficulties in hearing sounds which the individual wishes to hear, represents one of the commonest disabilities affecting some 20 per cent of the adult population. Different individuals with hearing loss will experience different disabilities according to the severity of their hearing loss, their lifestyle, their non-auditory disabilities and the social situation in which they live.

Within this chapter the system of classification used will follow that advocated by the World Health Organization (WHO, 1980). Applying that system of hearing we have the situation as outlined in Figure 17.1. The *aetiology* (e.g. infection, head injury, metabolic disease) will result in *pathology*, or pathological changes, which may occur anywhere in the auditory pathway from the outer ear to the auditory cortex.

These will result in a measurable deficit, or *impairment*, which may be reflected in an elevated threshold of hearing, impaired speech discrimination performance, abnormal frequency discrimination or a variety of other measurable psychoacoustical changes.

This impairment will in turn lead to the individual becoming aware that he has difficulties in hearing what he wants to hear under different circumstances, i.e. a *disability*. This may be reflected in difficulties in his hearing the television, carrying out a conversation or locating a bird singing in his garden. In many individuals such disabilities may lead to a change in the individual's life, withdrawal from social events, losing his job, or becoming dependent on others for his or her shopping, which then constitutes a *handicap*. Some individuals may have a handicap without a disability.

CAUSES OF HEARING DISABILITY

Hearing disability may result from problems in any part of the auditory system from the pinna (auricle) to the auditory cortex. Most commonly,

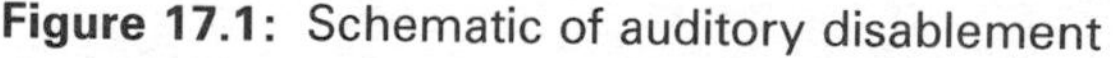

Figure 17.1: Schematic of auditory disablement

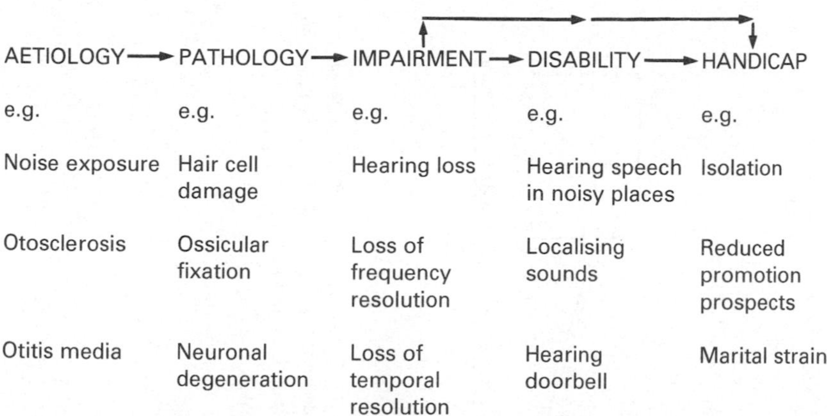

however, problems arise from the outer middle or inner ears rather than from the central pathways. Lesions in the outer and middle ear result in what is called a conductive hearing loss, essentially an attenuation of the input sound without any significant distortions. Damage to the inner ear where the mechanical energy of sound is transduced into nervous impulses, however, leads to significant distortions of the sound input in the time frequency and intensity domains, as well as a loss in hearing sensitivity. Disorders of the hearing nerve cause further distortions and hearing loss, but more rostral lesions within the auditory pathways result rather in more subtle auditory distortions and only rarely in loss of auditory sensitivity.

AETIOLOGY → PATHOLOGY → IMPAIRMENT → DISABILITY → HANDICAP
e.g.
e.g.
e.g.
e.g.
e.g.
Noise exposure
Hair cell damage
Hearing loss
Hearing speech in noisy places
Isolation
Otosclerosis
Ossicular fixation
Loss of frequency resolution
Localising sounds
Reduced promotion prospects
Otitis media
Neuronal degeneration
Loss of temporal resolution
Hearing doorbell
Marital strain

Figure 17.2 shows the main parts of the auditory system with the common causes of hearing impairment listed. In the outer ear, which extends from the pinna to the eardrum, by far the commonest cause of hearing loss arises from wax, with otitis externa stemming from allergies or infective causes being less common. In some elderly individuals meatal atresia may result in a collapse of the ear canal.

The middle ear, particularly the tympanic membrane and the ossicles, may be damaged by middle ear infections resulting from a variety of organisms. There may be a secretory otitis media (glue ear), acute otitis media and various forms of chronic otitis media, suppurative and non-suppurative. The latter usually stems from secondary infections through perforations of the tympanic membrane. Such perforations may be the sequelae of acute otitis media, blast injury or other forms of direct or indirect trauma.

The commonest non-infectious cause of middle ear hearing loss is otosclerosis, a genetic condition which generally shows itself in the 3rd and 4th decade of life and affects the stapes footplate, interfering with the transmission of sound through to the inner ear.

Figure 17.2: Schematic of the auditory pathway

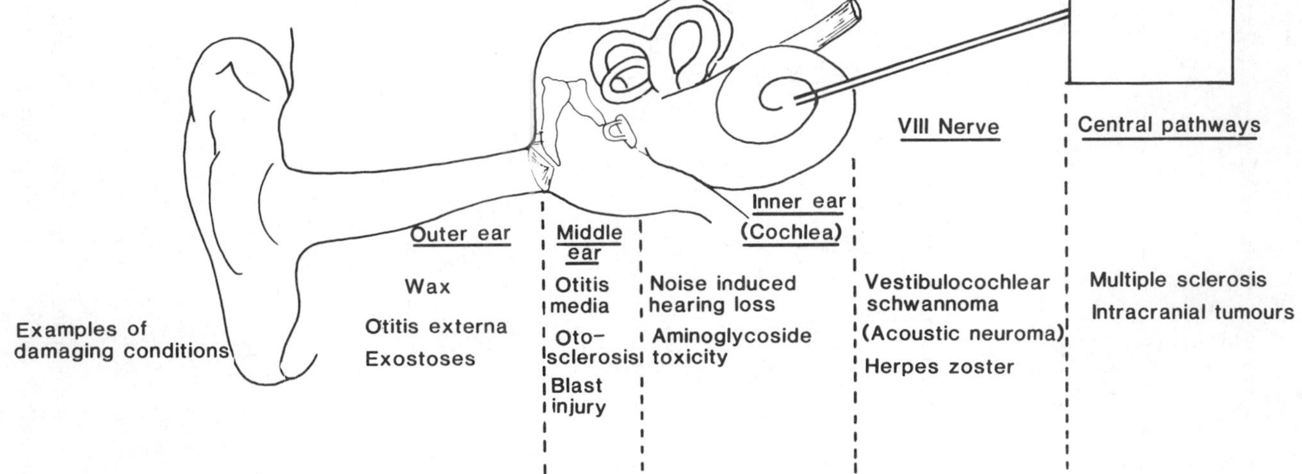

Inner ear (cochlear) hearing loss is caused by a great variety of conditions, local and systemic, many of which appear to be mediated by interference of the blood supply to the cochlea. More direct damage to the cochlea may come from certain infectious conditions, a labyrinthitis secondary to otitis media, meningitis, mumps, measles or syphilis. Traumatic causes may be direct head injury, or more commonly trauma to the hair cells of the cochlea coming from exposure to loud noises.

A variety of drugs may damage the inner ear. Those which have permanent effects are typified by the aminoglycoside antibiotics. Other drugs such as aspirin, quinine, loop diuretics and non-steroidal anti-inflammatory agents generally result in reversible hearing loss, but may potentiate other damaging agents and occasionally result in permanent damage themselves.

A number of families show late-onset genetic cochlear hearing loss, but in most other elderly individuals hearing loss is caused by a variety of disorders which compromise the cochlear blood supply. These include hypertension, diabetes, dyslipidaemias, arteriosclerosis and autoimmune conditions. In many patients the cochlear hearing loss is multifactorial.

Disorders affecting the neural auditory pathways and centres are generally common to other causes of intracranial damage, i.e. neoplasia, trauma, infection and vascular disorders. Two conditions which affect the VIII nerve, which have attracted much attention, are vestibulocochlear schwannoma (acoustic neuroma) and herpes zoster.

PREVALENCE

According to recent epidemiological studies (see for example Lutman and Haggard, 1983) some 15–20 per cent of the adult population suffer from an auditory impairment in their better hearing ear and an even greater proportion experience auditory disability. As always there are problems of definition of these, and the results of a number of studies and the prevalence of disability are summarised in Figure 17.3. From this figure it may be seen that the prevalence increases dramatically with age, and this is equally true of hearing impairment. Thus some 2 per cent of 20-year-old individuals show an auditory impairment, whereas some 80 per cent of 80-year-olds show an impairment by the same definition.

The prevalence of hearing impairment and disability is generally higher in males than in females. It is also greater in individuals from manual social classes than among white-collar groups.

The prevalence of hearing loss in children is complicated by the intermittency and seasonal variations in the common conditions of serous otitis media and acute otitis media. The prevalence of severe congenital hearing loss is, however, only of the order of 0.1 per cent of the population.

Figure 17.3: The prevalence of auditory disability with age, after Davis (in Lutman and Haggard, 1983)

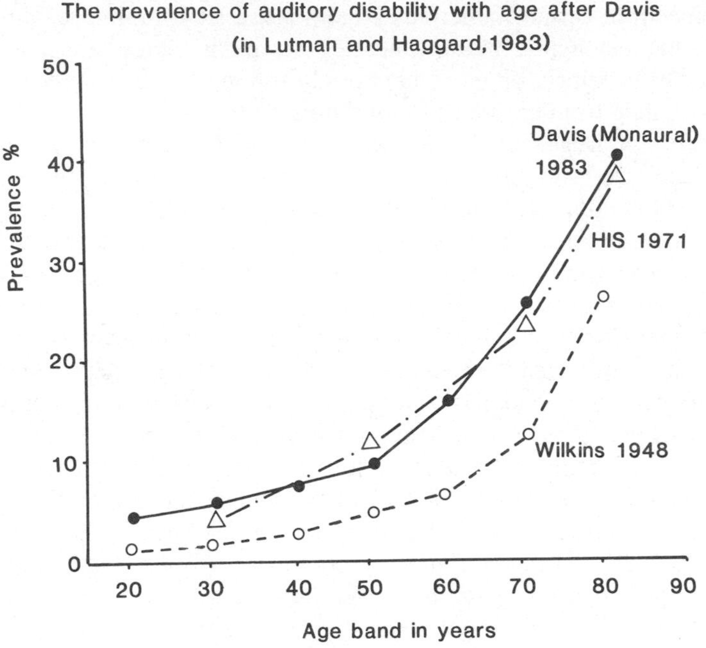

CONSEQUENCES OF HEARING LOSS

While there is an extensive literature on the consequences of prelingual hearing loss, until the past decade there has been a dearth of data on the effects of acquired hearing loss. The prevalence of anxiety and depression is some four times greater in the hearing-impaired population than among matched controls. There is some evidence that the problem is even greater among severely impaired individuals with poor auditory discrimination of speech.

Recent studies indicate no significant relationship between hearing loss and dementia in the elderly. They do, however, show some relationship between hearing impairment and loneliness, and a tendency for the individual not to go out and mix with others.

While hearing-impaired individuals experience difficulties in both work and domestic situations these result in no major effects on level of employment and marital status. There is, however, an increased likelihood of divorces/separations in individuals with severe acquired hearing loss, but the effects are relatively small and less consistent than those reported in the prelingually deaf (e.g. Schein and Delk, 1974).

MEDICAL AND SURGICAL TREATMENT

Overall the contributions of medicine and surgery to the treatment of hearing impairment are somewhat limited. Most emphasis must be put on either prevention or rehabilitation.

The important aspect of any medical therapy depends on early diagnosis. Once hair cell or neuronal changes reach a certain level they become irreversible and neither regenerates. However, early treatment in a variety of disorders, infectious and autoimmune, metabolic and vascular may lead to partial or complete recovery, and this emphasises the need for early and vigorous treatment. This is true particularly of cochlear artery vasculitis related to autoimmune disorders, hearing loss in dyslipidaemics and late congenital syphilis. In more long-standing cases the best that can usually be hoped for is prevention of the progress of the condition, and perhaps some alleviation of the secondary symptoms such as tinnitus.

Among the secondary problems there may be development of a secondary endolymphatic hydrops with various symptoms of fluctuating hearing loss, tinnitus, pressure sensation and vertigo. This should also be treated vigorously, although very few of the proposed treatments have withstood critical appraisal.

Surgical restorative treatment is restricted to middle and outer ear conditions, particularly the long-term consequences of otitis media and problems arising from otosclerosis. Otosclerosis may be well treated by carefully performed stapedectomies, but also it must be said that otosclerotic patients are ideal candidates for hearing aid fitting.

The treatment of chronic suppurative otitis media presents more of a problem both for the surgeon and for those concerned with hearing aid fitting. The latter ideally want a closed middle ear to which they can fit aids, as otherwise there is an increased risk of exacerbation of the infection. For the surgeon it is often difficult to eliminate completely the underlying infection prior to surgery, and the results are often poor except in the best hands. However, good results here can entail reconstruction of the ossicular chain and closure of any perforation.

AUDIOLOGICAL REHABILITATION

In most cases of hearing loss there will be persistent problems despite medical or surgical treatment. Alternatively, the condition may not be amenable to such treatment, or no definite aetiological diagnosis can be made. We are thus faced with the need for appropriate rehabilitative intervention.

Such intervention should be based on a problem-solving approach aimed at minimising disability and avoiding handicap. It is particularly important to approach this in a global way, considering in some detail the patient's needs and skills and then providing rehabilitative management appropriate to these.

In an effort to fit the management to the patient, and to take into account all relevant factors and possibilities, we have developed a management model of audiological rehabilitation (Goldstein and Stephens, 1981) which draws these aspects together. The overall process is summarised in Figure 17.4. This shows the same process in increasing complexity in the successive columns from left to right. The left-hand column indicates that

Figure 17.4: Audiological rehabilitation

Evaluation	Communication Status	Auditory Visual Speech and language Manual communication Previous rehabilitation Overall
	Associated Variables	Psychological Sociological Vocational Educational
	Related Conditions	Mobility Upper limb function Related aural pathology
Remediation	Integration and Decisions	Attitude modification Integration Categorisation
	Instrumental Help	Hearing aids Environmental aids Sensory substitution aids
	Strategy	Goal setting Philosophy/personality Tactics
	Ancillary	Psychological Medical Social services Employment support Educational services
	Communication Training	Information provision Skill-building Instrumental modification Counselling

the overall process of audiological rehabilitation may be split into two halves, termed Evaluation and Remediation. Thus it is important to know the details of the 'raw material' with which one is dealing, before beginning any rehabilitative therapy.

The middle column indicates that the Evaluative process is split into three sections of Communication Status, Associated Variables and Related Conditions. Communication Status comprises the basic aspects of communication abilities in different respects already possessed by the individual, together with components of his/her needs and potentials in these respects. Associated Variables is concerned with major factors which will determine the overall approach to be used by the professionals to overcome the problems experienced by the patient. Related Conditions, on the other hand, comprises those aspects of the patient's characteristics which may influence detailed elements of the instrumentation and other approaches to be adopted, rather than influencing the general approach.

The Remediation half of the model is likewise split into a number of sections; five in this case. These comprise an Integration and Decision section, pulling together the information acquired in Evaluation and making management decisions based on this, together with four directly remedial sections. The first of these, Instrumental Help, is concerned with selection of appropriate instrumentation, be it wearable hearing aid(s), environmental aids or sensory substitution aids. The next, Strategy, is concerned with a definition of desirable and achievable goals jointly by the patient and professional, together with a consideration of appropriate tactics to achieve these goals. Ancillary involves a consideration of other professionals who may have the skills necessary for specialist parts of the rehabilitative process such as employment retraining, special education and the like. Finally Communication Training, the ongoing remedial process, entails consideration of the needs for four components: information provision, skill-building, instrumental modification and counselling. This should all be tailored to meet the particular needs of the individual concerned.

EVALUATION

Communication status

This is concerned with different aspects of the communication abilities and difficulties of the individual comprising sections evaluating the various components individually, and finally in an integrated manner. Auditory is obviously the central component and may be subdivided into defining the individual's auditory disabilities or problems and measuring his/her auditory impairment. The former determines the overall direction that the rehabilitative process will take while the latter is critical to the detailed selection of instrumentation and the balance between auditory and visual aspects of the remedial process. It is concerned not merely with auditory threshold and speech discrimination measures, but also with measures of the dynamic range, binaural interaction and more sophisticated psychophysical measures which are becoming increasingly important in the selection of signal processing aids.

The Visual section deals with two major factors: the individual's corrected visual acuity and his speech-reading (lip-reading) ability. Correcting inadequately corrected visual acuity is the simplest and most effective way of improving lip-reading performance, at which most individuals have a reasonable degree of competence even if they are unaware of it. This testing also has a therapeutic role indicating to the patient that he possesses these skills, and highlighting the importance of using them.

Speech and Language is primarily concerned with productive performance. In addition it is important to be aware of what is the individual's maternal or dominant language, and to take this into account in any remedial programme. The speech productive skills split into components of phonetics/phonology which may change markedly as a result of certain patterns and types of acquired hearing loss, and syntax/semantics/pragmatics which are generally markedly abnormal only in the prelingually deaf.

This last group are generally the only users of Manual Communication, and it is important to determine whether or not the individual knows a manual system, which system it is, and his skills in this system. The vast majority of individuals with acquired hearing loss will neither know nor need to know such a system.

Many individuals seen in rehabilitation clinics will have had some previous rehabilitative help of one sort or another and, in Previous Rehabilitation, it is important to define what has been done before and to build on that, rather than merely repeating the mistakes of others.

Finally Overall pulls together these various components considered individually in the previous sections. It aims to look at the whole communication skills rather than merely the sum of the components. In its turn this is split into components of intersensory integration and to conversational processing, the latter using the patient's optimal mode of communication.

Associated Variables is concerned with four critical aspects of the patient, his lifestyle and life circumstances which critically influence the approach which the professional must take to his problems. These include Psychological, Sociological, Vocational and Educational factors. The former concerns particularly his attitude towards disability in general and his in particular, his approach to life, whether or not he is an outward-going or a shy withdrawn individual, and various cognitive factors. Sociological elements concern his lifestyle, whether he lives by himself or with others, and the attitude of the others to him and his disabilities. Vocational elements concern both the nature of his work and the attitude of others within his workplace towards his disabilities. Finally Educational factors, while most relevant to deaf or deafened children, may be a factor of all adults keen to acquire new information and/or skills, and are likely to constitute an increasing important aspect of life in the future.

Related Conditions are factors which have an influence on more detailed aspects of the rehabilitative process. The patient's Mobility and Upper Limb Function will influence particularly the choice of instrumentation to meet the patient's specific needs, taking into account his/her ability to use such aids appropriately. Related Aural Pathology is concerned with other aspects of ear disease which may particularly influence the choice of hearing aid and earmould type, and whether one ear, the other, or both, is to be fitted. Particularly important in this respect are the presence of otorrhoea (discharge) or tinnitus. In the majority of tinnitus sufferers with associated hearing loss, hearing aids constitute the single most effective way of suppressing the tinnitus.

REMEDIATION

Integration and management decisions

Once such information has been acquired it is important to pull it together and make the appropriate decisions on the management of the patient based on the relevant information. Overall we find that patients may be subdivided on the basis of their attitude towards the rehabilitative process and the degree of complication anticipated in their particular case. Many are highly motivated and prepared to follow any reasonable advice which they are given. Some of these may be regarded as straightforward, not requiring repeated counselling, and skill-building sessions. Others may have complicating factors, particular audiometric configurations, handling problems, poor previous management or severe hearing difficulties which may require a long-term and more complex rehabilitative approach. Some patients may genuinely want help but be opposed to a certain part of the rehabilitative process initially, e.g. hearing aids, which might be invaluable for their effective rehabilitation. It is important not to push that aspect of the rehabilitative process, but rather introduce it in an informal non-threatening context at a later stage of rehabilitation.

Finally some patients have been persuaded to come for help by their family, but in reality want no rehabilitation. It is important to recognise such individuals and provide rehabilitative and communicative advice, such as with regard to environmental aids, to the family. For the patient the best one can usually do is to leave the door open should s/he change her/his mind about help on a future occasion.

Instrumental Help — hearing aids play a pivotal role in the rehabilitative programme but, on occasions, may not be used. They constitute the only wearable approach to loss of auditory sensitivity, and have been considerably reduced in size. However, they do remain literally aids to hearing, and are incapable of fully overcoming the auditory distortions encountered by most hearing-impaired individuals, particularly the most common problem of hearing speech in a noisy environment.

The vast majority of hearing aids fitted now are head-worn, either behind-the-ear aids or in-the-ear/in-the-canal aids.

More sophistication or flexibility is usually available in behind-the-ear aids, although the canal aids have a number of acoustic advantages. Binaural hearing aids, an aid fitted to each ear, are advantageous to most patients with bilaterally symmetrical hearing losses and also to many individuals with asymmetrical losses. Body-worn aids are now generally fitted only to those individuals with inadequate handling skills to cope with head-worn aids, or those requiring a very high degree of amplification.

Environmental aids play an important part in the instrumental side of audiological rehabilitation and, in some cases, may be sufficient in themselves to overcome the patient's disabilities without the use of hearing aids. In most cases, however, they are complementary to the hearing aids. They may be divided into two groups: amplification devices and alerting/warning devices. The first cover telephone amplifier systems and devices to help the individual hear the television and radio. A great variety of both are available, some of which are designed to be used with the individual's hearing aid(s) and some of which are self-contained.

Alerting and warning devices are available to help the patient be aware that the telephone bell or doorbell is ringing, to awaken him in the morning, and to indicate to him that the baby is crying. Again a variety of systems and technologies may be used, although in this case most are independent of wearable hearing aids. Indeed the commonest difficulty for which they are needed, i.e. to overcome the patient's impaired discrimination of signals in noise, cannot be helped by current hearing aids. This is the individual's problem of hearing the door or telephone bell while watching the television. This problem may be easily overcome by the use of extension or extra-loud bells in the patient's living room, or by a sensory substitution system, linking the bells to the lighting system which then flashes when the doorbell is rung.

Sensory substitution aids. While sensory substitution is used in such alert/warning systems, for the profoundly/totally deafened, sensory substitution devices are needed to facilitate communication. Two major lines of approach are used for this very small group of patients: vibrotactile stimulation and electro-auditory stimulation (cochlear implants). The principle underlying the latter is the direct stimulation of the cochlear nerve, bypassing the defective cochlea. Such devices provide the patients with a supplement to their speech-reading (lip-reading), give them an awareness of environmental sounds and help them monitor their own speech. Some 'star' patients with the most sophisticated devices may also recognise a certain proportion of speech without visual input.

Strategy and goal setting

In the course of any rehabilitative programme it is essential for the therapist and the patient together to define a set of goals which the patient wishes to achieve, and also which are considered achievable, given his sensory defect. Once these have been agreed the therapist may then discuss appropriate tactics necessary to achieve such goals, taking into account the underlying philosophy/personality of the patient. This is important in order to define relevant hearing tactics for the individual. Hearing tactics essentially entail developing the skills of the patient in manipulating or modifying his environment (both human and inanimate) to facilitate his communication ability, and a wide range of approaches may be adopted to achieve such goals.

Ancillary entails obtaining other specialist help to deal with some of the patient's problems needing help beyond the skills of the audiologist. This may entail psychological and additional medical help, social service support, employment retraining and help, and specific educational advice. Some of this is briefly discussed below under the 'Special educational and vocational needs' headings.

COMMUNICATION TRAINING

While most of the earlier stages of the remedial process are essentially short-term activities, communication training may take place over days, weeks, months or even years. It may be performed on an individual or group basis, or a combination of the two. It may even take place within the patient's home, where this is necessary.

However it is implemented in practice, communication training essentially consists of four components: information provision, skill-building, instrumental modification and counselling. For each individual the balance and content of the different components must be decided according to needs and certain ones may be omitted altogether, although all four must be considered.

Information provision, be it about causes of hearing loss in general and the individual's in particular, mechanisms of hearing and hearing aids, or aims of different sections of the rehabilitative process, has the goal of helping the patient's adjustment and making him a more active participant in the rehabilitative process.

Skill-building may range from the banal to the sophisticated, according to the patient's needs. At one extreme the skill-building may entail teaching an elderly individual, with repeated practice, to fit an earmould in his/her ear. On the other hand it may entail training a patient fitted with a cochlear implant to discriminate between two meaningful sound patterns. In some patients it may entail the imparting of various skills by different members of the rehabilitative team. These may entail, for a brainstem-injured patient for example, speech production, speech recognition visually, auditorily and audiovisually; together with a range of hearing tactics.

Instrumental modification entails making adjustments to the characteristics of the patient's hearing aid(s) and earmould(s) to help him/her to cope better with difficulties experienced after the initial fitting. It may also entail the selection of appropriate environmental aids (e.g. TV or telephone aids) if it becomes apparent that the patient's hearing aid(s), even with optimal adjustment, cannot meet the patient's needs in these domains.

Counselling entails discussing the patient's problems, helping him/her to adjust to those which cannot be overcome and discussing ways of overcoming those more amenable to management. The counselling may extend to dealing with other non-auditory problems which the patient may encounter, and which may secondarily influence his auditory performance via changes in his mental state. It is, however, important here for the hearing health care professional to realise the limits of his expertise and involve other specialists, such as clinical psychologists, family therapists and social workers where necessary.

Special educational needs

Special education needs concern particularly children, and especially deaf children. However, young adults with acquired hearing loss and even older adults wishing to actively continue the learning process may have significant needs in this context.

While many general aspects of auditory rehabilitation, particularly good hearing aid fitting and appropriate hearing tactics, are important in this context, an important addition is in the use of FM radio or infrared-based aids. These entail the teacher/lecturer having a microphone and transmitter with the hearing-impaired student having a receiver directly linked to his hearing aid. Such a system gives the student a good and clear input of the teacher's speech regardless of which way he is facing, and maintains a favourable signal/noise ratio. This means for the student that the teacher's voice is not buried in the sounds emanating from the other pupils.

In addition it may be necessary for the student to obtain additional notes from the lecturer, sit sufficiently close to him to be able to read his lips, and, in extreme cases, have a lip-speaker or signer interpreting for him.

A valuable training system has been developed at the National Technical Institute for the Deaf in the USA, where the deaf students are trained with self-training video-recordings to learn individually to lip-read their future teachers in the vocabulary of the subject being taught (Simms *et al.*, 1982).

Special vocational needs (work)

These will depend very much on the nature of the individual's employment and the attitude of his employer. Again many aspects of this are merely an extension of an individual's needs in his more domestic everyday environment. However, particular problems require specific approaches.

The individual who has lost his ability to localise sounds, and has several telephones on his desk, may need telephone receivers with lights in the handpieces which light up when the particular phone rings. S/he may need a clip-on adaptor on the telephone to help him/her hear if s/he uses a variety of phones in different places rather than a built-in system for those with one telephone.

Nurses and doctors may need electronic stethoscopes and sphygmomanometers to help them auscultate their patients and measure blood pressure. All workers in dangerous places will need alternative signalling systems to the normal warning sounds, particularly if the patient is severely hearing-impaired.

Bank clerks and others who have to deal with patients through screens may need special amplifying or electromagnetic systems to help them hear their customers.

In other cases the technology may have to be modified and developed to meet the patient's needs. Appropriate hearing tactics and supportive colleagues and superiors are, however, essential for an appropriate and successful reintegration of the hearing-impaired patient.

In the employment situation, as with all other aspects of auditory rehabilitation, emphasis must be put on problem-solving, matching the technology and behavioural skills to be taught as closely as possible to the patient's abilities and needs.

ORGANISATIONS

Royal National Institute for the Deaf

105 Gower Street, London WC1. (Provides information on all aspects of hearing impairment; also organises certain residential schools)

British Association for the Hard of Hearing
6 Great James Street, London WC1N 3DA. (Information and meetings)

British Association of Deafened People
Longacre, Horsley's Green, High Wycombe, Bucks HP14 3UX. (Information and meetings)

Link Centre
19 Hartfield Road, Eastbourne, East Sussex, BN21 2AR. (Runs residential courses for deafened individuals)

REFERENCES

Davis, H, and Silverman, R. (1970) *Hearing and deafness*, 3rd edn, Holt, Rinehart & Wilson, New York

Goldstein, D.P. and Stephens, S.D.G. (1981) Audiological rehabilitation: management model. I. *Audiology, 20*, 432-52

Hinchcliffe, R. (ed.) (1983) *Hearing and balance in the elderly*, Churchill Livingstone, Edinburgh

Lutman, M.E. and Haggard, M.P. (eds) (1983) *Hearing science and hearing disorders*, Academic Press, London

Schein, J.D. and Delk, M.T. (1974) *The deaf population of the United States.* National Association of the Deaf, Silver Spring, Maryland

Sims, D., Walter, G.G. and Whitehead, R.L. (eds) (1982) *Deafness and communication*, Williams & Wilkins, Baltimore

World Health Organization (1980) *International classification of impairments, disabilities and handicaps*, WHO, Geneva

FURTHER READING

Thomas, A.J. (1984) *Acquired hearing loss*, Academic Press, London

Vognsen, S. (ed) (1976) *Hearing tactics*, Oticon, Copenhagen

Part 5

Neurological Disorders

18

The Young Adult with Neurological Disabilities

Ted Cantrell

There are so many apparently insoluble problems facing the fully healthy school-leaver that adding any severe disability must make the future very grim indeed for many disabled teenagers. Adolescence is a time of great emotional and physical change, where the dependent protected and cared-for 'child' has to learn to become an independent adult, free of parental and professional support or control, and with many crises of identity as a totally new and unknown life looms ahead. It is not helped by news reports of unemployment and threats of international warfare, especially when many of the employed adult population seem ignorant or unconcerned about such problems. Life is a struggle to break free from elders who always wish to advise, who threaten one's privacy, and who tend to treat one as a perpetual child. It is a time of no confidence dressed in bravado, and low status hidden in great energy.

If growing up is complicated by *spina bifida* or *cerebral palsy,* then becoming an adult is far more difficult. The 'perfect people' in society do not give the 'imperfect' a chance, they may focus mockery on the disabled, close friendships are difficult to make or keep, and mobility may depend on other people being free to help in transport. The worst public response to cope with may be pity and charity, sometimes the only way in which the able-bodied are capable of reacting. 'Childhood' status is prolonged excessively when physical needs require daily help from other people.

PREVALENCE OF NEUROLOGICAL DISABILITY

It is useful to try to get some idea of the frequency of different disorders causing disability by relying on community surveys rather than anecdote. A visitor to different centres could get conflicting opinions about the most common and important problems (spinal injury, cerebral palsy or phocomelia). Amelia Harris's survey (1971) attempted to get some idea of the broad categories of disease across the UK, and Wood (1978) calculated the approximate numbers of conditions that might be found in an average health district of 250,000 population (Table 18.1).

Several facts emerge from this table. Firtly, the enormous load placed on every health district to cope with elderly disabled may mean that the young get assistance only by special pleading from pressure groups. Balance of provision must be difficult to maintain, particularly in the group with arthritis. Secondly, the very serious acquired disease MS is already a big problem in the under-44 age group. Thirdly, in an average health district there may be 100 GPs, so the average family doctor is unlikely to have extensive experience of more than one to three disabilities in young adults from his own practice, although he or she may be the closest to the family coping with their problems.

In order to get some better idea of the incidence of different disorders affecting children, Wood (1978) examined Bradshaw's data on the 35,000 applicants for the Rowntree Family Fund. These could be biased towards families with the education and contacts to know about the Fund, but are interesting (Table 18.2). Neurological disorders account for a high proportion of the total, 42 per cent of the major physical disorder group, and probably (in a mixed disorder) a significant number of those with primary mental retardation. Damage to the CNS may therefore be significant in about 50 per cent of all severely disabled children.

Figures are not only difficult to find, but are likely to be changing. For instance, the number of spina bifida children now being operated upon at birth is reduced, as is the incidence generally as a result of alpha-fetoprotein estimates. The current 'bulge' of severe spina bifida young adults is likely to be a significant contribution to the numbers of young disabled well into the end of this century. Clearly it will be encouraging if similar preventive measures show results in reducing the numbers of cerebral palsy children being born, but it is possible that the epidemic levels of head injuries in

Table 18.1: Possible incidences of different disabilities in a health district (250,000 population)

Diagnoses	Total severely or very severely disabled	Age groups No. (16–44)	(No. 65+)
All arthritis	1,074	26	756
Cerebrovascular disease	427	6	316
Congenital disorders	102	61	9
Multiple sclerosis (MS)	96	27	13
Paraplegia	45	6	23
Mentally ill	29	5	13
Amputees	52	10	24
Totals	1,825	141	1,154

Table 18.2: Applicants for Rowntree Family Fund

Condition	Percentage	Group totals (%)
Mental diseases		
Down's syndrome Retarded	33	37
Mentally ill Autistic	4	
Sensory diseases		
Blind	2.7	8
Deaf	5	
Physical diseases		
Spina bifida	17	
Hemiplegia/paraplegia	17	53
Epilepsy Neurological disease	5	
Muscular dystrophy	2.8	
CVS diseases,	3.5	
etc	9.9	

the teenage and young adult population may be a very large group in the future. It is also possible that a new generation of brain-damaged or retarded children may result from those saved by the increased emphasis on intensive neonatal care for earlier stages of premature birth.

The total numbers of young people unable to look after themselves or cope alone with everyday tasks are shown in the Table 18.3 (from Wood), derived from Bradshaw's data, on disabled children.

Table 18.3: Young people unable to cope with everyday tasks (%)

Incontinent or urinary diversions	30
Need some help with toilet	77
Cannot walk independently (even with aids)	35
Parents' social life affected by the care of the child	78
Parents' earnings reduced by care of the child	40

These figures highlight another problem, namely a significant number of disabled young adults who are not able to live alone since they need some help with everyday living. Ideally, each one should be given an opportunity to be trained to live more independently, preferably before or during school, but this is not often possible when major energies are expended on trying to cope with school work, or when the policy of integration into open schools mean there is nobody skilled to help them learn to be independent.

The total number of people aged 16–65 who are dependent on the care of others is not easy to find, but data from Southampton suggest that 1 in 1,000 of the population is dependent on others due to physical disability (Cantrell *et al.*, 1985). It is possible that the numbers are higher, and this might show if the search was made in a truly house-to-house survey.

DISABILITY

The most important details of the disabled person's life are particular to those individuals who have been damaged. There is no 'typical spastic'. What counts most in the development of lifestyle are:

(1) *The outlook* or prognosis of the underlying conditions (static, improving, progressive or unpredictable)

(2) *The assets*: morale, strength of character and sense of humour of the individual, and what qualities or skills they have.

(3) *Personal objectives*: what sort of activities they wish to follow, but which may be limited (aims matched to ability).

(4) *Supports*: the availability of family, social or professional support in overcoming problems.

Although one could perhaps predict that 25 per cent of spina bifida adults are unable to walk freely, what matters more is how many have the energy and physical potential to learn to walk, will make every effort to do so, have a clear need to be able to, and can call on all the help they need to overcome the difficulties. For those who cannot readily achieve walking, the priority may be to accept this and adapt to other mobility patterns and goals. Two people with such a condition may therefore have an identical neurological condition (factor 1) but end up with totally different results due to differences in the other three variables. One may thrive on becoming a master chess player, the other become paralysed by depression because of all the things he cannot achieve.

Although it is essential to explore the disability problems of each person, it is equally important to look for abilities, strengths and potential, since these may be key factors in overcoming the limitations of the life they face. Anyone with a sense of humour can learn to laugh at himself and overcome feelings of inadequacy and deprivation. The person with any talent, academic, creative or practical, needs to find a support group and tutors who will bring that quality to its full capacity. The easily deflated, apathetic or depressed person will always be far more difficult to help.

PREDICTIONS (PROGNOSIS)

The major differences between disabled people depend on personality, prognosis and family characteristics. A careful medical investigation should be able to predict with some accuracy whether the young person's condition is:

(1) *improving*, with capacity to do better with great effort, special training or equipment;
(2) *static*, with little prospect of change;
(3) *deteriorating*, either as a likely result of neglecting special procedures (e.g. urinary infection testing) or because the disease usually becomes worse (e.g. muscular dystrophy).

It makes a great difference to any family to know that the latest in medical science is attempting to improve the condition. Equally, if the condition is deteriorating they need regular access to a specialist prepared to advise on the genuine value of any new advance they hear about in the media. It is an unbearable burden to live with a relative whose outlook contains no hope, and to be isolated from any professional person willing to listen and advise.

What is far more difficult to quantify and classify is the strength of character and personality of the disabled person and the main carer(s). These features are as important for long-term planning as the primary disease prognosis, but find little mention in medical records. In general, there are three categories of family to identify:

(1) *Stable*, where character, sense of humour, physical and mental resources are obviously good, a strong family where no reason for breakdown can be foreseen.

(2) *Potentially unstable*, where the home care may be adequate now, but past history suggests that pressure of a stressful situation will not be well tolerated.

(3) *Unstable*, where the home situation is already full of despair or neglect, or getting worse.

All disabled young people have in common the fact that there are several things they cannot do to the same level as their contemporaries. They will face *stigma* when their condition is easily visible (e.g. ataxia or callipers) and misunderstanding when it is invisible (e.g. fatigue, memory loss or deafness). Many will have to struggle hard to live away from relatives or to get regular care staff. Most will find post-school society more hostile and demanding than they expected, and certainly not the welcome relief they look forward to when they escape from school.

PAOM (PROBLEM- AND ASSET-ORIENTATED MANAGEMENT)

Lawrence Weed (1969) was instrumental in publicising a system of data organisation which has been debated widely and used by many (POMR, problem-orientated medical records). He stressed the need for any medical practitioner to define more precisely the specific disorders presented by a patient, so that elements of the whole could be tackled separately.

One difficulty with applying Weed's system to disabled people is that it concentrates on the negative side of a person; on what is wrong. As often used by medical people this may be restricted to medical comments (e.g. hypertension, poor visual acuity, hemiplegia), whereas it really should be a list that includes all disabilities, or practical outcomes of the condition (e.g. job impossible, reactive apathy, inadequate finance). Another difficulty is that the standard list does not include details of the family, or the context from which a person comes, or the people able and willing to be helpers in community life.

We are using in Southampton a Household Matrix System (Cantrell and Dawson, 1983) in which both positive and negative factors of importance are recorded for both the primary disabled person and the main helpers (see Figure 18.1). It is a simple, practical scheme for the management of any lifestyle, but it may be better when quantified, rather than descriptive.

It is clear from this example that the problems of this individual could be so great as to make totally independent life and employment difficult to achieve. Because of the range of personal assets it would seem likely that intensive further training (if wanted) might allow greater development of the personal abilities and lead to some opportunities for independent living

Figure 18.1: Example: PAOM = Problem and asset-orientated management

Name: AP ERSON (age 18)

Diagnosis: Cerebral palsy (diplegia and ataxia)

	Problems	Assets
Individual	Easily fatigued Slow Tendency to trip Awkward gait Slurred speech Ataxic hands	CSE 2 subjects Motivated to improve Almost ADL-independent Intelligent Interest in music Sense of humour
Family	Mother: backache Two younger children Low income	Supportive relatives Own house Father in regular work

and perhaps employment. The family side of the matrix indicates that home care will probably be available for as long as it is wanted, but that AP Erson will be competing for limited resources with two younger children whose needs are as yet undefined.

The matrix also highlights an important medical problem in the mother, since a history of backache identifies a recurrent condition that is likely to give more trouble if she has to do regular lifting. Hence independence training, especially in mobility and ADL (or activities of daily living) is of great importance.

If this example contained a less motivated person, totally dependent on others, with a single parent in difficult social circumstances, the whole balance of the family matrix would shift adversely (Figure 18.2).

Figure 18.2:

	Problems	Assets
I	++	0
F	++	0

If the underlying disease is one of physical and/or mental deterioration (e.g. MS), then the balance again is much more negative, and this will put far greater pressure on the family, with little prospect of relief in the future and a far greater likelihood of family breakdown.

ASSETS = POSSIBLE DREAMS

It is just as important to search for every possible interest, skill or potential in a disabled person as it is to look for problems, for two reasons. Firstly, it is the major guide to future development and to the building up of morale. However crazy (in physical terms) is the enthusiasm, it must be explored with the help of others with the same interest, as it could lead to something for which the disabled person wants to get up each day and strive. Without such dreams for the future the person becomes a 'case' or a 'client', an object that has to be looked after each day. In the PAOM example given earlier, the only immediate assets listed that were 'work-related' were music and CSE exams. It would make more sense to explore many more potential hobbies, seeking an enthusiasm to build on. If fully developed, a proper interest would mean that each day's activities have a direction and provide a reason to get through the mundane activities of self-care and mobility. Examples of assets which may be worth exploring to the extremes of potential are: music, gardening, academic work, fishing, painting, computing, driving, electronics, business, sports, nature studies, reading, sculpture, politics, craft work, writing, pottery, stamps, photography and sailing.

A second reason why assets are worth searching for is that they can often be a way of tackling some of the negative or problem areas. If a person cannot be bothered to go once more to the physiotherapy department to do repetitive exercises, or struggle once more with domestic work in OT, it may be because the activity is energy-sapping but unrelated to anything concrete in the future. Give disabled persons a clear vision of what they might do in the future, a 'possible dream', then it may make more sense for them to build muscles or learn to cook for themselves and be more independent as part of a wider plan.

DISABILITY MANAGEMENT — THE DOCTOR'S ROLE

It is essential that any doctor concerned with the planning of help for a disabled person has a comprehensive knowledge of the underlying medical condition, to allow prediction of future needs. If the GP is to be primary coordinator of this work, he (or she) must be given enough data from any relevant hospital consultant on which to base important decisions. If the condition is an obscure one, then the GP needs advice on what natural history to expect.

There is a second stage in diagnosis which the primary doctor needs to initiate, namely a medical analysis of each symptom/problem in order to take management one stage further. Table 18.4 shows how this analysis might proceed from the simple statement 'funny walk' or 'shyness' to a much more detailed understanding of why the problem arises and some solutions. Although this can be done by any GP or hospital doctor, it may be far better to bring in, at this stage, the expertise of other professionals to perform an in-depth assessment. The physiotherapist is much more used to analysing movement and gait, the speech therapist better at language/ speech disorders, and many other experts are relevant (e.g. occupational therapist, social worker, orthotist, psychologist, engineer).

An interested doctor prepared to assess the patient, analyse the problems and to build a continuing dialogue with other people who can answer them, makes for a comprehensive approach to the management of complex disabilities.

Table 18.4: Examples of disability problems

Problems	Analysis	Solutions
Shy	Could be real deformity/inabilities May be hypersensitive to feelings of others Could be in a hostile environment	Desensitisation training, PHAB clubs Counselling New training/working centre Education of the great British public
Funny speech	Regional accents or dysarthria? Dysphasia, breathing dyspraxia	Careful speech assessment and retraining
Funny walk	Any neuromuscular or arthritic cause General weakness or local problem Functional disorder	Detailed neuromuscular assessment Gait training, special equipment Confrontation with discrepancies
Poor school performance	Intellectually poor, concentration ↓ Intellectually good, frequently interrupted or changing schools Perception problems Totally low morale or expectations Sensory problems (vision/hearing)	Psychogenetic studies ? Intelligence Educational guidance on best training Special guidance for teachers/parents Intensive school/training Remedial teaching
Frustration	Sensible objectives — avoidable obstacles Unreasonable objectives — lacking insight Unavoidable obstacles in practical living	Awareness training Goal setting and careful self-monitoring Industrial/independence training — counselling
Skin sores	Immobility or insensitive areas Lack of skin care Poorly designed equipment (callipers, wheelchair, furniture)	Moving every 20 minutes Self-examination daily Better design of equipment
Isolation	Poor mobility, lack of self-movement No transport Not able to drive (epilepsy, vision, poor concentration, ataxia) Poor speech/hearing ability Pathological shyness, withdrawn person Unfriendly personality, hostile neighbours	Mobility retraining Mobility training centre Better public or private transport Speech or hearing therapy Counselling and independence training, PHAB Better access to work, pubs, clubs, houses, etc.

THE SOUTHAMPTON SURVEY (COMMUNITY CARE AND FAMILY SUPPORT)

In 1976 a start was made on a project to monitor the needs of heavily disabled people in Southampton, with a particular interest in looking at individuals and the families or helpers they relied on. The first 100 physically disabled people (ages 16–65) were then followed up for three years in order to see how they coped with the problems of living in the community (Cantrell *et al.*, 1985). Several important findings came out of this study, particularly relevant for the young disabled adult:

(1) Many people existed at home without regular contacts with any service, and often had answerable but unmet needs. It would probably be better if all such disabled people had regular visits from *some* statutory service (e.g. health visitors), or a chosen key worker.

(2) There was an extremely high rate of family breakdown seen (50 per cent approximately) because of the strains of looking after a person 24 hours per day, seven days a week. Admittedly there was a much higher prevalence of deteriorating disease than in the community (e.g. MS, 30 per cent), but the warning is there — home care is very hard work.

(3) Many relatives (50 per cent) had health problems of their own, and unless given regular support were liable to crack up under the strain of constant caring.

(4) The most essential quality of a disabled person that will determine the burden of home care is independence time; in other words the maximum amount of time that they can cope alone with all aspects of movement, self-care, toileting and activity. In 30 per cent of this series the maximum was two hours or less, a measure of very high dependency and strain on helpers. Clearly, independence time is made longer by the very determined person keen to do as much as possible for himself, but it does also increase with high morale, proper OT assessment and a well-designed house with essential equipment.

The major implication from this study is that no plans should be made for someone to leave hospital (or school) unless a careful study is made of the problems and assets of both the individual and the family members who are going to be involved.

RESOURCES FOR DISABLED PEOPLE OR PROFESSIONALS

It is easy to get the impression, when living with a severe disability, that one is isolated, and that there are few people to turn to; many professionals share this view. In reality, Britain is full of self-help, special interest and specialist groups of all shapes and sizes, willing to help with specific problems. What is lacking is a good contact between clients and resources.

Help for Health, a library-based information service in Southampton, received 5,000 enquiries from professionals and disabled people in 1984. It has details of at least 1,000 national bodies concerned with some aspect of disabilities, and over 2,000 local groups throughout Wessex. The Mental Health Foundation claim to have 10,000 groups on their lists, all involved in some voluntary or statutory work for people in need. Detailed studies in Wiltshire are producing amazing numbers of groups (about 6,000, including self-help, village halls, playgroups and social clubs). Many groups have been criticised by disabled people as basically amateur collections of patronising busybodies, but nearly always they are organised by people who are very keen to give their services, often highly motivated by having had to cope with a severe disability in their own families.

What is needed is better availability of information for anyone trying to solve a problem as to who there is locally (or nationally) who can offer help or solutions. It is possible to identify four levels in the information network, which all have an important part to play in the process of finding answers to disability problems (see Resources, Chapter 49).

(a) *Enquirers.* Any disabled person, or family, or any GP, health visitor, local professional or caring service may have problems they cannot answer.
(b) *Local information sources*
(1) Citizens' Advice Bureaux } in most towns and villages
(2) Public libraries }
(c) *Comprehensive resource centres.* These would be contacted by telephone or personal visits.
(d) *Professional advisers.* Any professional group working with disabled people, disabled people themselves and all voluntary or statutory groups and national fact-finding bodies (e.g. architecture, sport, work, holidays, etc.).

The information network really presents different qualities at each level (Table 18.5).

Table 18.5: Local information network

(a)	(b)	(c)	(d)
Disabled people	CAB	Help for Health	DLF Doctors Physiotherapists
GP teams	Public library	DIAL Equipment Demonstration Centres Housing Dept	Occupational therapists Speech therapists Social workers Disabled people Voluntary associations Architects Sportsmen DROs
Families			
Enquirers	Public access	Comprehensive resource centres	Professional advisers

(a) *Enquirers* are better informed if they are the sort of families (or doctors) who keep asking questions and keep trying to gain more information or knowledge. If they do not ask questions the whole network becomes irrelevant, since it is unusual for services to search out clients. In our survey of heavily disabled people in Southampton (Cantrell *et al.*, 1985) we found many families in difficulty because they did not know how to find answers for their unmet needs. There are many doctors who do not regularly attend meetings or show great keenness for new information, and their responses to patients' questions are either inspired guesses or unhelpful. A key worker would be particularly helpful in this group.

(b) *Public access.* In some areas the Citizens' Advice Bureaux and public libraries are beginning to advertise their willingness to channel the wide range of public enquiries to expert sources.

(c) *Resource centres.* These are only useful if they are truly open-access every day (eight hours/day) and carry a totally comprehensive bank of data that is easy to retrieve and up to date.

(d) *Professional advisers.* The main role of professionals is in their knowledge of a specific area of information, or special skills they have been trained in or gained by experience. The worst kind of professional (including the 'professional disabled person') is the type who pretends to know all the answers and refuses to recognise the skills and expertise of other colleagues. The ideal information network requires regular contact between experts who respect each other.

In the case-example (Figure 18.1 — PAOMR), the disabled person or parents might go initially to the public library for advice. They could be referred to the local 'DIAL', but the value of the help given would depend on how much the DIAL group regularly updated their information with all local or national professional groups.

SPECIFIC AND USEFUL RESOURCES (and see Chapter 49)

Special mention should be made of some types of resource group that are of particular relevance to the young disabled person:

(a) *Disorder-specific groups.* These offer a kind of practical expertise in the form of other families who have been through the same sort of trials and tribulations. Examples are the Spastics Society, Headway (for head injuries), or the Spina Bifida Association. These can offer help to the disabled, support for families, encourage independence, promote better research and lobby for improved services.

(b) *Social links.* It is essential to find local groups prepared to offer a place where young people can get to know each other informally, whether disabled or able-bodied. Many local clubs, sports centres and coffee bars are available to help remove the barriers of the shy and embarrassed generation, also allowing some release of energy through physical activities.

PHAB is the group that sponsors special meeting places between the physically handicapped and able-bodied.

(c) *Centres for independent living* are growing as the British response to the very political and successful American CIL movement. These groups can give enormous support to disabled people by their similarly disabled age group, and promote activity and self-confidence. Some have been so militant in their approach as to raise barriers, but when well led they can offer a great deal of help to young people who are trying to develop lives of their own in the community.

(d) *Sports clubs* exist in many places with special facilities or equipment for disabled people to use, if they wish, or times set aside for swimming, gym games, angling and many other activities. Much interest is being roused by special boats (e.g. *Lord Nelson*) and holidays or training courses for those who wish to sail.

(e) *Family replacement schemes.* A number of voluntary and statutory groups offer considerable help to those families who have to give daily assistance to a young person living in the community. The whole care attendant movement has proved to be of enormous value to many people, and was inspired by the original Rugby 'Crossroads' scheme. Many other systems now exist.

This approach means that healthy people can be paid to offer family replacement work, to give regular assistance to disabled people living alone, or temporary help at times of main-helper illness. They may give enough relief to relatives so that they can continue to manage the stressful work of long-term support for a disabled person. Their work is ideally supplemented by regular trips to a local day centre, assisted holidays, or planned cyclical relief admissions to a special unit (Lovelock, 1981).

Without family support schemes we have found evidence that many relatives crack up physically and mentally from the strain of regular and constant care, and this family breakdown is well worth preventing (Cantrell *et al.*, 1985).

Are case conferences useful?

The long-term planning of community care for any disabled person, particularly after leaving the unwelcome support of school, is a process that is full of complexity. So many statutory and voluntary organisations may be involved, and have no regular contact with each other. The result can be bureaucratic chaos, unless one person (key worker) makes sure that the others are in touch and that all know what is being done and needed. It is useful to meet occasionally for a case conference of those involved, but four cautions should be raised.

(1) *Expense* in travel and people's time can be massive if the meeting is not documented and prepared properly, or if people are ignorant about the kind of service offered by the others.

(2) *Personalities* can impede planning if any one member is striving to dominate the team, or if another person who does know a lot is too shy to speak before the rest.

(3) *Family* involvement is essential if the real customers are to be fully involved in community care.

(4) *Privacy* is threatened unless documentation and conversation are completely controlled.

Parents and professionals can easily be treated as adversaries if the young person is trying to break through the barrier of the child role to one of self-control and self-determination. It is also common to see the anger and frustration of the disability ('Why me?') transferred to hatred of the only people available who may be able to offer help or finance for some sort of independent life.

Rehabilitation units can offer help to young people by taking them into more neutral accommodation away from the familiar family strife and care patterns to a context where the whole lifestyle can be assessed and planned. this is ideally done in a unit which has an 'ordinary house' or bungalow attached, and where the whole 24-hour routine can be rehearsed (self-care, cooking, transport to the shops, social events and occupation) and counselling can be offered.

COMMON DISABILITY PROBLEMS

All young disabled people face the same myriad of problems that make adolescence a difficult period for all young adults. Many of these are made worse by immobility, obvious ataxia and speech disorders, and by visible features which make them incapable of merging into the general teenage fashion and behaviour patterns. They stand out as especially 'odd' at an age when everyone is acutely self-conscious and pretending not to be.

Some of the common problems of disabled people are discussed in other chapters of this book, and require only special mention because of teenage factors:

(a) *Education* (Chapter 40) is a major struggle where a local school is not designed for the wheelchair or unsteady walker, or where staff are unable to restrain the inevitable teasing or abuse from other students. There is always a debate about whether to learn the rules of the social jungle and keep in touch with the local community by risking the local school, or rather to commute to a distant special school that can make allowances for slow speech, awkward gait, perception problems and other sequelae of disabling conditions, but loses touch with the community.

(b) *Transport* (Chapter 47) needs individual assessment, initially by therapists and engineers, in order to find out how a young person can be trained to achieve maximum mobility. This should include the use of public transport or the chance to learn to drive.

(c) *Finance* is critical, but there is clear evidence that many disabled people do not get all the (minimal) benefits they are entitled to. It is essential that someone (a genuine expert) is given the task of making sure that the needs of any young disabled person and his family are studied with great care to see if anything else can be claimed. The *Disability Alliance Handbook* (annual) is a good guide for this.

(d) *Housing* (Chapter 39). If a person elects genuinely to stay with parents, then the design of the house and the space allocated need to be reviewed by an OT on a home visit.

If the client really wants to live away from home (not all do), then two other essential moves must be made. Firstly, the precise daily (or infrequent) needs he has for *personal* help from other people must be assessed, preferably on a 24-hour chart (Cantrell and Dawson, 1983) to see how long the total independence times are, and how often through the day help is needed. If two hours is the maximum independence time, then living-in or reliable on-call helpers have to be found.

Secondly, *buildings* are being provided by many councils and housing associations for disabled people. They take a long time to plan and set up; not all have personal care available; and no design exists which will automatically suit every handicap. CEH (Centre on Environment for the Handicapped) provides excellent advice from architects and disabled people on this subject.

(e) *Incontinence* (Chapter 29) is a distressing burden for the active teenager, and it is essential that some of the many satisfactory systems available are considered for any young adult facing this. It is of course much more difficult to find safe, acceptable answers for girls. Continence advisors may be helpful.

(f) *Sensory loss* in the skin anywhere is a potent cause of pressure areas, and needs careful education so that the person learns how to avoid trouble and how to examine the skin daily for signs of damage. A mistake leading to an ulcer can lead to weeks or months of frustrating hospital or bed care to heal up (Chapter 31).

(g) *Blindness* (Chapter 16) and *deafness* (Chapter 17) both have specific major implications requiring training and equipment for young people, and are best dealt with by people with special experience in this field.

(h) *Confidence* is commonly lacking in teenagers, or it may be diverted to aggressiveness or depression. Kept within a small family circle this may have little chance of resolution without a very relaxed and caring open relationship, and some opportunities for holidays away, special hobbies or opportunities for being adventurous (e.g. sailing courses) may make a major difference in allowing people to learn for themselves how to accept themselves in the company of others.

(i) *Smothering relatives or helpers.* It is a natural reaction of many parents, and of many other helpers, to overdo the caring for someone who has to struggle to cope, and to perpetuate the dependence status. This may be done from a sense of guilt or pity, and most families find it difficult to facilitate a smooth transition to a position where disabled sons or daughters are pushed to do more for themselves, take risks, make mistakes and gain maximum independence. If this is not achieved then, when the parent is ill or dies, the young disabled persons suddenly have to manage by themselves, in a much more hostile or difficult context.

(j) *Sexual development* (Chapter 30). It is totally wrong to assume that a disabled person does not develop normal sexual feelings (sometimes very powerful ones). It is common to assume that if these are not mentioned they do not exist. Anyone who has taken time to raise the matter in conversation with a young disabled person will find the floodgates opened for a series of strong unresolved feelings and many practical problems. For most doctors and health workers it is probably best to be able to ask the initial questions directing the patient to others with more training and time to deal with the detailed advice and counselling (e.g. Family Planning Association or Marriage Guidance Council). Some problems may need specific medical advice (incontinence, painful joints, paralysis, sensory loss, poor mobility, ataxia), but probably the majority of difficulties are caused by problems of embarrassment, how to relate to the opposite sex, how to express tenderness and affection, particularly if genital contact is difficult or impossible.

(k) *Isolation* is common because of difficulties in getting to the usual places where young people meet, the stigma of being ‘crippled’ or different, and the difficulty in being able to be spontaneous and go off with friends (camping, disco, parties, concerts, etc.). The impulse to go off as a group will be considerably inhibited if there are routines of care needed (e.g. catheter bags) or if mobility is impaired and others are rushing off (by foot, bus, train or hitch-hiking). Some disabled people are cheerful, outgoing, extrovert and popular and can ignore themselves enough to be able to mix well; the great majority lead lonely lives and may need help to meet others.

(l) *Anger* is a powerful response when a young person’s needs are frustrated by pain, immobility or other problems. Not only are they angry about having the condition that limits them, but they also can become aggressive about the things they cannot do and particularly with people who may want to help them (‘do-gooders’). This reaction is understandable and often unanswerable, and it is probably better if it is allowed some expression. Sometimes it is a call for help, and leads to better assessment and the resolution of some practical needs, but too often the anger raises antipathy or avoidance and prevents such answers being considered.

(m) *Menstruation.* For the teenage girl with disabilities there may be embarrassing problems about managing menstrual loss, particularly if periods are irregular. For some there is a need for a helper who is regularly available to help deal with this, although special equipment does exist for self-care which should be encouraged where possible.

IMPAIRMENT-SPECIFIC PROBLEMS

Cerebral palsy

This title encompasses a varied range of disabilities arising from congenital (or perinatal) brain damage and therefore may present at any spot on a range from intellectual/perceptual/speech disorders to the more visible hemiplegia/paraplegia/diplegia or ataxic movement difficulties. The special complications that need mention are:

(a) *Joint contractures* are common, particularly if a limb-stretching routine is not practised daily from early childhood. This approach minimises the short tendons, distorted limbs and painfully stiff joints; anyone who has dealt with untreated adults with CP is aware of the profound restrictions that occur from this disorder if neglected.

(b) *Osteoarthritis* may occur early because of distorted joints and the very hectic gait which throws body weight into joints and movements never designed for such repeated trauma. The neck and feet may be particularly affected and become painful, and so can hard-pressed hands. A variety of special equipment and shoes may be needed.

(c) *Speech* can be incoherent or simply difficult to understand. Most young adults want to talk endlessly, be easily understood and often commune with the noisy background of pop records. To tackle this with spastic distorted speech is a major disadvantage to building up new friendships and keeping up with the whole group. It can interfere with education. Some of the distortions are reducible if expert training of the mouth and desensitisation of the tongue are introduced and practised on first diagnosis (Chapter 15).

(d) *Stigma.* The public usually assumes that someone with funny speech and peculiar gait is mentally subnormal. It takes time to prove that one has intelligence and a sense of humour. Groups like PHAB do much to allow the real worth of the young person to emerge.

Spina bifida

Patients with spina bifida may be paraplegic and may often show early (or later) the serious complications of hydrocephalus and perception problems. Special disabilities are:

(a) *Renal failure* has to be carefully avoided by regular checking of incontinence appliances, looking for recurrent infections and periodic ultrasound and/or IVP studies. A standing frame routine can improve bladder drainage, and hence renal function long-term, and may be more reliable than the struggle to keep walking with the common retreat to wheelchair mobility (Chapter 29).

(b) *Perception problems* need identifying early because they may mask other learning abilities by giving the general impression of a slow learner. Preparation for employment (or hobbies) may require that greater training in practical skills is given to allow for visuospatial or verbal association difficulties. This is within the scope of the OT, but not always available in open schools, or in employment training centres.

(c) *Pressure sores* have been mentioned, but are usually a preventable disaster. Far more special equipment is now available to help avoid these (special beds, mattresses and cushions, alarms for the immobile, etc.) (Chapter 31).

(d) *Apathy and lethargy* are said by some to be the only retreat some people have from severe handicap. Careful OT, psychological and social evaluation are needed to make sure that these do not arise from perception problems, repressed anxiety, family stresses or an uninformed feeling of hopelessness about the future. It is also vital to make sure that the limited-ambition teenager is not being pressurised by over-ambitious and aggressive parents with unrealistic expectations.

(e) *Scoliosis* and decreasing chest/lung function can be a major difficulty when the whole spine develops curvatures and pulmonary function is compromised. Not only does this impede activity due to breathlessness, but people are much more prone to serious chest infections. Preventive bracing and physiotherapy given regularly from an early stage can minimise these effects, but surgery may be needed (Chapter 28) (Figure 18.3).

Deteriorating diseases

Some conditions, like MS and muscular dystrophy, will usually get worse. Such patients should be monitored regularly and repeatedly. The prospect of deteriorating can shatter all but the strongest of people. It is made easier if frank and open planning is available not only for present needs but for future needs. It helps to offer regular supported holidays (together or

Figure 18.3: Spina bifida with scoliosis convex to the left with rotation, special cushioning support was needed in the wheelchair. The feet may become very cold as well as swollen; soft thick footwear may be useful

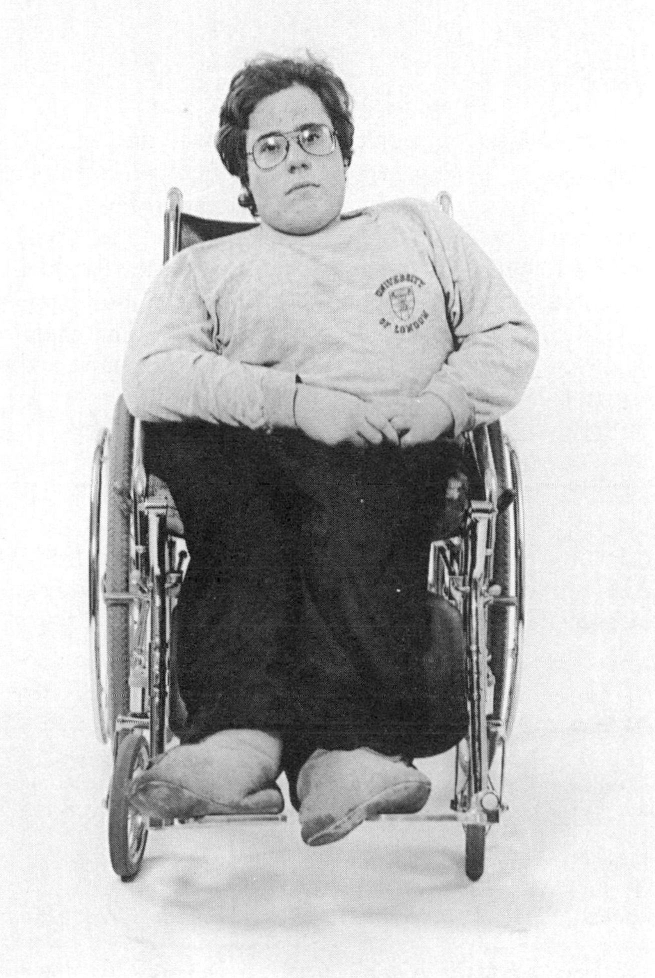

separately) so that all can live with each other without tearing themselves apart.

There must be one person to whom they can turn regularly or when needed to examine each new problem. We can recommend health visitors for this work from Southampton experience, since they are trained widely enough to be familiar with medical and social needs. Social workers can sustain only a limited case-load, and GPs tend to stick to short intensive sessions concerned with purely medical matters. It is essential for any family in this position that one key worker is identified who can maintain contact and is well accepted by the young person and the relative.

CONCLUSION

The needs of most disabled people can be analysed into a series of components in a problem list by any medical practitioner who listens well and uses common sense. Answers to such needs are not so easy, but if they are referred to different professions and resource groups, then suitable answers can usually be found. This process is more complete when the enquiry includes a search for motivating interests (or assets) and similar positive and negative factors for the family or main helper. The chapter explores some ways in which needs can be matched up with resources or answers. It concludes with some important reference books.

ACKNOWLEDGEMENTS

I am particularly grateful for detailed resources advice from Bob Gann (Help for Health) and Sue Farr (Aids Demonstration Centre) and also to the many disabled people who have taught me so much.

REFERENCES

Cantrell, E.G. and Dawson, J. (1983) Young disabled in the community. In J. Barbenel, C.D. Forbes and G.D.O. Lowe (eds), *Pressure sores*, Macmillan, London

Cantrell, E.G., Dawson, J. and Glastonbury, G. (1985) *Prisoners of Handicap*, RADAR, London

Harris, Amelia (1971) *Handicapped and impaired in Great Britain*, HMSO, London

Lovelock, R. (1981) *Friends in deed*, Social Services Research Intelligence Unit, Hampshire Social Services

Weed, L. (1969) *Medical records, medical education and patient care*, Case Western Reserve University

Wood, P.N.H. (1978) Size of the problem and causes of chronic sickness in the young. *J. Roy Soc. Med.*, *71*, 437-42

BOOK GUIDE

The New Source Book for the Disabled, edited by Glorya Hale, Heinemann, 1983.

A practical, well illustrated book dealing with many aspects of daily living, work and leisure, including many suggestions of aids and equipment.

Signpost — where to go for advice, information and help. RICA (Research Institute for Consumer Affairs), 1984. As the name implies, it directs you to further detailed help. Has a chapter on 'Aids to make life easier'.

Compass — the direction finder for disabled people. DIG (Disabled Income Group), 1984. Has a chapter on 'Aids, equipment and services', and detailed advice on finance and welfare benefits.

With a little help. Series of eight booklets. Philippa Harpin. Muscular Dystrophy Group of GB. An excellent series of booklets with many practical suggestions of use to many people with neuromuscular problems, not just MD. Very well illustrated.

Chapter 49, on Resources available, lists information and organisations to help disabled people.

19

Motor Neurone Disease

Richard Langton Hewer

INTRODUCTION

Motor neurone disease (MND) is one of those conditions which we all hope we shall never develop ourselves. It involves progressive weakness of the limb and bulbar muscles. The cause of the disorder is totally unknown, and no treatment is available to halt its inexorable progress. The majority of patients die within three years. Since the death of David Niven the disorder has become better known, and much has been written about it. Despite our therapeutic impotence, the disorder poses a major challenge to the competence of the medical and allied professions. Informed and compassionate management can undoubtedly ease the distress and discomfort of patients and their relatives. The object of this chapter is to show how this may be achieved.

WHAT IS MOTOR NEURONE DISEASE?

In MND degeneration occurs in the motor neurones, i.e. those that control certain specific components of muscle movement. The vast majority of the remaining portions of the nervous system remain normal.

There are two main groups of motor neurones. The first originates in the cells of the motor and pre-motor cortex and travels through the brain to terminate either in the brainstem or in the spinal cord, in close relation to the bulbar nuclei or the anterior horn cells. The second group of motor neurones have their origin in the brainstem or in the spinal cord and terminate on the muscle fibres. Thus four main structures are involved in MND:

(1) *The anterior horns of the spinal cord.* Degeneration of these cells results in wasting and weakness of muscles. The term 'progressive muscular atrophy' (PMA) is applied when muscle wasting and weakness predominate.

(2) *The corticospinal tracts.* These tracts lie in the lateral columns of the spinal cord and contain the long nerve fibres which originate in the motor and pre-motor cortex of the brain. Involvement of this structure produces 'upper motor neurone' signs in the limbs — weakness, spasticity, and extensor plantar responses. The term amyotrophic lateral sclerosis (ALS) is applied when these upper motor neurone signs predominate. In practice *there is usually a combination of upper and lower motor neurone signs* (i.e. muscle wasting with exaggerated tendon reflexes and spasticity).

(3) *The nuclei of the nerves to the bulbar muscles.* These nuclei are the counterparts of the anterior horn cells discussed above. For example, there may be degeneration of cells in the hypoglossal nuclei (situated in the medulla) producing wasting of the tongue. The term *bulbar palsy* is applied when wasting of bulbar muscles occurs.

(4) *The corticobulbar fibres.* These fibres (counterparts of the corticospinal fibres discussed above) contain the nerve fibres of cells which originate in the motor and pre-motor cortex. Involvement produces signs of 'upper motor neurone' involvement in the brainstem territory — for example, a spastic tongue which cannot be protruded, and an exaggerated jaw and facial jerk.

When upper motor neurone signs predominate, the term pseudo-bulbar palsy is applied. In practice *there are usually signs of both upper and lower motor neurone involvement (for example, a wasted but spastic tongue).*

The fibres in the spinal cord subserving sensation are not involved. Precisely why these particular areas are affected in motor neurone disease, is not known. Vision, hearing and intellectual function remain intact to the end.

HOW MANY CASES?

The annual incidence rate is 1-2 persons per 100,000 population, and the prevalence is about 6 per 100,000. Most patients are aged between 50 and 70. The disorder is usually sporadic, but in about 5 per cent of cases it appears to be familial — with an autosomal dominant mode of inheritance.

EARLY SYMPTOMS

The early clinical features vary considerably — depending upon which structures in the central nervous system are affected. Common early symptoms include the following:

(1) Wasting and weakness of one hand. This may produce difficulty in writing and doing up buttons.

(2) A 'foot-drop' due to weakness of dorsiflexion of one foot.

(3) Weakness of the proximal limb muscles producing difficulty with washing the hair and shaving if the arms are affected, and difficulty with mounting stairs if the legs are involved. In many instances there is spontaneous twitching of muscles (fasciculation).

(4) If upper motor neurone signs predominate there may be a complaint of stiffness in the legs and inability to walk fast.

(5) In about 20 per cent of cases the first symptoms involve the bulbar muscles, causing slurred speech and choking with fluids.

Later symptoms

Later in the disease the above symptoms become more troublesome and others develop. These problems are discussed below.

THE DIAGNOSIS

The diagnosis is made largely on clinical grounds, i.e. after carefully taking a history and examining the patient. Electromyography may be a useful adjunct. In general the diagnosis is easy for a neurologist to make in about 80 per cent of cases. In the remaining 20 per cent there can be substantial doubt, at least in the early stages.

Obviously the certainty with which the diagnosis can be made will influence what the patient is told. There is much to be said for obtaining a 'second opinion' if the diagnosis of MND is being seriously entertained.

THE PROGNOSIS

No treatment has been shown to alter the course of the disease. The majority of patients die within three years, but up to 30 per cent may survive five years or even more. The prognosis is particularly bad in patients who show dysphagia and choking at an early stage.

WHAT SHOULD THE PATIENT BE TOLD?

There has been some debate about precisely what the patient should be told (Carey, 1986). The following points need to be borne in mind:

(1) the majority of people have not heard of MND, and simply telling them the name of the disorder may be meaningless;

(2) no medical treatment will influence the course of the disease.

Our practice is to tell both the patient and spouse the diagnosis in general terms at an early stage once it is reasonably certain. We do not find it appropriate to spell out the future in great detail at this early stage. We consider that 'gradual dawning' is probably better than 'brutal telling' in most patients. As time goes on, and the patient becomes psychologically more receptive, more details can be given. Much sensitivity is required, and it is totally unsatisfactory for these delicate matters to be dealt with by inexperienced junior staff. However, it is important that each member of the team should be aware of what has been said.

PROBLEMS EXPERIENCED BY MND PATIENTS

The nature and range of problems experienced by MND patients and their families is very considerable, and much expertise is necessary in handling them. These will be discussed under the following headings:

(1) Mental distress.
(2) Bulbar problems.
  (i) Salivary dribbling
  (ii) Dysphagia
  (iii) Choking
  (iv) Dysarthria
(3) Pain.
(4) Poor sleeping.
(5) Weakness of the arms.
(6) Weakness of the legs.
(7) Respiratory insufficiency and breathlessness.
(8) Constipation.

(1) Mental distress

There is ample evidence that many patients and their relatives experience distress at various stages of the disease. Distress is sometimes related to fruitless consultations and lack of advice about the disease and its course. Some patients have been resentful that they are told half-truths, learning from others because 'the neurologist would not say plainly, and my family doctor was honest enough to say that he did not know' (Carus, 1980).

Particular 'crisis' points include the time at which the diagnosis is made, the point at which the patient has to give up work, the time at which a wheelchair has to be introduced, and when it is no longer possible to go upstairs and when permanent admission to hospital becomes necessary. There may be worries about dying from suffocation or from gradually worsening respiratory muscle paralysis, or in some other frightening way. Many patients fear the unknown.

Some patients experience emotional lability, exhibiting inappropriate laughing and crying. This symptom may sometimes be helped by the use of imipramine in a dose of 25 mg two or three times a day.

(2) Bulbar problems

Dribbling, dysphagia, choking, and dysarthria are particularly distressing symptoms. At any one time more than 50 per cent of MND patients will be experiencing some, or all of these problems (Newrick and Langton Hewer, 1984). The vast majority will do so eventually. These various problems can be a cause of social isolation due to the patient becoming embarrassed and friends being upset and sometimes frightened. In most instances the problems are due to a combination of both upper and lower motor neurone disturbance.

(i) Salivary dribbling

A normal person produces about two litres of saliva per day. This is swallowed automatically. Salivary dribbling is a common problem in patients with MND. There are a number of different causative factors, but there is no definite evidence that volume of saliva is increased. A reduction in the frequency of automatic swallowing is probably a major factor. Dribbling tends to be thought of, in the public mind, as being associated with mental disorder. The patient will require constant reassurance about this. Later in the disease he may fear that he may drown in his own saliva, but it seems unlikely that this ever occurs. The detailed management of the problem is discussed below:

(a) Oral candidiasis (thrush) is common and should be treated.

(b) Head position: many patients have weakness of the neck muscles and dribbling may occur when the head falls forward. This problem can frequently be controlled by appropriate posturing, including a reclining backrest and/or the provision of a collar.

(c) Stimulation of swallowing: automatic swallowing can sometimes be stimulated if the patient sucks sweets. Great care must be taken with this technique, especially if there is a tendency for choking to occur.

(d) Lip closure: weakness of the lips may make dribbling worse. Attempts to improve this can be made by, for instance, getting the patient to hold a spatula between the lips whilst he is otherwise relaxing, e.g. watching television.

(e) Cosmetic: the patient's blouse or shirt should not be allowed to become saturated with saliva. A false shirt front or polo-neck which could be changed frequently may be helpful. 'Bibs' can appear degrading.

(f) Medication: atropine 0.6 mg three times a day is frequently appropriate. Many of the antidepressant drugs also have an atropine-like action. It should be remembered that pyridostigmine (Mestinon) can increase the amount of saliva.

(g) Suction: some patients wake up in the middle of the night with a feeling that they are choking on their own saliva. The provision of a simple portable suction apparatus in this situation can be helpful, but both the patient and carer must be properly instructed in its use.

(h) Surgery: various operations have been tried. The most useful operation is bilateral division of the corda tympani via the middle ear. Surgery is not required in the vast majority of cases.

(ii) Dysphagia

Once again several different factors contribute to swallowing problems in MND. These include weakness of the masseter muscles (producing difficulty with chewing), impaired tongue mobility (making it difficult for a bolus to be formed), palatal weakness (resulting in reduced intra-oral pressure) and weakness of the pharyngeal muscles. In addition, there may be spasm of the pharyngeal muscle.

In each case a careful evaluation of the swallowing problem should be undertaken by taking a history and watching the patient eat and drink. In appropriate cases it may be helpful to undertake video-fluoroscopy. The patient's weight will need to be monitored.

The precise advice that is given to the patient will clearly depend on the result of the assessment. In each case the mechanism of swallowing should be explained to the patient, as should an account of what has gone wrong. The patient will need to be seen at regular intervals during the course of the disease, as the dysphagia, and attendant problems, will change with time. The following specific points need to be emphasised:—

(a) Diet: solids are often better tolerated than fluid. Foods that crumble should be avoided. Smooth, liquidised food may be required in the latter stages. However, in each case it will be necessary to experiment so that the texture of the most appropriate food can be found for each patient.

(b) Ice: spasticity can often be reduced for a few minutes by the local application of ice. The patient can be asked to suck ice cubes for ten minutes prior to a meal. Alternatively, ice can be applied to the outside of the throat.

(c) Medication: some clinicians find that Mestinon can be helpful, but in our experience this drug has been of doubtful use. Baclofen, in a dose of 20–60 mg a day, may reduce spasticity and can be tried. The actual swallowing of drugs needs to be carefully assessed, as some patients have great difficulty with swallowing larger tablets or capsules.

(d) Head position: it is important that the head and neck should be maintained in an appropriate position during meals. If the head is allowed to fall forwards, then swallowing will probably become more difficult. A collar may be required.

(e) It may be necessary to use a nasogastric tube during the latter stages of the disease. The modern narrow-bore tubes are more acceptable than the old-fashioned wide-bore Ryles tube. Indications for a nasogastric tube include frequent choking, repeated inhalation pneumonia, severe dehydration, severe weight loss, and taking an unacceptable time to eat a meal.

(f) Surgery: a number of different surgical techniques are available, but in our experience surgery is rarely required.

   (1) Cricopharyngeal myotomy: this procedure is only undertaken if there is demonstrable, consistent hold-up of food at the level of the cricopharyngeus muscle. The procedure is associated with a substantial mortality rate (Loizou *et al.*, 1980).
   (2) Oesophagostomy: this technique involves the insertion of a tube into the oesophagus via an incision on the side of the neck.
   (3) Gastrostomy: a tube is inserted directly into the stomach.

(iii) Choking

It is necessary to remember that choking and coughing are defence mechanisms which prevent aspiration into the air passages. The symptom can be very frightening.

Choking can occur in various situations. It most commonly occurs when the patient is drinking or eating. Occasionally it occurs at night if there is pooling of saliva at the back of the throat. This latter problem may be dealt with by the use of a sucker (see above).

Anxiety and panic will make choking worse, and therefore calm reassurance is necessary at all times. It is particularly important to avoid ingesting substances that trigger choking, including particularly: crumbly food, strong curry, whisky and brandy. If a severe bout of choking occurs the carer should be prepared to apply the 'hug of life'. It should be remembered that choking is probably an uncommon cause of death (Saunders *et al.*, 1981).

(iv) Dysarthria

Initially the speech may become slightly slurred, but ultimately many patients become totally unable to articulate. The first symptom is often a weak palate associated with nasal escape. Weakness of the lips may be a further important problem. In this early stage intelligibility may be improved by training, and by the supply of a palatal support. Some patients can compensate for the loss of speech by writing. However, many are too weak to write, and for these a communication aid will need to be provided. Recent experience in Bristol indicates that patients require as many as five or six different aids during the course of their illness. With the help of a competent speech therapist, who is familiar with communication aids, most patients can be enabled to communicate with their families up to the time of death (see Chapter 15).

(3) Pain

A recent study (Newrick and Langton Hewer, 1985) has shown that pain may occur in as many as 64 per cent of people with MND. Cramp in the limbs is common. Pain may be experienced in various sites, including the shoulders and back. The cause for this is frequently not obvious. Late in the disease, discomfort at night can be distressing, and can only be relieved by a change in position. It is particularly important that the patient is provided with a chair which fits his body, in which he can sit comfortably. If pain and/or mental distress become severe, then opiates should be used. Diamorphine in a dose of 2.5 mg initially is usually acceptable, and this dose can be gradually increased as necessary. Cramp may be helped by the use of quinine (in an initial dose of 300 mg at night).

(4) Poor sleeping (see Table 19.1)

Poor sleeping may itself result in depression and feelings of chronic tiredness. These feelings may also be experienced by the spouse, whose sleep is also liable to be disturbed, with the resultant risk of breakdown in his/her ability to cope. The management of insomnia requires careful assessment of the causes. The uncritical use of hypnotics should be avoided.

If the problem remains intractable it may be necessary to admit the patient to hospital or to a hospice for a short while in order to give the spouse some respite (see below).

Table 19.1: Facts contributing to poor sleeping in MND patients

Problem	Management
1. Inability to change position without help.	An electric turning bed may be helpful.
2. Pain (see above) and general discomfort.	It is important to make sure that the bed is as comfortable as possible. A small dose of diamorphine may be helpful.
3. Depression and anxiety.	Counselling; antidepressant drugs.
4. Frequency of micturition.	Nocturia is a common symptom in older people. Management includes fluid restriction during the previous evening.

(5) Weakness of the arms

Marked weakness of the proximal arm muscles produces difficulty with feeding, combing and washing the hair, and donning vests and shirts. Mobile arm supports, attached to the wheelchair, can aid feeding in some patients (see Chapter 45). Clothes may need adapting (for example, shirts and vests should be 'front opening').

Weakness of the hand muscles produces difficulty with a multitude of tasks including writing, doing up buttons, knitting and feeding. A wrist-drop support, the use of wide-handled cutlery, and velcro instead of buttons, may be indicated. Communication aids are discussed elsewhere (Chapter 15).

(6) Weakness of the legs

Difficulty with climbing stairs, standing and walking, together with falls (which may lead to fractures), are the principal results of weakness of the leg muscles. Leg oedema is an important secondary effect. The management includes housing modification (e.g. ensuring easy access to the toilet and to the garden) and the supply of a wheelchair (Chapter 43).

(7) Respiratory insufficiency and breathlessness

Respiratory insufficiency occurs ultimately in most cases. This is frequently, but not always, accompanied by a sensation of breathlessness. Nocturnal breathlessness may be helped by giving the patient several pillows so that he sleeps in a semi-recumbent position. Chest infections require treatment. Medication can worsen respiratory insufficiency, particularly large doses of diazapam or morphine.

Some patients require assisted ventilation particularly at night (Norris *et al.*, 1985). In occasional cases a tracheostomy may be performed and artificial ventilation instituted (Norris *et al.*, 1985), but this has not been undertaken in my own service. Distressing breathlessness should clearly be avoided, and we usually use diamorphine in small (e.g. 2.5 mg at a time) doses, which should be given regularly. The dose is increased as necessary.

(8) Constipation

Constipation is a frequent and distressing symptom in many patients. Contributing factors include weakness of the abdominal muscles, difficulty with maintaining a sitting position, decrease in intake of bulky foods and of fluids (in patients with dysphagia) and medication (particularly opiates and anticholinergic agents). Effective management involves, as always, making a careful assessment of the problem to find out precisely what has gone wrong. However, in many cases the problem remains intractable. Simple measures include increasing fluid intake with careful use of purgatives. Regular enemas may be required. Faecal impaction is common in the later stages of the disease. Manual evacuation by the spouse should be avoided if possible.

AIDS AND APPLIANCES

There is no doubt that the problems of MND patients can be eased considerably by the supply of effective aids and appliances. The most commonly needed pieces of equipment are listed in Table 19.2.

ORGANISATION OF CARE

There has been criticism of the way in which MND is handled (Newrick and Langton Hewer, 1984). The criticisms include lack of interest by doctors, insufficient psychosocial support, and long delays in the supply of equipment such as wheelchairs, which may be unsuitable when they do arrive. Patients clearly dislike attending clinics where they are seen by junior doctors who have no specific experience, or training, in the management of the disorder. The pattern is easily seen as being disorganised and uncaring.

Someone 'in charge'

The management of MND should ideally be coordinated by one person. The GP should clearly be involved, although he is unlikely to have much

Table 19.2: The principal aids and appliances used in motor neurone disease

Appliance	Indication	Type	Comments
Collar	Significant weakness of the neck muscles. This is particularly liable to occur when the patient is a passenger in a car. Pain in the neck and inability to look up are other indications.	Must be lightweight, not unduly bulky; washable and cosmetically acceptable.	Common problems include the supply of large, clumsy collars which are ill-fitting and ugly.
Wrist splint	Severe wrist and/or finger-drop with preservation of hand movement.	A lightweight splint cosmetically acceptable is needed. The 'Futuro' splint is usually acceptable.	
Mobile arm supports	Severe weakness of arm abductor muscles with some preservation of hand function. Some patients may be enabled to feed independently.	The support is usually attached to a wheelchair. The supports are supplied by the Artificial Limb and Appliance Centre.	The Artificial Limb and Appliance Centre does not always provide proper instructions.
Foot-drop supports	The tip of the shoe catches on the ground in walking. This may result in falls, with resultant fracture of long bones.	Lightweight moulded ortholene supports which fit into the shoe and extend up the back of the leg. Modular splints are often not satisfactory. A below-knee calliper is not usually appropriate because of its weight.	A delay of several weeks in the provision of these supports is common.
Wheelchair	(1) Frequent falls. (2) Inability to walk inside the house. (3) Inability to walk outside — e.g. to get to the garden, pub or shops. *Remember:* Many people only need a wheelchair occasionally.	(1) A simple 'Model 8' is suitable for many people. (2) An electric wheelchair may be required — particularly if the patient wishes to get to the pub or shops independently. (3) If the patient needs to sit in the chair for long periods a head-rest, proper padding, and leg supports are essential.	The provision of wheelchairs is frequently unsatisfactory. Specially adapted wheelchairs may take many months to arrive.
Armchair	All patients need to sit in a chair that is comfortable.	The chair should be well padded, the back should recline, there should be proper support for the head, and there should be some form of leg support.	Disabled patients may sit in an arm-chair for as many as 14–16 hours per day, and it is particularly important that the chair is comfortable and suitable.
Communication aid	Inability to speak intelligibly combined with inability to write.	A wide variety of aids are available. The most popular include the Canon Communicator and the Memowriter.	

experience of the disease. The District Department of Neurology is also in a position to provide continuity and support, although this frequently does not happen in practice. The hospices can offer much help (Saunders *et al.*, 1981).

We have previously suggested (Newrick and Langton Hewer, 1984) the concept of a 'key worker' who would work closely with the GP and hospital consultant. No proper evaluation of this suggestion has yet been undertaken. Our experience in Bristol has been that a speech therapist, working closely with a hospital consultant, can provide a satisfactory level of support. This arrangement seems particularly appropriate in view of the fact that the most intractable problems involve the bulbar musculature. Such support could probably also be given by a properly trained nurse, social worker, or remedial therapist.

In suggesting a 'model' way of dealing with MND, five arbitrary stages may be recognised:

(1) Early

At this point the patient will probably have little, or no, disability.

(a) The diagnosis should be made correctly and effectively.

(b) The patient should be told the diagnosis in general terms. The spouse should be present at this interview. They should be given as much information as seems appropriate in their particular case. They should be told that proper support will be given throughout the course of the disease, and that the general practitioner, the hospital consultant, and their supporting staff, will do everything possible to provide support.

Certain positive aspects of the disease need to be emphasised. Many patients are relieved to know that they have not got multiple sclerosis, and that the disorder is not usually familial. It is also worth emphasising that the majority of patients retain their intellectual faculties until the end, and that vision, hearing and continence are usually preserved.

(c) Because of the nature of the disease, we recommend that a second consultant opinion should usually be sought at this stage. Unnecessary diagnostic doubt should be avoided if at all possible.

(2) Stage of mild disability

At this stage the patient may need advice on employment, driving, and how to cope with home duties. The diagnosis will probably need to be further discussed.

(3) The stage of severe disability

It is at this point that considerable support is needed. It is particularly important that the various groups of workers should liaise closely together, avoiding overlap and underlap. It is all too easy for large numbers of medical and paramedical staff, working in the community and in hospital, to become involved with little or no overt cooperation between them. A 'key worker', if available, becomes particularly important at this stage. *It is absolutely essential that the patient and spouse should be able to get immediate advice and help if a crisis arises.*

Specific needs include the following:

(a) Intermittent admission to hospital. This may be needed in order to give the spouse a regular break, or if an emergency occurs (e.g. if the patient develops pneumonia, or if the spouse becomes unwell). As the terminal stages of the disease approach, more frequent admissions to hospital may be required.

It is particularly important that the ward staff should be properly trained in the management of the bulbar problems itemised above. Unless this happens the spouse may refuse to allow the patient to go into hospital.

(b) The effective provision of equipment and the undertaking of housing adaptations.

Equipment such as walking aids, commodes, and wheelchairs should be supplied as soon as possible after the need is demonstrated. It is necessary to anticipate the patient's needs. Delays of weeks or months are not acceptable. However, it is also important to avoid suggesting equipment which is not yet required (e.g. the premature provision of a wheelchair may upset the patient unnecessarily). Similarly, housing adaptations, e.g. to provide proper access to the toilet, or a stair rail to enable to patient to get upstairs, should be provided quickly.

A variety of equipment may be required, including wheelchair, a proper chair to sit in, a collar, a proper bed, and various types of communication aid.

(c) Complications. Complications should be avoided if possible. If they do occur they must be dealt with efficiently. They include limb fractures, fungal infections of the mouth, pressure sores, severe dependent oedema, uncontrolled pain, contractures, and breakdown in the health of the spouse.

(4) The terminal stage

The objective is to help the patient to die with dignity, and with the minimum of pain and distress. Many patients prefer to remain at home for as long as possible. We have found the policy of gradually increasing the amount of time spent in hospital to be satisfactory for many patients. Indeed, some patients still regard themselves as 'living at home' even when they only have a single home visit once a fortnight.

The principles of care at this stage have been discussed by Saunders, and include unhurried and sympathetic handling by staff, and the use of appropriate analgesic drugs (particularly diamorphine).

(5) After death

A major objective of management is to prevent the relatives from feeling guilty that they have failed to do everything possible. An interview with one of the senior doctors shortly after the patient's death may be helpful. Additionally, the key worker, or social worker, may remain in contact with the relatives for a few weeks, or even longer in some cases.

CONCLUSIONS

It will be seen from the above discussion that motor neurone disease (MND) presents a large number of quite complex problems. The efficient handling of the disease requires considerable knowledge, expertise, patience and sympathy. The present evidence appears to be that many patients with MND could be handled better. Because of the rarity of the disease it is suggested that management should ideally be centred on departments of clinical neurology. However, other organisations may well have an important role to play, and the lead being taken by the hospice movement is helpful and important. It is suggested that there should be a 'key worker' who would work closely with the neurologist and with the general practitioner. Other medical and paramedical staff are also involved, and the speech therapist, has a particularly important role in managing the distressing problems of dysphagia, choking, dribbling and dysarthria.

MND certainly presents a challenge to all those involved — doctors, nurses, therapists and social workers. We need to be constantly striving to improve the quality of care offered to our patients. This will involve monitoring the quality of care, and ensuring that defects are remedied. The task is certainly challenging, frequently frustrating, but potentially enormously worthwhile.

ACKNOWLEDGEMENTS

I gratefully acknowledge the help given by Dr P.M. Enderby in the preparation of this chapter.

REFERENCES

Carey, J.S. (1986) Motor neurone disease — a challenge to medical ethics. *J. Roy. Soc. Med.*, *79*, 216-20

Carus, R. (1980) Motor neurone disease: a demeaning illness. *Br. Med. J.*, *280*, 455-6

Loizou, L.A., Small, M. and Dalton, G.A. (1980) Cricopharyngeal myotomy in

motor neurone disase. *J. Neurol. Neurosurg. Psychiatry, 43*, 42-5
Newrick, P.G. and Langton Hewer, R. (1984). Motor neurone disease: can we do better? A study of 42 patients. *Br. Med. J., 289*, 539-42
Newrick, P.G. and Langton Hewer, R. (1985) Pain in motor neurone disease. *J. Neurol. Neurosurg. Psychiatry, 48*, 838-40
Norris, F.H., Smith, F.A. and Denys, E.H. (1985) Motor neurone disease: towards better care. *Br. Med. J., 291*, 259-62
Saunders, C., Summers, D.H. and Teller, N. (1981) *Hospice — the living idea*, Edward Arnold, London

ADDRESS OF ASSOCIATION

Motor Neurone Disease Association
38 Hazelwood Road, Northampton NN1 1LN. (Publishes much useful information for patients and professionals)

20

Stroke

Derick Treharne Wade

INTRODUCTION

In a typical British Health District of 250,000 people there will be about 1,500 people who have suffered a stroke, 750 of whom will have significant problems as a result of their stroke. Each year 400 more people will suffer an acute stroke, of whom approximately 200 will die within the year. In British acute hospitals, patients with acute stroke alone account for nearly 5 per cent of all expenditure in any one year.

Stroke is too common to allow all patients to be concentrated under the care of a few specialists, and too rare to allow all doctors to gain great experience. Instead, patients with stroke are managed by a wide variety of doctors, most of whom are not neurologists and many of whom may not be interested in stroke. Consequently some patients may receive sub-optimal care. This chapter hopes to remedy this state of affairs. It covers the major aspects of stroke management from the point of view of a doctor; other aspects are covered elsewhere. The main thesis of this chapter is that effective management depends upon close attention to clinical details; the use of standard measures; and good organisation including an audit of the service offered.

PRINCIPLES OF STROKE REHABILITATION

After stroke, patients present with a wide variety of problems needing solutions. The important components of good management are as follows:

(a) Accurate medical diagnosis, separating stroke from other causes of the stroke syndrome.

(b) Provision of immediate support and nursing care, together with specific treatment where appropriate.

(c) Knowledge of natural history of, and prognosis after, stroke.

(d) Thorough early assessment to identify all problems.

(e) The use of standard assessments familiar to all those involved.

(f) Active early intervention: to reduce complications; to enable 'natural recovery' to occur without hindrance; to teach adaptive techniques for overcoming any difficulties; to ensure that appropriate aids are given and used correctly; and possibly to encourage intrinsic neurological recovery.

(g) The involvement of: a coordinated team of helpers (therapists, social workers, doctors, etc.); who should be readily available to all patients wherever they are; and who should specialise in stroke care.

(h) Follow-up to monitor progress and the effectiveness of any intervention, and to identify any new problems.

(i) Foward planning, especially concerning major changes such as hospital discharge.

(j) Active early involvement of relatives, with stress upon providing information and emotional support.

(k) Always leaving a telephone 'life-line' for recovered or discharged patients to use, to ask for help and advice.

Some of these principles will be discussed within this chapter, but the detail is necessarily limited. Further information, and evidence for most statements, can be obtained from Wade *et al.* (1985).

DIAGNOSIS

The clinical diagnosis of stroke (in distinction to 'not stroke') is usually easy and reliable. It is important to establish that the onset was relatively sudden. One good way is to try to discover the time of onset of symptoms: if the patient or the family cannot fix the onset then doubt the diagnosis. Most strokes come on in under an hour, but some can evolve over a day or more. Further there may be some fluctuation during the first few days. The second important aspect of diagnosis is to ensure that there is no other reasonable explanation for the neurological deficit.

The conditions most commonly *misdiagnosed as acute stroke* are post-epileptic (Todd's) paresis, transient ischaemic attacks and non-specific alterations in consciousness. Tumours, subdural haematoma and other surgically treatable causes are rare, as is hypoglycaemia.

Diagnosis of the *type of stroke* (haemorrhage or thromboembolic) is unreliable on clinical grounds. Atrial fibrillation, for example, is as common in cerebral haemorrhage as it is in non-haemorrhagic stroke, and other clinical features are probably equally unreliable at distinguishing the type of stroke. Identification of cerebral haemorrhage is only of importance if the patient is already on anti-coagulant drugs, or if anticoagulation is being considered (see later). A computerised tomographic scan (CT scan), preferably done within 10–14 days, is the only reliable way to identify cerebral haemorrhage: lumbar puncture with simple inspection of the CSF cannot reliably exclude haemorrhage. It is unlikely that thrombotic and embolic strokes can be separated; indeed they probably overlap.

INVESTIGATION

There are four possible reasons for investigating a patient presenting with a clinical diagnosis of acute stroke. The first is to *exclude other causes* of the acute stroke syndrome. As stated above, clinical diagnosis is usually correct and the majority of other causes are revealed by the passage of time rather than by any test. Any patient suspected of having a cerebral mass needs a CT scan. A blood glucose test to eliminate hypoglycaemia would be wise in anyone on hypoglycaemic drugs (e.g. insulin, chlorpropamide).

The second possible reason for investigation is to establish *more detail* about the stroke, such as its site and size, or the presence of haemorrhage. This rarely affects management and is not useful prognostically in comparison with clinical prognostic indicators discussed later. The only type of stroke which may need identification is a cerebellar haemorrhage or infarction causing hydrocephalus, when surgical intervention might save life. In practice cerebellar haemorrhage is rare (less than 1 per cent). Moreover not all cases need surgical treatment, and so CT scan should be reserved for those cases where the clinical suspicion is strong (predominantly cerebellar symptoms/signs with little weakness), where someone is deteriorating, and where neurosurgical intervention is a realistic option.

Third, investigation could reveal some *underlying cause* for the stroke. For example, some strokes occur after myocardial infarction; the proportion is disputed but is probably less than 5 per cent of all strokes. The major preventable cause of stroke is hypertension, which is easily detected; anaemia and polycythaemia rubra vera are rare but treatable other causes. This avenue is only worth pursuing if management might be altered.

Enthusiastic searching for an occult cause is usually fruitless even in patients under 55 years. In most patients the cause is generalised arterial disease secondary to ageing, hypertension or diabetes. There is often other evidence of arterial disease. A few patients develop stroke as a recognised complication of a disease which has already been diagnosed, such as aortic valve disease. Very few have a hidden treatable cause.

The last reason for investigation is to detect some potential *complication of stroke*, preferably one which is treatable. For example, some patients develop hyperglycaemia (or maybe had undiagnosed diabetes). Other patients may become uraemic.

It could be argued that no 'routine' tests are needed. However, the risk and cost of some tests are so low as to allow one to perform them freely. In the uncomplicated case a full blood count, urea and electrolytes, and a blood glucose test soon after stroke would probably be enough. Other tests should only be carried out if indicated clinically.

A CT scan is normal in about 20 per cent of patients with stroke, and cannot 'prove' the diagnosis. It should be used in four circumstances: when there is serious suspicion that the patient has an intracranial mass (tumour, subdural haematoma, abscess); when it is important to exclude cerebral haemorrhage, notably when a patient is already on anticoagulant therapy or is about to be given some; when a cerebellar haemorrhage or infarction is suspected, particularly if the patient's level of consciousness is dropping and surgical intervention is possible; and when the patient's course is atypical, which would raise doubt as to the correct diagnosis.

Arteriography carries a morbidity approaching 10 per cent, with some 5 per cent being significant. It would be indicated if surgery to the carotid artery were contemplated, but this is not of proven benefit and often carries considerable risk. Arteriography has a very limited role in the investigation of stroke.

TREATMENT

No routine acute treatment has yet been proved to benefit all patients with stroke. This is scarcely surprising. For example, something suitable for thrombosis would probably worsen a haemorrhage. Unfortunately there are no reliable guidelines to select patients for specific treatments, and no proof that any treatment is effective even for selected patients. In particular there is currently no evidence that steroids (e.g. dexamethasone), intravenous dextran or mannitol, immediate anticoagulation with heparin, hyperbaric oxygen, naloxine or many other proposed drugs are of benefit. Some may be harmful.

The only ray of hope comes from a recent Swedish study (Strand *et al.*, 1984) which found that venesection followed by replacement of withdrawn blood with dextran led to a better functional recovery at three months. A further study is in progress to confirm this finding. If confirmed, this will have manor implications for the organisation of stroke care as it will necessitate more CT scans to exclude haemorrhage and a considerable increase in medical and nursing supervision over the first week.

Until there is proof that a treatment is safe and effective, and until there are simple guidelines to allow selection of suitable patients, it is wisest to restrain oneself from initiating active treatments such as anticoagulation. This applies even in the case of an apparently embolic stroke, and in a progressing stroke. The diagnosis of embolism cannot be made with certainty. Moreover anticoagulation can lead to haemorrhage into infarcted brain tissue.

Surgical intervention is only of benefit to patients with a cerebellar infarction or haematoma causing hydrocephalus with progressive deterioration in consciousness. There is no firm indication for arterial surgery at present. Evacuation of intracerebral haematoma has yet to be proven beneficial.

IMMEDIATE CARE

Together with diagnosis, the doctor's main early task is to ensure that satisfactory nursing care is available. Often this will require hospital admission but not inevitably so. If the patient and/or the family wish for home care and the general practitioner agrees, then this can be undertaken. The principles are similar, though the solutions to practical problems may differ.

Specific details are outside the remit of this chapter. Comatose patients will need the usual care. Consideration needs to be given to swallowing, as about 10 per cent of conscious patients choke on attempting to swallow in the first few days. Excretion may provide problems, usually overcome using a commode, pads and patience; early catheterisation should be avoided. Paralysis will necessitate careful positioning and handling of the patient as discussed elsewhere. Fear, both in the patient and in the family, should not be overlooked; explain what has happened.

SURVIVAL AND RECURRENCE: NATURAL HISTORY AND INTERVENTION

One-third of patients die within three weeks and about half will be dead within a year of their stroke. Death is most likely in those who are incontinent of urine for whatever reason. Other indicators of a poor prognosis include any depression or loss of consciousness, severe paralysis, and inability to look towards the paralysed side. Most of these patients die directly or indirectly from their stroke, but an appreciable number die from a further stroke or heart disease.

Considering early (three-month) survivors, about 16 per cent die each year, an increased rate when compared with age-matched controls. Some of these deaths can be attributed to the original stroke, but cardiac disease is the commonest cause followed by another stroke. Recurrent stroke (fatal or non-fatal) occurs in about 10 per cent of survivors each year. The major prognostic indicators of long-term risk of death and/or recurrent stroke are any manifestations of cardiac or vascular disease, such as major ECG abnormalities.

Control of hypertension even after a stroke may reduce the risk of death or recurrence. Before initiating treatment one should ensure that the raised blood pressure is not simply a response to the stroke. Unless there is independent evidence of hypertension it is wise to wait three weeks before diagnosing someone as suffering hypertension. Decisions upon the level of blood pressure warranting treatment are difficult; it is best to treat only those you would normally treat, using whatever criteria you usually use.

Aspirin probably reduces the risk both of death and of recurrent stroke. Dipyramidole (Persantin) as an addition to aspirin does not increase the protection, and it is no more effective than aspirin alone. The best dose of aspirin is uncertain, but 300 mg/day would seem reasonable. The duration of treatment is also unknown but, as the risk remains high for life, life-long treatment would seem logical. No other specific ways of reducing risks are known (American–Canadian Cooperative Study, 1985).

RECOVERY

Natural history

That most survivors of acute stroke show some recovery is well known. More recently the speed and extent of that recovery has been studied in detail, and it is now possible to give guidelines as to the natural history of recovery. It should be stressed that most of this information has been gained from groups of patients. Individual patients may not conform exactly to the general rules; prognosis is considered later. On the other hand, the rules about to be described probably apply to all types of loss seen after stroke.

About half of all recovery occurs in the first 14–21 days, with many patients making an apparently complete recovery in that time. This certainly applies to such physical activities as walking independently and being able to dress, and probably applies to recovery of language, visual field loss and sensation.

Four qualifications should be noted. First, this statement is based upon research conducted upon people who survived at least three months, and often longer. Therefore one cannot necessarily conclude that patients who are so severely affected that they are destined to die within a month or so are going to recover in the same way. Second, some patients may deteriorate (or even have a further stroke), which will tend to reduce the apparent rate of recovery in these studies based on groups of patients. Third, a proportion of patients will never lose independence in some spheres: for example, not every patient loses the ability to dress. Last, most studies have used a dichotomous classification, with patients being either dependent or independent. No account is taken of speed or ease of performance once independence has been achieved (Isaacs, 1971).

Recovery can continue for at least six months, with 2–9 per cent of patients making an appreciable recovery of independence between six months and one year. Published information on later qualitative improvements in performance is scarce. It is quite likely that patients continue to improve their performance in recovered functions for well over six months. In other words, few patients regain independent mobility after six months, but possibly walking becomes easier in those who have become independent.

Prognosis

Two questions arise after an acute stroke. Will the patient survive? If he survives, how good will his recovery be? Recent research suggests that a

Figure 20.1: Recovery of Barthel ADL scores: four groups on initial severity (Wade *et al.*, 1983; by kind permission of the Editor of *Journal of Neurology, Neurosurgery and Psychiatry*) (Table 20.3 shows the 10 items scored)

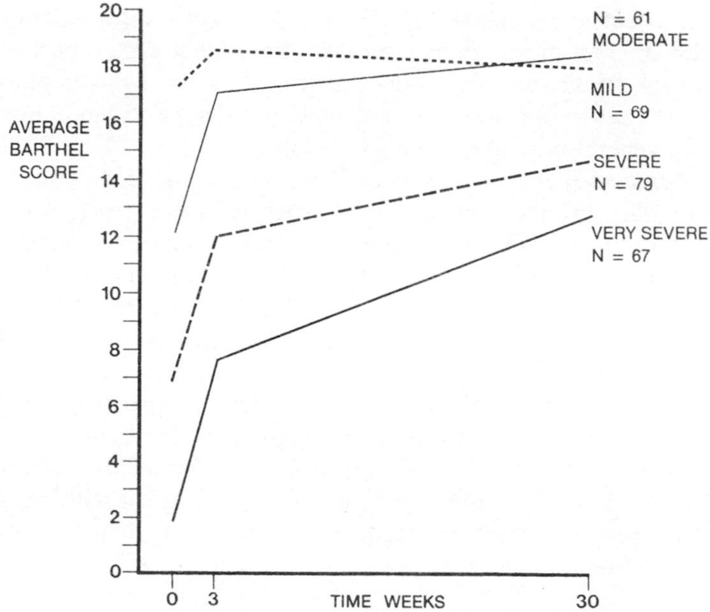

single observation at 24–48 hours can give good guidance. Patients who are incontinent of urine for whatever reason (e.g. in coma, unable to get attention of nurse, previously incontinent) are both more likely to die within the first six months and, if they survive, to be left seriously disabled and often needing long-term care.

An important distinction should be drawn between variables which are important in giving a prognosis, and variables which may influence rehabilitation. For example, urinary incontinence is important as a prognostic indicator but specific treatment of incontinence (e.g. using a catheter) is unlikely to influence outcome. On the other hand, apraxia is not a good prognostic indicator because it is uncommon. Nonetheless, if present apraxia may have a major influence on the pattern of rehabilitation.

When considering any particular function (e.g. speech, use of the arm) then the more severe the original loss, the less good will be the final outcome. For example, the first measure of language function taken at (say) three weeks is the major prognostic factor determining language function at six months. Similarly the best predictor of arm function is the initial severity of arm paralysis. In practice, urinary incontinence will allow an early estimate of overall recovery, but specific measures of each function will probably give a better indication of recovery in each individual ability.

ASSESSING THE PATIENT

Just as an accurate medical diagnosis precedes effective medical management, so effective rehabilitation depends upon accurate assessments. No single test or assessment can 'measure' stroke. Rather each aspect of stroke needs to be tested separately and interpreted in the light of other tests. Details of what to assess when, and how, are discussed later. First some important general principles need to be stated.

Use standard measures wherever these are available. Stroke management has been crippled by the wide variety of measures (still) used by therapists and doctors. Consequently there is no common language, inhibiting communication between team members. Physiotherapists (in Britain) are currently debating the form of a standard assessment, but until they reach some conclusion the assessments discussed here would form a reasonable basis.

Perform a thorough assessment: too often important problems are overlooked simply because no-one formally tests for them. A common example is the failure to recognise aphasia (this term will be used to cover all grades of language disturbance, and is synonymous with dysphasia). Obviously there is a limit to the detail which can be achieved, but each aspect should be covered.

> A 58-year-old woman, Mrs W, was discharged from hospital to her flat after a two-week stay in hospital, most spent attending for rehabilitation. She spent the first 24 hours at home in great distress as she was unable to find her way around the kitchen, could not use any equipment, and kept knocking against things. She could not read. No-one in hospital had detected her hemianopia and apraxia. After spending four weeks with her sister, she was able to return home.

Monitor progress, auditing the effectiveness of any interventions. One advantage the doctor has is his relatively objective involvement, seeing the patients less frequently than most others involved. Further, he has a wider perspective, and should be able to bring together and interpret all the information. By monitoring progress the doctor can evaluate whether any treatment initiated has had any effect. Moreover failure to progress might be due to some unidentified problem itself amenable to treatment.

Use appropriate assessments. For example, when screening for language loss soon after stroke, a short test should be used reserving more detailed assessments for those found to have aphasia. In addition the aspects needing assessment will change with time. For example, depression is an important long-term complication but does not need to be searched for within the first few days.

INITIAL ASSESSMENT

The first full assessment of any stroke patient should be carried out as soon as the diagnosis is certain and any immediate investigations and treatment have been completed. This will often be within 24 hours, and should not be delayed beyond three days if possible. Early assessment is useful for several reasons. It can identify otherwise undiagnosed deficits which may modify initial management. For example, it is quite common for mild aphasia to be unrecognised for several days or even weeks. Second, initial deficits might be of prognostic importance. Last, an early assessment provides a useful objective measure against which future progress can be gauged.

Two competing requirements influence the first assessment. On the one hand it is important to cover all likely areas of deficit, and not simply to concentrate upon those already diagnosed. On the other hand the assessment is constrained by the patient's clinical state, and the assessor's time and patience. The major functions which should be assessed are cognition, communication, motor and sensory function, and probably activities of daily living (see Chapter 6, Functional Assessment and Chapter 5, The Doctor's Assessment).

LATER ASSESSMENTS

Once the immediate crisis is over then it is important to assess the social background of the patient. This would include obtaining information on his lifestyle and abilities before stroke, assessment of his housing and the problems it might pose, and evaluation of the social support available. Emotional disturbance is common after stroke. While this is often recognised in the first weeks, it is not always taken into consideration later. It might be worth considering the use of formal assessment of mood as an adjunct to clinical judgement.

Good rehabilitation would probably include formal assessments at four weeks, six months and possibly one year after stroke. These assessments allow monitoring of general progress and can be used to audit the overall standard of care given to the generality of patients. In addition it is probably useful to interpolate assessments at one week after discharge from hospital and one month after the end of formal rehabilitation. These help to ensure that no major difficulties are left at these points.

Several advantages might accrue from a policy of routine follow-up. Deficiencies in the rehabilitation service are more likely to be identified and thus remedied. Patients may feel less abandoned. Staff will become more aware of the natural history of stroke, in particular that many people do make good recoveries. On the other hand, it has to be accepted that routine follow-up is expensive. Until evidence is produced to show that there are benefits, some doctors might prefer simply to discharge patients as soon as possible without follow-up, performing regular assessments simply on patients still under active rehabilitation.

COGNITION

Coma and confusion will affect about half of all patients in the first few days. A record of the lowest level of consciousness reached is useful for prognostic reasons — it is associated with an increased fatality rate and a less good outcome. A record of the current level of consciousness is important, especially to help interpret other findings (a confused patient may not cooperate with other tests). Last, a routine assessment of memory and orientation is useful in management.

The level of consciousness is best measured using the Glasgow Coma Scale (GCS) (Teasdale *et al.*, 1979) (Chapter 6). This assesses a patient's best response to stimulation in three sections: opening of eyes, verbal response and motor (limb) movement. Because patients with aphasia will score badly on the verbal section it is important to show the individual section scores, not simply the total. If brevity is vital, then the motor scale alone should be used. Memory and orientation should be tested using the

Hodkinson mental scale (Table 20.1); anyone scoring 0–6 has a significant disturbance (Hodkinson, 1972).

Other more detailed cognitive tests are available, but may not be needed. The Rivermead Perceptual Assessment should be used if there is any suspicion of neglect or other perceptual problems. It is available commercially, and has been well tested for validity and reliability. Specialised tests of memory, IQ and other cognitive functions exist but are rarely necessary (Bhavani *et al.*, 1983).

COMMUNICATION

Dysarthria (slurring of speech) occurs in at least one third of conscious patients in the early stages. This rarely causes a persisting difficulty with communication. Aphasia (language disturbance, also known as 'dysphasia') occurs in about a further one-quarter of conscious patients, and about 15 per cent of survivors are left with some aphasia. It is important to identify aphasia as soon as possible so that a speech therapist can identify a patient's capabilities thoroughly, thus allowing staff and relatives to communicate with the patient in the most effective manner (Chapter 15).

A recently developed test, the Frenchay Aphasia Screening Test (FAST), has been developed specifically for use with patients after an acute stroke. It is a reliable method of detecting aphasia, although certain precautions are needed in interpreting the results in patients with confusion or hemianopia. This test will soon be commercially available and should be used routinely after stroke if there is any possibility of aphasia (e.g. in all patients with right-sided weakness). The test covers expression, comprehension, reading and writing.

Aphasia needs only to be tested for once. If absent, then no further

Table 20.1: Hodkinson mental scale (from Hodkinson 1972)

(Score 1 for each correct answer)
Age of patient
Time now (to nearest hour)
Address. Given for recall at end of test: 42 West Street
Name of hospital (area of town if at home)
Year
Date of birth
Month
Years of First World War
Name of monarch (President in the USA)
Count backwards from 20–1 (no mistakes)

assessments of communication are needed. If present more complete assessment by a speech therapist is required, and she should perform routine follow-up assessments. This is discussed elsewhere.

MOTOR AND SENSORY TESTING

Although it is the most obvious manifestation of stroke, weakness is discussed third as testing depends upon adequate cognitive and communicative ability. Detection of weakness is not usually a problem, but describing its severity is often ignored. A simple rapid measure is the 'Motricity Index' which gives a 0 (total paralysis) to 100 (normal) score, reflecting the extent of paralysis in the arm and in the leg. Although less detailed than other available measures, it has the great advantages of brevity and simplicity (Table 20.2) (Demeurisse *et al.*, 1980).

Sensory testing is much more difficult, and often unreliable. The 'thumb-finding' test is probably worth performing routinely; it is a formal

Table 20.2: The 'Motricity Index' (after Demeurisse *et al.*, 1980)

The tests:

Arm:

(1) Pinch grip — 1" (2.5 cm) cube between thumb and index finger
(2) Elbow flexion
(3) Shoulder abduction

Leg:

(4) Ankle dorsiflexion
(5) Knee extension
(6) Hip flexion

Scoring:

Test	Score and criterion
1	00 = no movement
	33 = beginnings of prehension
	56 = grips cube, without gravity
	65 = holds cube against gravity
	77 = grips against pull, but weaker than other side
	100 = normal
2–6	00 = no movement
	28 = palpable contraction, but no movement
	42 = movement without gravity
	56 = movement against gravity
	74 = movement against resistance, but weaker than other side
	100 = normal

Totals (all range 0–100):

Arm score = total of tests (1 + 2 + 3)/3
Leg score = total of tests (4 + 5 + 6)/3
Total motricity score = (arm + leg)/2

test of proprioception, but also depends upon other cortical functions being intact. In this test the patient closes his eyes and the affected arm is moved passively to some posture. The patient is then asked to 'find his thumb', and put his unaffected hand to it. He should do so directly without feeling up his arm from the shoulder. Sensory neglect will probably cause poor performance on this test but can also be tested for using simultaneous touches to the hands (Lyle, 1981).

The other sensory modality which should be tested routinely is the visual fields. Confrontation testing using both individual and simultaneous stimuli (usually moving fingers) should be carried out to detect both complete hemianopia and visual inattention.

ACTIVITIES OF DAILY LIVING

Information about a patient's ADL function is central to the management of all disabling diseases, including stroke. No single scale has yet won universal acclaim, and each hospital uses its own. Adoption of a single scale through each hospital, district, region and country might advance stroke care significantly. The *Barthel ADL Index* has been used in more research than any other ADL index, and should be adopted as the standard. Its ten items are shown in Table 20.3 (Barthel and Mahoney, 1965).

More detailed information on individual aspects of function does not need to be recorded routinely, but measures do exist. They should probably be used selectively on patients who have particular problems. Anyone whose walking is affected should have his speed measured by timing him over a ten-metre walk using whatever aid is needed and walking at his own preferred speed. Two suitable measures of arm function are the Action Research Arm Test (Lyle, 1981) and the Frenchay Arm Test (Wade *et al.*, 1983).

SOCIAL AND EMOTIONAL ASPECTS

It could be argued that formal assessments are unnecessary in this field because the clinical (i.e. unstructured) approach is adequate and possibly more adaptable. This may be true in the hands of experienced and conscientious staff, but such people are relatively rare and even they may slip up on occasion. The use of a standard approach might ensure that all major areas were covered, and that other people involved in the team understand these aspects.

These are perhaps the most difficult areas to assess formally. The only short simple index of 'non-ADL' activities available is the Frenchay Activities Index (FAI) (Holbrook and Skilbeck, 1983; Wade *et al.*, 1986)

Table 20.3: The Barthel ADL Index (from Barthel and Mahoney, 1965)

Item	Categories
Bowels	0 = incontinent 1 = occasional accident 2 = continent
Bladder	0 = incontinent/catheterised and unable to manage 1 = occasional accident 2 = continent
Grooming	0 = needs help 1 = independent for face/hair/teeth/shaving
Toilet use	0 = dependent 1 = needs some help 2 = independent
Feeding	0 = dependent 1 = needs help, e.g. cutting, spreading butter 2 = independent in all actions
Transfer (bed–chair)	0 = unable 1 = major help, can sit 2 = minor help (verbal or physical) 3 = independent
Walking	0 = unable 1 = independent in wheelchair 2 = walks with help of person (verbal/physical) 3 = independent (may use aid)
Dressing	0 = dependent 1 = needs help, but does half 2 = independent (including buttons/zips/laces)
Stairs	0 = unable 1 = needs help (verbal/physical) 2 = independent
Bathing	0 = dependent 1 = independent

(see Chapter 6), which covers 15 different activities. Information on pre-stroke functioning should be gathered as soon as possible. At any time from six months on, a patient's performance on the FAI should be checked. An explanation should be sought for any reductions observed; often there will be an obvious case for stopping an activity, but it is quite common for the FAI to reveal unnecessary changes in lifestyle. For example, someone may not go shopping simply because no-one has 'given permission', even though he is quite capable.

About one-third of survivors feel depressed at any one time after stroke; some have clinical depression. The important point is to look for depression, particularly in relation to people who have restricted their lifestyle without good (physical) cause. Clinical diagnosis is not always easy, and the use of questionnaires might help. Several exist. One recent self-assessment questionnaire designed for use on hospital patients with physical disorders is the Hospital Anxiety and Depression (HAD) scale (Zigmond and Snaith, 1983). Although this has not yet been used with stroke patients, it could be a useful screening test for significant emotional disturbance later after stroke. It only has 14 questions, and this should enhance its acceptability (see Chapter 6, Table 6.5).

Housing is still more difficult to assess, and is covered in more detail elsewhere in this book. A problem-orientated approach is probably the simplest, considering six problems: number of living levels (one floor or two?), toilet arrangements, bathing, kitchen arrangements, mobility within the house, mobility out of and outside the house.

INTERVENTION

Texts on rehabilitation traditionally concentrate upon what to do to (or for, or with) the patient, yet this chapter has scarcely mentioned intervention. There are several reasons for this. First, most techniques are practical, being learnt most easily by experience with patients and not from books. Second, other chapters consider therapy. Third, there is little scientific evidence that any intervention necessarily improves upon natural recovery. Last, and most important, it is quite likely that the major defects in current practice relate to the organisation of care in its widest sense, and to not detecting remediable problems.

Although there is little scientific evidence to support most of them, the following actions are likely to be beneficial:

(a) Ensure rapid, early mobilisation (i.e. within hours or days). It is certainly not contraindicated and may be beneficial.

(b) Give good physical (nursing) care. This is vital to avoid such complications as bed-sores or contractures.

(c) Actively involve the patient, his family, all nursing and ward staff, and anyone else concerned with the patient. Even 'intensive therapy' can only occupy 5 per cent of a patient's waking hours. Therefore the need is for a rehabilitative milieu in effect at all times, rather than episodic 'treatment' in isolation from normal daily care.

(d) Maintain motivation and interest. Patients must be kept stimulated. Every achievement should be praised.

(e) Be pragmatic. Relate therapy to a patient's needs and abilities. Do not stop someone from walking in an odd way if it enables him to be mobile. The increase in morale outweighs most other considerations.

(f) Identify all relevant problems, not only difficulties arising from the stroke, but also any incidental disabilities such as arthritis, blindness or deafness.

(g) Use a uniform approach. All team members treating an individual patient need to use a consistent method, and their answers to questions (e.g. on prognosis) need to be consistent.

(h) Be curious. If someone is not progressing as expected, find out why. Patients who put clothes on wrongly, or get lost in the department may have visuo-spatial (perceptual) problems. Other patients lack drive, usually due to depression but sometimes specifically from frontal lobe damage.

Some particular aspects of intervention need discussing. As mentioned initially, all professional staff involved should work as a team, with as little demarcation as possible. All team members should work towards the same goal; consequently their distinct roles will overlap to a considerable degree. Each profession represented in the team should see each patient at least once, to assess whether their expertise is needed.

The approach to the patient should be sensible and not dictated inexorably by some all-enveloping theory. There is no evidence to support any particular approach (e.g. Bobath), and even the importance of 'positioning' has not been investigated scientifically. Each therapist should use the methods that s/he has most experience of, adapting the approach as necessary. Further, whatever the theoretical basis, it seems cruel to put a patient with hemianopia so that he cannot see the rest of the ward, or to place his belongings on the side he neglects. There is no evidence that this approach improves recovery.

Spasticity has been described as 'the fable of the neurological demon and the emperor's new therapy' (Landau, 1974). There is no evidence that regular use of antispastic drugs is useful. On rare occasions such drugs (baclofen, dantrolene) may be needed to reduce tone which is painful or obstructive, but they are unlikely to benefit patients who are still recovering. Spasticity reflects poor motor control, rather than causing it (Chapter 27).

One aspect of stroke care sometimes overlooked is the need for long-term social support. Too often patients who appear to have made a good recovery or a good adaptation to their residual disability are discharged only to fester at home, lonely and depressed. Most areas (of Britain and other countries) have various voluntary and state-run organisations (e.g. Stroke Clubs) which can provide help and support for people left with problems after stroke. Medical social workers are the usual source of information on this topic.

ORGANISATION OF A STROKE CARE SERVICE

An increase in the attention given to the organisation of services for stroke patients might well lead to a greater improvement in stroke care than any other single procedure. Most health care is based upon defined communities; in Britain these are the Health Districts which contain an average of 250,000 people. In other countries the communities may be larger or smaller, but only by a factor of two or three. The principles to be discussed could be adapted to most health care systems if wished.

The major requirements of the service are that it should make an accurate medical diagnosis; it should ensure a good standard of immediate nursing care wherever the patient is being nursed; it should identify and treat any medical conditions which need treatment; it should avoid causing complications; it should facilitate the process of recovery; it should provide emotional and physical support to the family and the patient; and it should utilise any available services to provide long-term support for patients needing them.

One way of fulfilling these requirements is to develop a group of people drawn from the many professions who may be involved in stroke care, this group specialising in the rehabilitation of patients with stroke (and probably other neurological diseases too). Primary medical care would not be the concern of this team, but the team should include a doctor who could give his expert opinion if requested. This team should be involved as soon as possible. Any individual patient should be seen by the same members of the group throughout his illness, particularly after discharge from hospital. The team should see all strokes from its community, and should audit the care given.

CONCLUSIONS

The most important advance in stroke research this century is probably the identification of hypertension as a major and treatable risk factor for stroke. In addition there has been a considerable increase in our knowledge of almost all aspects of the pathology and natural history of stroke. Unfortunately we have not yet found any certain way of either reducing the immediate brain damage or of increasing the neurological recovery. This apparently pessimistic state of affairs should not prevent the application of a good standard of care. This requires constant attention to detail, and is facilitated by the use of standard assessment procedures. The next major advance in stroke care could be the development of audited services which might improve rehabilitation dramatically, through ensuring that any defects are identified and thus remedied.

REFERENCES

American–Canadian Cooperative Study Group (1985) Persantin aspirin trial in cerebral ischemia. Part II: End-point results. *Stroke, 16,* 406-15

Barthel, D.W. and Mahoney, F.I. (1965) Functional evaluation: the Barthel Index. *Maryland State Med. J., 14,* 61-5

Bhavani, G., Cockburn, T., Whiting, S. and Lincoln, N. (1983) The reliability of the RPA and implications in some commonly used assessments of perception. *Brit. J. Occup. Ther., 46,* 17-19

Demeurisse, G., Demol, O. and Robaye, E. (1980) Motor evaluation in vascular hemiplegia. *Eur. Neurol., 19,* 382-9

Hodkinson, H.M. (1972) Evaluation of a mental test score for assessment of mental impairment in the elderly. *Age and Ageing, 1,* 233-8

Holbrook, M. and Skilbeck, C.E. (1983) An activity index for use with stroke patients. *Age and Ageing, 12,* 166-70

Isaacs, B. (1971) Identification of disability in the stroke patient. *Mod. Geriat., 1,* 390-402

Landau, W.M. (1974) Spasticity: the fable of a neurological demon and the emperor's new therapy. *Arch. Neurol., 31,* 217-19

Lyle, R.C. (1981) A performance test for assessment of upper limb function in physical rehabilitation, treatment and research. *Int. J. Rehabil. Res., 4,* 483-92

Strand, T., Asplund, K., Eriksson, S., Hagg, E., Lithner, F. and Wester, P.O. (1984) Randomised controlled trial of hemidilution in acute stroke. *Stroke, 15,* 980-9

Teasdale, G., Murray, G., Parker, C. and Jennet, B. (1979) Adding up the Glasgow Coma Scale. *Acta Neurochir. Suppl, 28,* 13-16

Wade, D.T., Langton Hewer, R., Wood, V.A., Skilbeck C.E. and Ismail, H.M. (1983) The hemiplegic arm after stroke: measurement and recovery. *J. Neurol. Neurosurg. Psychiatry, 46,* 521-4

Wade, D.T., Langton Hewer, R., Skilbeck, C.E. and David, R.M. (1985) *Stroke. A critical approach to diagnosis, treatment and management.* Chapman & Hall Medical, London

Wade, D.T., Leigh-Smith, J. and Langton Hewer, R. (1986) Social activities after stroke: measurement and natural history using the Frenchay Activities Index. *Int. Rehabl. Med., 1,* 176-81

Zigmond, A.S. and Snaith, R.P. (1983) The Hospital Anxiety and Depression Scale. *Acta Psychiatr. Scand., 67,* 361-70

The Frenchay Asphasia Screening Test and the Rivermead Perceptual Assessment are both available from NFER-Nelson, Darville House, 2 Oxford Road East, Windsor, Berkshire, SL4 1DF.

FURTHER READING

Jay, Peggy, *Help Yourselves — a handbook for hemiplegics and their families,* 4th edn, 1985. (A practical book that covers many of the everyday problems arising from hemiplegia)

Mulley, G.P. (1985) *Practical management of stroke,* Croom Helm, London/ Medical Economics Company, Oradell, New Jersey

ADDRESSES FOR INFORMATION

Chest, Heart and Stroke Association,
BMA House, Tavistock Square, London.

21

Parkinson's Disease and Other Forms of Parkinsonism

Lindsay McLellan

Parkinson's disease is a relatively common condition, having an incidence of approximately 20/100,000 and a prevalence of some 160–200/100,000. In the British population approximately 74/100,000 people are severely or very severely handicapped with Parkinson's disease and approximately half of these are in residential care (Fahn, 1986; Mutch *et al.*, 1986; Sutcliffe *et al.*, 1985).

The mean age at onset is 55 years and male to female ratio is 3:2. It is commoner in the elderly, some estimates suggesting that one in 10 of all those over the age of 80 have Parkinsonism. However, the diagnosis is often more difficult to make in elderly people, and many elderly people whose movements are slow, or whose balance is poor, may be suspected of having Parkinsonism on superficial assessment, but in fact do not have it.

Parkinson's disease starts insidiously and progresses gradually. Before the introduction of levodopa treatment, death would be expected some 12–15 years after the first symptom due to the complications of immobility, notably bronchopneumonia. Since the early 1970s the life expectancy has improved, and is probably normal in many cases though for the 10–15 per cent of cases who do not respond to treatment the prognosis is presumably unchanged. It is not yet clear, however, whether the subgroup which does not respond to dopamingergic therapy has a different natural prognosis from the rest.

Terminology

The terminology of Parkinson's disease can cause confusion. Parkinson's original description in 1815 is usually held to apply to the idiopathic progressive form of the disease and neurologists tend to reserve the term Parkinson's disease to this clinical entity, referring to all other clinical forms as Parkinsonism. The term Parkinsonism is also used to embrace the whole spectrum of neurological disorders in which bradykinesia is accompanied by one or more of the other classical clinical features of the disease.

There are, however, a number of rare conditions in which some of the clinical features of Parkinsonism coexist with further neurological deficits suggesting lesions in other parts of the nervous system. Since these conditions are identified by their additional features, they are grouped under the rubric of 'Parkinsonism Plus' (Fahn, 1986). This somewhat unsatisfactory terminology reflects the fact that the causes of Parkinsonsim are poorly understood, and the nature and distribution of the lesions responsible for it may be impossible to ascertain during life.

Causes of Parkinsonism

See Table 21.1.

Table 21.1: Causes of Parkinsonism

Cause or type	Characteristic clinical features	Course
Definite Parkinsonism		
Idiopathic	(Classical description)	Steadily progressive
Postencephalitic	Often other neurological signs; autonomic disorders common; oculogyric crises may occur	Progressive at first, may become clinically static for long periods
Drug-induced	Tremor often absent. Akathesia and/or orofacial dyskinesias may also be present	Parkinsonism resolves when drug is withdrawn
Striatonigral degeneration	No tremor, no response to anti-Parkinson drugs	Progressive
Toxic (MPTP)	History of narcotic abuse	Recovery is rare
Parkinsonism-like states (none responds to dopaminergic drugs)		
Alzheimer's disease	Dementia, prominent 10% have Parkinsonism-like features	Progressive
Intermittently raised pressure hydrocephalus	Incontinence and dementia also present	Variable, may improve with ventricular shunting
Hypertensive encephalopathy	Marked rise in blood pressure	Potentially reversible
Wilson's disease	Onset usually under age 30; often evidence of hepatic disease and encephalopathy; Kayser–Fleischer rings, family history	Progressive and fatal if not treated
Rigid forms of Huntington's chorea	Onset usually under 30 years; dementia present	Progressive
Parkinsonism plus (none responds to dopaminergic drugs)		
Progressive supranuclear palsy	Impaired downward conjugate gaze, ataxia of gait, dystonia of face and neck	Progressive
Multiple system atrophies	Other additional neurological signs	Progressive

CLINICAL FEATURES OF PARKINSONISM

Bradykinesia

The fundamental clinical disorder is bradykinesia. The diagnosis of Parkinsonism cannot be made in the absence of bradykinesia no matter what other clinical features are present.

Bradykinesia is a slowness of voluntary movement, referring both to the initiation of movement and to its execution. Its earliest manifestation in the hands is impairment in the performance of fine skilled tasks such as writing or handling delicate tools; later it may be increasingly difficult to button or unbutton clothing or to use a knife and fork effectively. The most sensitive clinical test for bradykinesia of the hands is to place the palmar surface of the wrist on a table and to drum the middle and index fingers alternately as fast as possible, ensuring that as one finger extends the other flexes concurrently and that these movements simultaneously reverse. In bradykinesia this sequence can only be performed slowly, and there is a marked tendency for both fingers to move together in the same direction or for each finger to make a succession of taps while the other fails to move. In the legs, bradykinesia presents as a difficulty in rapid movements of the feet (as in drumming or dancing) or a tendency to shuffle. As the disease progresses the patients finds it increasingly difficult to make a particular sort of mental effort or to respond to an external stimulus. In more severe cases a step that cannot be initiated voluntarily may be initiated in a reflex-like way by pushing the subject forward or rocking him from side to side. Such a stimulus can initiate a sequence of short steps ('festination') over which the subject has only a tenuous voluntary control, and he may continue to festinate forwards or backwards until he meets an obstacle or something to grasp hold of.

Formal studies of the nature of bradykinesia have shown that the simple reaction time may be normal, but that more complex responses in which a decision or choice has to be made are delayed. There is a characteristically slow build-up of muscle activation and the burst of activity achieved when attempting to perform a ballistic movement is of a lower amplitude than normal. Complex sequences (such as grasping with the hand at the same time as flexing the elbow) are conducted much more slowly than either component would be if undertaken singly. This has led to the suggestion that superimposing and sequencing of simple basic motor 'programmes' is defective in bradykinesia.

A number of clinical observations have suggested that visual cues may either help or hinder the ability to walk. Parkinson reported of his sixth case, 'it was observed by his wife, that she believed, that in walking across the room, he would consider as a difficulty the having to step over a pin'.

Patients with severe bradykinesia of gait tend to 'freeze' as they approach doorways and may be assisted by the presence of horizontal lines across the surface over which they are walking. It is uncertain whether these observations are best interpreted as signs of poor sensory-motor integration, or whether these visual cues simply facilitate or inhibit the complex process of voluntary initiation of movement by acting as targets. Some patients develop complex stereotyped mental strategies to reinforce their ability to initiate movement. Under extremes of emotional stimulation (such as immediate physical danger) the ability to move may for a few moments be restored almost to normal; similar short-lived periods of mobility sometimes occur in the first few minutes after waking from sleep.

Tremor

Tremor does not occur in all cases of Parkinsonism, and in an untreated patient, tremor unaccompanied by bradykinesia is *not* due to Parkinsonism. At least two types of tremor are seen. The most classical form is tremor 'at rest'; that is to say when the subject is awake but not having to move or maintain a posture so that the limb is relaxed. In the upper limb the classical picture is of a 'pill-rolling' tremor in which the forearm is partially supinated and the thumb extends as the fingers flex, mimicking the movement of rolling a small object in the palm of the hand. The tremor is rather slow, with a frequency of 4–5 Hz, and may be suppressed when a voluntary movement is made, returned after a few moments (in severe cases) even though voluntary activity continues. The second form of tremor is 'action' or 'postural' tremor brought out by maintaining a posture such as holding the arm out to the front. This resembles a physiological tremor but its frequency at 7–8 Hz is intermediate between resting tremor and physiological tremor, and coincides with the frequency of cog-wheeling described below. It is distinct from resting tremor. Finally some patients quite clearly have mild intention tremor as well, but by common consent this fact is ignored, since it is incompatible with the clinical categorisation of tremors as taught to medical students.

Rigidity

Rigidity is the term given to the 'plastic' or 'velocity-independent' resistance to passive stretch which is seen especially in the flexor muscle groups in the upper and lower limbs. In many cases the resistance is broken up into bursts of activity at a rate of 7–8 Hz (similar to the frequency of postural tremor). This can occur whether or not overt tremor is present, and is due to a specific and characteristic abnormality in the passive stretch response.

Rigidity expresses itself by altering the posture of the patient; since it is most pronounced in flexor muscles both upper and lower limbs (and the neck and trunk) tend to assume a flexed posture. In mild cases this tendency can be readily overcome by voluntary effort. Impoverishment of movement is much more likely to be due to bradykinesia than to rigidity, for the mechanism of reciprocal inhibition is unimpaired in mild and moderate rigidity so that there is little or no mechanical constraint by antagonist muscles during voluntary movements.

OTHER EARLY SIGNS OF PARKINSONISM

Parkinsonism may easily be missed when it is mild, and other signs helpful in diagnosis are a lack of facial expression and a reduction in associated postural movements — notably a failure to swing one or both arms when walking. Since the disease often starts unilaterally the first objective sign may be a discrepancy between the amount of swing in the two arms during normal walking.

OTHER CLINICAL FEATURES OF PARKINSONISM

Some of these are restricted to particular forms of the disorder such as post-encephalitic Parkinsonism.

Autonomic disorders

Postural hypotension and excessive seborrhoea are the two most common autonomic disorders. Postural hypotension tends to be accentuated by treatment, and this sometimes limits the dose of dopaminergic drugs that can be taken. These features are more common in post-encephalitic Parkinsonism than in idiopathic Parkinson's disease. More prominent disorders occur in some forms of 'Parkinsonism Plus' (Table 21.1).

Impairment of memory and cognitive function

These disorders are common in some of the diseases associated with Parkinsonism (see Table 21.1). In idiopathic Parkinson's disease there are subtle impairments of visuospatial function, associative learning and recent memory, and also in tests of order-dependent short-term memory (Mayeux, 1981).

The literature relating to dementia in idiopathic Parkinson's disease is confusing, partly because of the difficulty in allocating patients to this category and partly because of the confounding effects of increasing age. Thus the incidence of dementia is reported as 15 per cent in some series and as much as 90 per cent in others. In patients presenting below the age of 65 years the likelihood of subsequent dementia is probably 10–15 per cent.

The dementia associated with Parkinson's disease is accompanied by changes of behaviour, which shows dependency, tearfulness, indecision and passivity. There is a difficulty in shifting conceptual sets and a tendency to perseverate, suggesting a disorder of frontal lobe function. Depression is also common, occurring in approximately 25 per cent of patients and usually being reactive in type. The occurrence of dementia cannot be predicted, either from physical disability, nor from the presence of depression or impaired function on visuospatial tests. It is possible that impairment on tests of recent memory indicates a greater than average risk of developing dementia, but this is not firmly enough established to be clinically useful at present. These interesting observations indicate that functions other than physical functions are impaired in a number of patients with idiopathic Parkinson's disease. The value of the response to levodopa as a diagnostic tool has yet to be established.

Speech disorders

Speech disorders are present in the vast majority of patients with Parkinson's disease. One frequently finds dysarthria with hoarseness, decreased volume and a monotonous tone. Consonants may be imprecise and the full picture makes it difficult for the patient to gain and sustain the attention of the listener (Robbins *et al.*, 1986).

Associated pains

Nearly half of all patients with Parkinson's disease complain of somatic pains, and three-quarters of these complaints relate to sensations of muscle cramp or tightness in the neck, paraspinal muscles and calf muscles. Approximately 28 per cent of patients have painful dystonias of one or both feet, most of these being present in the mornings, though a few are related to times at which dopaminergic drug action is at its peak. Radicular pain occurs in approximately 14 per cent of cases. All these features are associated in time with the severity of bradykinesia and, to a lesser extent, rigidity. In addition, approximately 14 per cent have pains in the joints of the shoulders, hips and knees and ankles lasting several hours at a stretch. These joint pains are not related in time to fluctuations in the severity of bradykinesia or rigidity.

Social effects

The cost to the community is not inconsiderable, given the size of the problem. The social cost to the individual and the family can also be substantial; indeed the effect has been likened to premature social ageing, with increased periods of idleness and with predominantly passive leisure pursuits (Singer, 1973).

Allocation of patients with Parkinsonism into a clinical category

The classical picture of idiopathic Parkinsonism is easy to recognise. A patient in his late 40s to early 60s presents with a combination of the three cardinal signs, which are usually asymmetrical. There is an initial excellent response to levodopa, but as the disease progresses this response is increasingly difficult to maintain, as described below.

In all cases it is important to record the presence of a family history, a history of taking major tranquillisers (especially phenothiazines), exposure to narcotics or toxic chemicals, blood pressure measured in lying and standing positions, mental function and an assessment of urinary continence. In younger patients, under 35, a history of encephalitis should be sought and every effort made to exclude a family history of Huntingdon's chorea or Wilson's disease.

The diagnosis in elderly people can be much more difficult. Elderly people tolerate lower doses of dopaminergic and anticholinergic drugs, so that mental confusion may be induced at a dose too low to improve mobility. For this reason it may be impossible to establish whether the patient has a form of Parkinsonism that could respond to therapy or not.

Table 21.1 indicates the principal features characteristic of each form of Parkinsonism. One of the commonest difficulties is to distinguish Parkinsonism. Up to 50 per cent of patients with idiopathic tremor ('benign essential tremor') have a family history, and it was contamination of the Parkinsonism population by such cases that led to reports of an increased familial incidence of Parkinson's disease.

Idiopathic tremor is usually an action (postural) tremor but it can be indistinguishable from the tremor of Parkinson's disease. The cardinal feature is that bradykinesia is absent, but it can be hard to be sure about this if the tremor is severe. The course of idiopathic tremor is relatively benign, but a minority of patients are moderately severely disabled by it. There is an association between idiopathic tremor and torsion dystonia, some patients having features of both conditions.

Pathology of Parkinsonism

In idiopathic Parkinson's disease nerve cells in the substantia nigra degenerate, with the formation of Lewy bodies containing filamentous material in the perikaryon of some of the surviving neurones. Other pigmented nuclei are also affected, notably the locus caeruleus and the dorsal motor vagus nucleus. Degeneration may occur also in the innominate substance, the hypothalamus, the raphe nuclei of the rostral pons and midbrain and in the sympathetic ganglia. In post-encephalitic Parkinsonism the neuropathological hallmark is neurofibrillary tangles, predominantly in the substantia nigra. Lacunar infarcts in the basal ganglia may occur in cerebrovascular disease with atypical Parkinsonism.

Causes of Parkinsonism

The cause of Parkinsonism is unknown, although there have been suggestions that the premorbid behaviour of patients may be related to later development of the disease. Many cases of post-encephalitic Parkinsonism were produced by the pandemics of encephalitis lethargica in 1918 and 1922 but obvious post-viral cases are now very unusual. Phenothiazine drugs (which block dopamine transmission) can induce Parkinsonism with persistence of the Parkinsonism for up to two years. Recently a number of cases of acute, severe Parkinsonism have occurred in young people poisoned with MPTP (*N*-methyl-4-phenyl-1-1,2,3,6-tetrahydropyridine), a contaminant of inexpert attempts to manufacture diamorphine, which selectively destroys the nigrostriatal dopamanic neurones.

Mode of action of anti-Parkinsonism drugs

Anti-Parkinsonism drugs act by inhibiting cholinergic transmission or potentiating dopaminergic transmission, as outlined schematically in Figure 21.1. Dopaminergic transmission may be potentiated presynaptically by levodopa, which increases the concentration of dopamine in synaptic terminals, and by amantadine, which potentiates the release of dopamine when the terminal is depolarised. Dopamine in the synaptic cleft is normally taken back into the dopaminergic neurone or metabolised outside the neurone by oxidation. Oxidation can be suppressed by a dopamine-B oxidase inhibitor, selegeline, which prolongs the survival of dopamine in the synaptic cleft and increases its binding to postsynaptic dopamine receptors. Dopamine receptors can be activated directly by dopamine agonists such as bromocriptine, apomorphine, pergolide and lisuride.

Levodopa is metabolised to dopamine in many tissues of the body and

Figure 21.1: Simplified schematic diagram of neurotransmitter pathways thought to be involved in the treatment of Parkinsonism. − = Inhibition; + = excitation. Degeneration of dopaminergic nigrostriatal neurones disinhibits cholinergic neurones. This is counteracted by boosting dopaminergic transmission or inhibiting cholinergic transmission

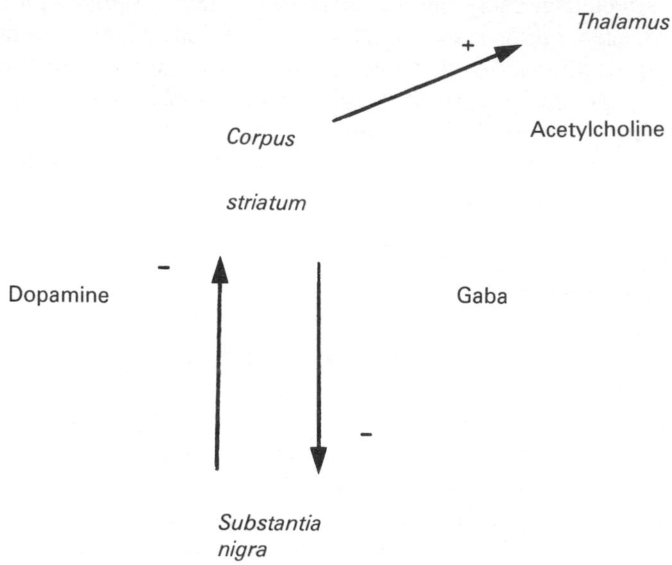

its unwanted effects upon automatic function, cardiac muscle and the chemotactic trigger zone in the area postrema of the fourth ventricle can be blocked by giving a decarboxylase inhibitor (such as benserazide or carbidopa), which also has the effect of stabilising the blood levels of levodopa in the cerebral circulation. Commercial formulations tend to include a combination of levodopa and decarboxylase inhibitor in a fixed proportion. This is a disadvantage for those who can tolerate only small amounts of levodopa, for toxic effects of levodopa appear before a dose is reached that contains sufficient decarboxylase inhibitor to provide full background inhibition of decarboxylase. In these circumstances fluctuations in the level of decarboxylase inhibitor can further destabilise the control of symptoms.

Levodopa cannot be infused intravenously because it is too irritant, but dopamine agonists such as lisuride have been used in an attempt to provide smoother control of unpredictable fluctuations in clinical state (described below).

TREATMENT OF PARKINSON'S DISEASE

Purpose of treatment

Phenothiazine-induced Parkinsonism is best treated by reducing the dose of phenothiazine, but some of the symptoms, notably tremor and rigidity, can be improved by adding anticholinergic drugs. In idiopathic Parkinsonism the purpose of treatment is to maintain normal activity without inducing side-effects. Treatment probably prolongs life, but only in so far as it suppresses symptoms; it does not modify the underlying pathological process. After treatment with levodopa has continued successfully for several years, a state is often reached in which the response to treatment is unstable; involuntary movements (dyskinesia) alternate with periods of severe Parkinsonism in a pattern that cannot be explained on the basis of changes in the blood level of levodopa. It is possible that prolonged treatment with levodopa itself induces changes in synaptic function leading to this unsatisfactory and uncomfortable state. A further aim of treatment is therefore to delay the development of this tendency to unpredictable fluctuations. There is no point in treating signs or symptoms if the patient is not inconvenienced by them.

Initial management

Treatment begins at the time of diagnosis when it consists of a full *explanation* of the nature and prognosis of the disease. If the symptoms are of recent onset it may not be easy to predict the time-course of deterioration in an individual patient, but patients are often encouraged by knowing that treatment is optional and that they are expected to exercise day-to-day judgement in the dose of any medication that it used. The patient must avoid obesity and take regular exercise. The patient should be informed that if necessary an occupational therapist can be consulted for advice about alternative ways of undertaking particular physical tasks, and about the selection and use of physical aids and adaptations.

Questions commonly asked by patients on learning the diagnosis are what is the cause of Parkinsonism, whether their way of life has contributed to the occurrence of the disease or will affect the prognosis, whether it is familial or transmittable, and whether any measures are available that will slow down the rate of deterioration.

Booklets such as those published by the Parkinson's Disease Society (Franklyn *et al.*, 1982) form a helpful information base for the patient and family at this stage, and such booklets should be routinely available in all clinics where the diagnosis is likely to be communicated to the patient. This also enables the patient to contact the Parkinson's Disease Society if desired. Follow-up consultation after intervals of a few days will normally be necessary to ensure that the patient has a clear understanding of the disease, and that the unavoidable stress of learning the diagnosis is not unnecessarily exacerbated by inadequate information or misinformation.

When should drug treatment start?

The purpose of treatment is to relieve symptoms, so the decision to start should always be negotiated with the patient. Mild symptoms may cause concern only until their cause has been diagnosed, and if the patient is certain that dexterity or mobility have not significantly declined then medical treatment can be postponed. However, it is not a good idea to wait until activities are seriously compromised, and the pattern of disease varies in every patient. Sometimes patients may deny symptoms because they do not associate certain difficulties they have experienced (like turning over in bed) with the obvious signs of the disease (such as tremor). It is therefore useful to go through the following checklist of functions with the patient: writing, using a knife and fork, eating soup with a spoon, using a small screwdriver; rising from a chair, walking through doorways; turning over in bed at night, getting comfortable in a chair, going for walks, and speaking in company.

Having identified a goal for treatment it is essential to adjust the dose until the goal is reached, and not simply to prescribe a set number of tablets as though treating an infection. Treating Parkinsonism is like treating diabetes — both the individual doses and the overall daily dose need to be titrated against the beneficial results and side-effects, and the requirements change as the disease progresses, which means that the dose should be reviewed regularly even in patients who appear stable.

Early drug treatment

There is some evidence that patients treated with levodopa alone in full doses from the onset of symptoms reach the stage of unpredictable fluctuation sooner than those who start treatment with a dopamine agonist such as bromocriptine. This evidence is not yet conclusive, for a significant minority of those who respond well to levodopa cannot tolerate bromocriptine, so that those who can tolerate it are a subgroup of the Parkinsonism population. A further factor is that dopamine agonists alone usually relieve the symptoms less effectively than levodopa or a combination of levodopa with a dopamine agonist. A common policy at the time of writing is therefore to start treatment with a combination of levodopa (plus decarboxylase inhibitor) and a dopamine agonist such as bromocriptine in modest doses. Levodopa should be used with great caution, and bromocriptine should not be used in patients who suffer from dementia or schizophrenia.

In people under the age of 65 it is usually safe to start with a levodopa preparation in a dose of 100–125 mg two or three times a day, together with bromocriptine 2.5 mg twice daily. The doses are then increased until either a satisfactory clinical response is obtained or side-effects occur. A definite response in newly diagnosed patients is usually seen with a dose of levodopa preparation of 100–125 mg three times a day and bromocriptine 5 mg three times a day. In people over the age of 70 the initial dosage should be smaller, and bromocriptine tends to be less well tolerated.

Dopaminergic drugs are the most effective treatment for bradykinesia but if the only symptom to trouble the patient is tremor, an anticholinergic drug such as trihexyphenidyl (benzhexol) or ophenadrine may suffice. The starting dose is 2 mg trihexyphenidyl or 50 mg orphenadrine twice daily,

Figure 21.2: Diagram showing mode of action of decarboxylase inhibition. Levodopa and a decarboxylase inhibitor are taken orally and absorbed by an active transport mechanism in the small intestine. The inhibitor does not pass the blood–brain barrier and enters the CNS only in the area postrema of the fourth ventricle (chemotactic trigger zone, *) where it reduces the generation of nausea and anorexia. Levodopa is converted to dopamine only in the shaded area of the CNS

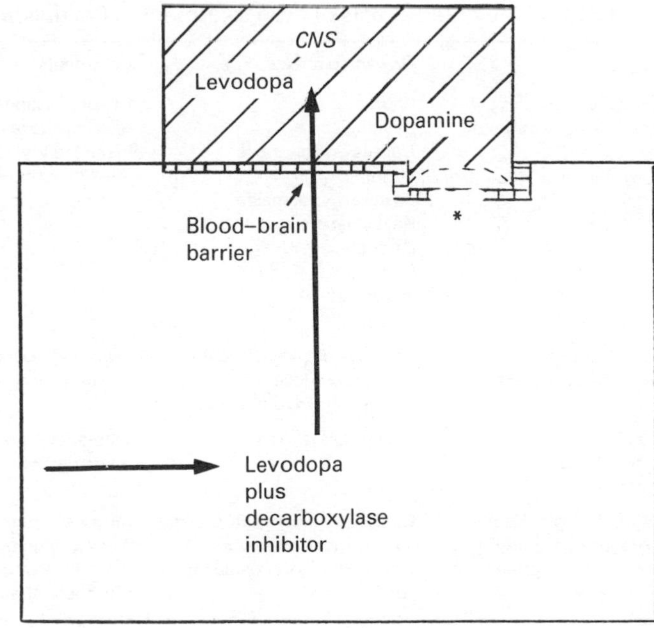

increasing to a total maximum daily dose of 15–20 mg trihexphenidyl or 600 mg orphenadrine.

The purpose of early treatment is to enable the patient to continue to function normally. Therefore all patients whose disability cannot be completely relieved will experience side-effects of drugs while the optimum dose level is being established. New side-effects may also occur as the disease progresses, or as a result of drug interactions, even though the dose has not been changed. For those reasons the recognition of side-effects is a vital skill for all those treating Parkinsonism to acquire; they are described in some detail here because they are such an important indicator in management.

Side-effects

The side-effects of these medications are summarised in Table 21.2. The most frequent side-effect of levodopa is *dyskinesia*, a movement disorder that overlaps both chorea and athetosis. All muscle groups may be affected, the face and cervical muscles being most commonly involved. The head may weave or duck from side to side and twitching movements affect the mouth and periorbital muscles; the tongue may repeatedly protrude involuntarily. Chorea also affects the shoulders, trunk and limbs.

Table 21.2: Unwanted effects of drug treatment of Parkinson's disease

Drug	Unwanted effects	Comments
Levodopa plus decarboxylase inhibitor	Chorea Dystonia Nausea and anorexia Flushing Postural hypotension Hallucinations Paranoia Confusion Insomnia Anxiety	Onset of action 30–45 minutes after oral dose and lasts 6–8 hours in mild (early) cases but only 30–120 minutes in brittle cases
Bromocriptine (dopamine agonist)	As above but greater tendency to cause confusion, flushing and postural hypotension	Lasts 3–6 hours. Less well tolerated in elderly people
Selegeline (dopamine B oxidase inhibitor)	Potentiates levodopa	Side-effects on fixed dose may appear after 7–14 days of use
Anticholinergic drugs (e.g. trihexyphenidyl (benzhexol), orphenadrine)	Confusion, dry mouth, blurred vision, impaired erection, exacerbation of prostatism, constipation	Must be withdrawn gradually over 3 weeks after prolonged use. Good for tremor or rigidity but much less effective for bradykinesia

Movements such as reading or walking may show bizarre trajectories with exaggerated high stepping or flexion movements, or tweaking movements of the hands and feet. Akathesia also occurs — that is, an irresistible desire to walk about, the commonest manifestations being compulsive standing from the sitting position, restless rapid walking, or continual crossing and uncrossing of the legs.

Patients themselves are often unaware of these movements even when they have become so prominent as to cause embarrassment to their companions. In more severe cases these movements tend to be accompanied by dystonia, which is painful. Dystonia is involuntary coactivation of many muscle groups including physiological antagonists, so that the limbs, trunk and face become fixed in a distorted posture that has a characteristic configuration. Thus the tongue may be continuously protruded, or the masseter muscles in spasm so that the mouth cannot be opened; the trunk stiff and twisted or flexed to one side, and the limbs held stiffly in the postures recognisable as characteristic of basal ganglia disease.

The second most common side-effect of levodopa is *confusion*, which may be accompanied by suspiciousness amounting on occasions to paranoia, visual hallucinations or (in severe cases) delusions. This occurs most often at high doses or in elderly people, but it is a side-effect that patients can successfully hide, and the patient's spouse or companion should be asked to watch for its appearance. It is important to ask patients specifically whether hallucinations have occurred, for they are characteristically reticent about them. The hallucinations are visual, not auditory; they often have a disturbing quality and are sometimes frightening.

Postural dizziness due to postural hypotension is seen in some cases of Parkinsonism, and this feature is always intensified by dopaminergic treatment, or may appear for the first time as a result of treatment. Sometimes the symptoms can be controlled by using fludrocortisone to expand plasma volume, but those who develop this complication are often elderly, and there is a risk of causing congestive cardiac failure by this means. When postural hypotension occurs it usually limits quite severely the dose of levodopa that can be tolerated.

The side-effects of anticholinergic drugs are well known and shown in Table 21.2. A side-effect of particular importance in elderly men is *hesitancy of micturition* which may be mistaken for prostatism since the prostate gland tends to be enlarged at this age. It is important to withdraw the drugs for at least a month before any prostatic surgery; prostatecomy for the side-effects of anticholinergic drugs usually produces incontinence. Anticholinergic drugs commonly cause confusion, especially in elderly people.

Anorexia and associated weight loss are commonly seen in people taking full doses of levodopa. They often do not complain of anorexia unless it is accompanied by nausea. Nausea can be reduced by taking levodopa with meals, but the therapeutic effect may also be impaired because of reduced absorption. Nausea can also be countered, of course, by reducing the dose of levodopa, or by adding domperidone to the treatment in a dose of 10 mg once or twice a day.

There have been some reports of *cardiac arrhythmias* being exacerbated by levodopa, especially after acute myocardial infarction. This side-effect is blocked by dopadecarboxylase inhibitor (such as benserazide 100 mg/24 hours) being given.

Later stages in treatment

In the early stages of treatment with levodopa the patient does not notice the onset of wearing off of each dose. However, as the disease progresses the dose has to be increased in order to achieve the same effect, and it becomes obvious that onset of the effect is 30–45 minutes after an oral dose. The dose may last for shorter and shorter periods of time, reducing from 6 to 8 hours to as little as 45–60 minutes in severe cases. As the dose increases so the risk of involuntary movements increases, occurring shortly after the time the plasma concentration of levodopa reaches its peak (1–1½ hours after an oral dose). In order to avoid peak-dose dyskinesia it is necessary to give smaller individual doses at more frequent intervals, and the regimen can become irksome. Smooth control of symptoms can be helped by using a programmable alarm watch. The night-time may be particularly uncomfortable, since high doses shortly before retiring tend to cause insomnia, while smaller doses wear off in the middle of the night.

A 'background cover' of anticholinergic drugs is very helpful in this situation, and also in cases where levodopa fails to suppress the tremor. Anticholinergic drugs have a longer duration of action; though most of their effect is gone after 24 hours, withdrawal after prolonged use may be followed by some deterioration in the Parkinsonism seven to ten days later.

Withdrawal of treatment

Both levodopa and anticholinergic drugs should be withdrawn slowly over two to three weeks.

Potentation of levodopa

As explained above, levodopa can be potentiated by the concurrent use of a dopamine agonist such as bromocriptine. Bromocriptine is useful in having a longer duration of action than levodopa, and therefore avoiding fluctuations in mobility. Its principal drawbacks are its rather greater tendency to cause confusion and postural hypotension. The action of levodopa can also be prolonged by the use of dopamine-β-oxidase inhibitor, selegeline. In a dose of 5–10 mg once or twice a day selegeline can reduce the overall requirements for levodopa by some 25–30 per cent but its use in 'complex fluctuators' (see below) is disappointing because of the difficulty in avoiding peak-dose toxicity. Other drugs such as amantadine have been superseded by these other treatments.

Drug interactions

Dopaminergic and anticholinergic drugs are safe to use with tricyclic antidepressants, benzodiazepine tranquillisers and analgesic drugs. Antihypertension drugs may be potentiated by levodopa.

Phenothiazines and tetrabenazine antagonise dopamine and can induce or accentuate Parkinsonism. This effect is dose-dependent but may take several months to subside and there are reports of symptoms persisting for as long as one to two years after prolonged treatment with phenothiazines. Antibiotics may alter the absorption of levodopa, destabilising a previously established regimen.

If the dose of levodopa is being limited by nausea, domperidone appears to be the dopamine antagonist with the least effect upon mobility, and is the drug of choice in the suppression of nausea.

Management of non-responsive cases and complex fluctuations

The above guidelines are sufficient for establishing drug regimens in most patients. However, 10–15 per cent of patients with idiopathic Parkinsonism do not show any clinical improvement with levodopa. In such cases it is important to ensure that the dose has been increased to the limit of tolerance, and to review the original diagnosis. Residual disability should be carefully assessed and dealt with as described below under general management.

A number of different patterns of fluctuations are described, usually starting some three to five years after the onset of treatment (Marsden *et al.*, 1981). The most common is end-of-dose dyskinesia alternating with periods of immobility as the dose 'wears off', and this is treated by taking smaller doses at more frequent intervals. It is often helpful for the patient to complete a diary hour by hour for several days since the requirements for oral levodopa alter during the course of 24 hours, being influenced also by a number of extrinsic factors, especially meal times since the effect of a single dose is attenuated if taken after or shortly before a meal. It is often necessary to regulate meal times and the amount of food (especially protein) in order to achieve smooth control.

As time passes the *therapeutic window* between immobility and dyskinesia becomes progressively narrower, and a second pattern of fluctuation may be seen in some 10 per cent of cases. This is diphasic dyskinesia, in which the patient passes through a brief period of dyskinesia while passing from immobility to mobility, and again as the dose wears off while passing back into immobility. This is best countered by moving the doses closer together while ensuring the peak-dose dyskinesia is avoided. Third, there are some patients in the later stages (including a very few quite early on in their response to treatment) who show dramatic fluctuations in their responses which are hard to relate to the timing and dose of medication ('complex fluctuators'). Periods of flaccid akinesia occur, which may result from excess rather than too little dopamine. Some of these difficulties probably reflect the fact that the threshold blood level of levodopa causing dyskinesia is now lower than the level required to restore mobility. Trials of continuous intravenous infusion of a dopamine agonist such as lisuride suggest that these fluctuations might be controlled if a sufficiently steady state could be maintained. However, the response threshold and therapeutic 'window' appear to change rather rapidly over several days of continuous infusion, and these techniques are currently unsuitable for normal clinical use.

An alternative approach has been to provide a continuous background cover of a full dose (for example 100–120 mg per 24 hours) of decarboxylase inhibitor and then to administer small oral doses (15–40 mg) of levodopa at frequent intervals (McLellan and Dean, 1981). This can be helpful especially when the patients' tolerance of levodopa has reduced the amount of combined preparation that can be taken to the point at which dopa decarboxylase is only partially inhibited. However, it may be necessary for levodopa and the decarboxylase inhibitor to be present in the gut at the same time to ensure optimal absorption.

Stereotactic thalamotomy

Lesions in the ventrolateral nucleus of the thalamus not only abolish contralateral tremor, but also abolish or greatly reduce levodopa-induced dyskinesia. Stereotactic thalamotomy is rarely performed now for tremor, because of the effectiveness of medication, although it can still be valuable for some patients with severe unilateral tremor. A few surgeons have used it to good effect in the management of intractable levodopa-induced dyskinesias, enabling a patient to continue to take a dose that abolishes bradykinesia. Previous thalamotomy does not impair the effect of levodopa upon bradykinesia (Knutsson *et al.*, 1972).

GENERAL MANAGEMENT

It is important to remember that many measures other than drugs can improve the quality of life in Parkinsonism (Shindler *et al.*, 1987). The future should be discussed with the patient so that realistic plans are made, and activities that depend on full mobility are not postponed until the progression of the disease has made them impossible. It may be necessary for the patient to plan for changes at work or for moving house; in Britain the Manpower Services Commission can provide funds and equipment to the employer of a physically disabled person to help them remain at work, and it is essential to inform the patient of this possibility (Chapter 41).

Physiotherapy and speech therapy

Regular physical exercise should be encouraged, and obesity avoided. The role of physiotherapy and speech therapy in Parkinsonism is controversial (Franklyn and Stern, 1981; Perry and Das, 1981). There is little evidence that bradykinesia can be improved by training, but there is considerable anecdotal evidence that periods of immobility (for example, being confined to bed after a limb fracture) leave the patient significantly more impaired than before, while regular spells of exercise promote a sense of physical confidence and well-being (Doshay, 1962; Gordon and Oster, 1974).

Very few objective trials have been undertaken, and they have mostly been small, technically unsatisfactory and inconclusive. A 'control group' who stays at home, while the 'treatment group' is spirited across London several times a week in a minicab (Robertson and Thomson, 1984) is of little value for comparative purposes. Negative trials of physiotherapy have tended to use very crude outcome measures, or to use refined measurements totally different from the functions that the therapy was designed to improve (Gibberd *et al.*, 1981). There is much anecdotal evidence that keeping patients on the move, physically active and socially involved helps to maintain mobility and communication, but there is no convincing evidence that the specific techniques employed by physiotherapists or speech therapists have any specific effects in Parkinsonism. By contrast, the encouragement provided by therapists in setting goals and specifying exercises may kindle interest and enthusiasm in the patients' relatives also, which probably helps to keep the patient active.

Speech therapists may be of help in teaching the patient strategies to deal with the rigidity and bradykinesia which underlie the articulatory disorder and are helpful in advising on the prevention of aspiration (Chapter 15). Robbins *et al.* (1986) discuss swallowing and speech. Videofloroscopy showed abnormal orophalangeal movements in six patients although only 50 per cent of the subjects admitted to any swallowing difficulty. They emphasised that it is the bradykinesia that causes the speech impairment, and also that the unrecognised swallowing problem causes aspiration which may not be noticed until the patient has a chest infection (Scott *et al.*, 1985).

A minority of people with Parkinsonism themselves develop mental strategies for initiating movement such as ritual preparatory movements or mental 'countdowns'. This has encouraged some therapists to employ the techniques of conductive education to improve mobility. This approach is worthy of research, but at present there is insufficient evidence to recommend it for the treatment of Parkinson's disease.

Walking

Bradykinesia poses unique problems for mobility. The inability to turn over in bed or to get out of bed can be helped by using an electrically operated cushion or 'sit-up' bed, since once the upper part of the trunk has been raised turning may be achieved more easily. The difficulty in rising from low chairs can be avoided by the use of firm higher chairs; spring-loaded chairs which catapult the patient upright are not well liked because of the likelihood of falling forwards, but electrically operated standing chairs which achieve the upright posture more gradually are better tolerated in the more severely affected subjects. Walking frames are difficult to use because a ballistic movement is required to lift and replace them; trolleys are more useful but the subjects' poor balance may allow them to run out of control. The most useful walker is a three-wheeled frame with two handles and a handbrake, that can also be folded for ease of transport (Chapter 46).

Falling over is part of walking, and a technique for getting up again is something that needs to be worked out for all patients whose ability to walk is becoming compromised. This is something that many physiotherapists include in their treatment programmes. Bradykinesia results in reduction of the swing phase and prolongation of the stance phase of walking. Walking speed is slowed (Knuttson, 1972), which is shown most simply by timing walking over a fixed distance. Physiotherapy helps to improve this (Gibberd *et al.*, 1981; Franklyn and Stern, 1981) which may lead to a reduction in shuffling and a more normal heel-strike toe-off gait.

Driving

The factors that impair the capacity to drive a car are the ability to depress the pedals fully in emergencies and to turn the steering wheel sufficiently fast. Power-assisted brakes and steering are helpful, and an automatic gearbox is an advantage. In those whose mobility is subject to frequent fluctuations it is important to time driving periods so that they fall within safe periods of mobility, and this often means that long journeys are impossible unless the driving is shared or separated into short segments. Confusion, poor concentration or dementia are all obvious contraindications to driving, and it is essential to check for these features with a patient's spouse or companion as the patient himself may underestimate their significance. In cases of doubt, formal assessment should be undertaken at a recognised disabled drivers' assessment centre. Oxtoby (1982) provided information on outdoor mobility; only 18 per cent of his series were able to drive, and public transport was mostly inaccessible (Chapter 47).

Occupational therapy

Where disability cannot be avoided by drugs, the help of an occupational therapist should be enlisted to assess the nature of practical difficulties encountered by the patient and to recommend alterations in clothing, the provision of special equipment, adaptations to the patients' houses and so on.

The attention of an occupational therapist can bring about very significant improvements in independence and lifestyle, especially when the therapist visits the patient in his own home. Bathing and feeding are the activities most widely helped (Beattie and Caird, 1980; Beattie, 1981). In a group of severely disabled patients living at home, less than half had ever seen an occupational therapist (Beattie and Caird, 1980) and a quarter of those who had seen one needed additional equipment. The equipment needs appear to increase by approximately 12 per cent a year as the disease progresses, so that routine visits every six months could be justified for many cases. This would be very likely to correct the 'gross underprovision of equipment' found by Beattie and Caird (1981), but their recommendations have not been widely adopted; in 1986 Mutch *et al.* reported that only 60 per cent of patients in the community were seeing their doctor regularly, and only 25 per cent had seen an occupational therapist. The data suggest that the dose of medication should be reviewed at minimal intervals of three months, and that disabled patients should be visited at home by an occupational therapist every six months.

It is important to recognise the response which is likely to be provoked in therapists, doctors and carers by the patient's facial immobility. Pentland

and co-workers (1987) have shown that such lack of smiling and movement bring forth a negative response on the part of the observer, which is likely to produce an unconscious bias against the patient with Parkinson's disease, even in the absence of any depression or dementia.

Hobbies and outside interests

The Glasgow survey of Manson and Caird (1985) showed much reduction of gardening and other social activities, patients restricting themselves to television, reading and more sedentary pursuits. There is clearly a problem of idleness and lack of interest in life.

The carer

The burden of care on the patient's spouse or companion may be heavy, particularly if the patient is suffering from dementia; the spouse too is likely to be of the age at which some degree of physical disability is common. An important priority for the physician is to ensure that the partner obtains regular periods of relief from care and supervision of the patient, in order to help maintain a cordial relationship between them and to reduce the risks of serious symptoms of stress and depression in the partner. In Britain, the Parkinson's Disease Society provides many patients and their families with valuable support, and associations or societies exist in the USA, Canada, Australia and several other countries.

REFERENCES

Beattie, A. (1981) Aids to daily living for the patient with Parkinson's disease. *Br. J. Occup Therp.*, *44*, 53-6

Beattie, A. and Caird, F.I. (1980) The occupational therapist and the patient with Parkinson's disease. *Br. Med. J.*, *280*, 1354-5

Doshay, L.J. (1962) Method and value of exercise in Parkinson's disease. *N. Engl. J. Med.*, *267*, 297-9

Fahn, S. (1986) Parkinson's disease and other basal ganglia disorders. In A.K. Asburg *et al.* (eds), *Diseases of the nervous system*, Heinemann, London, chapter 98 (pp. 1217-28)

Franklyn, S. and Stern, G.M. (1981) Physiotherapy in Parkinson's disease. In F. Clifford Rose and R. Capildeo (eds), *Research progress in Parkinson's disease*, Pitman Medical, London, chapter 51 (pp. 397-400)

Franklyn, S., Perry, A. and Beattie, A. (1982) *Living with Parkinson's disease*, Parkinson's Disease Society, London

Gibberd, F.B., Page, N.G.R., Spencer, K.M., Kinnear, E. and Hawksworth, J.B. (1981) Controlled trial of physiotherapy therapy for Parkinson's disease. *Br. Med. J.*, *282*, 1196

Gordon, V.C. and Oster, C. (1974) Rehabilitation of the patient with Parkinson's disease. *J. Am. Osteopath. Assoc.*, *74*, 307-15

Gotham, A.M., Brown, R.G. and Marsden, C.D. (1986) Depression and Parkinson's disease. *J. Neurol. Neurosurg. Psychiatry*, *49*, 661-8

Knuttson, E. (1972) An analysis of Parkinsonian gait. *Brain*, *95*, 475-86

Knuttson, A., Martensson, A., Myerson, B.A. and Risberg, A.M. (1975) The influence of a previous thalamotomy on the L-dopa effects on mono-manual dexterity in Parkinsonism. *Scand. J. Rehabil. Med.*, *5*, 130-3

Manson, L. and Caird, F.I. (1985) Survey of the hobbies and transport of patients with Parkinson's disease. *Br. J. Occup. Ther.*, *48*, 199-200

Marsden, C.D., Parkes, J.D. and Quinn, N. (1981) Fluctuations of disability in Parkinson's disease — clinical aspects. In C.D. Marsden and S. Fahn (eds), *Movement disorders*, Butterworths, London, chapter 7 (pp. 96-122)

Mayeux, R. (1981) Depression and dementia in Parkinson's disease. In C.D. Marsden and S. Fahn (eds), *Movement disorders*, Butterworths, London, chapter 6 (pp. 75-95)

McLellan, D.L. and Dean, B. (1981) Improved control of brittle Parkinsonism by separate administration of levodopa and benserazide. *Br. Med. J.*, *284*, 1991-2

Mutch, W.J., Strudwick, A., Roy, S.K. and Downie, A.W. (1986) Parkinson's disease: disability, review and management. *Br. Med. J.*, *213*, 675-7

Oxtoby, M. (1982) *Parkinson's disease patients and their social needs*, Parkinson's Disease Society, London

Parkinson, J. (1817) *An essay on the shaking palsy*, Sherwood, Nelly and Jones, London

Pentland, B., Pitcairn, T.K., Gray, J.M. and Riddle, W.J.R. (1987) First impressions of Parkinson's disease patients. Paper presented at meeting of Society for Research in Rehabilitation

Perry, A.R. and Das, P.K. (1981) Speech assessment of patients with Parkinson's disease. In F. Clifford Rose and R. Capildeo (eds), *Research in progress in Parkinson's disease*, Pitman Medical, London, chapter 48 (pp. 373-83)

Robbins, J.A., Logemann, J.A. and Kirshner, H.S. (1986) Swallowing and speech production in Parkinson's disease. *Ann. Neurol.*, *19*, 283-7

Robertson, S.J. and Thomson, F. (1984) Speech therapy in Parkinson's disease: a study of the efficacy and long-term effects of intensive treatment. *Br. J. Dis. Comm.*, *19*, 213-24

Scott, S., Caird, F.I. and Williams, B.O. (1985) *Communication in Parkinson's disease*, Croom Helm, Beckenham

Shindler, J.S., Welburn, P., Brown, R. and Parkes, J.D. (1987) *Measuring quality of life in Parkinson's disease.* Ciba Symposium (in press)

Singer, E. (1973) Social costs of Parkinson's disease. *J. Chron. Dis.*, *2*, 243-54

Sutcliffe, R.L., Prior, R., Mawby, B. and McQuillan, W.J. (1985) Parkinson's disease in the district of the Northampton Health Authority, UK. A study of prevalence and disability. *Acta. Neurol. Scand.*, *72*, 363-79

22

Multiple Sclerosis

George Cochrane

INTRODUCTION

Multiple sclerosis (MS) is one of the commonest neurological diseases affecting young adults in temperate climates. The prevalence rate in northern Europe is over 50 per 100,000 of the population. There is a female preponderance, 1.4 to 1. The disease most often strikes in the prime of life: in approximately 90 per cent the onset is between the ages of 17 and 50 years and the mean age of onset is 32 years. Few illnesses cause so much disability, suffering and disruption of the life of those affected and those close to them.

PATHOLOGY

MS is characterised by patches of inflammation, varying in size, random in distribution and time throughout the brain and spinal cord, but with a predilection for the optic nerves, the periventricular white matter, the thickly myelinated areas of the brainstem and close to the surface of the spinal cord.

The first sign of inflammation that can be seen microscopically is clustering of monocytes around a small vein; the monocytes having migrated from the circulation initiate an inflammatory reaction enhanced by lymphokines. Lysosomal enzymes attack myelin basic proteins, myelin is destroyed and fragments of antigenically active protein are released. Suppressor T-cells which reduce the immune response are fewer. Phagocytes become laden with lipid from destroyed myelin.

Partial demyelination leads to local slowing of conduction of nerve impulses and the refractory period after single impulse transmission is increased; the nerve is unable to transmit high-frequency trains of impulses, perhaps accounting for the loss of vibration sense in MS. Extensive demyelination ultimately destroys axons.

Within the first few weeks of an attack inflammation diminishes and attempts at repair begin. Oedema fluid is resorbed and there is substantial return of function; conduction that has been temporarily blocked is restored. In some lesions a few lamellae of new myelin form, but where demyelination has been extensive the loss of axons is irrevocable. Following neuronal damage the terminal fibres of undamaged neurones may sprout and replace damaged neurones at synaptic receptor sites. Previously dormant synapses may become active (McDonald, 1974).

EPIDEMIOLOGY

MS is limited in latitude, perhaps related to an environmental factor such as infection by a slow virus acting perhaps many years before the first attack of MS. With the exception of the Eskimos and the Japanese the prevalence of MS varies according to the distance from the Equator: in tropical countries MS is rare. In Great Britain the prevalence rate is 51 per 100,000, and 102 per 100,000 in the Orkney and Shetland Islands.

In addition there appears to be an inherited predisposition to MS. There is a 15-fold increase in the prevalence of the disease among the first-degree relatives of patients, and the risk increases with the closeness in the degree of relationship, but the low rate of concordance in monzygous twins precludes a simple genetic explanation. The histocompatibility antigens HLA A3 and B7 occur substantially more commonly in patients with MS. The prevalence of HLA A3 and B7 is known in many populations, and correlates with the prevalence of MS (Mackay and Myranthopoulos, 1966).

NATURAL HISTORY

The median survival may exceed 35 years (Kurtzke *et al.*, 1977). Many people remain well for many years. The course of the disease is variable and unpredictable. A few people die within two years of the onset, 10 per cent are independent 30 years later, but the rest have progressive disease over many years and finally become chair- and bedridden and die from bronchopneumonia or renal failure from chronic urinary tract infection. Many patients are confined to wheelchairs for several years. When swallowing becomes difficult and speech unintelligible, the skin broken and urine infected, death may come as a relief. MS is far ahead of other diseases in leading to admission to Cheshire Homes and Younger Disabled Units, affecting nearly half of the residents.

Four common patterns of the disease are:

(1) intermittent relapse followed by remissions, but with each attack the remissions are less complete and substantial disability ensues over 10–20 years;

(2) a benign course with infrequent attacks and long periods of remissions;

(3) a progressive deterioration without regression;

(4) a rapid deterioration with numerous relapses and severe incapacity within two years of the onset.

DIAGNOSIS

There is no specific test for the disease, the diagnosis being based on the recognition of lesions at two or more distinct sites in the white matter of the CNS and the history of relapses and remissions. The signs depend on the sites of inflammation. Common first symptoms are defective vision and pain in one eye due to retrobulbar neuritis, weakness and tiredness of one or more limbs due to involvement of a corticospinal tract, paraesthesiae from a lesion in the spinothalamic tract or urgency of micturition. Usually the symptoms abate within a few weeks and a period of remission follows, lasting only a month or two or many years.

The diagnosis is supported by exclusion of other diseases, physiological tests and characteristics of the cerebrospinal fluid.

VISUAL EVOKED POTENTIALS

The normal latency of these potentials is 100 milliseconds, but frequently in MS there is appreciable delay, the waveform is broad and its amplitude reduced. In clinically definite MS abnormality rates in different series are between 75 and 97 per cent (Blumhardt, 1984). Abnormally delayed responses are not specific for demyelinating disease.

CEREBROSPINAL FLUID

Immunoelectrophoresis of CSF shows that over 95 per cent of those with MS have an oligoclonal pattern of IgG due to localised synthesis of IgG by lymphocytes. In 50 per cent the ratio of kappa and lambda light-chains is raised in CSF and normal in serum.

CLINICAL FEATURES

The disease may present with urgency of micturition, blurred vision and alteration of visual field, diplopia from extra-ocular palsy, weakness, sensory perversion, ataxia, vertigo, dysarthria, facial palsy or facial pain like trigeminal neuralgia. Internuclear ophthalmoplegia from demyelination in the medial longitudinal fasciculi causes ataxic nystagmus, greater in the abducting eye with poor adduction of the other eye. Long tract motor or sensory signs and Lhermitte's sign of electric shock-like sensations down the back and in the limbs on flexion of the neck are other presentations. Each symptomatic attack develops over a few days and begins to remit after two to six weeks. The scattered demyelination may affect nerve fibres anywhere in the hemisphere, brainstem and spinal cord.

Corticospinal tract involvement causes hyperreflexia, clonus, loss of abdominal reflexes, extensor plantar responses and exaggeration of the tendon stretch reflexes. Weakness is asymmetrical and in the upper limbs is mainly in extension at the elbow, wrist and fingers and in the lower limb in dorsiflexion and eversion of the foot. Paraparesis and spasticity may be accompanied by sudden involuntary jerks of the legs. Exaggerated withdrawal responses may cause painful flexor spasms.

Cerebellar dysfunction causes incoordination, ataxia and dysarthria. In health the cerebellum facilitates the discharge of impulses to the intrafusal fibres of the gamma system. Deprived of the influence of the cerebellum the intrafusal fibres remain flaccid, there is loss of tonic stretch reflexes, the inbuilt regulation of muscle activity is lost and voluntary activity takes place through the alpha neurones alone. The features are muscular hypotonia, diminished or pendular tendon reflexes, fatiguability of muscles and abnormal rate and force of movements. In cerebellar dysarthria the voice tends to be loud and the speech is jerky and explosive; the syllables tend to be separated yet words are indistinct for the consonants are not properly formed. Titubation or continuous rhythmic tremor of the head and trunk may be so severe as to make willed movements impossible. Jerky horizontal nystagmus is made more obvious by lateral deviation of the eyes. Vertical nystagmus is evidence of a lesion in the brainstem. Touching the nose or putting the heel on the opposite shin examines for disturbance in the amplitude of movements (dysmetria). Intention tremor demonstrates disturbance of coordination of movements (dyssynergia). Inability to perform rapid alternating movements, such as pronation and supination, shows disturbance in the rhythm and speed of alternating movements (dysdiadochokinesia). Speed of grasp and release of the hand grip shows disturbance in the speed of starting and stopping movements (dyschronometria).

Bladder dysfunction is very common, and precipitancy of micturition may be an early sign of the disease. The major abnormality is uninhibited detrusor activity, 'detrusor hyperreflexia'. If the sphincter is relaxed there is urgency and incontinence. If the sphincter fails to relax there is delay in starting micturition and retention. Occasionally the bladder is atonic and the bladder neck may be normal or flaccid.

Sensory disorders of paraesthesiae and dysaesthesiae are almost invariable at some stage of the disease. Proprioceptive loss contributes to ataxia. Vibration sense is usually diminished at the ankles. A distinct sensory level is sometimes found in the trunk.

Pain is common in MS from muscle spasms, spasticity or trigeminal neuralgia.

Intellectual and emotional changes suggest demyelination in periventricular areas and frontal lobes. The irrational euphoria is well known, but anxiety and reactive depression are as common. Patients with MS may be tense and lack confidence, and perform more poorly than expected. Conversion symptoms may occur and a mistaken diagnosis of hysteria may be made. In two-thirds of patients with established disease there is intellectual deterioration, varying from mild loss of memory to profound dementia which is common in the later stages. The extent of organic disorder can be explored by tests of memory, reasoning, criticism, attention and concentration. More than any other disabling disease, MS causes unhappiness within the family, particularly between marriage partners with the breakdown of marriage.

Sexual dysfunction. More than half of those with MS admit to diminished libido, and in men there is commonly failure of erection, loss of ejaculation, decreased genital sensibility and failure of orgasm. In women there is often lack of vaginal lubrication and unpleasant vaginal dysaesthesiae which may cause vaginismus or refusal. In a Finnish study 91 per cent of males and 72 per cent of females admitted change in their sexual lives (Lilius *et al.*, 1976). Later in the disease, paresis, spasticity, ataxia, defective vision, loss of self-esteem, dependence, anxiety and urinary incontinence are additional barriers.

TREATMENT OF MS

There is no cure, but there are endless opportunities for treatment and at different times in its whole course many people contribute, in hospital, at home and in support services, self-help groups and vocational guidance. Good coordination of services is essential.

The first consultation begins a relationship which embraces knowledge of the patient and family, and establishes a bond of trust which is the foundation of care for a very long time. Once the diagnosis is clear the patient must be told: the telling requires gentleness and may perhaps be done gradually. The truth may come as a shock, and little that is said thereafter may be comprehended, or it may be met with denial or anger. It is well that the person closest to the patient is there. The opportunity may be given for a further discussion a few days later when the strategy of management may be explained. A second opinion may be offered, together with selected literature with information about the local branch of the Multiple Sclerosis Society.

GENERAL ADVICE AND DIETS

The patient should be determined in self-care, take regular exercise, stopping short of exhaustion, avoid emotional stress as far as possible and eat a normal diet and weigh regularly, neither to be too fat nor too thin.

As the blood level of linoleic acid has been found to be abnormally low, and reduced still further during acute episodes, there is continuing interest in treatment with polyunsaturated fatty acids. Linoleic acid may be immunosuppressant and necessary to maintain the integrity of myelin against immunological challenge. It also prevents the sludging of platelets and lowers the level of cholesterol.

Polyunsaturated fatty acids can be taken in the form of sunflower seed oil, 15 ml twice daily, or corn oil. Linoleic acid and linolenic acid, in the oil of the evening primrose, have been shown to protect laboratory animals from experimental allergic encephalomyelitis. To produce the same effect as taking sunflower seed oil 30 ml daily, patients would have to take daily 192 capsules of evening primrose oil! An economical diet excludes fats that are solid at room temperature and substitutes soft margarine. There is no evidence in favour of gluten-free diet, nor of gluten enteropathy in MS.

DRUG TREATMENT

1. Treatment with immunosuppressants

Since it has been postulated that MS is an autoimmune disease, the use of *ACTH and corticosteroids* as immunosuppressants is reasonable and may have an anti-imflammatory effect. ACTH has no therapeutic advantage over steroid analogues and the responses of different individuals to ACTH are variable. Patients in an acute relapse appear to improve more quickly following a short course of ACTH or glucocorticoids than without these agents, the effect of which is to reduce IgG synthesis within the CNS (Tourtillotte *et al.*, 1980). There is a tendency to use large doses of steroid, such as dexamethasone, in the first five to ten days of an acute episode. Single high-dose pulses of intravenous methylprednisolone, 0.5–1 g daily for five days, have been used to produce clinical improvement (Buckley *et al.*, 1982), but the value remains unproven. Reduction of oedema can be seen in resolution of optic papillitis and in computerised axial tomographic scanning of the brain. Continued treatment with ACTH or corticosteroid brings nothing to MS but complications.

Azathioprine in a dose of 2.5–3 mg/kg per 24 hours is usually well tolerated but has attendant risks of bone marrow suppression, hepatic impairment, infection, nausea and vomiting. Hitherto the results of controlled trials (Mertin *et al.*, 1982) suggest but do not confirm that azathioprine may slow the course of the disease and reduce the rate of relapse.

2. Treatment with immunostimulants

Since MS may be due to diminished rather than increased immunity, treatments directed to stimulating the immune system by *transfer factor*, *levamisole* and *interferons* have been tried, but none has proved effective (Jacobs *et al.*, 1981).

3. Drugs in the management of symptoms

Vitamin B_{12} is often used as a placebo and may boost morale: there is no evidence that B_{12} is lacking or that it may in any respect alter the course of the disease.

Spasticity occurs frequently in MS, may restrict mobility, hinder perineal toilet, make sitting uncomfortable and lead to contractures which only surgery can correct. Spasticity may be painful as well as paralysing. It may call for treatment (Chapter 27), but the major disadvantage of treatment with spasmolytic drugs is that loss of rigidity of the legs in extension may take away the ability to stand and walk. Extensor spasticity may be useful: flexor spasticity is not. *Diazepam*, *baclofen* and *dantrolene* all have a place in the management of spasticity in MS and their prescription will be decided in each individual by the balance of beneficial and undesired effects.

Quinine bisulphate 300 mg at bedtime may relieve nocturnal leg cramps.

Intrathecal 5 per cent phenol in glycerine should be restricted to relieving spasticity in flexion in those who are already incontinent; 0.5–2 ml is injected intrathecally when pain and flexor spasms are severe (Liversedge and Maher, 1960).

Carbamazepine. Trigeminal neuralgia and other lancinating pain respond well to carbamazepine 100 mg twice daily increased until the best response is achieved, usually around 800 mg daily. Plasma concentrations should be monitored when high doses are given. Toxic effects are dizziness, drowsiness, rash, visual and gastrointestinal disturbance and rarely leucopenia. Carbamazepine controls paroxysmal brainstem epilepsy, the features of which are recurrent fleeting attacks of giddiness, diplopia, dysarthria and ataxia. Epilepsy caused by focal inflammation and occurring in 6 per cent of patients with MS may be controlled by carbamazepine, phenytoin or phenobarbitone.

Psychological changes

These are common, distress the patient and relatives and may cause more suffering than the physical effects. Treating depression can alleviate some of the miseries of MS. Emotional support is needed for the patient and those who are directly involved. Reactive symptoms call for experienced counselling, which may be provided by the doctor, nurse, health visitor, psychologist or social worker. Often endogenous depression is present as well, and calls for the prescription of an antidepressant which may have additional sedative properties, such as *amitriptyline*, or not, such as *imipramine*.

Urinary dysfunction

Frequency, urgency and urinary incontinence are common, occurring in up to 90 per cent of patients at some time during the course of the disease. Urinary symptoms interfere with social, sexual, vocational and psychological functions and may cause patients to be house-bound.

There are three common causes of bladder dysfunction

(1) Failure to store urine because of hyperactive detrusor muscle with bladder of small capacity and residual volume under 100 ml. The treatment is an anticholinergic to relax the detrusor muscle so that a larger amount of urine may collect before the urge to micturate is experienced.

(2) The bladder may fail to empty because the detrusor muscle is underactive or the sphincter hyperactive, the bladder capacity is normal or large and residual urine greater than 100 ml. The treatment is intermittent catheterisation.

(3) There may be both hyperactive detrusor muscle and hyperactive sphincter with failure to empty, and the treatment is intermittent catheterisation and anticholinergic medication.

Anticholinergic drugs

Propantheline bromide (Probanthine) 15 mg t.d.s. one hour before meals and 30 mg at night, increasing to 120 mg daily, diminishes the amplitude and frequency of contractions and increases the bladder's capacity, but unwanted effects may be dry mouth, dilated pupils, blurred vision, difficulty in swallowing and constipation. *Emepromium bromide* (Cetriprin) 200 mg t.d.s. or q.d.s. acts similarly, but must be avoided if there is any oesophageal lesion, and taken with water to prevent oesophagitis. *Imipramine* 25–100 mg at night and other tricyclic anti-depressants are anticholinergic. *Oxybutynin chloride* 3–5 mg t.d.s. is probably the most effective.

Urinary infection is common and may cause increased spasticity, stones, pyelonephritis and ultimately renal failure. The urine should be cultured frequently, and infections treated as they occur. Long-term prophylaxis may be prescribed as *co-trimoxazole* 480 mg every 12 hours, *nalidixic acid* 500 mg b.d. or *hexamine hippurate* 1 g daily. If the bladder cannot be emptied properly it may be impossible to maintain sterile urine. A 24-hour micturition chart records the times and quantities of intake and voiding. Other investigations are estimation of blood urea, intravenous urography, radio-isotope renal scan and residual urine determinations, measuring of the residual urine after micturition by catheterisation and in specialised centres cystoscopy and urodynamic studies (Cochrane and Leacock, 1984).

Bladder neck resection by endoscope may be necessary in patients in whom cystoscopy shows obstruction at the bladder neck. In men urine may be drained by urinary condom connected to a bag. The condom is changed daily. Condoms are available in different sizes and secured by adhesive or loose restraint. For women the choice has lain between intermittent catherisation, indwelling catheter, urinary diversion by ileal conduit, and incontinence pads (Cochrane and Wilshere, 1984).

Intermittent self-catheterisation relieves total or subtotal urinary retention and is suitable for those who have a competent sphincter and a bladder capacity of over 200 ml. Intermittent catheterisation every four hours during the day has the advantages of freedom from indwelling catheter and reduced incidence of urinary tract infection. For women the most commonly used is the Scott catheter of stiff plastic with rounded tip.

Indwelling catheters should not exceed 16 FG, the balloon should be 5–10 ml and for women a female catheter should be used. Latex catheters should be changed every two weeks but expensive silicone or silastic catheters may not need to be changed for three months. Bladder washouts, as an aseptic procedure using normal saline or tap water at body temperature, prevent blockage. Leakage around the catheter may be due to blockage, overstretching the urethra by the use of a large-diameter catheter, or bladder spasm in response to irritation caused by infection or by the catheter and balloon. If the urethra has been overstretched the correct action is to recatheterise with a *smaller* catheter and allow the urethra to recover, using additional protection with pads for a time.

Constipation

Constipation may aggravate urinary incontinence and spasticity and regular defaecation should be achieved by plentiful addition of bran: a stimulant laxative may be used occasionally. The lower bowel must be emptied and defaecation can be helped by a rectally administered laxative, such as *bisacodyl* suppository. It may be necessary to stimulate complete evacuation of the rectum using a finger.

Vertigo

Vertigo caused by inflammation in the brainstem may be relieved by an antihistamine, such as *cinnarizine* 15–30 mg t.d.s. or *betahistine hydrochloride* 8–16 mg t.d.s. or a phenothiazine derivative, such as *prochlorperazine* 20 mg initially then 10 mg t.d.s.

REMEDIAL THERAPY

Physical treatment is directed at reducing spasticity, controlling movements, regaining sensation and achieving, as far as possible, independence in everyday activities. The evil consequences of immobility are joint stiffness, contractures, venous thrombosis, pressure sores and physical and mental decay. Both pressure sores and contractures increase spasticity and must be prevented. Contractures are witness of poor management. Periods of immobility must be kept very short: patients can ill afford to be off their feet even for a day.

Attention should focus upon necessary functional activities. Movements depend upon the controlled position of the head, trunk and limbs. Postural control may be lost when there is interruption of the flow of afferent information from the eyes, vestibular organs, skin, muscles, tendons or joints, if there is disturbance of central interpretation and integration and when there is interference in the motor pathways. Physical treatment is directed at enhancing appropriately each of these stages. The physiotherapist makes and must maintain contact with the patient over the many years that the disease persists and not, as has been usual, for two or three hours a week for a limited period.

Effective treatment is directed at performing functional activities with numerous repetitions. New skills need to be reinforced and consolidated by practice. Most physical treatment can and should be self-administered and patients are taught the relevance of functionally orientated exercises, receiving verbal and written instructions from the physiotherapist.

Fatigue is a frequent and depressing feature and provoked by raising the body temperature. Periods of exertion should be short and interspersed with periods of rest, even in the early stages of the disease when patients may undertake strenuous exertion. Hydrotherapy in a heated pool may exhaust and weaken, but swimming in an ordinary pool may enable and strengthen movements.

Spasticity may be reduced by physiotherapeutic management techniques such as vibration, reflex inhibitory positions to control muscle tone and slow stretching after applying cold in the form of ice pack or towel immersed in chipped ice or water. Treatment should be directed to the flexors of the elbows, wrists and fingers and in the lower limbs to the adductors of the hips, hamstrings and calf muscles. Stretching must be applied slowly and steadily: a sudden stretch augments spasticity by exciting stretch reflexes. Lying prone helps to stretch the flexors at the hips and knees; patients may learn to stretch other groups of muscles (Bobath, 1978) (Chapter 27).

Ataxia due to loss of cerebellar regulation of muscle activity is resistant to physical treatment and can rarely be reduced. By assiduous practice in postural control the patient strives to achieve precision by watching, feeling, rhythm and repetition. Movement strategies are only learned by voluntary movements. Cuffs weighted by lead attached to the wrists or ankles, or weights on the head, have been employed, but seldom with enough advantage to persist. Instability may require use of an appropriate walking aid — stick, frame, rollator, kitchen trolley or wheelchair (Chapters 43 and 46).

Muscle weakness is treated by progressively resisted exercises in patterns of movement which are functional, and this is the principle underlying the techniques of proprioceptive neuro-muscular facilitation.

In later years, when disability is caused by weakness, spasticity and incoordination, choices must be made about the best aids for mobility and personal care, orthoses, hoists, self-propelled or powered wheelchairs, seating for comfort, performance and inhibition of spasticity and electronic devices for communication and control of immediate environment (Chapter 48).

When the use of a wheelchair becomes necessary flexion contractures are not far behind unless standing, prone lying, stretching and splinting are practised diligently. Contractures may be tackled by serial plasters, use of turn-buckle orthoses or reversed dynamic slings, but sometimes only tenotomies and capsulotomies will achieve correction to relieve painful spasms, facilitate nursing and allow the patient to sit with comfort (Dickson, 1976). Excess weight gain must be prevented by attention to diet.

OTHER TREATMENTS AND ALTERNATIVE THERAPIES

Treatment by *hyperbaric oxygen* has been promoted by the charity Action for Research into Multiple Sclerosis (ARMS) with dramatic increase in the number of people being treated, rarely under controlled conditions. The two controlled trials which have been published provide insufficient evidence to prove efficacy (Mertin and McDonald, 1984; Barnes *et al.* 1985).

SEXUAL INTERCOURSE, PREGNANCY AND MENSTRUATION

Sexual counselling is important to both partners, and advice may be offered on sexual stimulation, coital positions and alternative methods of sexual activity. Advice must be available on contraception: a low-oestrogen oral contraceptive has no adverse effect on the disease. Pregnancy may be deferred until the disease has been in remission for two years. Two factors must be considered — the increased risk of relapse, particularly in the first three months after delivery, and the added responsibilities and work of rearing a child. Termination of pregnancy because of MS is not usually warranted.

Women confined to wheelchairs are irked by menstruation; many prefer vaginal tampons to sanitary pads. Painful periods may be suppressed by uninterrupted taking of a low-dose oestrogen contraceptive. Alternative treatments are danazol 200–400 mg daily, which inhibits pituitary gonadotrophin secretion, hysterectomy or radium-induced menopause.

PRESSURE SORES

Late in the course of the disease pressure sores are common, yet like flexion contractures of joints they are preventable. Causative factors include urinary incontinence and infection, widespread paralysis, loss of sensation, asymmetry of posture, diminished intellect, reactive depression and reliance on others. Prevention demands: (i) regular inspection, (ii) careful washing and drying of the skin, (iii) meticulous management of incontinence, (iv) frequent changes of position and night-time turning, (v) attention to general health, (vi) correction of anaemia, and (vii) the use of special mattresses and cushions to distribute the load more evenly over a larger surface area, and to allow ventilation for cooling and evaporation of moisture. The principles of treatment of pressure sores are simple but their practice is demanding. The patient must be placed to avoid any pressure on the ulcer, whilst equal care is taken of all other areas at risk. Relief of pressure is much more important than any dressing which may be applied, and thought must be given lest the dressing should interfere with granulation and regrowth of epithelium (Chapter 31).

EMPLOYMENT AND VOCATIONAL GUIDANCE

MS strikes most individuals at the peak of earning and family responsibilities, and they need advice about continuing or changing the work for which they have been trained. Their worries are concerned with physical demands, the weight of responsibilities of the job, whether the nature of the work will have any adverse effect on the disease and whether they will be able to meet their financial commitments now and in the future. The leading reasons for unemployment are disturbance of gait and movements through spasticity and incoordination, impaired vision and difficulties in travelling, especially in those engaged in semi-skilled or unskilled work. Higher education, professional and managerial work and having held the post for more than two years favour employment continuing 20 years after the onset of the disease (Scheinberg *et al.*, 1981). Registration with the Manpower Services Commission as a disabled person brings the advantages of the disablement resettlement officer helping with placement and retraining if necessary, greater security of tenure, provision of special equipment necessary for work, sometimes partial relief from the costs and difficulties of travelling and possible financial assistance to the employer to undertake alterations that are essential to the employment of a disabled person (Chapter 41).

COMMUNITY CARE

Most people with MS live at home throughout their illness, coming into hospital only for short periods for medical or surgical treatment of complications. Later, when the burden of care is so heavy by day and night that the companion must have respite, the patient may be admitted to hospital at intervals.

Eligibility must be considered for Attendance Allowance, Invalidity Pension, Severe Disablement Allowance, Supplementary Benefit, Rate Rebate and Mobility Allowance. The cooperation of the social worker ensures that benefits which are due are claimed and received.

Environmental control equipment may often be useful: either the Steeper Control or Possum Controls PSU 3 may be supplied on free loan by the DHSS at the request of the District Medical Officer acting on the advice of the Regional Environmental Control Assessor (Chapter 48). Such controls enable people who have the will, need and ability to operate a switch, to summon aid and use essential electrical apparatus for communication, comfort or security. It is the wish of most people to live at home, and when resources are scarce shifting the balance towards care in the community becomes increasingly important (Cochrane, 1983).

PROGNOSIS

Every patient and relative will be anxious to know what will be the outcome, but in a disease which is so variable it is impossible to give an accurate forecast. The mean number of fresh attacks is 0.4 a year and the median survival is 35 years. A *favourable* course often follows retrobulbar neuritis as the sole first sign, a long remission after the first attack, slight motor disability during the early years and attacks with only sensory symptoms which remit. *Unfavourable* signs are progressive disease from the onset without remission, relapse within six months of the first attack and the early occurrence of disease of the brainstem with cerebellar dysfunction and motor disability. The relapse rate and changes in the Kurtzke disability score are two guides to the rate at which the disease is progressing (Kurtzke, 1965).

REFERENCES

Barnes, M.P., Bates, D., Cartlidge, N.E., French, J.M. and Shaw, D.A. (1985) Hyperbaric oxygen and multiple sclerosis: short term results of a placebo controlled double-blind trial. *Lancet, 1*, 297-300

Blumhardt, L.D. (1984) Do evoked potentials contribute to the early diagnosis of multiple sclerosis? In C. Warlow and J. Garfield (eds), *Dilemmas in the management of the nuerological patient*, Livingstone, Edinburgh, pp. 18-42

Bobath, B. (1978) *Adult hemiplegia: evaluation and treatment*, 2nd edn, Heinemann, London

Buckley, C., Kennard, C. and Swash, M. (1982) Treatment of acute exacerbations of multiple sclerosis with intravenous methylprednisolone. *J. Neurol. Neurosurg. Psychiatry, 45*, 179-80

Cochrane, G.M. (1983) Aids in the home. *Br. J. Hosp. Med., 29* (2), 121-6

Cochrane, G.M. and Leacock, A.F. (1984) *The management of urinary and faecal incontinence and stomata; a guide for health professionals*, Oxfordshire Health Authority, Oxford

Cochrane, G.M. and Wilshere, E.R. (1984) *Incontinence and stoma care: equipment for the disabled*, Oxfordshire Health Authority, Oxford

Dickson, R.A. (1976) Reversed dynamic slings; a new concept in the treatment of post-traumatic elbow flexion contractures. *Br. J. Accident Inj., 8*, 35-8

Jacobs, L., O'Malley, J., Freeman, A. and Ekes, R. (1981) Intrathecal interferon reduces exacerbations of multiple sclerosis. *Science, 214*, 1026-8

Kurtzke, J.F. (1965) Further notes on disability evaluation in multiple sclerosis with scale modifications. *Neurology, 15*, 654-61

Kurtzke, J.F., Beebe, G.W. Nagler, B., Kurland, C.T. and Auth, T.L. (1977) Studies on natural history of multiple sclerosis (No. 8): early prognostic features of the later course of the illness. *J. Chron. Dis., 30*, 819-30

Lilius, A.G., Valtonen, E.J. and Wikstrom, J. (1976) Sexual problems in patients with multiple sclerosis. *J. Chron. Dis., 29*, 643-7

Liversedge, L.A. and Maher, R.M. (1960) Use of phenol in relief of spasticity. *Br. Med. J., ii*, 31-3

McDonald, W.I. (1974) Remyelination in relation to clinical lesions of the central

nervous system. *Br. Med. Bull.*, *30*, 186-9
Mackay, R.P. and Myranthopoulos, M.C. (1966) Multiple sclerosis in twins and their relatives. *Arch. Neurol.*, *15*, 449-62
Mertin, J. and McDonald, W. (1984) Hyperbaric oxygen for patients with multiple sclerosis. *Br. Med. J. (Clin. Res.)*, *288*, 957-60
Mertin, J., Rudge, P., Kremer, M., Healey, M.J.R., Knight, D.C. and Compston, A. (1982) Double-blind controlled trial of immuno-suppression in the treatment of multiple sclerosis: final report. *Lancet*, *2*, 351-4
Scheinberg, L., Holland, N., Larocca, N., Laitin, P., Bennett, A. and Hall, H. (1981) Vocational disability and rehabilitation in multiple sclerosis. *Int. J. Rehabil. Res.*, *4*(1), 61-4
Tourtillotte, W.W., Baumhefner, R.W., Potrin, A.R., Ma, B.I., Potrin, J.H., Mendez, M. and Syndulko, K. (1980) Multiple sclerosis de novo C.N.S. IgG synthesis: effect of A.C.T.H. and corticosteroids. *Neurology*, *30*, 1155

FURTHER READING

Learning to Live with MS
R. Dawie, R. Povey and G. Whitley. MS Society, 1981. (Has a short section with suggestions for some practical problems and addresses of where to obtain further help)

INFORMATION

Multiple Sclerosis Society
25 Effie Road, Fulham, London SW6 1EE

Action for Research into Multiple Sclerosis
11 Dartmouth Street, London SW14 9BL

23

Paraplegia and Tetraplegia (Non-traumatic)

John Goodwill

Tetraplegia refers to paralysis of all four limbs due to involvement of the cervical cord. Paraplegia refers to paralysis of the legs due to a lesion below this level. Either may be complete or partial, affecting sensation, motor function, sexual, bladder, bowel and autonomic functions. Spinal injury patients are usually treated in special centres but often return later to a general hospital, and the many non-traumatic 'medical' spinal patients are often treated entirely in a general hospital so it is important that the principles of treatment are known outside the special centres. There are very many causes of spinal pathology; the following list is not exhaustive and excludes spinal injuries.

Spina bifida

Tumours:

- Primary: extradural (mostly benign), e.g. neurofibroma, meningioma; intradural, e.g. glioma
- Secondary carcinoma (most often from bronchus, breast). This may be spread from a deposit in the vertebral body or it may be extradural.
- Myeloma
- Lymphoma

Vascular causes:

- Spinal artery thrombosis
- Dissecting aortic aneurysm
- Bleeding from vascular malformation

Bone causes e.g.

- Paget's disease
- Cervical myelopathy in rheumotoid arthritis or spondylosis
- Primary bone tumours (rare)

Infections:

- Osteomyelitis of vertebral body (pyogenic or tuberculous)
- Syphilis, epidural abscess

Post-infective

- Transverse myelitis, e.g. herpes simplex or zoster, measles, etc.

Primary neurological diseases:
Multiple sclerosis (Chapter 22)
Familial paraplegia
Syringomyelia
Other chronic spinal cord degenerations
Myelopathy due to radiation

INVESTIGATIONS OF ADULT-ONSET NON-TRAUMATIC PARAPLEGIA/TETRAPLEGIA

(1) Clinical history and full examination, both neurological and of other systems, may show evidence suggesting the cause of the spinal cord lesion.

(2) Appropriate blood tests and X-rays considering the possible pathology listed above.

(3) Neurophysiological tests, e.g. visual evoked responses if multiple sclerosis (MS) is a possibility.

(4) Local X-rays where a spinal level is noted on motor and/or sensory examination, followed by CT scanning, magnetic resonance imaging, and/or myelography using a water-soluble contrast medium. If a spinal block and/or tumour is found surgery is usually indicated to determine the pathology and to decompress the spinal cord. The latter will probably also apply even when the cause is a secondary deposit, because the quality of the patient's life may be improved; the surgical approach must be such that the spine is not rendered unstable, and is usually followed by radiotherapy once the scar has healed.

TREATMENT

Non-traumatic spinal cord lesions may develop over hours, days, weeks or even years depending on the underlying pathology which should be treated as far as is possible. These patients are often cared for on general wards instead of in a special centre or in a rehabilitation ward; such facilities will prevent many complications and produce a more independent and fitter patient.

The lesion(s) may be partial or complete, it may be an isolated illness incident as in transverse myelitis, fluctuating as in MS, steadily progressive as in the various spinal cord degenerative conditions, or part of a disease involving other body systems. Clearly the treatment will vary, management being simpler if the lesion is partial but more complicated if the patient has other disabilities, particularly where there is intracranial involvement as in MS with intellectual damage.

Prognosis as to mortality will depend on the primary cause of the spinal cord lesion, the management of its results and the prevention of complications.

Prognosis as to function and independence depends on the level of the lesion, whether it is complete or incomplete, the age and physical fitness of the patient and his motivation, and on the underlying pathology as mentioned above; i.e. whether it is reversible as with a benign tumour or whether it is progressive as in MS or familial paraplegia.

(1) General health

Hypertension, anaemia or diabetes are common coexisting conditions in the age group of many 'medical' spinal patients who are older than those with traumatic lesions. If the patient is paraplegic the management of these conditions is no different from usual, except that there may be undue sensitivity to drugs used in hypertension. For the tetraplegic patient the possibility of producing hypotension is greater. If tetraplegia is due to MS or rheumatoid arthritis (RA) then coexistent ataxia or joint problems add to the arm and hand disability due to the spinal cord lesion, and may make the patient heavily dependent on others. Untreated anaemia, diabetes or a protein-deficient diet will encourage the development and persistence of pressure sores, while a diet poor in calcium and/or vitamin D will cause osteomalacia and make the leg bones even more likely to fracture. It is thus important to consider the patient's general health as well as the spinal lesion.

A coordinated approach from all the staff is essential to prevent complications from occurring, e.g. pressure sores not only give chronic skin problems but also delay mobilisation and independence, because the prolonged bed rest required will cause muscles to atrophy and may allow contractures to develop.

It is helpful to consider the management of the spinal lesion under the following headings:

Skin care
Bladder care
Bowel care
Sexual function
Oedema, venous stasis, autonomic and other complications
Indoor mobility
Outdoor mobility
Activities of daily living (ADL)
Work and recreation
Counselling and adjustment to disability

(2) Skin (see also Chapter 31)

Causes of pressure sores (often several of these are concurrent)

Anaesthetic skin with immobility. *Pressure* may cause skin ischaemia when it is *prolonged* above 15–30 minutes and above 30–40 mm of mercury, which compresses capillaries. It is the combination of these two factors which is important (Daniel *et al.*, 1981; Nola and Vistnes, 1980).

Injury to the skin by rubbing on a hard surface; this causes *shearing forces* (Bennett *et al.*, 1984).

Faecal and/or urinary soiling.

Infection of the broken skin.

Poor general health of the patients e.g. fever, anaemia, uraemia, diabetes, other illnesses.

Prevention (acute stage)

The anaesthetic areas below the lesion can develop pressure sores *within half an hour*, especially if sharp objects are left under the patient causing high local pressure, and any or all of the above factors are present. Prevention of pressure sores is achieved by nursing the patient on a firm even mattress of such construction that pressure is evenly distributed, e.g. Vaperm mattress. The patient is *turned every two hours* from the back onto one side and then the other side, with a turning chart kept on the end of the bed to prevent confusion when nurses change. *The development of redness which takes longer than ten minutes to fade* indicates that pressure has been kept too long on that part of the skin; the time on that part must be reduced or the patient supported on firm pillows or foam packs to relieve pressure. The areas most at risk are over bony prominences such as the greater trochanter of the femur, ischial tuberosity, sacrum, heel, malleoli or over the medial side of the knees, which are kept apart by a small pillow. In tetraplegic patients the scapulae and elbows are also areas to be protected. Manual turning of the patient even without a spinal injury requires at least two nurses every two hours, so it is easier to use an electrically operated bed such as the Egerton bed in which the patient can be turned and repositioned by one nurse (Figure 23.1) (Noble, 1981). Alternatives are a low-loss air bed, a water mattress, or a net bed. When turning the patient care must be taken to avoid shearing forces on the skin.

Treatment of pressure sores

The sore must be kept free of any pressure and any general health problem treated. Superficial sores will heal with clean dressings and relief of pressure. For deeper sores dead tissue must be removed down to clean living tissue, which will then granulate, allowing a small ulcer to heal completely. If the ulcer is larger the granulation and shrinkage in size of the sore may allow direct surgical closure without a skin flap. Any local appli-

Figure 23.1: Egerton electric turning and tilting bed (Mark 2). The patient can be turned from supine to half-right or half-left; the whole bed can be tilted head down or feet down. (Egerton Hospital Equipment Ltd, Tower Hill, Horsham, West Sussex RH13 7JT)

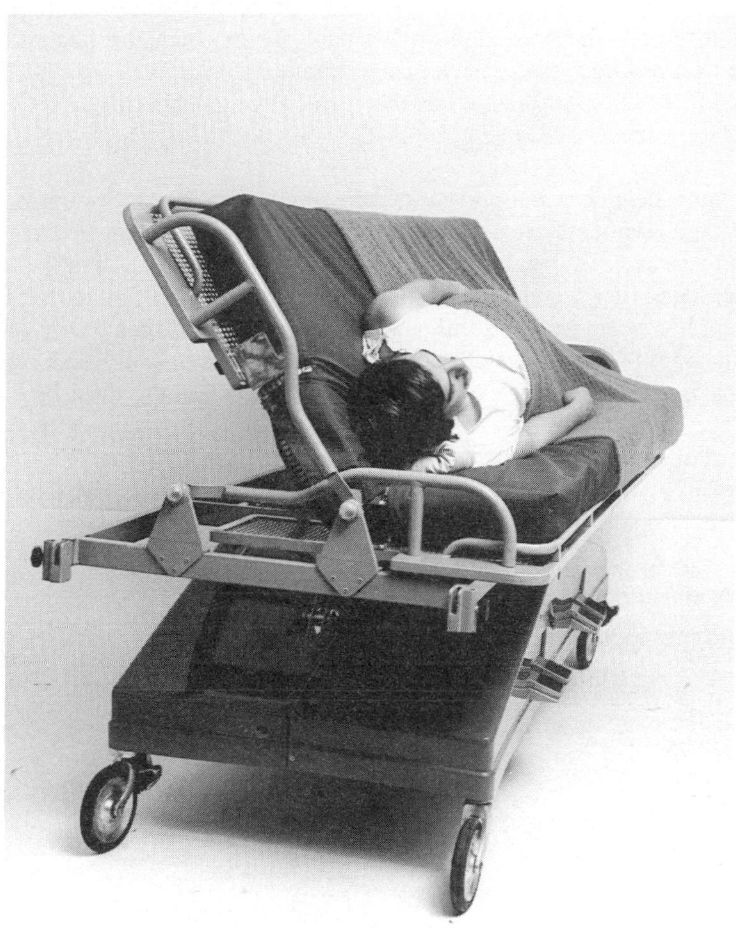

cation is less important than these measures. All sores are open wounds and so are infected, although antibiotics are only used for deep spreading infection, which may include anaerobic bacteria. The aim is to prevent sores, but if one does develop any resulting scar needs to be mobile, as a tight scar adherent to the underlying bone will be a persistent source of skin breakdown (Chapter 31).

Surgery. For deep persistent sores the whole skin ulcer is excised down to clean living tissue. If the sore is over the trochanter or ischial tuberosity simple excision and closure may be possible, but infection in the underlying bone requires its removal, and if the defect is large a full-thickness skin or myocutaneous rotation flap is used for skin cover (Minami *et al.*, 1977). Over the sacrum the defect after excision of dead tissue often requires a rotation flap; if the area high up the back from which the flap has been rotated cannot be closed easily, any resultant defect is covered with a split skin graft, which is satisfactory as this is not a weight-bearing area (Vyas *et al.*, 1980; Turner, 1985) (Figure 23.2).

Long-term skin care and prevention of sores. This is the responsibility of the patient, who must learn to examine the skin daily, particularly over pressure areas.

If redness of an area of skin persists for more than ten minutes after pressure has been removed this suggests incipient skin breakdown and the patient should not bear weight on that area until this has subsided, if necessary staying in bed for a few days. Wheelchair cushioning must be consid-

Figure 23.2: A man of 69 years admitted with almost complete C6 tetraplegia due to vertebral osteomyelitis. The sacral sore required a full-thickness rotation skin flap; hip and knee contractures required surgical release. He slowly recovered with antibiotics and walked with orthoses. After four months he walked using only a stick

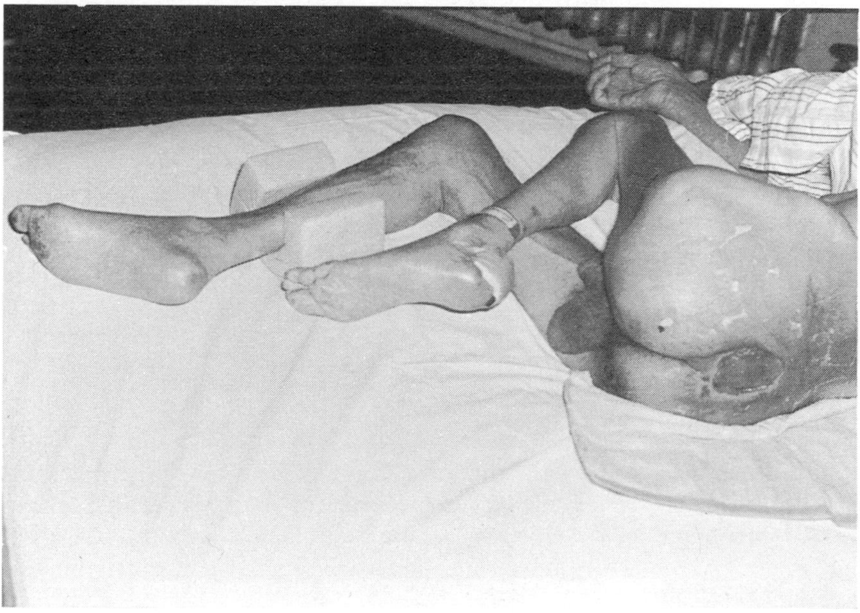

ered individually for each patient; it aims to support the patient evenly, to distribute pressure over as large an area of skin as possible, and to provide a firm platform for mobility and all other activities (Chapters 42 and 43). Close attention to skin cleanliness is essential. The patient who spends prolonged periods in a wheelchair is taught to shift his position at least every 10–15 minutes and to lift himself with his arms by pressing down on the armrests or wheels, although there is no direct relationship between the frequency of push-up pressure relief and the occurrence of pressure sores (Merbitz *et al.*, 1985). With a complete lesion above C6 causing the absence of triceps function this will not usually be possible, making adequate seating and weight distribution even more important (Seymour and Lacefield, 1985; Patterson and Fisher, 1986).

Complications of pressure sores occur due to infection spreading to underlying bone, joint or other tissues causing anaemia, protein loss and possibly blood spread of infection elsewhere in the body. Amyloidosis only occurs with long-standing untreated sores. The presence of sores will increase spasticity and the likelihood of contractures, limit the patient's mobility, independence, employment and life expectancy.

(3) Bladder

The eventual aim of bladder treatment is to have a continent bladder with the lowest possible residual urine volume (preferably not more than 50 ml), which is free from infection and calculi, so preventing back-pressure on the kidneys, ascending infection and renal failure. If continence is not possible then the urinary drainage system used must be a closed system in the male; for the female this may not be possible (England and Low, 1985).

After an acute spinal cord lesion there is urinary retention requiring a catheter. Every catheterisation must be done using a strict aseptic technique. In a general hospital without a rehabilitation ward a self-retaining catheter is usually used (12–14 FG with a 5 ml balloon). This can be left in place for four weeks if it is made of silicone. The catheter should be clamped for two to three hours once daily to help to maintain bladder capacity. In the male patient the penis should be bent upward and the catheter taped to the abdomen to prevent pressure by the catheter on the urethra at the peno-scrotal junction and the danger of infection and peri-urethral abscess. In the female patient the catheter is taped to the medial side of the thigh.

If a special ward is available then an intermittent catheter programme is possible, draining the bladder with a thin soft catheter (12 FG) every six hours. The urine volume should be *no more than 500 ml*, over-stretching of the bladder delays return of function. Fluid intake is restricted to 1.5 litres daily.

Intermittent catheterisation is continued until voluntary voiding returns (if the spinal cord lesion recovers), or voiding is possible by suprapubic tapping, abdominal straining or expression. A catheter is still passed after voiding to ensure that the bladder is empty, and only when the residual urine is getting less is the frequency of catheterisation reduced, being stopped when the residual is below about 100 ml. The eventual aim is a residual of less than 50 ml, preferably none. Frequent urine cultures are done, and any infection is treated promptly as indicated. An alternative is a small suprapubic catheter which avoids repeated urethral instrumentation. This may be useful where there are not any facilities for intermittent catheterisation or if there is urethral infection already, but if it blocks and cannot be cleaned repeated bladder puncture is needed (Namiki *et al.*, 1978).

With any means of urinary drainage, blockage of the catheter and an over-distended bladder may cause autonomic dysreflexia. An indwelling catheter, whether used for a few weeks or long-term, can block with deposits of calcium salts, the rate of deposition varying from one patient to another. The problem is exacerbated by immobility, which causes loss of bone salts with increased renal excretion. Calculi will predispose to bladder and kidney infections, but the incidence of these may be reduced by a high fluid intake (2–3 litres daily), except if the patient is being managed with an intermittent catheter programme immediately after onset of the spinal lesion when fluid is restricted to 1.5 litres daily. Acidification of the urine by the use of oral ascorbic acid or the use of a urinary antiseptic such as hexamine may reduce urinary infections, but the most important long-term measure is to ensure complete bladder-emptying.

When a permanent indwelling catheter is used, as in severe MS, bladder infection often becomes chronic, and then antibiotic treatment is only used where the infection becomes symptomatic, especially if there is fever. Blood cultures are essential because a Gram-negative septicaemia will cause severe systemic effects and possibly collapse, requiring intensive parenteral antibiotics and maintenance of fluid balance.

Most 'medical' spinal patients have a gradual onset of neurogenic bladder symptoms: urgency, frequency, incontinence or retention. For the male patient who has persistent *incontinence* external sheath drainage to a leg bag is used, but for the female patient long-term catheter use may be needed as in MS, unless the leakage is small enough to be contained by absorbent pads. An alternative for the women is diversion to an ileal-loop bladder. When *retention* of urine is the problem, possibly with overflow, then self-catherisation three or four times daily is possible for a woman or a man, providing there is good hand function. Relief of obstruction at the external sphincter or bladder neck by surgery may be indicated, especially if there is evidence of back-pressure. This particularly applies to the male patient (Golji, 1980). *For nocturnal dribbling* self-catheterisation last thing at night may keep the patient dry, and may be combined with oxybutinin or imipramine at night. For all patients a bladder retraining programme is the most important part of bladder management (Merritt *et al.*, 1982; Abramson, 1983; Jarvis, 1981). Bladder and incontinence problems, including the use of drugs and the value of urodynamic studies, are discussed in detail in Chapter 29.

An artificial sphincter has been introduced recently for the patient with an atonic bladder and minimal detrusor activity. It may be used where there is satisfactory bladder capacity and no evidence of back-pressure. For the patient with retained excitability of the sacral nerves, stimulating electrodes implanted on the S234 anterior nerve roots may be used to allow bladder-emptying when it is convenient for the patient, while maintaining continence at other times (Brindley *et al.*, 1986).

(4) Bowels

Bowel activity is reduced with an acute cord lesion, the stomach may become dilated requiring a nasogastric tube while the bowel action decreases also. After a few days small enemas may be used as required; as soon as possible the patient is started on a regular bowel pogramme. Bulk in the diet is needed and the bowel is evacuated daily or on alternate days at the same time of day, often most conveniently after breakfast. Two glycerine suppositories are used, and will often produce a bowel action after 20–40 minutes; if needed an oral laxative can be used the night before, e.g. Senokot two to five tablets depending on the patient's reaction to a trial dose. Oral lactulose 10 ml twice or three times daily may also be useful. Most 'medical' spinal patients have increasing constipation with slow onset of the spinal lesion(s), so it may be necessary to clear the bowel with repeated enemas before the patient can be started on a regular bowel progamme.

Adequate fibre in the diet is essential but weight gain must be avoided. Eventually the aim is for the patient to control his own bowels, using suppositories and/or laxatives as needed; some patients find that digital stimulation of the rectum with a gloved finger will produce a reliable bowel action. The patient must learn the effect of variations in his diet and in his use of laxatives or suppositories on the maintenance of a regular bowel action, with continence at other times.

The higher tetraplegic, or patient with other severe disabilities, will continue to require nursing assistance and may need manual evacuation of the bowel. Providing the bowel is emptied daily, or on alternate days, the patient is usually continent at other times so that a normal wheelchair life is possible. Those with flaccid paraplegia at cauda equina level may continue to have some incontinence of faeces, whereas those with hyperactive reflexes will usually be continent due to spastic contraction of the sphincter (Melzak and Porter, 1964).

(5) Sexual function (see also Chapter 30)

The woman

With acute onset of 'medical' paraplegia the periods usually continue, but there may be amenorrhoea for a few months as often occurs after spinal cord injury. However most 'medical' spinal patients have a slow onset of their spinal cord lesion. Before intercourse the woman may retain or remove the indwelling catheter if used, and the bladder should be emptied. Fertility is retained, and even in complete paraplegia normal delivery is possible; if the lesion is complete the patient may not feel the onset of labour so hospital admission well before this time may be advisable (Robertson, 1972). The major problems in the woman are related to the patient's self-image and feelings of unattractiveness and depression due to the disability. If she can see herself as a normal person, albeit as one perhaps in a wheelchair, then sexual problems and resulting marital breakdown are less likely. Counselling is all-important for the patient and her husband.

The man

Again there are the feelings of depression and loss of self-image as in the female, but in addition there may be inability to obtain or sustain an erection, and the usual position for sexual intercourse with the man above is difficult for the severely disabled man. The other possible positions, and the counselling of men and women patients on sexual problems of disability, are discussed in Chapter 30, and staff must be aware that patients need encouragement to discuss these matters. It is important to emphasise that fulfilment in a relationship is not related to physical sexual prowess. Normal erection and ejaculation depends on the integrity of parasympathetic pathways from S2–4 and sympathetic efferents from the T11 to L2 segments. In partial paraplegia due to medical causes there is rarely a major physical problem, unless the spinal lesion completely destroys these segments producing flaccid paraplegia and inability to obtain an erection, or the patient is also a diabetic with neuropathy causing impotence. If this occurs silicone sponge or inflatable penile implants are possible. With a complete lesion higher up producing a spastic lesion a reflex erection may be obtained by the patient stimulating these reflexes below the level of the lesion, intercourse then being possible; however the patient can develop autonomic dysreflexia during intercourse, causing a dangerous rise in blood pressure (see below). With complete lesions male fertility is greatly reduced but fatherhood is still possible, and the management is as for those with spinal injury. However many 'medical' spinal patients have partial lesions and also are older than those with spinal injury, so fertility is less important than the ability to have normal satisfying sexual intercourse, which maintains the sexual identity of both partners.

(6) Oedema, venous stasis, autonomic and other complications

Immobility due to a spinal lesion causes *venous stasis* whether the cause is trauma or 'medical'. Providing there is no danger of bleeding from the cause of the spinal lesion, or from a coexisting active ulcer, the patient with an *acute lesion* should receive anticoagulation until he is mobile. There is a distinct risk of thromboembolism, which even persists longer-term, but it is highest shortly after the onset of the illness. With slow-onset spinal lesions there is less risk, and long-term anticoagulants are not used.

Oedema is due to impaired venous and lymphatic return, aggravated by dependent legs. Elevation of the legs while resting will reduce this. Elastic stockings may help but are difficult for the patient to put on. Diuretics are not useful. The feet and lower legs get cold with immobility so that warm shoes and clothing are helpful measures. Clearly only the patient with a partial lesion will feel the cold feet, but cold oedematous feet make the skin more liable to breakdown with minor trauma.

Disorders of autonomic function may occur if there is interruption of the thoracolumbar sympathetic outflow (T1–L2) and are most frequent in complete lesions above T4. Such problems are usually only seen with the acute-onset complete lesion, causing gastric dilation which may require a nasogastric tube, and hypotension when the patient starts to move towards the upright position. The 'medical' patient can gradually start sitting up within a few days of the cord lesion, unlike the spinal-injured patient who must wait for the bones of the spine to become stable. The patient is placed horizontally on a tilt table, the angle of tilt gradually being increased towards the vertical over several days, or a few weeks if the lesion is high or the patient is elderly. While in bed the patient spends increasing periods sitting up at an increasing angle, until he can sit safely and start wheelchair activities.

Autonomic dysreflexia occurs most often in complete traumatic lesions above T6 due to isolation of the autonomic nervous system from modification by higher centres (Lindan *et al.*, 1980). Many 'medical' spinal patients have incomplete lesions, and so this complication does not occur often. The usual precipitating causes are a full bladder, possibly due to a blocked catheter, bowel distension due to faeces and/or gas, or it can occur during sexual intercourse. There is vasoconstriction, the blood pressure rises causing headache and even a stroke due to haemorrhage, the pulse slows and sweating occurs above the level of the lesion. Treatment is by sitting the patient up, draining the bladder by catheter, and the use of alpha-adrenergic blocking drugs or TNT. Caution is needed in the use of these drugs and prevention is much preferable. The likelihood of this complication occurring decreases with time (Erickson, 1980).

Myositis ossificans (heterotopic ossification) is rarely seen in 'medical' spinal patients, unlike traumatic cord lesions where it may occur round paralysed joints, particularly the hip and knee joints, usually in the patient who has developed pressure sores or persistent urinary infection. It may cause swelling and redness with later limitation of joint movement which impedes the patient's overall mobility. A radioisotope bone scan may show soft tissue abnormality up to six weeks before the ossification is seen on X-rays (Freed *et al.*, 1982).

Because of the increased osteoblastic activity there is a rise in blood level of alkaline phosphatase, which only gradually subsides. Surgical excision of the abnormal ossification is occasionally tried if there is severe joint limitation due to it, but it must be delayed for 18–24 months until the osteoblastic activity has subsided, and the alkaline phosphatase has returned to normal.

Fracture of the femur or tibia may occur with minimal or no trauma, the bones of the paralysed legs being osteoporotic. This is commoner in women than in men, particularly in older patients, the paralysis adding to the normal bone thinning that occurs with age, especially in post-menopausal women. The fracture is pain-free unless the spinal lesion is partial, and the first sign may be bruising or bone deformity. Healing is usually satisfactory in plaster but skeletal traction or internal fixation may be required. The enforced immobility increases the risks of other problems such as pressure sores, and may increase spasticity. If the limb is totally anaesthetic then great care is needed in applying plaster because any areas of excess skin pressure will not be felt by the patient, and a sore will easily develop. Fortunately many 'medical' spinal patients have partial lesions with retention of some sensation.

Pain occurs in from 14 to 45 per cent of spinal cord-injured patients depending on the series, but is not often a problem in 'medical' spinal patients. Weight-bearing on the arms in a paraplegic patient can cause joint pain and osteo-arthritis of the shoulder, elbow and wrist. Back pain may be caused by poor posture and wheelchair cushioning, especially if the patient becomes overweight. In this older group of patients disc degeneration and spondylosis is common, and may require treatment by physiotherapy, or a collar or corset, depending on the level of the pain. Persistent severe pain may require other treatment such as transcutaneous nerve stimulation (TCNS) (Chapter 7).

Chest infection is more common with tetraplegic than paraplegic patients, the immobile obese patient being most at risk. Symptoms may be mild until the patient is severely ill. Fever and rapid breathing may not be obvious until late, and early symptoms may be only increased lethargy and sleepiness. A high index of suspicion on the part of the doctor, and early use of antibiotics, are essential.

(7) Mobility

Care of joints and prevention of contractures

With acute-onset spinal lesions the affected limbs are flaccid at first; physiotherapy is used to move the joints through a full range of movement daily and thus prevent contractures as muscle tone returns. With slower onset, as in progressive spinal cord pathology, spasticity is often severe, constant effort from patient and therapist being needed to prevent contractures. *The hip* tends to become flexed and adducted, *the knee* flexed and *the foot* goes into equinovarus. In the arm the stiff adducted *shoulder* is the most common problem. These joints need to be moved daily, at first by the therapist but later by the patient and his family. It is this constant moving of the joints through their full range of movement that delays or prevents contractures. A daily period of prone lying will help to stretch the knees and hips; in this position the ankles must be kept at right angles and *not placed in plantar flexion.* It must be combined with positioning of the patient in the chair or wheelchair in a functional upright position; slumping down or to one side will only aggravate spasticity, produce contractures and make pressure sores more likely to occur. For the patient who can stand but not walk, a standing frame used daily will ensure that the leg joints are all stretched fully each day, and also help boost the morale by putting the patient in the normal upright human posture. If contractures have developed surgical release should be considered (Chapter 28).

Spasticity

The neurophysiological mechanisms of spasticity are discussed in Chapter 27, together with its possible treatment by drugs and/or nerve block injections with phenol. It is caused by the underlying spinal cord pathology but will be aggravated by increased afferent input to the spinal cord due to:

(1) bladder irritation from retention, infection or calculi;

(2) loaded bowel due to constipation;

(3) skin pressure sores or ingrowing toenails;

(4) pressure from tight clothes or orthoses (which may not be noted by the patient if that area of the skin in anaesthetic);

(5) joint contractures;

(6) poor positioning in the wheelchair.

Treatment is by elimination of these factors, sometimes by drugs such as baclofen or dantrolene or by the use of blocking injections of phenol into the motor points of muscles, peripheral nerves or occasionally intrathecal block. Nerve roots may be blocked as they exit from the spinal foramina; this allows a more specific effect than intrathecal block.

The physical treatment of spasticity is all-important. The muscles are slowly and repeatedly stretched to prevent contracture and the patient positioned upright in a standing frame or sitting upright in a wheelchair — poor posture aggravates spasticity. At first the physiotherapist does this, but in time the patient and his family must take over responsibility for this (Bromley, 1985), learning from the therapist exactly how it is to be done (Figure 23.3). Thus it is necessary for the carer as well as the patient to learn handling and transferring techniques while the patient is in hospital and during trial days and weekends at home.

Muscle strength

If the lesion is at T12 or below, the abdominal muscles are functioning, and walking becomes a useful activity using elbow crutches and orthoses

Figure 23.3: Spastic equinus feet in paraplegia. The deformity was fixed due to inadequate stretching and a poor position in the wheelchair. The feet should be positioned flat on the footrests

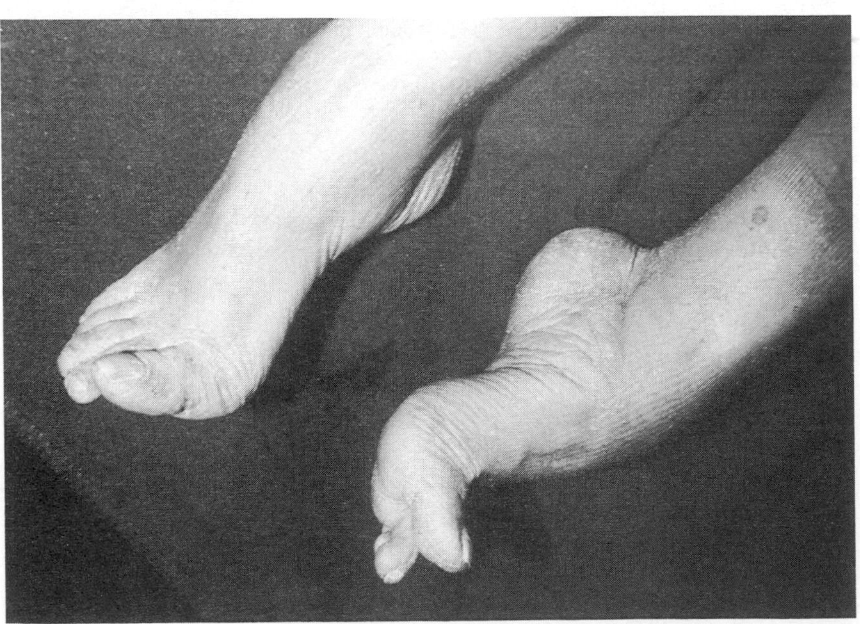

(Chapter 45). Above that level it is possible, but energy consumption in walking increases as the level of lesion rises, and above T8 most patients prefer to use a wheelchair for all activities. 'Medical' paraplegics are older than those with spinal injury and more readily take to wheelchair mobility, providing the wheelchair prescription and support is correct (Chapter 43).

Physiotherapy aims not only at preventing contractures of paralysed muscles and joints but also at strengthening the functioning muscles. The arms need to be strong enough either for wheelchair propulsion and transfers, or to use elbow crutches for walking. With the latter the shoulder girdle is supported, allowing the pelvis to be lifted and the leg to swing through; this is carried out by the remaining spinal and abdominal muscles and also by the latissimus dorsi which are attached below to the pelvis but which have a cervical innervation and so are preserved. Much effort is required from the patient; the staff will show him what to do but only he can make the continued effort required to regain mobility and independence.

The walking patient has to be taught how to get up from and get into a chair, how to fall when maintenance of balance is not possible, and then how to get up from the floor either to chair or onto crutches (Bromley, 1985). If the patient is partially or wholly in a wheelchair he needs to learn how to transfer sideways onto bed, toilet or into a car; independent transfer should be possible up to lesions at the level of C7, but many 'medical' spinal patients have other problems so that it is often only those who are paraplegic, rather than tetraplegic, who can transfer independently. For the severely disabled a hoist may be needed (Chapter 44).

(8) Outdoor mobility

The paraplegic should be able to propel his wheelchair for short distances outdoors, but if the environment is hilly or rough, or the patient has an energy-restricting disorder of the heart or lungs in addition to the locomotor problem, then an outdoor powered chair is needed (Chapter 43). The better chairs that will easily go up and down kerbs are expensive, but the Mobility Allowance can be used to help cover the cost, possibly using a cheap hire-purchase scheme available through Motability (Chapter 37).

Driving is the real means of maintaining independence. For the paraplegic independent transfer into and out of the car should be taught, together with the means of folding the wheelchair and getting it in and out of the vehicle (Chapter 47), but for the older tetraplegic this is usually not possible without help. Driving is straightforward for the paraplegic using automatic transmission and hand controls. For the low tetraplegic at the C8 or T1 level this is also possible, but it is more difficult, and the car conversion more expensive, when the lesion is higher. Above C6 level driving is not a practical possibility. The non-driver who cannot transfer to the car, even with help, will probably need an electric-powered chair for everyday use. For car transfer a hoist may be used (Chapter 44) or the patient may sit in his wheelchair and drive into the back of a specially modified van, with a raised roof, rear ramp, and rear suspension that can be lowered to allow rear access. An alternative is a special power chair designed to be lifted by an electric motor into the passenger side of the car with the normal seat removed (Chapter 47). Often limitation of outdoor mobility is as much due to local environment, non-availability of helpers or lack of finance as due to the disability itself. Many Social Services departments run special transport for the disabled, but the level of independence gained by the car driver is much greater, and may enable the patient to retain or find work, particularly if the patient has a lower-level lesion.

(9) Activities of daily living

Most paraplegics should become independent in self-care; putting on shoes, socks, trousers, or tights and skirt may be difficult, requiring training from the occupational therapist. Often dressing the lower half of the body is more easily done on the bed than in a chair, and most patients find it easier to do this once they have had the morning bowel action and washed themselves. Orthoses take time to put on, so many patients decide that their time and energy would be better spent on other activities, and so do not use them. For the paraplegic transfer down into a bath may be possible but difficult, and whatever the level of the cord lesion, many patients find that a shower is easier, a firm seat being fixed in the shower for this purpose, or a mobile shower/toilet chair being used. It is advisable to have toilet and shower (or bath) in one room, which will allow more room to manoeuvre the wheelchair.

For the tetraplegic everyday activities of washing, dressing, etc., pose greater problems; with a lesion at C8 or T1 almost complete independence is possible, but with higher lesions it becomes progressively more difficult. At the C7 level (and with some at C6) the patient can transfer to and from the wheelchair, can do a few activities such as shaving, washing the upper half of the body and eating, but will find other activities more difficult or impossible. It is often better for him to spend his time and energy on useful work or hobbies rather than spend a long time on self-care activities which are very difficult to achieve and cause extra fatigue. The amount of care available at home will determine this. Malick and Meyer (1978) provide an excellent account of what can be achieved to improve arm and hand function in the tetraplegic patient by the use of dynamic orthoses, but this will generally apply more to the traumatic patient than to the 'medical' spinal cord patient.

Surgery may be of value to improve function in the arm or hand providing useful sensation is retained and the spinal lesion is static (Chapter 28).

Domestic activities. For the ambulant disabled a perching stool may be used in the kitchen, but most will function from a wheelchair requiring kitchen work surfaces to be 80 cm high, cupboards, window locks and taps, etc., to be accessible from the chair and for the whole of the home to be on one level with doors wide enough for wheelchair access. Preferably the door sets should be 90 cm. Goldsmith (1976), in his book, details these and other design requirements for wheelchair housing, and this can usefully be studied by the patient and the carer as well as the staff.

(10) Work and recreation

Any spinal patient, whether with MS, transverse myelitis or other medical conditions, will need to decide where he wishes to direct his energy. Clearly a paraplegic can carry out all sedentary activities and some tetraplegic patients can do likewise. In practice most 'medical' tetraplegics only have a partial cord lesion, medical lesions producing complete tetraplegia often being fatal due to the underlying disease (such as MS, or rheumatoid cervical myelopathy). With partial tetraplegia limitation of arm and hand function may reduce opportunities, but typewriter or computer keyboards can be used with a stick held in or attached to the hand. If work is possible with suitable modifications to the work situation and/or the work environment such as toilet access, then the Manpower Services Commission of the Department of Employment can provide funds for these modifications, and help may be provided initially for transport to and from work (Chapter 41). Work and income produce more independence than any amount of social support. The ability to drive independently, or ready access to transport, will be necessary if the patient is to work. For recreation activities transport is almost equally important, and for the tetraplegic modification of the activity and/or the provision of aids or arm orthoses may be required (Ford and Duckworth, 1974). Besides indoor sedentary interests available to all spinal patients the paraplegic or low tetraplegic patient can engage in many sports such as archery and swimming. He can fish, providing the wheelchair is suitably anchored so that the fish does not win, and can pursue other outdoor activities such as gardening, and possibly birdwatching (see resources, Chapter 49).

(11) Counselling and adjustment to disability

Medical spinal cord lesions cause feelings of anxiety, depression and doubt about the future, as do those due to trauma; but where the cause of the condition is not clear, as with transverse myelitis, then anger and frustration may be even greater. Even if not expressed, these feelings are there, often combined with a grieving reaction from the patient and relatives for the lost functions and future potential, so that the younger the patient the more angry he may be. The attitude of the staff and close relatives is all-important, honesty is essential and slowly the patient must learn the truth about future prospects of what can and cannot be achieved with rehabilitation, *the aim being eventual adult acceptance of reality.* However, the patient cannot be told too much too soon, and the staff should appreciate the 'coping mechanism' of that particular patient; it may be denial for the first few weeks in order to minimise depression. This applies equally to the 'medical' and to the injured patient. All should realise that certain times are particularly stressful for the patient and his family — perhaps the first time he moves about in a wheelchair, the first visit home, or an outing to a familiar place. The whole family participates in the management programme in which staff can help by concentrating on all the functions that remain, rather than on those such as walking that have been lost. Talking with other patients who have learnt to live a full life with a disability is invaluable. The family may accept the real situation before the patient does, and all will find that the reality of a wheelchair life requires adjustment. The patient should first leave the hospital or rehabilitation centre with a staff member, for this is the time when a patient becomes acutely aware of his disability and changed relationship to others who need to understand that he is still the same person. Outings are gradually increased in length, with the patient spending weekends at home and then gradually adjusting to a new lifestyle. Continuing support is necessary for the physical and psychological effects of a spinal cord lesion. A 'package' of community care must be agreed before the patient is discharged, which will include community nursing, home help, modifications to the home, etc. The general practitioner needs to be involved in these discussions from an early stage. After discharge the patient needs to have easily available contact with the staff who have been treating him through this devastating episode in his life, so that counselling or medical treatment is available without delay. Many 'medical' spinal patients will have progressive or fluctuating lesions such as MS, so that adequate follow-up is even more essential.

REFERENCES

Abramson, A.S. (1983) Neurogenic bladder: a guide to evaluation and management. *Arch. Phys. Med. Rehabil.*, *64*, 6-10

Bennett, L., Kavner, D., Lee, B.Y., Trainor, F.S. and Lewis, J.M. (1984) Skin stress and blood flow in sitting paraplegic patients *Arch. Phys. Med. Rehabil.*, *65*, 186-90

Brindley, G.S., Polkey, C.E., Rushton, D.N. and Cardoza, L. (1986) Sacral anterior

root stimulators for bladder control in paraplegics: the first 50 cases. *J. Neurol. Neurosurg. Psychiatry*, *49*, 1104-14
Bromley, I. (1985) *Tetraplegia and paraplegia; a guide for physiotherapists*, 3rd edn, Churchill Livingstone, Edinburgh
Daniel, R.K., Priest, D.L. and Wheatley, D.C. (1981) Aetiologic factors in pressure sores: an experimental model. *Arch. Phys. Med. Rehabil.*, *62*, 492-8
England, E.J. and Low, A.I. (1985) Long-term management and prevention of urinary tract disease. In Sir G.M. Bedbrook (ed.), *Lifetime care of the paraplegic patient*, Churchill Livingstone, Edinburgh, pp. 94-105
Erickson, R.P. (1980) Autonomic hyperreflexia: pathophysiology and medical management. *Arch. Phys. Med. Rehabil.*, *61*, 431-40
Ford, J.R. and Duckworth, B. (1974) *Physical management for the quadriplegic patient*, F.A. Davis, Philadelphia
Freed, J.H., Hann, H., Menter, R. and Dillon, T. (1982) The use of three phase bone scan in the early diagnosis of heterotopic ossification. *Paraplegia*, *20*, 208-16
Goldsmith, S. (1976) *Designing for the disabled*, Royal Institute of British Architects, London
Golji, G. (1980) Urethral sphincterotomy for chronic spinal cord injury. *J. Urol.*, *123*, 204-7
Jarvis, G.J. (1981) A controlled trial of bladder drill and drug therapy in the management of detrusor instability. *Br. J. Urol.*, *53*, 565-6
Lindan, R., Joiner, E., Freehafer, A.A. and Hazel, C. (1980) Incidence and clinical features of autonomic dysreflexia in patients with spinal cord injury. *Paraplegia*, *18*, 285-92
Malick, M.H. and Meyer, C.M.H. (1978) *Manual on management of the quadriplegic upper extremity*. Harmaville Rehabilitation Centre, Pittsburgh
Melzak, J. and Porter, N.B. (1964) Studies on the reflex activity of the external sphincter in man. *Paraplegia*, *1*, 277-96
Merritt, J.L., Lie, M.R. and Opitz, J.L. (1982) Bladder retraining of paraplegic women. *Arch. Phys, Med. Rehabil.*, *63*, 416-18
Merbitz, C.T., King, R.B., Bleiberg, J. and Grip, J.C. (1985) Wheelchair push-ups: measuring pressure relief frequency. *Arch. Phys. Med. Rehabil.*, *66*, 433-8
Minami, R.T., Hentz, V.R. and Vistnes, L.M. (1977) Use of vastus lateralis muscle flap for repair of trochanteric pressure sores. *Plas. Reconstr. Surg.*, *60*, 364-8
Namiki, T., Ito, H. and Yasuda, K. (1978) Management of the urinary tract by subprapubic cystostomy kept under a closed and aseptic state in the acute stage of the patient with a spinal cord lesion. *J. Urol.*, *119*, 359-62
Noble, P. (1981) *The prevention of pressure sores in persons with spinal cord injuries*, World Rehabilitation Fund, New York
Nola, G.T. and Vistnes, L.M. (1980) Differential response of skin and muscle in the experimental production of pressure sores. *Plast. Reconstr. Surg.*, *66*, 728-33
Patterson, R.P. and Fisher, S.V. (1986) Sitting pressure–time patterns in patients with quadriplegia. *Arch. Phys. Med. Rehabil.*, *67*, 812-14
Robertson, D.N.S. (1972) Pregnancy and labour in the paraplegic. *Paraplegia*, *10*, 209-12
Seymour, R.J. and Lacefield, W.E. (1985) Wheelchair cushion effect on pressure and skin temperature. *Arch. Phys, Med. Rehabil.*, *66*, 103-8
Turner, A. (1985) Decubiti. In Sir G.M. Bedbrook (ed.), *Lifetime care of the paraplegic patient*, Churchill Livingstone, Edinburgh, pp. 54-65
Vyas, S.C., Binns, J.H. and Wilson, A.N. (1980) Thoraco-lumbar sacral flaps in the treatment of sacral pressure sores. *Plast. Reconst. Surg.*, *65*, 159-63

FURTHER READING

Bedbrook, Sir G.M. (ed.) (1985) *Lifetime care of the paraplegic patient*, Churchill Livingstone, Edinburgh

Fallon, B. (1975) *So you're paralysed*, Spinal Injuries Association, London. (A handbook for the newly paralysed patient)

Grundy, D., Russell, J. and Swain, A. (1986) *ABC of spinal cord injury*, British Medical Journal, London

24

Head Injury

Peter Eames

INTRODUCTION

The size of the problem

In comparison with some rehabilitation problems (stroke, for example), head injury is not common. However, it particularly afflicts young adults, especially males, and so its *economic* impact is of great importance. An as yet unpublished epidemiological study from the West of Scotland found that head injury was responsible for an annual loss of some 4,000 working days per 100,000 of the population.

The *incidence* of head injuries of all degrees of severity presenting at hospital casualty departments in the UK each year is of the order of 1,500 per 100,000, a total of about 825,000 (a fall of about 15 per cent since the introduction of compulsory seat-belts). About 130 per 1,000 are of Moderate Severity (see below) and will be followed by little lasting physical disability, but significant cognitive disorder; about 17 are Severe or Very Severe, being followed by some degree of *permanent* physical and cognitive disability. This amounts to nearly 14,000 Severe injuries in the UK each year. These, of course, are the *survivors.*

The *prevalence* of persisting disability from head injury is less clear. The most recent figures are those from the West of Scotland survey, which estimated a prevalence of 1 per 1,000 of the population — an average of about 250 per Health District, or two on each GP list.

Causes

The commonest cause is the motor vehicle. Until the recent seat-belt legislation the rise in the incidence of head injuries closely paralleled the rise in the number of vehicles registered. Less frequent causes are assault, falls, and work accidents. Penetrating missile injuries remain rare in the civilian population.

Some other causes of *brain* injury may produce results which are similar: subarachnoid and intracranial haemorrhage, some forms of encephalitis, and the very diffuse insults of hypoxia, ischaemia and hypoglycaemia, may produce patterns like those of head injury, involving a combination of diffuse and localised damage.

THE BREADTH OF THE PROBLEM

The nature of the insults in closed-head injury

In order to understand the breadth of the disturbances of function produced by head injury it is necessary to understand the mechanics. Most head injuries are produced either by a blow to the head causing it to move very suddenly through space, or a sudden arrest of movement. This class of injury is known collectively as 'acceleration/deceleration injury', and causes a very abrupt transfer of kinetic energy to the head. The disposition and 'tethering' of the brain within the skull restrict its movements to quite small excursions, and the result is a brief but very rapid *oscillation* of the brain about the axis of the brainstem. (Since this is the site of centres controlling the state of consciousness, the distortion of the brainstem leads to loss of consciousness. It should be noted that very severe and destructive injuries to the brain caused by slow crushing usually do *not* disturb consciousness.) The lesions produced include diffuse shearing of fibres, and microhaemorrhages causing localised destruction of neurones. The oscillation leads to two other kinds of damage. First, pressure waves of centrifugal force travel outward from the central parts, again producing diffusely scattered lesions, this time maximally at the cortical–subcortical junction. Second, the more or less 'pointed' parts of the surface (particularly the poles and orbital surfaces of the frontal lobes, and the anterior and medial temporal lobes) undergo repeated buffeting against the adjacent skull and tentorial edges, resulting in bruising (contusion). Contusions are also common on the cortical surface subjacent to the blow ('coup injury') and diametrically opposite ('contre-coup'). It may also happen, especially with blows to the lower part of the head, that the brainstem is directly contused, either by the rim of the foramen magnum (medulla), or the tentorial edge (midbrain), and this leads to rather distinctive 'brainstem syndromes', often involving very prolonged coma.

The degrees of diffuse and contusional damage depend on the magnitude and duration of oscillation, which in turn are determined by the amount of energy associated with the blow. (Paradoxically, therefore, skull fractures can be protective, since some of the energy is diverted into breaking the bone.)

These are the immediate or 'first injury' results. In a proportion of victims there follow so-called 'second injuries'. These include haemorrhage (extradural haematoma, from rupture or shearing of meningeal arteries outside the dura, acute subdural haematoma from bleeding arteries in the lacerated brain, subacute subdural haematoma from venous bleeding, and intracerebral haematoma from bleeding deep in the substance of the brain), fluid collections (acute hygromas), and localised or global brain swelling (which is commonest in children and adolescents). As well as causing localised damage, these all raise intracranial pressure, and may produce brainstem injury through 'coning'.

Other 'second injuries' come from the effects of hypoxia and ischaemia, from surgical shock, inadequate airway, or cardiorespiratory arrest, sometimes due to coincidental chest injury.

Effects on consciousness

Any blow to the head involving significant transfer of kinetic energy disturbs consciousness, and post-mortem studies have shown that even the slightest of such disturbances causes destruction of cells in the brainstem. These phenomena are subsumed in the word 'concussion'. Nearly always there is some disruption of memories of the immediate past: most typically the approach of the accident is recalled, but not the blow itself. With increasing severity of injury, the extent of this *retrograde amnesia* increases, though even in the severest cases it rarely extends more than a few months. (Very extensive retrograde amnesias are nearly always psychological in origin.) The relationship with severity is not very accurate, however, and the duration usually shrinks during recovery.

There is then (depending on severity) a period of full unconsciousness — *coma.* Whether this occurs or not, there is a following period during which the victim may appear confused (although in mild cases, and towards the end of the period, appearances may be entirely normal), but when no memories are stored. Once this has passed it can be measured as the period for which the person lacks continuous day-to-day memory, and it is referred to as the period of *post-traumatic amnesia* (PTA).

After very severe injuries there may be a continuing severe disruption of memory function, so that PTA cannot be measured in this way. In such cases the best measure comes from identifying the time at which the individual ceased to seem confused to observers.

Severity

Ritchie Russell showed that there is a general relationship between outcome (and therefore some aspect of severity) and the duration of PTA. Later research showed that the correlation was mainly with the amount of *diffuse neuronal damage* to the brain. It is important to note that the definition of PTA on which the measure is based is 'the period from the time of the injury to the restoration of continuous day-to-day memory'. (It is *not* the period to the 'first memory', which is frequently an island of memory.)

Ritchie Russell's categories of severity based on this measure are as shown in Table 24.1.

Table 24.1: Ritchie Russell's categories of severity

Severity	PTA
Mild	< 1 hour
Moderate	> 1 hour < 24 hours
Severe	> 24 hours < 7 days
Very Severe	> 7 days

Although this traditional measure of severity remains serviceable, the correlations are not very accurate. Moreover, with improved survival from catastrophic injury it has become apparent that not all 'Very Severe' injuries carry the same prognoses; yet beyond a week or so, PTA estimations become increasingly inaccurate, partly at least because significant persistence of disorders of memory function is increasingly common.

Another potential measure is the duration of *coma*. There is a problem with the definition of coma, since this was traditionally described in a wide variety of subjective terms. The Glasgow Coma Scale (Brooks, 1984) has made possible the use of a *numerical* definition, and this should have solved the problem. However, the use of the scale is still (13 years on) far from universal, and in hospitals where it *is* used, recordings tend to lapse too soon, and scores are rarely extracted from the record sheets.

There is a further difficulty. PTA and coma can give good measures of the severity of *diffuse* damage, but do not necessarily relate to localised damage, which may nevertheless dictate outcome (as with large destructive lesions of the linguistic cortex, or localised brainstem lesions). Moreover, 'second injury' damage shows a rather poor relationship to these measures, yet contributes greatly to outcome.

It seems likely that PTA and coma will continue to be used (and refined) as helpful measures of the severity of diffuse neuronal damage, since this underlies many of the persisting *cognitive* deficits of moderate and severe injury. But at the same time, some of the recognisably distinct patterns of damage (primary and secondary brainstem lesions, for example) will probably be incorporated into a wider concept of severity.

Effects of injury on function

What does the brain do?

The key to understanding the range of effects of injury to the brain is to remember, first, that head injury produces *both* widespread localised lesions *and* diffuse neuronal damage, and second, that the brain is involved in *everything* that we perceive, think, know and do.

Minor injuries

The less severe the injury, the more the effects are likely to be restricted to those of the concussive damage. In practice this means greater or lesser degrees of disturbance of *attention* (and therefore some aspects of *memory* and *thinking*), *fatiguability* (which is the minimal form of drive deficit), *irritability, noise intolerance,* and often *dizziness* (or even frank vertigo) from subtle disturbances of vestibular connections. Mild disruption of the control of eye movements may lead to transient *diplopia,* often without visible strabismus.

However, each injury happens to a particular brain, with its own pre-existing characteristics and quirks, and sometimes very mild injuries produce surprisingly disproportionate effects. Just as some skulls are more prone to fracture than others, some brains have areas whose structural organisation is defective (as seen in the neuropathology of some epileptogenic lesions, and of brains of individuals with developmental learning disabilities). Such areas may suffer significant functional disruption after mild injury — hence the small incidence of post-traumatic epilepsy even after head injuries which do not appear to disturb consciousness.

More severe injuries

The more severe the diffuse injury, the more obvious will be disruptions of attention and drive. Moreover, contusions of the cortex will be more likely, and so a wide range of deficits may be seen — more or less transient *hemipareses, dysphasia, perceptual disorders, frontal lobe syndromes,* and, of course, later, *epilepsy.* With brainstem contusions, *drive disorders* and all forms of *movement abnormalities* may be seen.

The olfactory nerves are particularly vulnerable, and *anosmia* is common after all degrees of injury. (This includes loss of sense of flavour, so that most people will complain of — or admit to — loss of both smell and 'taste'.)

If the skull is fractured there may be localised destruction of cortex. If the base is involved, cranial nerves may be sheared, and in particular there may be degrees of *deafness*, *visual field defects*, or *eye movement disruptions.*

With intracranial haemorrhage there is a wide range of possible localised lesions of functional systems. Often there will also be distortion and damage in the brainstem, and the same is true if brain swelling develops. (It is worth remembering that the brainstem houses the origins of most of the cranial nerves, and acts as a funnel through which sensory, motor and coordinational connections are made between the brain and most of the body.)

All these 'effects of brain injury' are disruptions of *brain functions.* Most of the things patients complain about are '*person functions*'. In the analysis of life problems, however, and in the design of rehabilitation endeavours, it is important to identify the brain system malfunctions first, and then try to apply remedial measures to them in such a way as to re-create effective integrated 'person functions'.

Deficits and disorders

Movement

With a relatively pure cortical lesion, as might follow a contusion of the motor cortex, there is weakness, but little change in tone (which is reduced, if anything). Such deficits are common, but almost always transient.

Movement disorders which persist may result from intracerebral haematomas (when pure spasticity is usually the dominant feature). But almost always, movement is disrupted by head injury in very complex, mixed ways. The severest problems come from brainstem lesions, where pyramidal damage leads to weakness and spasticity, cerebellar connections are disrupted leading to dystaxic incoordination, and extrapyramidal nuclei and tracts are damaged, producing rigidity, slowness, delayed initiation of action, and a variety of involuntary movements. Similar confusing combinations of deficits can result from severe diencephalic damage coupled with cortical lacerations and diffuse white matter lesions. 'Weakness' is often an unsatisfactory description, since the patient can often develop near-normal power in a movement, if given a minute or two of continuous encouragement and effort. 'Spasticity' is almost always an inadequate word, since disorders of tone are mixed. A useful term (and assessment approach) was introduced by the Chessington group (Evans *et al.*, 1977) to get around this problem: dynamic interference by abnormal tone (DIAT). The measures involve the ability to isolate movements at the different joints of the limbs.

When the brainstem is injured there may be problems of balance. Again, these are rarely simple. Balance depends not only on vestibular and midline cerebellar functions (though undoubtedly the most disruptive is dysbasia from lesions of the vermis and flocculonodular lobes), but also on the ability to initiate and modulate movements of trunk and limbs rapidly, and this is impaired by both pyramidal and extrapyramidal deficits.

One particular extrapyramidal disorder is the so-called red nucleus or peduncular tremor. It deserves special mention because it is often misidentified, is extremely disruptive of both upper limb efficiency and locomotion, and is not uncommon after very severe injuries associated with high brainstem lesions. This is a coarse, irregular, variable tremor, often of alarming amplitude, usually affecting only the shoulder muscles (but passively transmitted to the rest of the arm, the trunk and often the leg and head as well). Typically it makes its appearance some weeks or months after injury (unlike the cerebellar intention tremor with which it is usually confused, and which is present from the beginning).

The highest levels of movement deficits are the dyspraxias, in which simple movements may be unimpaired, but either cannot be synthesised into more complex actions (motor or speech dyspraxia, which result from cortical lesions), or can be used only on direct command ('motor inattention'), or only as incidental or automatic movements (ideational dyspraxias, usually from subcortical associational or commisural lesions). Closely related are curious disorders of volitional movement (and action, and even behaviour) which may be seen with some basal ganglia lesions. Some dyspraxias are very specific, and may be seen in isolation (both after brain injury and as developmental anomalies); examples are running and dancing dyspraxias, and an inability to smile, except on purpose.

Skills

Most activities called 'skills', whether motor skills like riding a bicycle, personal care skills like brushing the teeth, domestic skills such as making a cup of tea, occupational skills, or community skills like using public transport, involve *all* of the functional systems of the brain. The more specific deficits there are, the more difficult will such skills be to perform in the smoothly integrated forms which we recognise as being within the range of normality.

Communication

As with hemiparesis, dysphasias (expressive, receptive or mixed) caused by contusion are usually transient, although minor residual word-finding problems may persist. If the cause is brain laceration or intracerebral haematoma, however, the dysphasia is unlikely to show much recovery, or even response to treatment, once any associated brain swelling has subsided. It is necessary therefore to remember that language is only one aspect of communication. Moreover, all aspects of language need to be examined, since some patients cannot speak, but can understand, read, and write (aphemia).

More commonly, there may be a disorder of *speech* with or without disorder of language. Such problems range in severity from mild but irritating dysarthria to complete anarthria (as in severe brainstem damage), and in nature from cortical aphemia or speech dyspraxia, through 'pseudobulbar' disorder from bilateral hemispheric or diencephalic lesions, to brainstem combinations of spastic (pyramidal), scanning (cerebellar) and dystonic (extrapyramidal) dysarthrias.

There is more to communication than words. Areas of the 'non-dominant' cortex homologous with the linguistic areas of the 'dominant hemisphere' are now known to subserve the functions of the perception, analysis and output of *non-verbal aspects of language.* These include not only gesture, but also intonation and affective colouring — features of spoken language which can radically alter the meaning imparted by words. These functions may be disrupted alone, or together with verbal functions. They are important not only for communication of meaning, but for the whole arena of social skills.

An important recent finding is that a large proportion of head injury victims show evidence of pre-existing developmental learning disabilities. (The most comprehensive study found that 20 per cent of a consecutive series had been diagnosed as dyslexic during their educational careers, and a further 40 per cent had evidence of unexpectedly poor scholastic achievements (Santa Clara Med., 1982). It seems that developmental learning anomalies must be considered a risk factor for head injury. There are obviously important implications for language rehabilitation.

Social skills

One of the achievements of social psychiatry has been to recognise that there is a range of behaviours and performances which are necessary for the establishment and maintenance of interpersonal and social relationships, that are learned during development, and may be lost as a result of mental illness. What has been less readily appreciated is that these same 'social skills' are often disrupted by head injury. The most important deficits involved seem to be those of non-verbal language, and those of social inhibition (such as are disturbed by orbital frontal lesions). However, disturbances of appreciation or control of rhythm, and deficits of facial motility, may contribute. Whereas in psychiatric practice the usual pattern of deficit is one of homogeneous loss, head injury more often produces patchy areas of deficit, and this poses great challenges in the application of the techniques of social skills training.

Perception

Sensory deficits such as deafness, ocular blindness or large field defects rarely escape detection. Less obvious ones (including anosmia, ageusia and astereognosis) often need to be looked for, and can have significant impacts on 'person function'. Even more elusive are the disorders of high-level perception, yet they are usually even more disruptive, both in themselves and because, if they are not recognised, the odd behaviours to which they may lead may be misconstrued as 'just psychological' or, even worse, 'lack of motivation'. With auditory dysgnosia all sounds (not only speech sounds) may be difficult to identify. Visual dysgnosia may mean that, whilst the patient can recognise and describe the component features of what he sees, he is unable to see 'wholes', and thus to identify, recognise, or extract meaning from complex visual stimuli — which is what the real world is largely composed of. Less subtly, visual (or somatosensory) hemi-inattention results in the inability to perceive from right and left fields simultaneously: as an example, this can have as devastating an effect on driving ability as a full hemianopia, yet the patient is completely unaware of the deficit. There are many very subtle disorders of perception which can have profound and puzzling impacts on everyday performance, and the reader is strongly advised to become acquainted with them by reading Oliver Sacks' book *The man who mistook his wife for a hat* (Sacks, 1985).

Cognition

'Cognition' encompasses such functions as attention, memory, thinking, problem-solving and judgement, as well as language and number. Number has specific cortical mechanisms for its handling, just as language does. The organisation of thinking and acting ('behaviour') depends on the frontal lobes, which are crucial also to the exercise of judgement. Speed and flexibility of thinking depend also on the number of associational channels available, and since this is depleted by diffuse neuronal injury, it is diminished in proportion to the severity of diffuse head injury. Such deficits can interfere disastrously with everyday performance, yet are not revealed by the usual forms of psychological testing.

Memory disturbances are the *rule* after head injury, and are produced by three different mechanisms. Memory function proper is diminished by lesions of the diencephalon or of the medial temporal structures: damage in the language hemisphere disturbs mainly verbal memory, whilst in the 'spatial' hemisphere it is non-verbal memory which is most affected. (In head injury the typical finding is a combination.) Lesions of the connections between the memory mechanisms and other temporal structures or the frontal lobes, or between the frontal lobes and the diencephalon, disrupt 'attention': this is a complex set of functions, but some aspect of attention is certainly crucial for the organisation of information in such a way as to transfer it to memory storage in a form, and with appropriate 'labelling', which will allow efficient access and retrieval. Since even minimal head injury has some deleterious effect upon attention mechanisms, *attentional* disorders of memory are the commonest single complaint met with in this condition (a good deal more common than their nearest rival, headache). Finally, patients with significant lesions of the frontal cortex, whose performances on tests of intelligence and memory have long since returned to normal, still showing devastating disorders of 'memory' in everyday life, the deficit being in the ability to impose *order and organisation* on information, which is a prerequisite for orderly storage.

Arousal and drive

Drive is best thought of as an enduring characteristic of the individual, concerned with the persistence and gusto with which activities are pursued. *Arousal*, on the other hand, is a fluctuating state, and has two distinct aspects. One concerns the level of consciousness (or *alertness*), and interacts with the individual's drive level: for example, people of high drive can become drowsy. The other concerns *emotional arousal*, which can vary independently of alertness. (Perhaps the best-known pathological example is the agitated, overactive but confused, drowsy state seen in belladonna poisoning, and very similar mixtures of low alertness and high arousal are seen in the post-traumatic confusional period.)

After severe brainstem damage a very long period of coma is likely to be followed by a very long stage of gradually improving underarousal; once normal diurnal levels of alertness are achieved there is usually a further long period of reduced drive, associated with, and ultimately outlived by, marked fatiguability. (In severe diffuse injury a similar sequence is seen, but the time span is usually over just a few weeks or months, rather than years.)

A purer type of drive deficit is seen after medial frontal lesions (and this is recognisably the same as is found after anterior cerebral artery strokes).

Drive disorders have considerable implications for the very complex problem of *motivation*. Different goals and objectives have different values (or degrees of desirability) for different people, partly because of individual differences in 'taste', partly because of different previous experiences. At any particular time the level of motivation a particular person has towards a particular goal depends on the prevailing balance between the intrinsic factors of drive and value and the extrinsic factors of the degree of difficulty and the amount of effort required to achieve the goal. A reduction of drive level through neurological effects of head injury, with perhaps a reduction (as a result of diencephalic damage) in the ability to experience pleasure (dyshedonia), is bound to reduce the tendency to exert effort towards a goal. We should remember, also, that the 'goals' in rehabilitation are often *our* goals, and we have no business making loose judgements about our patients' 'motivation' — rather it is our business to manipulate these factors in motivation as best we can in the patient's favour.

Behaviour and personality

Much confusion stems from a failure to distinguish between these two words. They differ in the same way as do 'arousal and drive', or 'mood and temperament', or even 'weather and climate'. The importance of making this particular distinction is that it is widely believed (quite rightly, for the most part) that 'personality' cannot be changed. 'Behaviour', on the other hand, can be changed.

The most troublesome behaviour disorder after head injury is *aggression*, and several different varieties must be distinguished. In the early stages of recovery most aggression is driven by *confusion*, and compounded by the alien surroundings of the acute hospital ward. As confusion resolves, the commonest problem is one of general *irritability*, which very slowly settles, over days, weeks or months. The most disruptive and distressing form of post-traumatic aggression (especially for the families of the victims), however, is the very explosive, often dramatic and destructive, but usually brief outburst behaviour of the *episodic dyscontrol syndrome* (EDS). This appears typically some months after injury, though it may be delayed for several years. This syndrome has many similarities with epilepsy (delayed onset, paroxysmal pattern, brief duration, dysthymic after-effects, and responsiveness to anticonvulsant drugs), and although conclusive evidence on its nature is not yet available, it is also referred to as 'limbic epilepsy'. Outbursts may be unprovoked, but are more often triggered by trivial frustrations (and curiously almost never by substantial provocation), in much the same way as the reflex epilepsies.

Closely related, and often associated, are intermittent deficits of impulse control, and also paroxysmal (and usually contextually incomprehensible) mood changes — sudden depressive or hypomanic states which may last from minutes to a few days, beginning and ending as though 'switched on or off'. Intermittent impulsive aberrations of sexual behaviour may also occur (and need to be distinguished from so-called 'sexual disinhibition').

These dyscontrol syndromes are most clearly associated with medial temporal lesions affecting limbic structures. They have been said to be rare, but it is apparent that reports have described only the socially most severe (involving murder or rape, for example) and the socially most apparent (those which appear outside the family circle). In fact at least a third of individuals attending a routine head injury follow-up clinic show evidence of this sort of disorder. It is interesting, therefore, that emerging studies with magnetic resonance imaging show that the commonest cortical lesions after even moderate head injury are contusions in the anteromedial temporal lobes.

Finally, it must be remembered that a few individuals will have been habitually aggressive, or even nasty, and only rarely does a head injury improve them.

Hypothalamic lesions may give rise to behaviour disorders related to alterations of specific drives. With sexual drive the usual problem is hyposexuality. A quite frequent disorder is a sustained increase in 'feeding behaviour', in which, although the subjective feelings of hunger and satiation are usually normal, the patient is driven almost continuously to want to find food, and to eat. Not only does this lead to significant obesity, it also often provokes considerable conflict between the patient and the family, who very reasonably try to exert outside control on the 'self-damaging behaviour'.

Personality changes are changes in the pervasive and consistent modes of action and interaction shown by the individual. Clearly, drive disorders result in changes of one aspect of personality. The more obtrusive disorders of personality after head injury, however, are those of the so-called 'frontal lobe syndrome'. The main difficulty with this term is that there are several features of frontal lobe dysfunction, some apparently contradictory, and it is best to think in terms of frontal lobe syndromes. There are three main groups of features. Orbitofrontal damage is particularly associated with the most obvious constellation, comprising *social disinhibition* (the tendency to say and do things which are usually *thought*, but inhibited because they are socially undesirable), persistent fatuous humour, and self-centred childish attitudes and behaviour. Inappropriate sexual behaviours are often given specific mention, but this is seldom justified. The severest of such behaviours is inappropriate (i.e. more or less public) masturbation. Much more common are socially unacceptable sexual propositioning, excessively personal discussion or remarks, and persistent badgering of individuals who can reasonably be seen as sexually or romantically attractive to the patient. In other words, these are straightforward problems of social disinhibition, and the sexual content derives from the prominence of sexual drive in young adults.

Medial frontal damage produces a lack of drive, but particularly a lack of spontaneity and initiative.

Dorsolateral frontal lesions affect planning, judgement, flexibility and adaptability, the ability to think and construe in abstract terms, and the ability to suppress previous responses (deficits of which lead to perseveration, more especially of actions, but also in speech).

It is often said that a characteristic feature of the frontal lobe syndrome is a lack of insight. Whilst it is usually true that the dorsolateral syndrome includes a definite lack of realistic self-judgement and self-criticism, patients with the orbitofrontal syndrome are nearly always quite aware of the inappropriateness of their uninhibited and self-centred behaviour. This is not easily apparent, however, since they also know that they are unable to control it, and usually 'brazen it out' by claiming that there is nothing amiss. But with sensitive inquiry it is possible to uncover their self-awareness, and the distress they actually feel.

Epilepsy

Post-traumatic epilepsy (PTE) is defined as epilepsy appearing for the first time following head injury. There are difficulties in identifying those in whom fits occur purely as a consequence of the injury: in the population at large there is an annual incidence of epilepsy of about 0.06 per cent. Since there is a prevalance in the UK of about 0.6 per cent, some people with epilepsy are likely to suffer head injury, and indeed may be more at risk than are those without epilepsy. Curiously, however, a family history of epilepsy appears not to increase the risk of PTE significantly.

It is necessary to distinguish between *early* and *late* PTE, the former being defined as epilepsy appearing within the first week after injury. The relationships between the two are somewhat confusing. The incidence of each is about 5 per cent in those who suffer at least some degree of concussion. Early epilepsy carries a relatively good prognosis, in that only a quarter of those who have fits in the first week go on to have later fits. On the other hand, early PTE is a high *risk factor* for late PTE, since only about 3 per cent of those without it develop fits later.

There are two other factors which significantly predict late PTE, namely depressed fracture (15 per cent) and intracranial haematoma (35 per cent). Combinations of these three factors lead to even higher risk rates.

Late PTE arises most commonly in the first year after injury (over 50 per cent). Thereafter the incidence gradually declines, but only 80 per cent have their first fit within four years. Focal fits are very common (40 per cent), and the mechanics and pathology of head injury suggest that the great majority of fits arise from a focal origin, the probability of generalised phenomenology being determined by the individual's constitutional convulsive threshold.

The importance of PTE cannot be too strongly stated: in long-term follow-up series, overall outcome of social functioning and psychological adjustment is very significantly worse in patients who develop late epilepsy.

'Disease, illness and predicament'

Professor David Taylor of the University of Manchester (Child and Adolescent Psychiatry) has for many years used this 'model' to remind us that all pathological change occurs in a context. We know a good deal about the neuropathology of head injury ('the disease'), and we can both infer and observe the functional deficits it produces in the individual ('the illness'). But our understanding of the full impact of the head injury on the person and his life ('his predicament'), and of the needs and prognosis for rehabilitation, depends on careful consideration of the patient's personal history, personality, family, and occupational, domestic and social 'ecological niches'.

We must also remember that the patient's family is 'injured', too. Family members should be involved in assessment of the patient (they will often have insights and be able to make observations which are not possible for the professionals involved), as well as in treatment, from the earliest stages.

Not only will this enhance our understanding, it will also help the family to cope with their distress, by ensuring that they have full and accurate information about the state of their relative and about head injury in general, and by giving them real, practical and explicitly valued ways of helping. Such involvement allows the exercise of a degree of control over the family's attitudes and approaches to the patient, thus helping to minimise later factitious dependency.

ASSESSMENT AND REHABILITATION

Continuity

Although there is some advantage in considering assessment and rehabilitation separately, it must be appreciated that they are merely stages and aspects of one continuous process of constant reassessment and redirection of management efforts.

In the early stages of recovery, and especially with mild and moderate injuries, formal reassessments are usually appropriate at intervals of a week or two. After the first month or two they are more useful and informative if made every two to three months.

Principles of assessment

Breadth and the team

Since the potential spectrum of disorders includes all cerebral, and therefore all personal, functions, the breadth of expertise needed in assessment and rehabilitation demands a large team. The following disciplines are *central* to the process: nursing; medicine (with a strong neuropsychiatric flavour); neuropsychology; behavioural psychology; social work (with both practical and counselling aspects); physiotherapy; speech therapy; occupational therapy (with physical, ADL and social aspects); industrial rehabilitation; and, of course, the family. A helpful addition is a teacher with experience in special education. For cognitive retraining there is a need for psychology technicians to avoid swamping of the neuropsychologist's time.

This mixture can reasonably be described as a 'multidisciplinary team'. However, in practice such teams tend to operate from and in their respective departments, and much therapeutic power is lost in this way. Patients will often perform quite differently with different members of such a team, and usually this will be unknown except perhaps at the time of team assessments. Many functional skills need simultaneous use of several sorts of therapeutic techniques for optimal training. All of these needs are best met by *interdisciplinary team* organisation, in which 'the department' is the whole team, and the work setting is the head injury rehabilitation unit. Where this is not achievable, because of the lack of an appropriate physical unit, the minimum requirement is that the team identifies itself as a committed team, and meets regularly, not only for 'assessments', but also informally.

In a team of this size, responsibility for some tasks may be unclear, and they may be overlooked or forgotten. One solution is to include in the team someone whose main function is coordination. Another helpful structure is to have one member of the team specifically responsible for the *overall* management of each patient. This also makes liaison with the family easier, and less prone to misunderstanding or manipulation.

Funnelling and follow-up

Patients with severe injuries will progress naturally from acute care to inpatient rehabilitation. Those with mild or moderate injuries, however, are either not admitted at all, or spend only short periods in hospital, and may be lost to follow-up. Recently, initiatives have been described from Edinburgh and Bristol, in which the responsibility for decisions about admission of the head-injured are vested in a single medical team. This has increased the efficiency of decision-making, and reduced admissions by up to 50 per cent. It also makes it possible to channel those who do not need admission, but are at risk of debilitating minor symptoms, to the Head Injury Follow-up Clinic.

Expectations and the influence of severity

The first step in the assessment of the head-injured patient is to establish the severity of the injury, and the pattern of disorders. This makes it possible to predict the areas of functioning in which deficits are *likely*, so that problems will not be overlooked. The information on which judgements of severity (especially of diffuse injury) depend is rarely clearly available in hospital notes, and the earlier the rehabilitation specialist can be involved, the more accurately can this information be acquired.

Recording information

Any information recorded should be useful, simple and concise, easily accessible (otherwise it is unlikely ever to be used), and be displayed so as to be rapidly and accurately understandable (and wherever possible, this will mean graphically). Since many disciplines are involved in assessment, and need to share information as far as possible, there is a need for a common language and common formats. Each assessment needs a terse précis of each area, and an overall summary.

Principles of rehabilitation in head injury

Starting early, continuing late

It is generally assumed that the sooner after injury rehabilitative efforts begin, the more effective they will be. Curiously, little evidence has been available on this question until some systematic studies in the past few years, but these support the intuition. If the team becomes involved with the patient as soon as acute surgical interventions are completed, thus ensuring a comprehensive and coordinated approach from the beginning, it is far more effective than simply referring the patient to the various therapeutic departments when the primary carers think it advisable.

Because of the practice of managing the head-injured alongside patients suffering from a wide range of acute locomotor disabilities, periods of treatment have tended to be short. Studies have begun to appear showing continuing gains in social recovery and independence over much longer periods, and it is becoming apparent that the severest injuries can benefit from rehabilitation which continues intensively for a year or more.

Minor injuries and preventive rehabilitation

Head injuries which cause concussion, but do not demand admission, often lead nevertheless to symptoms which can be distressing and disruptive to work and social life. Many of these can be resolved by simple explanation, reassurance and counselling (of both patient and relatives). This applies especially to the headache, dizziness and irritability of the 'post-concussional syndrome'. Prediction and explanation of fatiguability, with firm advice on progressive graded effort in order to overcome it, and a gradual return to work, can make all the difference between success and the loss of a job.

Social psychology and rehabilitation design

Rehabilitation is concerned with moving from illness and disability towards independence in the ordinary world. This will be most easily achieved if the unconscious (as well as the conscious) attitudes of both victim and treaters are working in that direction. We are rarely and only dimly aware of our attitudes, yet they play a large part in determining our behaviour and motivation, and are significantly affected by cues in the environment. Hospitals and the usual trappings of medical and paramedical treatment are strong signals of *illness*, and illness is a legitimate reason for dependency and rest. The routines of hospital life are second nature for the rehabilitation professionals, but they are not features of the ordinary world for most patients. Moreover, the tacit atmosphere of 'looking after' and 'doing to' the patient is counterproductive to the aims of rehabilitation. It is apparent that much more attention needs to be given to the social psychology of rehabilitation, but it seems likely that the aims will best be served by increasing the real-life ordinariness of rehabilitation settings.

Drug treatments and the head-injured

The head-injured patient already has enough problems, without the addition of unforeseen (but foreseeable) 'side-effects', and *all* drugs for *any* indication must be given careful thought before being prescribed. (As an example, antihistamines may be useful for hay fever, but they often intensify attentional and arousal deficits, they may induce or exacerbate agitation, and they are potentially epileptogenic: a topical preparation is likely to be preferable.) There are two useful slogans: 'Avoid drug treatments if you can' and 'Think pharmacology!'.

In planning treatment it is worth remembering that drugs usually produce their effects much more quickly than do physical therapies — antispasticity agents are a good example. It makes sense to try any drug treatment first, since this gives the possibility of advancing the therapist's starting point.

The management of specific problem areas

Abnormalities of tone

The priority in the earliest stages after injury is to prevent contractures. The primary treatment method is the physiotherapist's skill in passive exercise, and for maximal efficiency the skill needs to be passed on, through careful training, to other members of the team, notably nursing staff and family members. Preventive splinting or casting may also be needed. Antispasticity drugs may be useful, but it must be remembered that baclofen is usually sedative in effective doses, and dantrolene may take weeks to become effective.

Increased tone often persists, and once the patient is conscious and able to cooperate there is a wide variety of physiotherapy techniques to try. Because of the complexity of abnormalities of tone, there is no established knowledge about 'the best treatment', and therapists should be encouraged to experiment, and to be inventive — provided, of course, that inventiveness is accompanied by the collection and recording of objective measurement, and evaluative research. Techniques already shown to have some value include serial casting, the Bobath approach, PNF, icing, and the application of electro-acupuncture to points located over spastic muscles. The use of Peto's conductive education techniques is being explored in a number of centres, with promising results in the control of movement, and with the added advantage of the simultaneous fostering of group identification, social skills, and the reintegration of complex activities. (This is a set of group techniques based on three well-established psychological principles: analysis of tasks into small steps; verbal monitoring of behaviour; and feedback of results.)

Walking

Here again, the eclectic use of a wide variety of techniques is needed, to try to establish the most effective treatments. Walking may be disrupted by paresis, abnormal tone, dystaxia, dysbasia or bradykinesia, and it is necessary to tease out the component deficits in each case. The hydrotherapy or swimming pool appears to have a particular place: walking in chest-high water tends to magnify the difficulties, but seems in some way to 'clarify the problems' and thus accelerate relearning. Imaginative use can be made of inflatables and tilt-boards in the retraining of balance and of saving responses.

Sometimes orthotic devices are helpful. As a general rule it is desirable to regard them as provisional in head injury rehabilitation, in order to avoid the possible inhibition of recovery and relearning. (In much the same spirit, no patient should be provided with a personal or customised wheelchair unless lengthy and intensive rehabilitation has demonstrated a very low probability of the achievement of independent walking.)

For many patients the duration of rehabilitation is determined by the needs of cognitive, social and occupational training, rather than by physical disability. An interesting result of this is the finding that it is often possible, through continuing physiotherapy, to improve the appearance of locomotion, as well as its functionality. Since social reintegration is greatly helped by the elimination of *apparent* abnormality ('cosmetics'), this is certainly a worthwhile goal.

Achieving independent walking is often seen by the patient as the most important goal. Indeed, it can be *too* important a goal, in the sense that, in ordinary life, walking is actually a *means* rather than an end, and it is well worth trying to preserve this perspective during rehabilitation by integrating locomotion training with other activities.

Manual skills

Work on defects of power, tone, coordination and sensation in the upper limbs, employing the established skills of occupational therapists and physiotherapists, is obviously an important platform for the restoration of manual skills. But once again it is necessary to go about this in contexts in which manual skills are actually required in everyday life. A helpful setting is the 'arm class', in which the OT and physiotherapist provide (and teach) specific techniques, but other staff conduct pertinent activities — eating, playing games ('I spy', 'Pass the parcel', board games, and so on), computer-based cognitive training, rhythm and gesture training, even basic social skills training.

There are two specific disorders which may sometimes be helped pharmacologically. The very disruptive peduncular tremor is often significantly reduced (though rarely abolished) by propranolol (80–240 mg b.d.). (This tremor often responds dramatically well to thalamotomy, but selection of patients for operation is difficult, because the rather unpredictable effects of other brain lesions may lead to prolonged disturbances of arousal, or to exacerbation of frontal lobe deficits of organisation and abstraction.) In a few cases cerebellar dystaxia may improve if cholinergic activity is enhanced by the use of lecithin or choline chloride (though the latter is often unacceptable because it can cause the patient to exude a fishy or uriniferous odour).

Speech

The development of techniques for the treatment of the dysarthrias has lagged behind the more interesting field of dysphasia, but recent years have seen the publication of schedules of objective assessment, and treatment approaches are being refined.

Many post-traumatic speech disorders lead to boring and colourless delivery and, as with walking, it is important to know that very prolonged intensive therapy can achieve hitherto unexpected improvements in prosody and intonation, which greatly enhance the patient's social acceptability.

Swallowing

This is the area where combined treatment by speech therapist, physiotherapist and nursing staff is essential. An important step is to establish whether the swallowing difficulty affects primarily solids or liquids or both, since the easier should be worked on first. If the patient is tolerating a nasogastric tube, treatment can be given with it in place — this adds to the difficulty, and thus tends to make the task at hand more definite. Icing techniques (ice-cream and ice-water particularly) are extremely helpful as a prelude to graded exercises aimed first at individual bulbar movements, and then at more complex integrated patterns. A variety of 'primitive reflexes' can be brought into play to model the movements required (for example, stroking upwards over the larynx stimulates reflex swallowing), and PNF techniques are also helpful. In severe brainstem injury the process is often very slow and painstaking, and serial measures of time taken and quantities swallowed are helpful to provide morale-boosting evidence for both patient and therapists.

Communication

Patients are people, and people *want* to communicate. Anarthria and severe dysarthria make this impossible, and are slow to improve, even with intensive treatment. Full use should therefore be made, as early as is cognitively possible, of alternative means of communication, including the growing array of electronic aids. At the same time, however, it should be recognised that people want not just to communicate, but to speak. A common frustration for the therapist is that the patient rejects the aid. A helpful practice is for the therapist to *begin each session* with exercises aimed at the speech musculature, before going on to training time with the communication aids.

Non-verbal language also may require retraining, and this is best dealt with in sessions devoted to the basic level of social skills training (q.v.).

Language

Most frank dysphasias either recover spontaneously, or are severe and show little response to therapy. However, there is a middle group which show slow but long-continuing response, in spite of little or no tendency to spontaneous improvement. (As with a number of head injury deficits, this has become apparent as a result of the practice of prolonged intensive rehabilitation over the past few years. Many rehabilitation units, especially in North America, have had referred to them patients whose injuries occurred several years previously, and who would be considered 'static' by traditional standards. Since all varieties of therapy tend to be deployed with all patients, it has been possible to see the effects of treatment in those who would previously not have been considered worth treating.)

Reading and writing skills can also be retrained. To avoid too much frustration it is as well to try to identify, through examination of the patterns of neuropsychological deficits as well as from the personal and educational history, pre-existing abnormalities in these areas. This is not to say that they cannot be helped, but progress is likely to be slower than with purely post-traumatic disorders.

Activities of daily living and domestic skills

The analysis of deficits and retraining of skills and routines in these areas are not significantly different for the head-injured than for other groups. There are three special points worth noting.

The behavioural, emotional and motivational fragility and unrealistic self-judgement of the head-injured often make them less than enthusiastic about ADL retraining. As with an unruly school class, much of the therapist's time and energy has to go into making sessions attractive. For this reason it is particularly cost-effective to use group techniques, which draw on peer-group pressures, competitiveness, and social rewards. (The techniques of conductive education again seem to be particularly helpful.) At the same time it should be standard practice in the rehabilitation unit that patients are ultimately *responsible* for their own self-care, nursing and other staff being available only as *assistants* — helping, but not 'doing for'. Every effort should be made to incorporate ADL and domestic retraining into real contexts — doing one's laundry in preparation for a weekend at home, for example, or cooking goodies for a party.

Social skills

Social skills training (SST) is not simply situational role-play. It consists of a set of well-researched, formalised techniques covering basic (eye-contact, personal space, gesture, and so on), interpersonal (approach, interruption, assertiveness, for example) and situational skills (shopping, interviews, eating out), and is usually organised into 'courses', so that gradual progression up these levels can be achieved.

The techniques (Wilkinson and Canter, 1982), are well known to clinical psychologists, and to many OTs who have worked in psychiatric settings. However, they can be learned and used by anyone, and there is great advantage in head injury work, where the whole span of deficits may contribute to social skills deficiencies, if *all* members of the team are involved in SST sessions (though not necessarily all at once!). Moreover, SST workshops are a valuable way of bringing the team closer together.

Cognition

In the past decade cognitive training has been the principal growth industry of head injury rehabilitation. Unfortunately, though many psychologists have produced training systems (most relying on microcomputers), almost none have mounted adequate studies of their effectiveness. There is thus little information about which method is best for which deficit in which sorts of patients. Such evidence as there is suggests that attention deficits can be retrained such that improvements are generalised to all activities, but that memory training improves only the actual memory performances trained. As a result the treatment of memory disorders has developed in the directions of 'prosthetics' (the use of aids such as alarm watches, diaries and notebooks) and of learning strategies to circumvent the memory difficulty. Graded training in problem-solving appears to be useful, but methods for the retraining of more specific cognitive (e.g. language and number) and perceptual skills are so far less clear (Wilson and Moffat, 1984).

There is often a mismatch in either direction between the abilities demonstrated by formal test procedures, and performances observable in day-to-day activities. Mention has already been made of the severe practical memory problems seen in patients with frontal lesions who score normally on formal tests of intelligence and memory. One also sees patients who perform appallingly on standard tests of intelligence, memory and attention who nevertheless establish and use accurate memories of people and events in day-to-day living. These puzzles are being actively pursued in research, but for the time being they bedevil formal assessment, and dictate the need for observational assessments by the entire team.

Largely because of attempts to find treatments for the degenerative dementias, various drugs are becoming available which may improve cognitive processes, though few have as yet been systematically tried in the head-injured. Although reports are conflicting there is evidence that vasopressin may be helpful in memory disorders, especially those which depend on attentional deficits. Some of the disagreement may result from the use of different preparations, the two most associated with positive reports being lysine–vasopressin (Syntopressin nasal spray) and DDAVP (as insufflated nasal drops). In those cases where good results are claimed, the regime is for a low dose administered twice a day in a single course of about a month. So-called 'nootropic agents' (piracetam and oxiracetam) are not generally available, but are undergoing clinical trials.

Finally, measures which improve arousal (alertness) and drive inevitably improve cognitive performance.

Arousal and drive

Undoubtedly the single most important measure for the improvement of underarousal is the avoidance of drugs which have sedative or tranquillising effects. This means not only major tranquillisers and long-acting hypnotics, but also most of the anticonvulsants commonly used for the prevention or treatment of epilepsy (Chapter 25).

Loss of drive and spontaneity from frontal lobe lesions is difficult, if not impossible, to treat. Very occasionally, stimulant drugs may give a modest improvement, but neither general stimulation nor systematic behaviour modification has any lasting effect. Bromocriptine may be of use.

For the underarousal and lack of drive associated with brainstem lesions, however, there is more possibility of success. Some patients show at least a partial improvement with vasopressin, though stimulant drugs such as the amphetamines have little more than a brief transient effect. Many patients fail to experience the normal unpleasant responses to vestibular stimulation, and will show a delayed but cumulative increase in drive and alertness if exposed to this on a regular (once or twice daily) regime. The technique is extremely simple: the patient sits in a 'secretary's chair', and is spun round at a speed of about half a revolution per second for several minutes, the direction of spin being reversed at the end of a minute. The duration of need for the treatment is unclear. If it is suspended after a few weeks there is usually a gradual loss of drive after the second week. Some patients have been found to become ordinarily sensitive to the stimulation, which therefore has to cease, and in these circumstances the enhanced drive level appears to persist. This has occurred after a year or more of treatment, and the same phenomenon has been reported, with similar time relationships, in developmentally disordered children.

When the drive level improves it may happen that disorders of control over behaviour worsen, but the individual also becomes more responsive to behaviour modification (reinforcement techniques), so that there is considerable net gain.

'Behaviour disorder'

If treated soon after their initial appearance, all of the various features of the EDS are very likely to be abolished, or at least improved, by the use of carbamazepine (400–600 mg b.d.) (see also 'Epilepsy' section). Such behaviours tend to elicit highly reinforcing responses from staff and relatives alike, and this inappropriate reinforcement increases and perpetuates the behaviour disorder (which is most often misinterpreted as some kind of response to the emotional stresses of injury). Where the behaviour has been present for some time, therefore, there is a need for some kind of behavioural treatment as well, the most effective being behaviour modification in a context of token economy (Eames and Wood, 1985a,b). Combination with carbamazepine is advisable, since the behavioural approach alone may produce only marginal improvements.

Increased feeding behaviour can be difficult to treat, and seems unresponsive to behaviour modification. Sometimes the drive can be reduced by the use of L-dopa.

Personality change

When frontal lobe disorders are of mild or moderate degree they usually diminish over time, and provided the patient and family are given explanations, and the support of regular follow-up, the outlook is likely to be good.

More severe disturbances are likely to be permanent. Drug treatments have no effect unless doses of major tranquillisers are used which are sufficient to produce persistent sedation — clearly not a desirable result. However, despite the uniformly poor response of spontaneously occurring personality disorders, it has been found that post-traumatic personality changes can be successfully and lastingly treated by consistent behaviour modification in a controlled setting (token economy). Interestingly, as the general quality of behaviour improves, so there is less and less evidence of 'lack of insight'.

It should be noted that when disorders of personality are clearly related to pre-accident personality traits, there is little chance of improving them with this or any other treatment approach.

Epilepsy

Since the development of PTE has such a large effect on social viability, it is generally agreed that protection should be given to patients with one or more of the three major risk factors (early epilepsy, depressed fracture and intracranial haematoma) even though there is insufficient evidence to know whether prophylactic anticonvulsant medication is effective. But given the doubt, it is important to ensure that no harm comes from the treatment: all major anticonvulsants, except sodium valproate, carbamazepine and clobazam, have significant deleterious effects on cognitive and affective functioning (Trimble and Thompson, 1983). The latter two are considered to be more effective than valproate in controlling focal epileptogenic disturbances, and clobazam has been associated with a high relapse rate after about six months. Thus carbamazepine is the drug of first choice for both prophylaxis and treatment of PTE.

Broader issues

The family

The family is at great risk of severe stress disorder: it also represents a powerful force (for good or ill) in the subsequent recovery of the patient. It should be enlisted as an ally. Support is also now available from 'Headway', the National Head Injury Association (address is at end of chapter). Local support groups include head injury victims, their families, and rehabilitation professionals. The central organisation has been involved in advising on the procedures for setting up new groups, in liaison, and more recently adopting a higher profile to press for improved rehabilitation facilities. It is also trying to develop appropriate long-term residential accommodation. 'Headway' deserves the involved support of rehabilitation professionals; moreover there is much that *we* can learn from *them.*

Studies in Glasgow (Brooks, 1984) indicate that the greatest burdens on families come from behavioural, emotional and cognitive disorders. There is a high casualty rate in marital relationships (whereas marital breakdown is no more common among victims of spinal injury than in the general population). This is probably not preventable, but sympathetic support can reduce the suffering associated with it.

Return to the community

Patients are usually discharged from hospital because of pressure on beds and the dearth of rehabilitation facilities, and this means a return to a home ill-prepared (by attitude or expectation), ill-equipped to cope with the many problems which arise, and with little support for patient or family. In spite of the difficulties, no patient should be discharged without careful thought about the independence, cognitive and behavioural implications, and about further rehabilitation plans, including work assessment and ultimate accommodation.

Work

Ideally the interdisciplinary team should carefully assess the patient's skills and work potential, in order to avoid inappropriate referrals (see Chapter 41). If the patient is unsuitable, some form of regular 'work-like' placement is needed, whilst further rehabilitation measures are pursued. Inactivity is a severe impediment to the recovery processes which can otherwise continue.

Driving

Some patients, usually after mild or moderate injury, are phobic about driving or being driven. Most will respond to traditional specific treatments for phobic anxiety states provided that they are not delayed.

After severe injury, most patients wish to resume driving, but often are medically unfit to do so (see Chapter 47). The greatest impediment is epilepsy. Physical disability can usually be circumvented by vehicle modifications. But disturbances of vision, particularly large field defects, visual hemi-inattention, and marked disruptions of binocular vision or horizontal visual scanning, are complete bars.

Driving, especially in traffic, is an extremely complex skill, requiring rapid perception and recognition of visual information, rapid and flexible responses and adaptations of forward planning, and so attentional deficits may preclude it. The more severe the diffuse head injury, the more severely are these functions impaired. However, practical performances can sometimes be unexpectedly efficient and the best course in such cases is comprehensive assessment (Chapter 47).

Follow-up

The most pressing reason for research is that almost all we know of long-term outcomes — our only basis for prognosis in individual cases — comes from a small number of studies, none of which examined the effects of rehabilitation. Ideally, therefore, *all* patients should be followed up indefinitely. This may be logistically difficult, but all should be followed up at least until they are stably occupying a satisfactory 'niche', and family burdens have been eased as far as is possible.

PREDICTION OF OUTCOME AND NEEDS

Outcome

We lack adequate data for accurate prognostication, and currently expectations of outcome are distorted by the awfulness of the early post-injury clinical picture and lack of appropriate rehabilitation facilities. Nevertheless there is evidence that physical and practical disabilities improve over many years (Roberts, 1979) that early and prolonged rehabilitation improves outcome (Eames and Wood, 1985b; Santa Clara Medical Center, 1982) and that behaviour and personality changes can be treatable (Sacks, 1985).

Predictions of outcome are important for planning, but also because they affect expectation, and therefore the enthusiasm with which rehabilitation is undertaken. Current evidence must be allowed to colour expectations, whilst further research is pursued.

Needs

Specialists in the rehabilitation of spinal cord injury can predict both needs and outcome for the patient on the day of admission, because the damage is irreversible. Rehabilitation involves making life liveable *in spite of the effects of the damage*, mainly through aids.

The aims after head injury are quite different. Outcome depends certainly on the degree of recovery (which is only roughly predictable), and probably on the quality, breadth and duration of rehabilitation (and at present we are unable to predict even the availability of this). Rehabilitation involves attempts to *restore function to the organism*, whilst aids are viewed as temporary, or items of last resort once maximal rehabilitative effort has ceased to produce further change.

How, then, are we to predict *needs*? One important answer is that most individuals suffering moderate injuries will need at least a few weeks, and those with severe or worse injuries months or years, of intensive rehabilitation, if they are to achieve the best outcome possible for them. Thus 'needs' are not specifiable in terms of bungalows or gadgets, but in terms of the availability of rehabilitation and treatment.

For many patients, injury will mean loss of the ability to work, perhaps permanently, and so financial support of some sort is vital. This need will depend on prior commitments.

Apart from prolonged, intensive, comprehensive rehabilitation, perhaps the only area of need we can come near to predicting for the severely head-injured is that of long-term accommodation, though even then the prediction can be made only rather late in the day. A very few, whose injuries are so severe that they never really regain awareness, will need permanent total nursing care. A slightly larger number will suffer, because of the particular nature and distribution of lesions in their brains, one or other of the odd behavioural syndromes necessitating permanent total tolerant care. A rather larger group will so stress their families as to be rejected by them, and will need long-term care in nursing homes and the like. But the great majority will be able to soldier on, in often unsuitable but coping family settings. This is the group for whom we must have some hope that *adequate* rehabilitation may help them achieve a greater degree of personal independence, and a lesser magnitude of burden on their families.

REFERENCES

Brooks, N. (1984) *Closed head injury: psychological, social and family issues*, Oxford University Press, Oxford

Eames, P. and Wood, R. (1985a) Rehabilitation after severe brain injury: a special-unit approach to behaviour disorders. *Int. Rehabil. Med.*, 7, 130-3

Eames, P. and Wood, R. (1985b) Rehabilitation after severe brain injury: a follow-up study of a behaviour modification approach. *J. Neurol. Neurosurg. Psychiatry*, *48*, 613-19

Evans, C.D., Bull, C.P.I. and Devonport, M.J. (1977) Rehabilitation of the brain-damaged survivor. *Injury*, *8*, 80-97

Roberts, A.H. (1979) *Severe accidental head injury*, Macmillan, London

Sacks, D. (1985) *The man who mistook his wife for a hat*, Duckworth, London

Santa Clara Valley Medical Center (1982) *Severe head traumas: a comprehensive medical approach* (collaborative). Institute for Medical Research, 751 South Bascom Avenue, San José, California 95128; November

Trimble, M.R. and Thompson, P.J. (1983) Anticonvulsant drugs, cognitive functions, and behaviour. *Epilepsia*, *24* (Suppl. 1), 555-63

Wilkinson, J. and Canter, S. (1982) *Social skills training manual*, John Wiley, London

Wilson, B.A. and Moffat, N. (1984) *Clinical management of memory problems*, Croom Helm, London

INFORMATION

Headway

200 Mansfield Road, Nottingham NG1 3HX. (Headway publishes a range of pamphlets for families, which give excellent outlines of many of the problems of head injury victims. They are very useful, too, for rehabilitation staff.)

25

Epilepsy

Jolyon Oxley

> 'Living with epilepsy', he said, 'is like playing Hamlet standing on a trap door which can open suddenly at any moment. When it does, you fall into a black hole, only to come round after a few minutes with your face smashed in and your pants wet. But unlike the theatre, this audience has seen everything. Sometimes they laugh; others are embarrassed; most, I guess, feel pretty helpless.' He looked up and smiled. 'You say that I won't have another fit if I take these tablets, but you can never be sure. I hate that bit of me that you call "epilepsy".'

This chapter attempts to analyse the handicap due to epilepsy in order to help disentangle some of the complex problems. But, as professionals, we must never forget the 'what it's like' factor which has just been described so graphically.

As about 1 in 20 of us will have a fit at some point in our life there is a need for everyone to know something about epilepsy and the impact that it may have. Epilepsy is not a subject just for specialists.

SOME FACTS ABOUT EPILEPSY

The prevalence of active epilepsy (defined as someone who has had a fit in the past two years and/or is still on treatment) is about 1 in 200. Therefore there are some 300,000 people in the UK known to have active epilepsy, but by no means all of these continue to have seizures.

Epilepsy is a very common disorder affecting people of all ages, races and social groups. It varies enormously in severity, presenting some people with seemingly insuperable obstacles to daily living and others merely with a few occupational restrictions. Because epilepsy affects so many people in so many ways, it is vitally important not to generalise about 'epilepsy' but to consider the people who have epilepsy and their individual abilities and needs.

There are no very detailed figures from the UK, but the USA Government Commission on the control of epilepsy and its consequences identified four major categories as follows:

Category 1 — inactive epilepsy requiring no ongoing treatment (34 per cent)
Category 2 — patients with mild epilepsy requiring occasional treatment (26 per cent)
Category 3 — patients with active epilepsy requiring ongoing medical treatment (36 per cent)
Category 4 — patients requiring institutional care (3 per cent)

Of those under active care (i.e. Categories 3 and 4) the identified associated disabilities were: none 23 per cent; intellectual 48 per cent; behavioural 54 per cent; neurological 10 per cent.

Patients in Categories 3 and 4 will feature most prominently in hospital outpatient departments and require a wide range of medical and social services. Nevertheless, patients in Categories 1 and 2 also require expert attention, information and counselling about the many problems the epilepsy can present.

ANALYSING THE HANDICAP

From this brief introduction it is clear that knowing someone has 'epilepsy' tells us very little about the individual. The disability which may stem from epilepsy can be looked at in a number of ways, but in simple terms it can be divided into (1) the primary handicap — fits and their treatment, (2) associated handicaps, (3) secondary handicaps.

Primary handicap

The fits

Seizures have a number of characteristics which cause problems.

Unpredictability: it is probably this quality more than any other that causes the difficulties. Even if fits appear to be completely controlled no guarantees can be given that another one will not happen at any time.

It is sometimes easier for the person to cope if the seizures have an established pattern, e.g. only at the time of menstruation or only in the early morning. The occurrence of a prolonged aura (or characteristic warning period) does help to avoid injury or having a fit in a public place.

Physical damage: Although some types of seizures, such as absences and complex partial seizures, are not commonly associated with physical injury, generalised seizures in which the person falls abruptly to the ground may result in intracranial bleeding, and repeated minor injuries may result in facial disfigurement and progressive neurological and intellectual deterioration.

Lack of control: unlike some conditions in which patients can avoid situations which exacerbate their symptoms, most patients with epilepsy do not have this degree of control over their condition. Some feel that their seizures are brought on by particular foods, stress, excitement, etc. With the exception of highly specific environmental stimuli such as some flashing lights, attempting to control the fits by avoiding such situations is not usually successful in the long run.

Disruption of daily routine: if seizures occur during the day disruption may occur to schooling, domestic and social life and employment. Clearly seizures that only occur during sleep are much less of a problem, although if they are severe or frequent they can produce disabling symptoms on wakening (confusion, headache, fatigue, etc.).

Associated signs and symptoms: the disability can be considerably increased if the seizure is accompanied by injury, confusion with automatic behaviour, prolonged post-ictal sleep and incontinence.

Negative reaction in others: seizures occurring unexpectedly may provoke anxiety and even hostility in onlookers. The cumulative effect of this may contribute to the secondary handicaps which are discussed below.

Treatment

It may seem unusual to consider treatment as part of the handicap. However, for those patients whose seizures are completely controlled taking tablets may be the only reminder of their disability. This can lead to frustration and non-compliance with treatment. Unfortunately the guidelines for withdrawing medication are not clear-cut. Many paediatricians are keen to do this after a seizure-free period of two or three years because of the possible adverse long-term metabolic and cognitive effects of drugs. Physicians who treat adults, on the other hand, tend to be more cautious because of the inevitable loss of a driving licence and possible threat to employment should seizures recur. Unfortunately the EEG is of little value in predicting the outcome of withdrawing therapy, and the pros and cons of so doing must be discussed at length. In patients whose seizures continue, treatment can add to the handicap if it is inaccurately or inappropriately prescribed. All antiepileptic drugs (AEDs) have side-effects, some of which may be subtle and not lead to obvious clinical signs. Rational therapy will, however, maximise control and keep side-effects to a minimum.

Associated handicaps

The same disease process that produces the epilepsy may also produce other disturbances of brain function, the nature of which often depends on which part of the brain is affected. Associated handicaps may be divided into four classes.

Physical handicaps

If there is a localised injury to the brain involving the motor cortex then a monoplegia or hemiplegia may result, as well as epilepsy. Such patients are prone to simple partial motor fits, sometimes with secondary generalisation, and these may be difficult to control because of the underlying structural lesion. Sensory disturbances in the affected limb(s) may also be troublesome.

Brainstem dysfunction is also seen in some patients with severe epilepsy. Symptoms such as ataxia, dysarthria and nystagmus can be caused by drug intoxication, but may also be due to the cumulative effect of frequent head injuries.

Higher function (cognitive) deficits

Focal cognitive deficits, such as dysphasia and defective visuospatial skills due to localised brain damage, may be more prominent immediately after a fit. However, some of these problems may not be obvious on routine clinical testing and formal psychometric evaluation may be necessary to pinpoint these difficulties. Their identification may help with long-term management. Some patients, particularly with temporal lobe epilepsy, complain of memory difficulties. There is no easy solution to this problem, but improving fit control and rationalising treatment may help. Formal testing sometimes fails to reveal significant memory impairment, however, and some patients may have a word-finding difficulty instead. The impact that epilepsy may have on learning is considered in more detail later in this chapter.

Mental handicap

The majority of people with epilepsy have normal intelligence. However, the presence of severe epilepsy from an early age is often accompanied by some intellectual impairment. In addition, if the fits result in frequent injuries to the head and are uncontrolled over a long period, a further decline in intelligence may occur. It is also true that people who are already mentally handicapped have about 30 per cent risk of developing epilepsy. Its severity varies widely, but in many the fits can be controlled easily, and the guidelines for treatment are the same as for everyone else. Certainly all the necessary facilities for diagnosis and management should be made available, and a regular review of medication is important.

There may, however, be additional problems. The mentally handicapped patient may find it difficult to cope with changes in treatment, and the physician may find it more difficult to assess side-effects if the patient's verbal abilities are poor. As drug intoxication can produce behaviour problems rather than the more conventional signs, it is important to keep drug treatment to a minimum, at the same time as controlling the fits wherever possible. This will at least allow people with mental handicap to make the most of their abilities, and will make it easier for them to live as independently as possible.

Psychiatric problems

This is a very complex subject. It is often difficult to identify those problems that are directly due to the same brain disturbance that produces the epilepsy (associated handicap) from those that arise as a person attempts to cope with living with epilepsy in our society (secondary handicap). Psychiatric disorders of various kinds are quite common in people with intractable epilepsy, and the majority can be treated in a conventional way. Some special points need to be considered, however.

(*a*) *Antiepileptic drugs*: in toxic doses these can produce psychiatric disturbances such as depression and psychosis. Serum AED levels should be checked in anyone with epilepsy presenting with psychiatric problems.

(*b*) *Psychotropic drugs*: although phenothiazines and tricyclic antidepressants are said to be epileptogenic, they are normally quite safe in people with epilepsy taking AEDs.

(*c*) *Peri-ictal disturbances*: some patients have stereotyped mood changes (agitation, tension or depression) before or after a fit, and a very few have a severe psychotic disturbance with hallucinations and delusions, usually after a group of fits. This is normally self-limiting and the best method of treatment is prevention, i.e. improvement in fit control.

(*d*) *Sexual difficulties*: these are commonly due to difficulties with interpersonal relationships. However, both fits and drug treatment may interfere with sexual function and expert assessment will be required before appropriate treatment can be given.

(*e*) *Pseudo-seizures*: reassessment involving prolonged EEG monitoring will be required if a person diagnosed as having epilepsy is thought to be having pseudo-seizures. Undoubtedly some patients with genuine epilepsy also have pseudo-seizures, but the treatment for these two problems is very different, as AEDs are contraindicated in patients who only have pseudo-seizures.

(*f*) *Personality problems*: it has been suggested that there is a particular personality common to people with epilepsy. There is little evidence that this is true of people with epilepsy as a whole, although certain unusual characteristics are sometimes seen in patients with temporal lobe epilepsy.

Although the features may be due in part to the intrinsic cerebral disturbance which causes the seizures, other factors such as adverse social circumstances and inappropriate drug treatment are sometimes important.

Secondary handicaps

This term is used to describe those extra problems that may arise as a result of a person having fits and living in our society. If the epilepsy is completely controlled at an early stage the secondary handicaps will be minimised, and may only amount to a few occupational restrictions (see Table 25.3). On the other hand if fits continue, a number of other problems may arise in many areas of daily living.

Although the majority of people with epilepsy live fully integrated lives within the social setting of their choice, a few feel that they are subjected to discrimination. Much of the social prejudice no doubt stems from ignorance and the fact that many successful people with epilepsy choose to hide it, and therefore do nothing to modify society's unrepresentative image of the condition. Ignorance, however, is not only confined to 'other people', and all too often the person's knowledge of his own disability is limited to 'I am an epileptic'. There is an urgent need for health education programmes so that people can deal positively with the problems that living with epilepsy may bring.

PROVIDING SOME SOLUTIONS

Accurate diagnosis

The essential element to accurate diagnosis is a detailed eye-witness account, supported by appropriate EEG investigation. Without this information the diagnosis of epilepsy should not be made, and it should certainly never be made by merely excluding other conditions. Sometimes the attacks themselves remit, and so establishing a diagnosis may seem less important. However, if this is left in doubt, problems may well arise later in life when the time comes to apply for a driving licence or a job.

It seems self-evident that making a diagnosis correctly is a central part of good management. There is evidence, however, that a small number of patients with seemingly intractable epileptic seizures do not have epilepsy at all, and the attacks are really 'pseudo-seizures'. The majority of these are psychogenic (functional or hysterical) and sometimes they supersede those due to epilepsy. This can lead to a complex management problem which often requires detailed reassessment, including expert clinical observation and EEG monitoring. Even in patients who undoubtedly have epilepsy, seizure classification is sometimes inadequate and may lead to unnecessary treatment failure. The commonest error is confusing complex partial seizures and absences in children which may look very similar clinically. Terms such as 'petit mal' and 'grand mal' should not be used, and all patients' seizures should be classified according to the International League Against Epilepsy classification (for a simplified version see Table 25.1).

Accurate treatment

In this short chapter the treatment of epilepsy cannot be reviewed in any detail, but a number of clinical points will be highlighted. Although antiepileptic drugs are the mainstay of treatment, a few patients can be helped dramatically by neurosurgery. Usually this is only considered in those who have a single focal EEG abnormality which is responsible for the seizures,

Table 25.1: A simplified classification and description of the more common epileptic fits

(i) Generalised	
The epileptic discharge is widespread throughout the cerebral cortex at the onset of the fit	
(a) Absences:	
Simple	Brief interruptions of consciousness often with flickering of the eyelids
Complex	Brief interruptions of consciousness with other signs such as jerking of the head, arms and trunk; may be serial
(b) Myoclonic jerks	May accompany absences as above, but may be severe causing the person to fall
(c) Atonic	Sudden loss of consciousness leading to the person crumpling to the ground
(d) Tonic	Sudden stiffening of the body with loss of consciousness which may cause a heavy fall; injuries are common
(e) Tonic–clonic	Stiffening of the body with loss of consciousness followed by rhythmical jerkings of the trunk and limbs.
All generalised fits except simple absences may be accompanied by incontinence of urine.	
(ii) Partial (or focal)	
The epileptic discharge is localised to one part of the brain, but sometimes may become generalised by spreading away from the site of origin.	
(a) Simple partial	Usually there is no loss of consciousness and the fit consists of isolated twitching of a group of muscles or a discrete sensory disturbance in one part of the body
(b) Complex partial	These commonly originate in the temporal lobe, with impaired consciousness, confusion and semi-purposive movements. Sometimes they are preceded by characteristic aura, comprising a rising sensation which starts in the epigastrium. Other psychic symptoms such as panic, fear and olfactory hallucinations may occur
(c) Secondarily generalised	The fit may begin as in (a) or (b) but develop into a generalised tonic–clonic seizure.

and when adequate drug treatment has failed. However, in suitable patients the possible benefits of surgery (usually partial removal of one temporal lobe) should be considered at an early stage, before many of the secondary handicaps have developed.

But before prescribing any treatment, the physician needs to answer a number of questions:

(a) Is the diagnosis established beyond all reasonable doubt?

(b) Are there situations which are likely to trigger further fits, which should be avoided, such as irregular sleep or high alcohol intake?

(c) Is treatment necessary?

(d) Does the patient understand the nature of treatment for epilepsy and wish to take it?

(e) What is the treatment of choice, taking into consideration all the circumstances?

(f) Are there facilities for monitoring treatment?

The primary objective of treatment is to control the fits completely. If this is achieved the risk of secondary handicaps will be minimised. In about 70 per cent of cases complete control is possible with monotherapy (single drug treatment) and only a minority will require combination therapy. Whether monotherapy is used or not, the benefits of keeping the number of drugs and daily doses to a minimum (rational therapy) are considerable. Compliance will improve, side-effects and long-term adverse effects will be reduced and maximum fit control will be achieved. Treatment should never be initiated with combination therapy, but the single drug of choice will depend partly on the seizure type and partly on considerations of possible toxicity including teratogenicity.

There are six drugs commonly used to treat epilepsy, as well as a number of others which have specialised uses. These include benzodiazepines for emergency use, ACTH for infantile spasms and pyridoxine for pyridoxine-dependent seizures. Other remedies such as hormones, diuretics, other vitamins, herbal remedies, homeopathy and biofeedback may be tried as a last resort, but are not reliably effective. Some important clinical points about using the major drugs are set out below.

Phenytoin

This is a well-tried drug which is inexpensive, particularly as the BP preparation. It is effective against all forms of generalised seizures (except simple absences), and focal seizures with or without secondary generalisation. Phenytoin is metabolised in the liver but has non-linear kinetics so that the dose has to be adjusted very carefully. Serum level monitoring is essential to achieve optimum control and avoid toxicity. The drug has a long half-life which is serum level dependent and adjustments to dose should only be made every two to three weeks unless loading doses are used. The long half-life means that once-daily dosing is possible. It is not essential for every patient to have a phenytoin level in the 'therapeutic range' (10–20 μg/ml or 40–80 μmol/l) but if fits continue, and the serum level is low, an increase in dose may well be beneficial. Acute toxic effects include drowsiness, unsteadiness, slurred speech and nystagmus. Not all patients will experience these side-effects with serum levels above the therapeutic range but, if these symptoms occur, phenytoin should be discontinued completely for 24–48 hours and then resumed at a slightly lower dose (25 or 50 mg less per day). Phenytoin has been blamed for producing a whole host of chronic adverse effects including acne, hirsutes, osteomalacia, folate and IgA deficiency. There is evidence, however, that when given on its own at an appropriate dose, these adverse effects are not such a problem. Some, including low folate and low serum and urinary calcium, are probably of little clinical significance and routine replacement therapy is not indicated. Enlargement of the gums, which is seen fairly often, is not a contraindication to phenytoin therapy, and gingivitis can be prevented by careful oral hygiene. Excision of gum tissue may occasionally be needed. Phenytoin is possibly the most teratogenic AED but maternal well-being is also important during pregnancy. So if fits are well controlled, discontinuation of phenytoin is not usually recommended. However, perhaps this drug should be avoided altogether in women who may become pregnant.

Carbamazepine

This drug is effective against generalised seizures (except absences) and focal seizures with or without secondary generalisation. It is usually well tolerated, although skin rashes and neutropenia sometimes occur early in treatment. If only a mild depression of the neutrophil count occurs, treatment can usually continue. The earliest sign of acute toxicity is diplopia, which can be remedied by reducing the daily dose slightly or rearranging the dosing schedule. Unsteadiness, nausea and sleepiness may occur with high serum levels (above 45 μmol/l). Dose adjustments are easy to make as the drug has linear kinetics and a short half-life (10-18 hours) when given with other drugs. If high doses are used (above 1200 mg daily) the drug may have to be taken three or four times a day, but otherwise twice-daily dosing is satisfactory. Carbamazepine is probably one of the least teratogenic AEDs, although reduced fetal head circumference has been reported.

Sodium valproate

This drug is effective against all types of generalised and focal seizures. Although carbamazepine has been said to be the drug of choice for focal seizures, most studies have suggested that phenytoin, carbamazepine and sodium valproate are all equally effective. Primary generalised tonic–clonic seizures are, however, easier to control than focal seizures, which may prove drug-resistant. Sodium valproate is usually well tolerated but may cause drowsiness if given in too high a dose. Other adverse effects include thrombocytopenia, hair loss, weight gain and hepatic damage. This latter has caused concern, particularly among paediatricians, as a number of children have died probably as a result of valproate therapy. However, such cases are rare and largely confined to multiply handicapped children, some of whom also took enzyme-inducing drugs. Although serial liver function tests are recommended when treatment with sodium valproate is started, they are of little predictive value. Close clinical monitoring is prudent. Serum valproic acid levels are not a great help to clinical management, as there does not appear to be a correlation between serum levels and efficacy, but clinical studies suggest that dosing once or a twice a day gives good results. Fetal neural tube defects have been attributed to valproate therapy.

Ethosuximide

This compound is only effective against simple absences which are accompanied by regular spike-and-wave EEG paroxysms. It is usually well tolerated but may cause nausea and anorexia. Because of the concern about valproate hepatotoxicity, ethosuximide is still regarded by some paediatricians as the drug of choice for absences in children.

Phenobarbitone and primidone

These two related drugs should be considered to be second-line treatment because they produce sedation and adverse cognitive and behavioural effects. Undoubtedly there are people taking these drugs who are both well-controlled and without serious side-effects. But if a patient appears sedated, or is difficult, aggressive or moody, then consideration should be given to discontinuing them. Withdrawal fits may occur but the risk will be minimised if the patient is covered by another drug with an adequate serum level, and if reductions are made slowly (30 mg of phenobarbitone or 125 mg of primidone every four weeks).

Benzodiazepines

These drugs have a special role in the emergency treatment of seizures. Intravenous diazepam remains the drug of choice for terminating a fit, but both the oral and rectal route can be effective. The value of these drugs, when given on a long-term basis, is limited by sedation and the development of tolerance to their anticonvulsant action. They are of value, however, in managing myoclonic epilepsy, but withdrawal seizures may be a problem if treatment with a benzodiazepine is stopped.

Information and counselling

The diagnosis of epilepsy may have a profound impact on a person's life and the scope of this may not be apparent immediately. The experience of seizures occurring out of the blue may be disturbing enough, but the aftermath in which the driving licence is lost and employment and social life threatened may be a very difficult time indeed. The managing physician must be available to provide support during this period, and it is far more constructive to take time to alert patients to the potential consequences and their possible remedies rather than just letting them find out the hard way. The responsibility for providing such counselling lies with the physician, but the help of other professionals including teachers, careers advisors, social workers and advisors from voluntary organisations should be sought when appropriate. A number of the areas of concern listed in Table 25.2 can be dealt with by providing accurate intelligible information, for example about the driving licence regulations. Others, such as pregnancy and inheritance, require detailed knowledge about the individual patient as well as the ability to communicate constructively about complex and

Table 25.2: Counselling checklist

Diagnosis and its implications
Prognosis
The need for and nature of treatment
Self-care
The impact of fits on others
Telling other people
Problems at school
Careers
Leisure
Getting and keeping a job
Driving
Contraception and having a child

sometimes uncertain issues. Clearly not all the matters listed will be relevant to all patients, and some may only become relevant at a later time. For this reason the successful management of epilepsy, particularly in those cases which prove resistant to early drug treatment, requires a long-term commitment, which, with the present arrangement of health services, can be difficult to provide.

A STRATEGY FOR HABILITATION

The term 'habilitation' rather than rehabilitation is used deliberately as some of the secondary consequences of epilepsy begin at an early age and many can be prevented.

The needs of a particular patient will very much depend upon the age at which the epilepsy first starts, the frequency and severity of seizures, their response to initial treatment and the presence of other handicaps, if any. Patients therefore require a detailed individual assessment, but the outline given below may be a useful guideline to some of the problems that can be encountered. With all age groups a rapid response to treatment will substantially reduce the handicap due to epilepsy.

Epilepsy starting in childhood

Prognosis

The commonest form of seizures in very young children are febrile convulsions affecting 3 per cent of children. They often require no treatment and usually have no long-term effects. Indeed, the overall prognosis for children who have non-febrile fits is good, particularly so for simple absences and benign focal seizures which commonly remit as puberty approaches. However, the prospect for total seizure control may be less certain in children in whom there is other evidence of cerebral impairment. If the fits remit completely, and there are no associated handicaps, the child should not be restricted in any way apart from the inconvenience of having to take tablets. On the other hand, if seizures continue, particularly during waking hours, difficulties may be encountered at school in terms of learning, recreation and the development of social skills. In particular the following points should be considered:

(a) Frequent major fits may lead to poor school attendance, particularly if a child is removed from school inappropriately every time a fit occurs.

(b) Frequent absence seizures, which may be difficult to detect, can impair learning.

(c) Children with more severe epilepsy may have episodes of disorganised brain activity, not sufficient to cause a fit, but which may impair performance and learning.

(d) Although the majority of children with epilepsy are of average intelligence, it is also true that children with mental handicap have a high incidence of epilepsy.

(e) If the epilepsy was caused by some localised injury to the brain, this damage may also cause other educational problems, such as poor verbal skills if the dominant half of the brain is affected or poor practical skills if the non-dominant side is involved.

(f) Incorrect or excessive drug treatment can also impair school performance, particularly if it makes the child sleepy. However, drugs should not be blamed for everything, and it is often difficult to distinguish between the effects of drugs and those due to ongoing epileptic activity in the brain.

(g) The child may have a poor self-image and inadvertently be fulfilling low expectations expressed by parents and teachers. Behaviour problems seen in some children with epilepsy may be related directly to the epilepsy, but are also commonly due to difficulties in relationships within the family and with other children.

Many of these additional problems can be overcome by a positive attitude on the part of parents and teachers, and close liaison between all the professionals involved with the child. The advice of an educational psychologist should be sought if there are learning problems, and a few children with more severe difficulties can benefit from expert residential assessment where learning, behaviour, seizures, EEG discharges and AED levels can be monitored closely. Whereas the vast majority of children with epilepsy are educated in ordinary schools, a few children in whom the epilepsy is very severe, or those who are multiply handicapped, will benefit from residential schooling on a longer term basis.

Family reaction

The impact that a child's epilepsy will have on the normal dynamics of a family will very much depend on the severity of the epilepsy, the speed with which it can be controlled, the presence of other handicaps, the integrity of the family structure and the quality of the support and counselling provided at the time of initial diagnosis. Children with any disability can be overprotected by their parents, but this is particularly common if they have seizures which are accompanied by injury. Although this is a perfectly understandable reaction, it is usually counterproductive to the child's emotional development. Taking risks is an important part of growing up, and blanket restrictions on children with epilepsy are unacceptable. Almost all activities, including swimming, climbing, riding, cooking and laboratory work, are possible provided there is adequate supervision. Individual assessment is essential with support and counselling from members of the primary health care team and hospital and school personnel. This is very important if childhood epilepsy continues into adolescence without the seizures remitting, to prevent families from becoming increasingly disillusioned.

Epilepsy in adolescence and early adult life

Prognosis and medical management

Many of the considerations for childhood epilepsy are also applicable to epilepsy starting during adolescence. Diagnostic difficulties may be encountered in distinguishing seizures from simple faints, particularly those which end in convulsive movements, aggressive outbursts or other acting-out behaviour and anxiety states including panic attacks.

Drug treatment is mostly straightforward, but particular consideration has to be given to the possible adverse cognitive, behavioural and cosmetic effects. If seizures are completely controlled, early consideration should be given to withdrawing therapy after 2 or 3 years freedom from seizures. This should be considered before the young person is aged 14, so that if seizures do recur treatment can be re-introduced to prevent problems with career opportunities or obtaining a driving licence.

Personal development

In adolescents whose seizures remit quickly, and who are otherwise not handicapped, there should be no particular problems in reaching their full potential. Nevertheless, a few careers will be barred if fits have occurred since attaining the age of 5 (see Table 25.3). So accurate careers guidance

Table 25.3: Barriers to employment

1. *Fits only before the 5th birthday*
   — no restrictions (except train driver, guard or track worker with London Regional Transport)
2. *Any fits after the 5th birthday* (whether or not they are now controlled with or without drugs)
   — jobs requiring HGV, PSV, commercial aircraft pilot's licence are barred; also train driver with British Rail
   — unlikely to be accepted by Fire Brigade, Police, Armed Services and Merchant Navy
   — professional driving is officially discouraged
3. *Fits still occurring*
   — in addition to above, problems may be found in teaching in state schools; nursing; child care; working at heights, near water, with machinery; working alone for long periods

Notes
1. These are guidelines only, and exceptions may well be made.
2. Employees who develop epilepsy may be able to retain their job under certain circumstances.

at an early stage is important in order to prevent disappointment and frustration.

On the other hand the adolescent who continues to have seizures while awake may encounter problems in many areas, not the least of which are limited career opportunities and the inability to drive. The extent of the problems will depend upon a number of factors including the frequency and severity of seizures, but often more importantly on the existence of other handicaps and the attitude of the persons concerned and their families. Just as children need to take risks and learn from that experience, so adolescents need to assert their independence, a process which often causes parental anxiety even if the young person is not handicapped in any way. The occurrence of seizures may make this a genuinely hazardous process, but often the fear of what might happen is a more powerful and negative influence than experience based on what has happened.

Parental anxieties about the young person's sexual development, emotional relationships, marriage and future childbearing may not be readily voiced, but ample opportunity to explore these matters should be provided by the physician and other professionals who are involved. It is essential that the young adult with epilepsy, as with other disabilities, takes on responsibility for self-care, including coping with seizures and medication, and also does not blame every failure on the epilepsy. This is perhaps particularly crucial when looking for work, which is currently difficult enough for young people without a disability. The presence of active epilepsy undoubtedly does constitute a major handicap, and expert assistance may be required from the specialist careers advisors for the handicapped and Disablement Resettlement Officers at Job Centres. Young people with epilepsy should be encouraged to obtain academic qualifications as good as, if not better than, their peers and to take full advantage of further and higher education as well as the various employment schemes for young people provided by the Manpower Services Commission (MSC).

Special help

Sometimes the mainstream of medical, employment and social services cannot deal adequately with the complexities of epilepsy in a young person. In such cases residential assessment and rehabilitation in one of the assessment units for epilepsy may prove very worthwhile as a full multidisciplinary team will be in operation. Ideally referral should be made before the problems are too entrenched, and longer-term support by local services will often be necessary. The number of people who require special accommodation simply because of their epilepsy is very small, but those whose seizures are very frequent, or who have other handicaps, may require supervision on a long-term basis. This can be provided at home, in a community unit run by a local authority or voluntary organization, or in one of the larger residential Epilepsy Centres. There are advantages and disadvantages to all of these provisions.

Epilepsy in adult life

Adults with a lifelong history of seizures often cope remarkably well with the problems that this presents. It is clearly important for the managing physician to be absolutely sure that all avenues have been explored in an attempt to control the fits, and that the medication is rational and not producing unnecessary adverse effects. Providing they have the necessary skills and work experience many people in this situation can be successfully employed and live in the social setting of their choice. Women with epilepsy who wish to have children require special counselling and medical supervision before and during pregnancy, and sometimes extra support in caring for the baby.

Sadly some adults with intractable epilepsy encounter a whole host of problems in all aspects of daily living, and these will represent a challenge to the medical and social services. The managing physician may not be able to relieve the problems by controlling the seizures but is nevertheless pivotal in coordinating effort from other professionals and in providing long-term support.

In people whose epilepsy starts in adult life the prognosis and the problems that may stem from the epilepsy must be carefully distinguished from those of any underlying cause. Seizures may only be a small part of the disability caused by a stroke, severe head injury or brain tumour, but their rapid control can be an important factor in minimising any disability. Nevertheless, the loss of a driving licence (see Table 25.4) and thereby the threat to some jobs is a very serious consequence of the diagnosis which may, as a result, be a rejected by the patient (Chapter 47). Although the driving licence regulations cannot be waived in the light of individual circumstances, many employers will, if necessary, assist the person to remain in his existing job, or offer redeployment. Retraining schemes are available at the MSC's Employment Rehabilitation Centres, and support from trade unions should be enlisted if an employer appears to be unsympathetic. The managing physician may need to work closely with the firm's occupational health service, which can play a crucial part in supporting an employee with epilepsy in the workplace.

The adult who develops epilepsy will, in all probability, already have the necessary experience and skills needed for independent living, and is therefore not as vulnerable to the social problems as the younger person with epilepsy who may be denied the opportunity of obtaining these essential attributes. Nevertheless seizures, particularly if uncontrolled for a long time, can have a devastating effect on self-esteem and personal relation-

Table 25.4: Laws on driving and epilepsy

These are legal restrictions to which no exceptions can be made. They include all epileptic disturbances including myoclonic jerks, auras and fits which result from changes in medication on medical advice

The licence holder must declare the epilepsy to DVLC

Ordinary licences
Provided all other requirements are met:
(1) a licence can be granted if a person has not had any fits while awake for 2 years, with or without medication
(2) a licence can be granted to a person who continues to have fits *only while asleep* 3 years after the first sleep fit

HGV, PSV, commercial pilot's licence (also applies to taxi driver)
(1) these licences will not be granted to anyone who has had a single fit following their 5th birthday
(2) if a licence-holder has a single fit, the licence will be lost indefinitely

ships. Time should be taken, at an early stage, to provide counselling and information about epilepsy and its implications. Unfortunately many of the services that are available are not particularly well geared to assisting people who are economically and socially intact.

CONCLUSION

Epilepsy should not represent a severe disability to the majority of people who develop this condition. An accurate diagnosis, effective treatment and counselling can substantially reduce the impact that epilepsy may have, but despite the expertise and services that are available some people are still denied these vital ingredients. In addition there are a minority of people whose seizures remain intractable to treatment, and in some the disability will be severe. The ingredients to good management mentioned above are still vitally important to this group, and much can be done to prevent further negative factors such as low self-esteem, overprotection, poor educational achievement and a lack of living and employment skills from making the handicap even worse. For those who have already developed these secondary handicaps, assessment and rehabilitation is available at the assessment centres for epilepsy where many of these complex problems can be disentangled and habilitation programmes implemented. A very few people with epilepsy will nevertheless require a sheltered living environment where medical and social support can be provided on a long-term basis.

FURTHER READING

Treatment

Richens, A. (1982) Clinical pharmacology and medical treatment. In J.P. Laidlaw and A. Richens (eds), *A textbook of epilepsy*, 2nd edn, Churchill Livingstone, Edinburgh, pp. 292-348

Pregnancy

Dalessio, D.J. (1985) Seizure disorders and pregnancy. *N. Engl. J. Med.*, *312*, 559–63

Psychiatric Problems

Reynolds, E.H. and Trimble, M.R. (eds) (1982) *Epilepsy and psychiatry*, Churchill Livingstone, Edinburgh

EEG monitoring

Binnie, C.D. (1983) Telemetric EEG monitoring in epilepsy. In T.A. Pedley and B.S. Meldrum (eds), *Recent advances in epilepsy*, vol. I, Churchill Livingstone, Edinburgh, pp. 155–78

Employment

Epilepsy and employment symposium (1986) (eds) F. Edwards, M.K. Espir and J. Oxley, Royal Society of Medicine, London, International Congress Series No. 86

Education

Children and young people with epilepsy — an educational package for teachers (1985) National Society for Epilepsy, Chalfont St Peter, Bucks SL9 0RJ

Other facts

NSE Leaflet series: *Explaining epilepsy*, National Society for Epilepsy leaflet series. *The Epilepsy Reference Book* (1985) P.M. Jeavons and A. Aspinall, Harper & Row, London

J. Laidlaw, A. Richens and J. Oxley (1988) *A textbook of epilepsy* (1988), 3rd edn, Churchill Livingstone, Edinburgh

26

Less Common Neurological Diseases

John Goodwill

Only a few of the less common diseases are discussed here; they are of numerous types, and many are genetically determined, the offspring either suffering from, or carrying, the disease. The functional problems will depend not only on the natural history of the condition but also on the social and psychological condition of the patient, as well as the family and environment in which he lives. Some of the diseases discussed occur mainly in childhood, but some patients survive to be disabled adults; without understanding of the childhood care it is not possible to adequately treat them as adults. Although the underlying pathology cannot be treated much can be done by sympathetic assessment of the disability and a functional approach used to provide appropriate care, advice and aids or equipment. If an attitude of hopelessness develops it will spread to other family members with resulting family, marital and other problems (See Chapter 5, Assessment; Chapter 30, Sexual problems).

Hansen's disease is not discussed, and because poliomyelitis is now uncommon in Western Europe only a few notes are included, together with suggestions for further reading.

MUSCULAR DYSTROPHIES

The two commoner types of X-linked muscular dystrophies are Duchenne and Becker, their management has been reviewed by Gardner-Medwin (1980) and Fowler (1982). The severe *Duchenne type* starts in boys between the ages of one and five years with progressive muscle weakness and the frequent occurrence of contractures and scoliosis. Patients eventually die from respiratory problems, not usually surviving beyond the age of 20–22 years; cardiac involvement also occurs. As with other progressive diseases much time is needed for discussion with the patient, parents and siblings to get the best out of life. The activities of siblings may be restricted by the disabled brother and depression, aggression or overprotection may occur. The boy must be encouraged to exercise as much as possible, including swimming and sports, if he is still strong enough. Physiotherapy helps to maintain muscle strength, and stretching of joints through their full range of movement reduces the occurrence of contractures which occur particularly in the leg joints. Light plastic night splints may be useful in preventing equinus. Later in the disease contractures may also occur in the elbows, wrists and fingers. As the muscles weaken, making walking difficult, lightweight above-knee orthoses may help the boy to continue walking for six to 30 months longer, but tenotomy of the tendo achilles and possibly of the iliotibial bands is usually needed first (Gardner-Medwin, 1979; Spencer and Vignos, 1962; Heckmatt *et al.*, 1985). Surgery and bracing of the legs must be used together, and the feet should be plantigrade.

Osteoporosis occurs. This prediposes to fractures particularly of the lower end of the femur but these heal satisfactorily. Sticks or crutches help to maintain walking but a wheelchair is usually needed by the age of ten or eleven years. Within one or two years further weakness requires the use of an electric wheelchair, the supply of which should not be delayed (Chapter 43). It is not helpful to force the boy to expend all his limited energy on the propulsion of his chair so that he is too exhausted to pursue enjoyable activities.

Kyphoscoliosis is frequent, although those who develop hyperextension of the spine with lumbar lordosis do not usually develop severe kyphoscoliosis or pelvic obliquity (Wilkins and Gibson, 1976). It seems reasonable to try and maintain extension of the spine and lumbar lordosis with a moulded polypropylene or block leather jacket although orthotic management of the scoliosis does not necessarily prevent progression (Seeger *et al.*, 1984). Spinal stabilisation may be needed (Gibson *et el.*, 1978). The wheelchair cushion should be on a firm supporting base, if necessary with side cushions to keep him upright in the wheelchair and thus to maintain the arms in a functional position. A moulded seat is another means of holding the boy in a good position but this restricts movements (Chapter 43). When the arms are too weak to lift food to the mouth, or to use a pen or keyboard, mobile arm supports (MAS) may allow these functions to be achieved by counterbalancing the weight of the arms (Chyatte *et al.*, 1965; Haworth *et al.*, 1978; Yasuda and Bowman, 1986). Details of MAS and their adjustment are given in Chapter 45. An electric typewriter and a computer/word processor help to maintain useful interest in life. There is also the need to maintain purposeful education and outside interests within the limits of the increasing locomotor handicap. This becomes even more important in later teenage, when the boy knows he is getting very weak and may have seen an elder brother progressing in this way. There is also a non-progressive intellectual deficit with a mean IQ between 75 and 85, the verbal score usually being lower than the performance score (Karagan, 1979).

The Becker type of dystrophy starts in boys usually between the ages of five and 15 years, it progresses much more slowly and walking may be possible into the 20s and 30s with a mean survival to 42 years (Gardner-Medwin, 1980). The problems and solutions are partly similar to those of the Duchenne type, but because the patient will survive into his 30s or 40s he will become an independent adult and need advice on wheelchair, housing, hoists, adaptations to the house, car, etc. (Chapters 39, 44 and 47). While the basic disease is untreatable that does not apply to the patient, for whom much can be done with the right technology and a positive attitude to assessment and advice about the problems. Not uncommonly the patient has been told that he has Duchenne type dystrophy in childhood, and has been led to expect a much worse prognosis than is the fact. In adult life such a patient may well be resentful of the health professionals for allowing this to happen; this makes advice more difficult. Clearly these patients are capable of sedentary work for many years (Chapter 41).

Facioscapulohumeral muscular dystrophy occurs equally in the two sexes, usually starting in adolescence or early adult life. Weakness of facial movement as well as causing lack of expression causes obvious difficulty with playing wind instruments. The common early difficulties are due to limb girdle weakness causing inability to do heavy work. Modification of the working environment, in conjunction with the Disablement Resettlement Officer from the Department of Employment, may enable the patient to continue working — financial support for required modifications being provided, or early job resettlement should be considered (Chapter 41). Driving may be impaired due to arm weakness, but usually power steering and brakes with automatic transmission will remove the problem until late in the course of the disease (Chapter 47).

Weakness of the legs may require below-knees plastic orthoses for foot-drop, and also the use of walking aids (Chapter 46). As the condition is only slowly progressive it is usually many years before the patient requires a wheelchair because of severe hip and knee weakness. The latter cannot be supported by knee orthoses because by this time the arms are too weak to use walking aids. However, once a wheelchair is needed it may be difficult to propel because of weak arm muscles. A few patients find it easier with the large propelling wheels at the front, but others use the usual rear propelling wheels, gaining extra purchase by hooking their arms under the pushing handles on the back of the chair. When these problems arise the need for an electric wheelchair is near; however, this may remove the last trace of exercise that the patient does. The power control may be mounted on the armrest, but it may have to be modified or positioned more centrally (Chapter 43).

Progressive arm weakness may cause the patient to support one elbow with the opposite hand in order to lift the arm up for some activities (see

Figure 26.1). If glenohumeral abduction is preserved, but there is weakness of scapular muscles causing instability of the scapulothoracic joint, the scapula can be fixed to the thorax (Copeland and Howard, 1978; Ketenjian, 1978). A higher, broader arm rest may be fitted to the wheelchair to support the arm in a better functional position for eating, shaving, etc. Later a *mobile arm support* (MAS) can be used to counterbalance the weight of the arms so that even Grade 2 (out of 5) shoulder movement and elbow flexion is sufficient to give useful function (Chapter 45). Writing may be difficult and an electric typewriter, possibly with a computer/word processor, may be helpful if correctly positioned. As weakness progresses an electric bed and environmental control equipment are needed to maintain some independence (Chapter 48).

Limb girdle muscular dystrophy occurs in either sex starting in teenage or early adult life. The condition only progresses slowly, but usually after

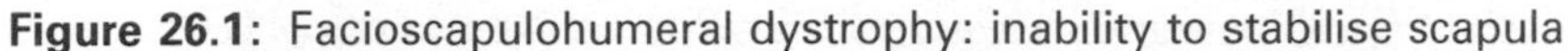

Figure 26.1: Facioscapulohumeral dystrophy: inability to stabilise scapula

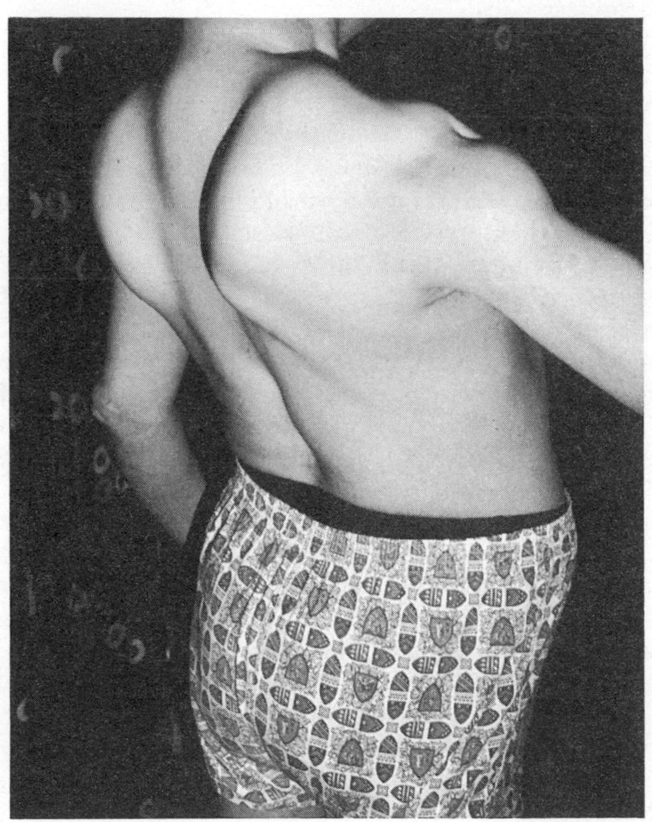

15 or 20 years the patient is disabled. The practical problems and solutions are similar to those with facioscapulohumeral dystrophy.

Myotonic dystrophy begins in teenage or early adult life, with weakness of muscles in the face, hands and forearms, later involving the feet, proximal limb muscles, the pharynx and larynx. The facial expression becomes blank, dysphagia and dysarthria occur, and walking becomes increasingly difficult. Besides the failure of muscle relaxation and progressive muscle weakness, there is premature frontal baldness in the male, atrophy of the gonads, cataracts and cardiac involvement, the last also occurring in some other dystrophies. Patients eventually die of respiratory infection, but cardiac dysrhythmia may also occur. Practical help is needed in the supply of below-knee orthoses for drop foot, appropriate advice on car and work modification and later about a wheelchair, most patients being unable to walk within 15–20 years of diagnosis. An additional problem with this condition is dementia, which may make it difficult for patients to accept or understand advice, less able to take initiative in overcoming their own disability problems and so less rewarding for staff to treat; this last factor is a problem with any condition in which patients are likely to be rather passive and unresponsive.

SPINAL MUSCULAR ATROPHIES (SMA)

Clinical heterogeneity within the spinal muscular atrophies (SMA) has long been a source of confusion for questions of prognosis and genetic counselling (Pearn, 1980). In his review of 240 patients different modes of inheritance occurred with different types. Most had their onset early in childhood although the Kugelberg–Welander type may appear later in childhood and the patient may well live into middle adult life. The distal type of SMA has some similarities to Charcot–Marie–Tooth disease, and again the patient survives for many years. There is also an adult-onset type of SMA which occurred in 8 per cent of this series at a median age of 37 years and again progresses slowly. This must be distinguished from motor neurone disease. Thus although many patients with SMA die during childhood one sees some young or middle-aged adults with this progressive neurogenic weakness for whom rehabilitation offers a real prospect of improvement in everyday function. The limb and limb girdle muscles are involved, as well as more distal muscles, but those of the face are spared. It is always important to distinguish this disease from a muscular dystrophy.

The problems are somewhat similar to those in Duchenne muscular dystrophy, and include the problems of prevention and treatment of scoliosis. Here we are concerned with those that either survive or have the onset in adult life. Weakness of hand muscles makes manipulation of everyday objects difficult; larger handles on cutlery, etc., may help. As arm weakness progresses to become a major problem the patient has usually ceased walking and a fixed or mobile arm support may be needed on the wheelchair as in muscular dystrophy. Physiotherapy is used to prevent contractures of the hand or shoulder; it is less of a problem at the elbow, and is also needed to stretch the leg joints. Tight tendo achilles easily occurs; a night splint may help but contracture there, or at the knee or hip, is rarely an indication for surgical release. In adults with SMA progression of the weakness is usually slow. They may be helped by below-knee orthoses but, as with limb girdle weakness in muscular dystrophy, by the time the knees are weak enough to require supporting by orthoses the arms are usually too weak to use walking aids, and so a wheelchair is required. If the proximal arm and shoulder muscles are greatly weakened the chair will need to be electrically driven (Chapter 43).

Later on these young disabled adults will also be unable to transfer in and out of the wheelchair, so require house modifications, hoists and also a care package of Social Service and Health Service staff to come in at regular times during the day to take some of the strain off the family. Usually it is the patient's mother who eventually does much of the caring for the patient at home. However, she is usually elderly by this time, and without support the patient will require admission to an institution. A recent review of SMA (Eng *et al.*, 1984) reviews the problems in children, but there is little published on the management of these patients in adult life. The spinal deformity problems in children are reviewed by Hensinger and MacEwen (1976), but by the time one sees these patients as adults the management of spinal deformity is by wheelchair cushioning and possibly a moulded seat. Schwentker and Gibson (1976) reviewed orthopaedic aspects of SMA in children. Ten of their 130 patients had required surgery for lower limb deformities but again release surgery in the adult for the hip, knee or tendo achilles is rarely indicated.

CHARCOT–MARIE–TOOTH DISEASE

This type of hereditary motor and sensory neuropathy usually starts in childhood or teenage with symptoms of weakness of small hand muscles or of difficulty in walking. Pes cavus, clawing of the toes and scoliosis are associated. There is slowly progressive muscle weakness spreading up the leg to just above the knees, and also weakness of small hand muscles which slowly spreads to those of the lower forearms. The former weakness causes difficulty in walking, with dropped feet noted during the swing phase of gait. In this situation a below-knee ortholon or polypropylene orthosis may be helpful (Chapter 45). These are moulded to the shape of the calf and foot, are put on under the sock and go easily into the shoe without showing. If there is also instability of the hindfoot during stance phase, which is not controlled by a polypropylene orthosis, then a below-knee double-upright metal orthosis with ankle stops is needed.

The pes cavus may cause problems of shoe fitting, particularly for women, as extra depth in the shoe is required; if necessary the shoes are specially made with insoles providing support behind the metatarsal heads and under the arch of the foot. Neuropathic joints may occur in the hindfoot but these are usually pain-free, requiring only strong leather shoes or boots with moulded insoles. Scoliosis may be the first aspect of the condition noted, in which case the patient must be reviewed by an interested orthopaedic surgeon and regular scoliosis X-rays taken to assess whether the curve is increasing or stationary, bracing and/or surgical treatment being used as for idiopathic scoliosis. In a series of 69 patients with CMT, 7 had kyphoscoliosis, 2 were mild, 2 required bracing and 3 needed spinal stabilisation (Hensinger *et al.*, 1976).

Although the hands are involved early in the disease, the patient is not usually disabled by this until later in the disease. Weakness of thenar muscle causes difficulty in opposition of the thumb which may require an orthosis to support the thumb in a functional position (Chapter 45). In general the very slowly progressive nature of the condition allows the patient to adapt. There may be interference with occupations or hobbies requiring intricate hand movements such as playing a musical instrument, and for those interested perhaps a keyboard is easier than strings or woodwind intruments.

HEREDITARY ATAXIAS

Friedreich's ataxia is the most common of this group of disorders. It starts in childhood or early adult life. Besides involvement of the cerebellum it causes atrophy of the dorsal columns of the spinal cord as well as the spinocerebellar and, sometimes, the corticospinal tracts. Pes cavus and kyphoscoliosis are associated, as with Charcot–Marie–Tooth disease, and require the same management. A wide-base ataxic gait is an early symptom which is little influenced by physiotherapy. The patient will need walking aids, especially later as the ataxia is worsened by proprioceptive loss. Dropped foot due to weakness of foot dorsiflexor muscles causes foot dragging during swing phase of gait, correctable by a below-knee orthosis. Intention tremor in the hands, and some dysarthria, occur later, causing difficulties with work and other everyday activities.

GUILLAIN–BARRÉ SYNDROME

This acute demyelinating polyradiculoneuritis causes ascending muscle weakness and sensory loss which may involve the respiratory muscles and require assisted ventilation. About 7 per cent of patients die, and a further 16 per cent suffer residual disability (Hughes and Winer, 1984); in another series (Winer *et al.*, 1985) eight out of 71 died (11 per cent), all these patients having a severe neuropathy. Failure to improve within three weeks of onset, or the need for assisted ventilation, were poor prognostic signs (Eberle *et al.*, 1975). Muscles are weaker in the legs than the arms, and besides the possible need for ventilation, treatment in the acute stage is directed at stretching of the weak muscles to prevent joint contractures, especially of the ankle, knee or hip.

As strength gradually improves resisted exercises are started to restore muscle strength; the patient is mobilised on a tilt table so that he is only slowly brought into the upright posture, otherwise postural hypotension may occur, partly due to voluntary muscle weakness and partly due to autonomic dysfunction. Flaccid foot-drop requires plastic below-knee orthoses, and if quadriceps weakness is present the orthoses must extend above the knee (Chapter 45).

Wiederholt *et al.* (1964) in a review of 97 patients reported 6 deaths; 61 patients had complete recovery within one year but 12 patients had incomplete recovery, mainly having persistent distal leg weakness. Ten had recurrences or relapses of the illness; the remainder were recent cases or were lost to follow-up. Löffel *et al.* (1977) reported 3 deaths in a series of 123 cases with complete recovery in 57 per cent, but 22 per cent had persistent motor signs, again mainly in the legs, 2 patients had minimal facial weakness and 4 children showed slight ataxia due to CNS involvement. In a recent series 51 out of 71 patients had some difficulty with walking when reviewed one year after onset of the illness (Winer *et al.*, 1985).

It is therefore clear that, even when the patient has survived the acute stage of the illness, he may still require prolonged physiotherapy with the use of orthoses, walking aids and car modifications (Chapters 45, 46 and 47). The residual disability may require changes in lifestyle, work and social activities, and even with good recovery and no relapse fatigue may persist for 12–18 months.

OTHER PERIPHERAL NEUROPATHIES

Whether these are due to metabolic or endocrine disorders, deficiencies or toxic agents, most do not present a problem of rehabilitation but of drug or other management of the primary disease. A few, such as those with persistent alcoholic neuropathy, develop foot-drop sufficient to require below-knee orthoses. There have been outbreaks of severe paralysis due to toxic agents such as triorthocresyl phosphate, some of these patients having widespread persistent paralysis comparable to that seen after poliomyelitis. They require prolonged physiotherapy to prevent contractures, to increase the muscle strength and restore function. Orthoses may be required to support the knee and/or ankle. Some patients poisoned by this chemical have been persistently paralysed and required a wheelchair, but apart from this, severe paralysis due to neuropathy is uncommon.

Diabetic neuropathy can cause problems of pain management (Chapter 7), and in the feet, especially when combined with peripheral vascular disease, ulcers and infection occur, these being largely preventable by adequate attention to footwear (Chapter 45). The most common cause of neuropathy is Hansen's disease, which is not discussed further in this book, although as in diabetes attention to footwear can prevent some problems.

POLIOMYELITIS

Poliomyelitis is due to any one of three serologically distinct viruses, which produce an identical clinical condition. It is now uncommon in Western countries although frequent in other parts of the world, probably about 500,000 cases occurring annually worldwide. Frequently there is no paralysis of muscles, but when it occurs about 80 per cent is confined to the legs (Ward, 1983), a similar figure of 54 out of 76 patients being found in a recent survey in Tanzania (Cross and Webber, 1985). An excellent recent review of 3,000 new patients with paralytic poliomyelitis found the usual male: female ratio of 1.3: 1.0, and 18 per cent of their patients were over nine years of age. 404 patients required surgery and 2,210 needed orthoses and/or special shoes (Rastogi *et al.*, 1983).

In the acute stage of the disease, in addition to maintaining ventilation, the aims of treatment are the same as for other causes of flaccid paralysis:

(1) to maintain skin viability and prevent pressure sores;

(2) to maintain muscle length and prevent contractures;

(3) to increase muscle strength: (a) in partially paralysed muscles, (b) in normal muscles to compensate for other weak muscles;

(4) to provide appropriate orthoses, walking aids, wheelchairs, etc.;

(5) to consider surgery for residual paralysis, where it can help to reduce functional disability and restore function.

In the UK we still have patients with residual paralysis, especially of the legs, who require orthoses, car modifications, or even surgery for increasing deformity (Chapters 45, 47 and 28). It is clear that some patients develop increasing disability many years after maximum functional recovery from the acute stage, which occurs up to 6 years from onset. These late problems occur at a mean time of 26 years later, causing increasing difficulty with mobility, activities of daily living, work and social activities due to fatigue, muscle weakness, joint and/or muscle pains, all of which require renewed medical attention (Halstead *et al.*, 1985; Halstead and Rossi, 1985; Holman, 1986). Some patients show a late decline in respiratory function (Alcock *et al.*, 1984).

To discuss this subject adequately would require a whole chapter, so the reader is referred to other texts.

REFERENCES

Muscular dystrophies and spinal muscular atrophies

Chyatte, S.B., Long, C. and Vignos, P.J. (1965) Balanced forearm orthoses in muscular dystrophy. *Arch Phys. Med. Rehabil., 46*, 633-6

Copeland, S.A. and Howard, R.C. (1978) Thoraco scapular fusion for facioscapulohumeral dystrophy. *J. Bone Joint Surg., 60b*, 547-51

Eng, B.D., Binder, H. and Koch, B. (1984) Spinal muscular atrophy; experience in diagnosis and rehabilitation management of 60 patients. *Arch. Phys. Med. Rehabil., 65*, 549-53

Fowler, W.M. (1982) Rehabilitation management of muscular dystrophy and related disorders. *Arch. Phys. Med. Rehabil., 63*, 322-8

Gardner-Medwin, D. (1979) Controversies about Duchenne muscular dystrophy. Bracing for ambulation. *Dev. Med., Child Neurol., 21*, 659-62

Gardner-Medwin D. (1980) Rehabilitation in muscular dystrophy. *Int. Rehabil. Med., 2*, 104-10

Gibson, D.A., Koreska, J., Robertson, D., Kahn, A. and Albisser, A.M. (1978) The management of spinal deformity in Duchenne muscular dystrophy. *Orthop. Clin. North Am., 9*, 437-50

Haworth, R., Dunscombe, S. and Nichols, P.J.R. (1978) Mobile arm supports; an evaluation. *Rheum. Rehabil., 17*, 240-5

Heckmatt, J.Z., Dubowitz, V, Hyde, S. A., Florence, J., Gabain, A.C. and Thompson, N. (1985) Prolongation of walking in Duchenne muscular dystrophy with lightweight orthoses; review of 57 cases. *Dev. Med. Child Neurol., 27*, 149-54

Hensinger, R.N. and MacEwen, G.D. (1976) Spinal deformity associated with heritable neurological conditions; spinal muscular atrophy, Friedreich's ataxia, familial dysautonomia and Charcot–Marie–Tooth-disease. *J. Bone Joint Surg., 58a*, 13-24

Karagan, N.J. (1979) Intellectual functioning in Duchenne muscular dystrophy: a review. *Psychol. Bull., 86*, 250-9

Ketenjian, A.Y. (1978) Scapulo-costal stabilization for scapular winging in facioscapulohumeral muscular dystrophy. *J. Bone Joint Surg., 60a*, 476-80

Pearn, J. (1980) Classification of spinal muscular atrophies. *Lancet, 1*, 919-22

Schwentker, E.P. and Gibson, D.A. (1976) The orthopaedic aspects of spinal muscular atrophy. *J. Bone Joint Surg., 58a*, 32-8

Seeger, B.R., Andrew, D.A., Sutherland, M.B. and Clark, M.S. (1984) Orthotic management of scoliosis in Duchenne muscular dystrophy. *Arch. Phys. Med. Rehabil., 65*, 83-6

Spencer G.E. and Vignos, P.J. (1962) Bracing for ambulation in childhood progressive muscular dystrophy. *J. Bone Joint Surg.*, *44a*, 234-42
Wilkins, K.E. and Gibson, D.A. (1976) The patterns of spinal deformity in Duchenne muscular dystrophy. *J. Bone Joint Surg.*, *58a*, 24-32
Yasuda, Y.L. and Bowman, K. (1986) Mobile arm supports; criteria for successful use in muscle disease patients. *Arch. Phys. Med Rehabil.*, *67*, 253-6

Guillain–Barré syndrome

Eberle, E., Brink, J., Azen, J. and White, D. (1975) Early predictors of incomplete recovery in children with Guillain–Barré polyneuritis. *J. Paediatr.*, *86*, 356-9
Löffel, N.B., Rossi, L.N., Mumenthaler, M., Lutschg, J. and Ludin, H.P. (1977) The Landry–Guillain–Barré syndrome. *J. Neurol. Sci.*, *33*, 71-9
Hughes, R.A.C. and Winer, J.B. (1984) Guillain–Barré syndrome. In W.B. Mathews, and G.H. Glaser (eds), *Recent advances in clinical neurology, 4*, Churchill Livingstone, Edinburgh, pp. 19-49
Wiederholt, W.C., Mulder, D.W. and Lambert, E.H. (1964) The Landry–Guillain–Barré-Strohl syndrome or polyradiculoneuropathy: historical review, report of 97 patients, and present concepts. *Proc. Mayo Clin.*, *39*, 427-51
Winer, J.B., Hughes, R.A.C., Greenwood, R.J., Perkin, G.D. and Healy, M.J.R. (1985) Prognosis in Guillain–Barré syndrome. *Lancet*, *1*, 1202-3

Poliomyelitis

Alcock, A.J., Hildes, J.A., Kaufert, P.A. and Bickford, J. (1984) Respiratory poliomyelitis: a follow-up study. *Can. Med. Assoc. J.*, *130*, 1305-10
Cross, A.B. and Webber, R.H. (1985) A poliomyelitis survey the simple way: the Tanzanian experience. *Br. Med. J.*, *291*, 532-4
Halstead, L.S. and Rossi, C.D. (1985) New problems in old polio patients: results of a survey of 539 polio survivors. *Orthopaedics*, *8*, 845-50
Halstead, L.S., Wiechers, D.O. and Rossi, C.D. (1985) Results of a survey of 201 polio survivors. *South Med. J.*, *78*, 1281-7
Holman, K.G. (1986) Post-polio syndrome. The battle with an old foe resumes. *Postgrad. Med. (Minneapolis)*, *79*, 44-53
Rastogi, S., Agarwal, A.K., Sipani, A.K., Varma, S. and Goel, M.K. (1983) A clinical study of post polio infantile paralysis. *Prosthet. Orthot. Int.*, *7*, 29-32
Ward, N.A. (1983) Poliomyelitis: a review. *Tropical Doctor*, *13*, 21-8

FURTHER READING

Bossingham, B.H., Williams, P and Nichols, P.J.R. (1979) *Severe childhood neuromuscular disease; the management of Duchenne muscular dystrophy and spinal muscular atrophy*, Muscular Dystrophy Group of Great Britain, London
The Physically Handicapped Child (1984) ed. Gillian McCarthy, Faber & Faber, London
Disorders of voluntary muscles (1981) ed. J.N. Walton, Churchill Livingstone, Edinburgh

27

Spasticity

David Marsden

INTRODUCTION

The term spasticity is derived from the Greek word spastikos which means to draw or tug. The clinician detects spasticity as a characteristic resistance to passive movement of a joint. At first, as the joint is passively extended or flexed, a mounting resistance is encountered, which is more marked the more rapid or sudden the stretching movement. After a certain range of passive movement, this resistance diminishes and the stretched muscle relaxes, more or less completely. This waxing and waning of resistance as the joint is moved through its range of action distinguishes spasticity from extrapyramidal rigidity, which consists of a constant resistance to passive movement throughout the range of joint movement (so-called lead pipe rigidity.)

The patient experiences the consequences of spasticity when attempting to move. Muscles become unnaturally stiff, often causing the limb to move into an abnormal or awkward posture, and the movement itself is executed clumsily. Some patients with severe spasticity may experience spontaneous muscle spasms, either in the form of repetitive clonus, or as flexor or extensor mass contractions or spasms.

Spasticity occurs when the 'parapyramidal' corticospinal motor pathways are damaged. Lesions of the 'pyramidal tract' in the medullary pyramid do not cause spasticity, but produce the Babinski response, or extensor plantar response, and abolish the contralateral abdominal reflexes. Lesions of the 'parapyramidal' pathways in the internal capsule spare other motor systems arising in the brainstem, such as the rubrospinal, vestibulospinal and reticulospinal pathways. Spinal cord lesions destroy not only corticospinal 'parapyramidal' pathways, but also these various bulbospinal systems. Accordingly, spasticity due to capsular lesions, which almost always are due to stroke, differs from that produced by damage to the spinal cord. However, after acute damage to either the internal capsule or the spinal cord, there is a phase of cerebral or spinal shock.

Cerebral and spinal shock

Immediately following a stroke or acute spinal cord injury, the affected limbs are flaccid, and the tendon jerks are absent. This cerebral or spinal shock persists for days or weeks, and the longer the limbs remain flaccid the worse the prognosis. However, with time, muscle tone gradually returns and spasticity appears.

Cerebral spasticity

The spasticity that gradually develops after a capsular hemiplegia has a characteristic distribution. In the arm it is the flexors that become spastic, and the extensors become selectively weak, so that the arm is held flexed and pronated across the chest, with the fingers over the thumb into the palm. In the leg, it is the extensors that become spastic, while the flexors become weak, so that the leg is held extended, with the foot plantar-flexed and inverted.

This hemiplegic posture is typical of damage in the internal capsule, but also may be produced by large cortical lesions, which inevitably destroy not only the motor cortex (Area 4), but also adjacent areas such as the supplementary motor cortex in the pre-motor area (Area 6). Very discrete lesions of the motor cortex alone (Area 4) may produce a weakness without spasticity. In addition, such discrete lesions of the motor cortex usually produce weakness focused on one limb or part of one limb, particularly the hand, and equal in both flexors and extensors. This different pattern of cortical weakness distinguishes it from that of hemiplegic weakness.

Spinal spasticity

Flexor spasticity gradually emerges over the first one to six months after the end of spinal shock. After flexor synergies appear, extensor synergies also gradually emerge, but more slowly. Eventually, in most cases, extensor spasticity predominates. There is considerable individual variation in the time course of these changes, and in the relative predominance of flexor as against extensor spasticity. Flexor spasm usually is provoked by noxious stimuli, such as those induced by urinary retention, infection and calculi, obstinate constipation, and breakdown of the skin. Paraplegia in flexion usually is the result of inadequate care of the bladder, bowel and skin, and most commonly is seen in those without a reliable automatic bladder and with bedsores. Extensor spasticity, on the other hand, is promoted by proprioceptive impulses from muscles and tendons provoked by appropriate physical therapy.

PATHOPHYSIOLOGY OF SPASTICITY

Spasticity is due to the sum of the consequence of exaggerated stretch reflexes and overactive anterior horn cells in the spinal cord. The former are dependent upon the activity of fusimotor gamma neurones driving muscle spindles and intact dorsal roots which carry the spindle input to the cord (gamma spasticity). The latter is independent of spindle input, but results from unbridled spontaneous anterior horn cell activity (alpha spasticity).

In most patients, gamma spasticity exceeds alpha spasticity. Usually there is no spontaneous activity in spastic muscles at rest, but stretch provokes a reflex electromyographic (EMG) response, the magnitude of which increases approximately linearly in proportion to the velocity of the stretching movement. In most patients the EMG response ceases when the movement stops, and slow stretch evokes no response. These observations indicate that spasticity is due to exaggerated responses in dynamic Group I afferent fibres from primary muscle spindle endings, but the static response of Group II fibres from secondary endings also contributes. For example, stretch of fixed velocity produces a reflex response in the hamstrings which progressively increases as the muscle is stretched, whereas that in quadriceps progressively diminishes as that muscle is stretched. Clearly, receptors signalling muscle length facilitate flexor reflexes and inhibit extensor reflexes in spasticity, and Group II muscle afferents exhibit just these properties. Such secondary spindle afferent input appears to facilitate flexor action, but inhibits extensor activity. The latter appears to be responsible for the clasp-knife phenomenon of mounting resistance to passive stretch of spastic muscles, followed by collapse of such resistive force once the critical length has been passed.

Group II afferent input from secondary muscle spindle endings are grouped together with input from cutaneous and deep pain receptors as flexor reflex afferents, which facilitate flexor motor neurones and inhibit extensor motor neurones. The spinal effects of flexor reflex afferent input are enhanced by corticoreticulospinal input but are inhibited by pathways from the pontomedullary reticular formation that travel in the dorsolateral funiculus of the spinal cord (the dorsal reticulospinal system). Capsular hemiplegias destroy the facilitatory corticoreticulospinal pathways, but leave the inhibitory bulbospinal pathways intact, thus favouring inhibition of flexor reflex afferent activity and evolution of extensor tone, especially in the leg. Spinal lesions, on the other hand, also destroy the bulbospinal inhibitory pathways, so that unbridled flexor reflex activity tends to dominate, causing flexor spasticity, particularly if there is excessive nociceptive input from bladder, bowels or skin.

The Babinski response, which arises from damage to direct corticospinal 'pyramidal' pathways, may be reinforced by additional flexor withdrawal of the whole leg when there is additional damage to the bulbospinal pathways, as in spinal cord lesions.

Finally, spinal reciprocal inhibition is disturbed in those with cerebral spasticity due, for example, to capsular hemiplegia. Reciprocal Ia inhibition normally leads to suppression of activity in the antagonist muscle when the agonist is stretched, via a disynaptic spinal pathway involving an interneurone. In capsular hemiplegia reciprocal inhibition of extensors by flexors is suppressed, while that of flexors by extensors is enhanced, particularly in the leg. This balance tends to favour extension of the leg, and overcomes the minor degree of enhancement of flexor reflexes produced by capsular hemiplegia. In contrast, this imbalance of reciprocal inhibition is not evident in spinal spasticity, which is dominated by the consequences of flexor reflex activity, unless the latter is prevented by scrupulous attention to care of bowels, bladder and skin, and by reinforcement of extensor synergies by proprioceptive facilitation.

FUNCTIONAL CONSEQUENCES OF SPASTICITY

The disability produced by spasticity varies considerably from patient to patient, and spasticity may be beneficial to some. In particular, those with stroke may utilise extensor spasticity in the leg to turn it into a stable prop on which to walk, while those with partial spinal lesions also may depend upon spasticity to keep the legs extended so as to bear the weight of the body (spastic crutches). In general, spasticity may aid function in the legs, but never that of the arms.

Frequently it is difficult to apportion relative blame for motor deficit between spasticity and weakness. In the case of the leg, removal of spasticity by drug therapy in those with partial spinal lesions often causes more disability, for removal of the prop of the spastic limbs reveals that they are too weak to support the weight of the body. Similary, in children with cerebral palsy, spasticity may be unimportant relative to profound disturbances of postural mechanisms due to additional damage. Such children cannot use their spastic limbs because they cannot stabilise their trunk and neck adequately.

Despite these caveats, however, spasticity can cause considerable disability in many patients, particularly in those with stroke, severe head injury, disseminated sclerosis, spinal cord compression or trauma.

Spasticity interferes with arm function by preventing extension of the fingers and wrist, and by distortion of normal movement patterns as a result of breakdown of normal reciprocal inhibition of antagonists in the case of cerebral spasticity. It is unrealistic to expect return of fine manual function in those with capsular hemiplegia, particularly if there is any sensory loss. However, the flexor synergies of the hemiplegic arm can be valuable to support weight, steady objects and carry with a simian grip, provided they are not rendered useless by spasticity.

Spasticity of the legs leads to scissoring of the thighs, and forced plantar-flexion and inversion of the feet on walking. In those with severe spinal spasticity, flexor or even extensor spasms may cause great pain, and may make nursing and self care extremely difficult, and sometimes impossible. Severe flexor and adductor spasms of the legs in the female make bladder and bowel care a great problem, and virtually prevent any sexual activity. Flexor spasms, which frequently are triggered by movement, may make it impossible for the paraplegic to transfer from wheelchair to bed or lavatory, so destroying their independence. For all these reasons prevention and treatment of spasticity may considerably alleviate disability.

PREVENTION OF SPASTICITY

In the discussion on the pathophysiology of spasticity, emphasis was placed upon the capacity of nociceptive stimuli to make established spasticity much worse. Now there are good reasons to believe that such stimuli may provoke the development of spasticity. In the phase of cerebral or spinal shock, repeated afferent input into the spinal cord is likely to establish the connectivity and density of synaptic sprouting that follows anterior horn cell denervation. For this reason, every attempt must be made to avoid those nociceptive stimuli known to favour the development of spasticity, particularly the flexor spasticity that may appear after spinal injury.

In those with established spasticity, spasm may increase during urinary tract infections, urinary retention, faecal impaction, deep vein thrombosis, and many other intercurrent illnesses. Brief reversible exaggeration of spasticity may occur if clothes are too tight, catheters become blocked, leg bag straps are fastened too tightly, or wheelchair cushions become too soft or wrinkled. Remedying such causes of nociceptive stimulation rapidly decreases spasticity. More chronic exacerbations of spasticity may be provoked by renal stones, chronic pyelonephritis, muscle and joint contractures, and frank muscle tears or ligamentous strains.

Accordingly, great attention should be given to the care of the bladder, bowel and skin during the acute phase of cerebral or spinal cord injury, in order to minimise the eventual level of spasticity.

In addition, evidence is accumulating to suggest that proprioceptive facilitation in the early stages of cerebral or spinal shock may reduce the eventual degree of spasticity and, in the case of spinal spasticity, may assist the valuable development of extensor synergies.

Accordingly, physical therapy designed to maintain joint mobility and to emphasise helpful extensor synergies may be valuable in prevention of subsequently disabling spasticity.

TREATMENT OF ESTABLISHED SPASTICITY

Spasticity may be attacked by a range of methods from simple commonsense measures to complex neurosurgical procedures.

Simple measures (avoid nociceptive input and stretching)

Patients with established spasticity should be educated to look for simple causes of nociceptive input if their spasticity worsens. Rigorous attention to bladder, bowels and skin often lessens spasticity dramatically.

Of all the many physical therapies advocated for spasticity, prolonged stretching seems to be of the greatest importance. Besides preventing joint and muscle contractures, stretching diminishes spasticity, and its effect may persist for many hours thereafter. Stretching of spastic muscles can be done by the patient, or by their family, at home. The aim should be to produce prolonged sustained steady stretch of all spastic muscles at least once, but preferably twice, each day.

Drug treatment

Three drugs are used extensively to treat spasticity: diazepam, baclofen, and dantrolene sodium. Each of these drugs acts in a different way and, accordingly, may be used to treat spasticity in different circumstances.

Diazepam. Benzodiazepines such as diazepam increase presynaptic inhibition in many areas of the brain and spinal cord, probably by facilitation of γ-aminobutyric acid (GABA) neurotransmission. Benzodiazepines enhance the coupling between activation of the GABA recognition site and the ionophore site responsible for the membrane changes of inhibition induced by GABA. Experimental observations suggest that diazepam does increase presynaptic inhibition of stretch reflex mechanisms in those with partial cord injuries, but it appears to have no effect on those with total cord transections. In addition, diazepam has proved surprisingly ineffective in cerebral spasticity; it is of little benefit in capsular hemiplegia.

The dosage of diazepam required to reduce spasticity (4–40 mg/day) often produces unwanted effects. Most important are drowsiness, fatigue and unsteadiness. Occasionally diazepam may cause depression, physical dependence and seizures on drug withdrawal.

Diazepam is of greatest value in those with spinal spasticity due to partial cord lesions, provided it does not cause too much sleepiness. Unfortunately, many such patients depend upon their spastic legs to take their weight, so that the effect of diazepam in reducing spasticity makes walking more, rather than less, difficult. Whether the drug will be of benefit to individual patients can only be established by trial and error.

Baclofen. Baclofen is a derivative of GABA, but it acts in a different manner from its parent neurotransmitter. Baclofen appears to reduce the presynaptic release of excitatory neurotransmitters such as substance P, and it also directly acts postsynaptically to reduce the firing of both alpha and gamma motoneurones.

Baclofen appears to diminish both cerebral and spinal spasticity, irrespective of whether the latter is partial or complete, so is of value in those with both capsular hemiplegia and spinal cord disease.

Baclofen initially may produce drowsiness, nausea and light-headedness, but these unwanted effects usually disappear as the dose is built up slowly to that required to reduce spasticity (15–80 mg/day). High doses of baclofen occasionally may provoke hallucinations, a toxic confusional state, or even seizures, but such events are rare if dosage is increased slowly and kept to the minimum required to produce benefit.

Dantrolene sodium. Dantrolene sodium depresses the release of calcium ions from the sacrcoplasmic reticulum, thereby decreasing excitation-contraction coupling between electrical stimulation of the muscle membrane and activation of the contractile process. This action probably affects not only the extrafusal muscle fibres, but also the intrafusal fibres so as to diminish spindle discharges. Because it acts at the muscle, rather than on the central nervous system, dantrolene should aid all forms of spasticity.

Unfortunately, dantrolene has been found to cause hepatic injury in approximately 10 per cent of patients, and occasional deaths due to liver necrosis have been reported. In addition, it may produce nausea, vomiting and diarrhoea, and also can cause severe muscle weakness.

Despite these problems, dantrolene (100–600 mg/day) may be of considerable help to some patients with spasticity, provided regular monitoring of liver function is undertaken.

Even though these three antispastic drugs are available, spasticity frequently remains severe enough, and causes sufficient disability, to warrant consideration of one of the many destructive operative techniques which can reduce muscle resistance. Therse vary from the simple techniques of motor point block to more complex neurosurgical operations.

Nerve or motor point blocks

The motor points of individual muscles, or the nerves supplying them, can be identified by manipulation of a stimulating Teflon-coated needle, and then destroyed by injection of phenol (5 per cent). The technique is time-consuming but simple and effective, providing the critical muscles responsible for spastic disability can be identified. These vary from individual to individual. However, motor point block of hip adductors and calf muscles may prevent 'scissoring' and equinus deformity in selected patients. Likewise, motor point block of wrist and finger flexors may allow the hand to open and motor block of biceps may allow elbow extension. The effects of motor point block may last for a month to as long as two years.

Tenotomy and neurectomy

Permanent relief of the consequences of spasticity may be achieved by the relatively simple means of tendon lengthening operations, or by selective nerve avulsions.

Lengthening of the Achilles tendon or tenotomy of the thigh adductors provides sustained release from equinus deformity or 'scissoring' of gait. It is of particular value when contractures are present.

Neurectomy or nerve avulsion will not relieve resistance due to contracture, but obturator neurectomies may help adduction spasm of the thighs.

Intrathecal neurolysis

Intrathecal injection of 5 or 7 per cent phenol in glycerin, or absolute alcohol, can be used to destroy nerve roots of the cauda equina. Glycerin is heavier than cerebrospinal fluid, so can be manipulated around selected roots by careful positioning of the patient. Alcohol is lighter than cerebrospinal fluid, so is more difficult to control, but its effects are longer-lasting.

Unfortunately, although some degree of selectivity for interference with the stretch reflex arc sometimes can be obtained by such techniques, there is a risk of non-specific damage to the reflex arcs of the second and third sacral segments, which may lead to urinary and even faecal incontinence. For this reason, the technique usually is restricted to relief of spasticity in those already incontinent or catheterised. The method can be employed to convert a spastic but incontinent bladder into a lower motor neurone bladder, so as to reduce retention and reflux.

Other surgical procedures

Division of posterior nerve roots (posterior rhizotomy) initially reduces spasticity, but has been abandoned because spasm returns after a few months, and because of the inevitable breakdown that occurs in anaesthetic skin. Anterior rhizotomy produces a flaccid paralysis, but is technically more difficult, and the resulting muscle wasting exposes bony points leading to bed sores due to loss of padding. Total excision of the transected cord segment (cordectomy) has similar disadvantages. Myelotomy (dividing the cord in half sagittally to sever reflex pathways) does not relieve alpha spasticity. None of these neurosurgical techniques is in use in most centres.

Likewise, dorsal column and cerebellar stimulation should be regarded as experimental procedures at present.

CONCLUSIONS

Cerebral and spinal spasticity are due to release of intrinsic spinal cord mechanisms from their normal supraspinal controls. The details of cerebral and spinal spasticity differ owing to the existence of bulbospinal motor pathways which are preserved in cerebral spasticity, but destroyed in spinal spasticity. The most striking and important difference between the two is the presence of flexor spasticity and spasms in the legs after spinal injury.

The development and severity of spasticity, and in particular of flexor spasms in the legs, depends upon the extent of nociceptive input from bladder, bowels and skin. Flexor spasticity and spasms probably can be reduced or prevented by proprioceptive facilitation provided by physical therapy, particularly by regular muscle stretching.

The treatment of established spasticity depends upon avoiding nociceptive input, a programme of regular muscle stretching, judicious use of drug therapy (diazepam, baclofen or dantrolene sodium, each of which acts differently), and resort to operative procedures such as motor point block, tenotomy, neurectomy, or even intrathecal injection of phenol or alcohol in selected cases.

NOTE

This chapter is reprinted, with minor modification, from *Rheumatology and Rehabilitation*, eds H. Berry, E. Hamilton and J. Goodwin (Croom Helm, London, 1983).

FURTHER READING

Calne, D.B. (1976) The pharmacology of spasticity. In H.L. Klawans (ed.), *Clinical neuropharmacology*, vol. 1, Raven Press, New York

Delwaide, P.J. and Young, R.R. (1985) *Clinical neurophysiology in spasticity*, Elsevier, Holland

Dimitrijevic, M.R. and Nathan, B.W. (1967) Studies of spasticity in man. 1: Some features of spasticity. *Brain, 90*, 1-30
Lance, J.W. (1980) The control of muscle tone, reflexes and movement. *Neurology, 30*, 1303-13
Lance, J.W. and McLeod, J.G. (1981) *A physiological approach to clinical neurology*, Butterworth, London
Landau, W.M. (1974) Spasticity: the fable of a neurological demon and the emperor's new therapy. *Arch. Neurol., 31*, 217-19
Young, R.R. and Delwaide, P.J. (1981) Drug therapy: spasticity. Part 1. *N. Engl. J. Med., 304*, 28-33
Young, R.R. and Delwaide, P.J. (1981) Drug therapy: spasticity. Part 2. *N. Engl. J. Med., 304*, 96-9

28

Surgery in Neurological Disability

Timothy Morley

Surgery will be unnecessary for most patients with neurological disability. Yet for a few it may result in substantial gains, may prevent or correct deformity, or may enable therapists to train the patient to a higher level of function. Sometimes this gain may be quite specific; a person unable to write may be enabled to do so and thus hold down a job. On other occasions the benefit will accrue mainly to the carer, making nursing of the heavily dependent patient less arduous or perhaps preventing pressure sores. The present chapter is not exhaustive, but is written to illustrate the use which may be made of surgery in common situations. Timing may be crucial.

A skeletal deformity may be caused by many factors, including:

(a) paralytic muscle imbalance,

(b) spastic muscle imbalance,

(c) shortening of structures crossing a joint.

The aim should always be to prevent deformity by physiotherapy, stretching and splintage. Sometimes deformity develops despite every effort. In this event surgery may have to be considered.

The aims of surgery should be:

(a) to improve function, remembering that this can only work within the confines of the neurological condition;

(b) to prevent further deformity when conservative measures fail;

(c) to allow the maintenance of hygiene;

(d) to improve cosmetic appearance.

The indications for surgery and the type of surgical intervention in neurological disability can cause considerable disagreement; this is mainly due to a lack of objective preoperative assessment, resulting in inappropriate surgery (Chapter 6). The situation is also made worse by the lack of careful objective follow-up.

Neurological disability can be divided into flaccid or spastic paralysis, the latter being responsible for the majority of unpredictable results.

FLACCID PARALYSIS

Disability and deformity in flaccid paralysis result from the unopposed pull of muscle, or from total paralysis resulting in a flail deformity in which joint position is solely the result of body weight and gravity. The surgical approach is either tendon, or occasionally muscle, transfer, or by stabilisation of a flail joint by arthrodesis.

Tendon transfers

In selecting tendons for transfer the principles originally laid down for the treatment of poliomyelitis still remain valid.

(1) The muscle to be transplanted must be strong enough for its new function, remembering that it will lose a grade of power when transferred, and should be at least grade 4 initially.

(2) The transferred tendon should be inserted as close as possible to the paralysed muscle being replaced.

(3) Transfer through tunnels in fascia or bone may cause adhesions and should be avoided.

(4) The nerve and blood supply to the muscle need to be protected.

(5) The joint on which the tendon transfer acts should be mobile and free from deformity.

(6) The muscle excursion should remain unchanged as far as possible.

(7) Agonists are preferable to antagonists. Antagonists may work voluntarily but rarely in a functional pattern, and require extensive retraining.

Bearing in mind these principles, the results are both predictable and valuable. Excluding poliomyelitis, flaccid paralysis results from traumatic lower motor neurone lesions, a variety of cord compressive lesions and from peripheral neuropathies. Due consideration should be given to the long-term prognosis and, if progressive, the rate of progression and also the pattern should be borne in mind. There is no point in transferring a muscle which is almost certainly going to become involved in the paralytic process.

Operations round the foot and ankle are the most frequent and rewarding. *Clawing of the toes* can be treated by joint excision and fusion, or if the toes are still mobile by Girdlestone's flexor/extensor tendon transfer (Taylor, 1951). The commonest foot deformities which need surgery are *cavovarus and equinovarus.*

If there is no osseous deformity then procedures such as the transfer of extensor hallucis longus into the neck of the first metatarsal (Jones, 1916) or extensor digitorum longus into the third cuneiform may be justified. Equinovarus deformity may be appropriately treated by lengthening the tendo achilles, plantar fasciotomy and either lengthening or transfer of the tibialis posterior.

The common peroneal nerve is particularly prone to damage in its subcutaneous pathway at the knee. Despite the fact that anterior transfer of tibialis posterior tendon breaks all the rules, by being brought through a fascial plane and being an antagonist, results are often gratifying.

Surgical intervention in the knee or hip is rarely required.

In the upper limb there may be useful procedures following *spinal cord injury and tetraplegia.* Decisions on tendon transfers are dependent on

Figure 28.1: Foot showing clawing of the toes on the left; these are mobile and can be treated by tendon transfer

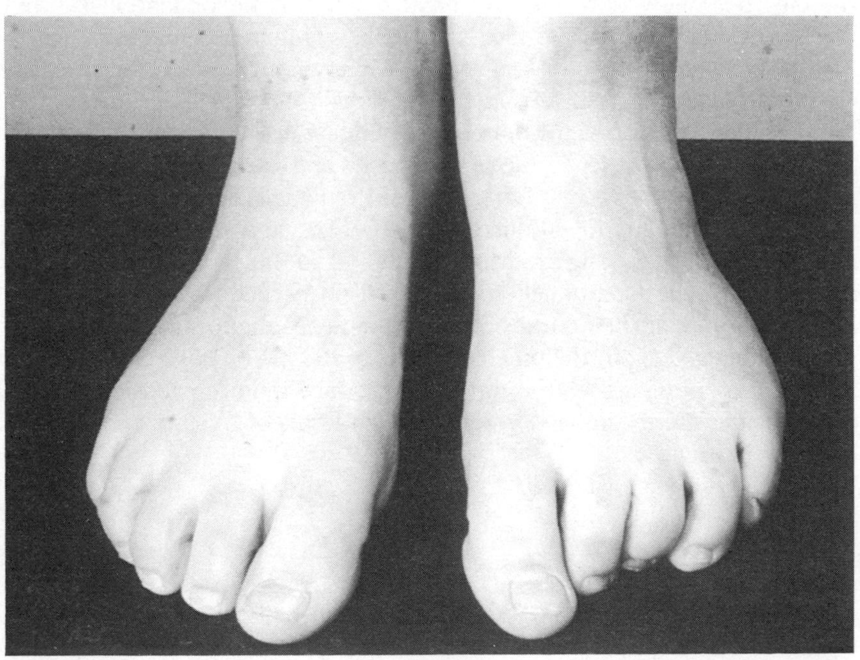

Figure 28.2: Cavus deformity of both feet associated with pain under the metatarsal heads

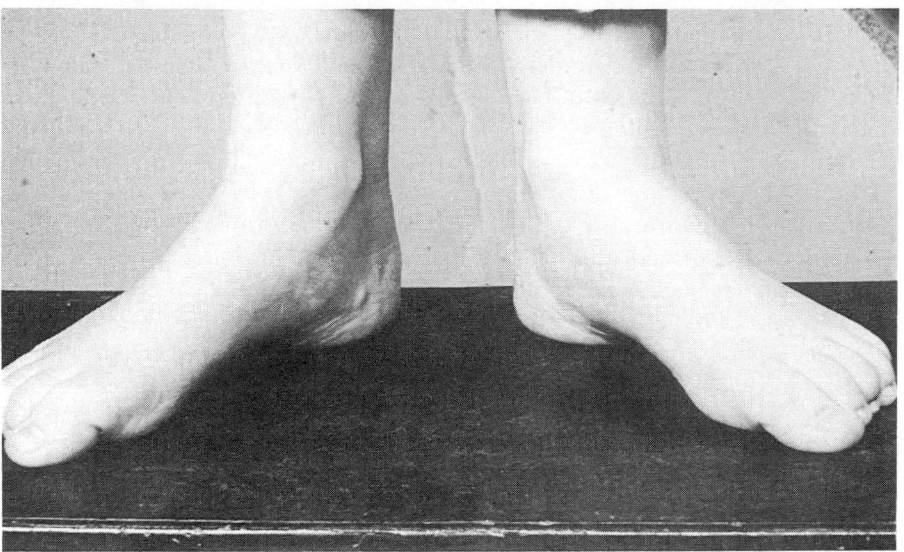

adequate sensation and proximal control. *C5/6* lesions retain extensor carpi radialis longus (ECRL) and brevis, and brachioradialis. In the event the only possible way to improve hand function is flexor tendonesis with transfer of brachioradialis to the flexor pollicis longus.

If extensor carpi radialis longus is not long enough, active wrist extension is achieved by transferring brachioradialis to ECRL, and doing an interphalangeal fusion of the thumb, with a flexor pollicis longus tendonesis. When the lesion is at *C6/7*, the same muscles are working plus flexor carpi radialis and pronator teres. Extensor carpi radialis brevis is transferred to flexor pollicis longus to produce thumb flexion, and then extensor carpi radialis longus to the long extensors of thumb and fingers to produce extension. *For C7 T1* the Bunnell (Bunnell, 1949) procedure is worth doing, flexor carpi radialis being transferred to the flexor digitorum profundus to produce finger flexion, the brachioradialis to the flexor pollicis longus and the flexor carpi ulnaris to the thumb to produce thumb extension. Procedures such as these can be very rewarding in terms of function, despite the lack of sensation.

Joint stabilisation

Joints which have either fixed deformity or are flail cannot be treated by tendon transfer. In this case arthrodesis may be considered. Examples of

Figure 28.3: Brachial plexus injury in a young man involving C7,8 T1 with inability to flex the fingers, but active extension of the wrist. C5,6 distribution was spared but there was some wasting associated with disuse

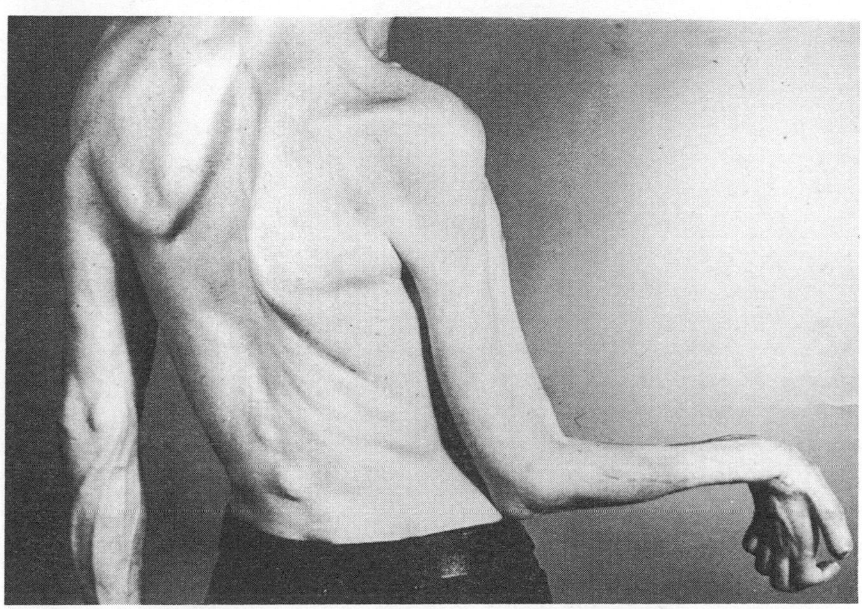

this are fixed clawing of toes treated by interphalangeal arthrodesis, or cavovarus deformity treated by triple arthrodesis (talocalcaneal, talonavicular and calcaneocuboid). Flail joints such as ankle and shoulder may be fused in the position of function.

THE SPINE

Deformity in the spine, secondary to neurogenic lesions, is essentially similar in both flaccid and spastic conditions.

A neurogenic curve is typically a long C curve with a tendency to associated kyphosis. In adults, because the ribs afford some form of protection, the deformity is most marked in the lumbar area and may be associated with severe pelvic tilting.

The deformities so produced cause:

(a) loss of sitting balance;

(b) difficulty with seating;

Figure 28.4: Typical neurogenic scoliosis. The curve was treated by segmental spinal instrumentation and fusion

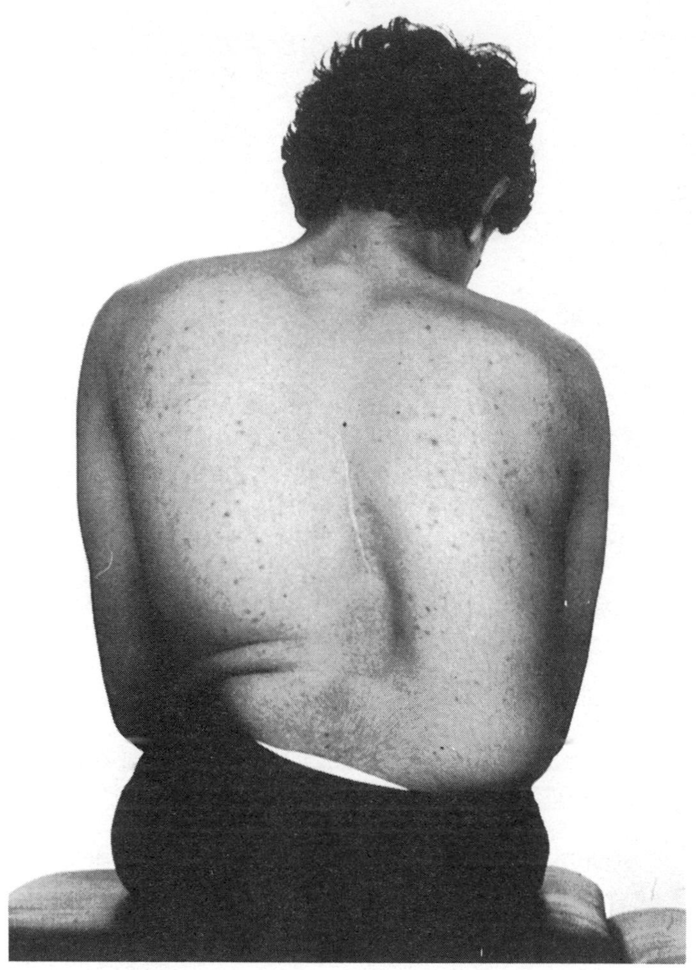

(c) skin pressure sore problems;

(d) cardiorespiratory failure;

(e) difficulty with controlling the hips;

(f) loss of body image, particularly in adult spina bifida;

(g) renal obstruction and problems with urinary diversion;

(h) increasing neurological signs.

Adults developing neurological disability rarely develop spinal curvatures, because growth has ceased. But children develop kyphoscoliosis with neurological disability such as spina bifida, and may need continuing treatment for this in adult life.

The basis of surgical treatment, when required, is that the correction must be complete, and instrumentation and fusion must be extensive, including both the front and back of the spine, and it must extend over the whole length of the deformity.

SPASTIC PARALYSIS

Because of the unpredictable results, there remains disagreement about the overall value of surgery in adult spastic paralysis. This unpredictability is due to difficulty with assessment of muscle control, patterns of weakness and individual muscle weakness (Roper, 1982).

Surgery can be complicated by associated soft tissue contractures requiring extensive soft tissue release, or correction may be lost. Arthrodesis is more difficult to achieve, and with osteotomies union may be delayed with subsequent loss of correction.

Postoperative rehabilitation is difficult because the simplest surgery may upset patterns of function. There may be loss of correction, and the patient may find it difficult to cooperate with attempts at rehabilitation.

The commonest causes of spastic disability in adults are stroke, multiple sclerosis or head injury. The incidence of stroke in the UK is 2 per 1,000 of the population per year, so there are half a million people suffering from neurological disability from this one cause alone. The initial prognosis may appear poor because intercurrent complications and associated diseases are common and the average age is high, so relatively few patients are considered for surgery. These factors are less marked following severe head injuries, which are more prevalent in young males.

The aim is to start conservative treatment as soon as possible, and surgery is usually only considered once the patient has achieved a steady neurological state and any residual deformity or obstructive spasticity has been identified. There is a complex interaction of normal muscles, spastic muscles, stretch reflexes and reflex action. These are difficult to evaluate on routine clinical examination but by watching the patient walk, by discussion with therapists and by video-record there has been improvement in analysis of typical patterns of action, with a greater understanding of the effects of surgery. Assessment has also been aided by selective peripheral blocking of nerves and the use of dynamic electromyography. With a head-injured patient one may consider surgery earlier on, where it is clear that spasticity and/or contracture will impede recovery of function.

Surgery consists of:

(a) release of tendons;
(b) lengthening and thus weakening muscles;
(c) occasional tendon transfer;
(d) neurectomies;
(e) soft tissue release;
(f) bony operations, with osteotomy or joint fusion.

Generally surgery is more useful in the lower limbs. Operations are divided into two main types.

(1) for the severely disabled chairbound patient,
(2) for the ambulant disabled.

(a) The severely disabled chairbound patient

In cases where there is severe hemisphere and/or spinal cord damage leaving primitive reflex arcs, surgery may be of value in aiding nursing care and in the maintenance of simple hygiene. In these circumstances the problems are usually hip adduction and flexion, and knee flexion. For the hip, release should be of the iliopsoas and the adductor muscles, with obturator neurectomy and sometimes release of the anterior capsule of the hip joint. Knee flexion contracture is treated by ham-string tenotomy, sometimes augmented by posterior capsulotomy of the knee joint, followed by serial plastering or reverse traction.

(b) The ambulant disabled

Surgery may be indicated where there is usable reflex activity, or when the muscles have usable voluntary control but function suffers from interference from excessive spasticity or from contracture.

The commonest deformity in these patients is *equinovarus.* This is caused by a relative overaction of the plantar flexors and invertors over the power of dorsiflexion and eversion. The Silfverskiold test to differentiate equinus caused by gastrocnemius or soleus is unreliable, and here the use of dynamic electromyography is useful (Perry and Waters, 1975). In most instances the tendo achilles requires lengthening. This may be done by the percutaneous slide with the tendon being divided percutaneously through half its bulk, medially–proximally and anteriorally–distally. The ankle is then forcibly dorsiflexed against the spastic muscles (White, 1943). If the equinus is very severe then the tendon can be lengthened by the open slide method; if there is varus at the heel the tibialis posterior may be divided or elongated at the same time (Roper *et al.*, 1978).

For foot varus which cannot be controlled by bracing, and where tibialis anterior is strong enough to allow clearance in the swing phase of gait, split tibialis anterior transfer may allow the brace to be discarded. Part of the tibialis anterior tendon is detached from its insertion and passed through a bony canal in the lateral tarsus.

Clawing of the toes, where these are still mobile, can be corrected by Girdlestone flexor to extensor tendon transfer. The severe clawing of the toes caused by imbalance of the intrinsic muscles of the foot is a more difficult problem and there is no satisfactory answer.

The commonest problem in *the knee*, in the ambulant patient with spasticity, is a persistent stiff leg gait. Selective tenotomy of one or two heads of the quadriceps based on electromyographic criteria improves knee flexion, but usually only by about 20° (Waters *et al.* 1979). Knee flexion contracture is less usually a problem in the ambulant and rarely needs surgical treatment. If required hamstring tenotomy is used followed by serial plastering or reverse traction.

The hip deformity is usually a flexion/adduction deformity, causing a scissoring gait. This is treated by adductor release from the public bone. If the scissoring is very marked then anterior obturator neurectomy is added. For the non-ambulant, when surgery is to improve hygiene, then the ileopsoas may require releasing also.

THE UPPER LIMB

In the upper limb the most frequent pattern of deformity in the patient with spasticity is flexion of the fingers and thumb; the latter may also be adducted. Flexion of the wrist with pronation of the forearm, flexion of the elbow and adduction, internal rotation of the shoulder.

In the arm the object of treatment is the production of an active range of movement sufficient to allow grasp, reach and, if possible, fine hand movements. This requires relatively normal sensation to be really useful. The results of surgery in the arm are not as good as in the leg where walking is usually the objective, a simpler goal to achieve.

In *the shoulder* the deformity of adduction in internal rotation is not a problem amenable to surgery. Painful subluxation often occurs, but does not follow a clear pattern which can lend itself to surgery.

The elbow rarely produces a flexion deformity severe enough to warrant surgery. Where anterior release is tried with lengthening of biceps the deformity usually recurs. Commonly there is sufficient range for everyday use.

The hand deformity consists of flexion of the fingers and a flexed adducted thumb. In addition the sensation is often reduced, and therefore even restoration of some grip does not always give useful function.

The thumb in palm deformity may be corrected by transferring flexor carpi radialis into the long thumb extensor, which is in turn re-routed from Lister's tubercle towards the radial aspect of the first metacarpal. In a very severe deformity it may be necessary to strip the first dorsal interosseus, divide the adductor tendon and lengthen the long flexor tendon of the thumb, before either doing a tendon transfer or alternatively inserting a bone block between the first and second metacarpals.

The finger deformities are either (1) flexion at metacarpophalangeal and *proximal* interphalangeal joints, or (2) metacarpophalangeal and *distal* interphalangeal joint flexion with the proximal interphalangeal in extension (the intrinsic plus hand) the latter deformity may be treated by intrinsic release (Figure 28.5). If the flexed fingers are associated with a straight wrist, wrist flexion may permit some finger extension and allow the hand to open enough for grasping objects. *If the wrist is also flexed* then the flexors of wrist and fingers require lengthening either by a slide at the proximal origin or at the wrist (Inglis and Cooper, 1966). If there is no wrist function, apparent tendon lengthening may be achieved by shortening the forearm and doing a Nissen–Brockman fusion. The lower end of the radius

Figure 28.5: Intrinsic contracture of the fingers due to stroke causing spastic right hemiplegia

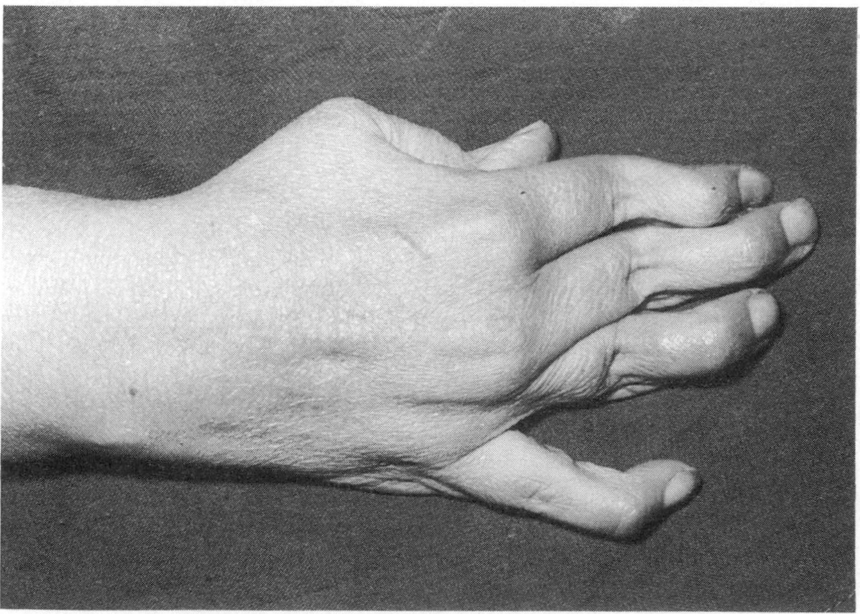

is shaped into a chisel and this is inserted into the carpus.

Because hand function is so complicated, function can really only be finally assessed one to two years after surgery. In addition to useful sensation the patient requires determination and intelligence to cooperate with rehabilitation.

It should not be forgotten that many patients find the spastic position of the upper limb very distressing, as the disabled hand is seen by all. Even with no useful functional improvement, surgery may be helpful to improve the appearance of the hand and so improve the patient's self-image.

Surgery of adult neurological disability is understandably not straightforward, but it must not be forgotten that a relatively small improvement in function can radically improve lifestyle and function. With advances in the preoperative assessment and postoperative treatment gratifying results can be achieved.

REFERENCES

Bunnell, S. (1949) *Tendon transfers in the hand and forearm.* American Academy of Orthopaedic Surgeons, instructional course lectures, Vol. VI, Ann Arbor

Inglis, A.E. and Cooper, W. (1966) Release of the pronator origin for flexion deformities of the hand and wrist in spastic paralysis. A study of 18 cases, *J. Bone Joint Surg., 48A,* 847-57

Jones, Sir Robert (1916) The soldier's foot and the treatment of common deformities of the foot. Part II: claw foot. *Br. Med. J., 1,* 749-53

Perry, J. and Waters, R.L. (1975) *Orthopaedic evaluation and treatment of the stroke patient.* Part II. 1a, American Academy of Orthopaedic Surgeons, instructual course lectures, Vol. 24, Mosby & Co., St Louis

Roper, B.A. (1982) Rehabilitation after a stroke. *J. Bone Joint Surg., 64,* 156-63

Roper, B.A., Williams, A. and King J.B. (1978) The surgical treatment of equinovarus deformity in adults with spasticity. *J. Bone Joint Surg., 60B,* 533-5

Taylor, R.G. (1951) The treatment of claw toes by multiple transfers of flexor into extensor tendons. *J. Bone Joint Surg., 33b,* 539-42

Waters, R.L., Garland, D.E., Perry, J. and Habig, T. (1979) Stiff legged gait in hemiplegia, surgical correction. *J. Bone Joint Surg., 61A,* 927-33

White, J.W. (1943) Torsion of the achilles tendon, its surgical significance. *Arch. Surg., 46,* 784-7

Part 6

Care and Treatment

29

Urinary Incontinence

James Malone-Lee, Mandy Fader and Christine Budden

Urinary incontinence at any age after early childhood is a personal catastrophe that demands an effective remedy that can be provided with confidence. Nowadays our understanding of the pathophysiological problems associated with the development of incontinence enables us to offer solutions that are effective and simple to apply. In order to appreciate the nature of the problems involved it is important to understand some of the functional neuroanatomy, and related pharmacology, of the bladder and urethra.

Anatomy (Figures 29.1 and 29.2)

The smooth muscle of the bladder, termed the detrusor, funnels at the bladder neck to be continued into the urethra as longitudinal fibres forming a tube. In the male these fibres are inserted into the verumontanum, but in the female they terminate at the distal urethra. The contraction of this group of fibres results in a rise in bladder pressure associated with a shortening of the urethra. The trigone forms a triangular base-plate with its apex at the bladder neck and base running between both ureters. Muscle fibres run from the ureters into the trigone and at the apex trigonal muscle fibres are continuous with those of the urethra. Contraction of the muscle of the trigone results in funnelling of the bladder neck. There are some fibres which originate in the detrusor and are inserted into the external surface of the trigone distally. These fibres will pull the distal surfaces of the trigone apart and thus open the bladder neck (Brocklehurst, 1978).

The internal urethral sphincter is fully developed in the male and forms a circular collar continuous with the prostatic smooth muscle. This sphincter is not present in the female. It functions to prevent the retrograde flow of semen during ejaculation and its failure to function is associated with passing milky urine after ejaculation, and with infertility. Despite this primary function the internal sphincter still needs to relax during normal micturition (Gosling *et al.*, 1981).

Figure 29.1: Diagrammatic representation of the male lower urinary tract

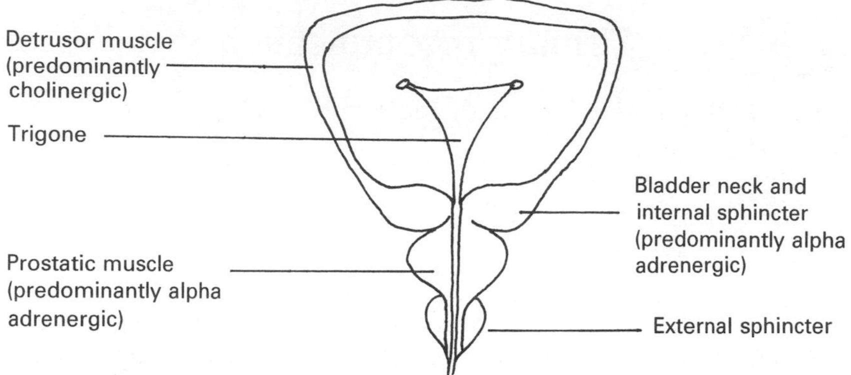

Figure 29.2: Diagrammatic representation of the female lower urinary tract

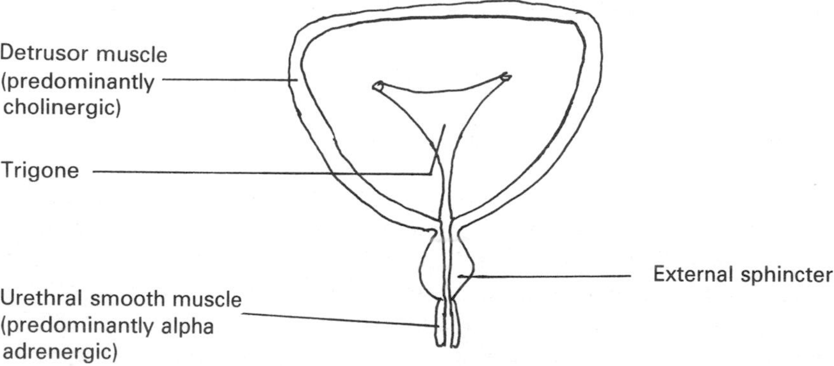

The external urethral sphincter is present in both sexes, and is the site of maximum urethral resistance (Griffiths, 1980). It produces a rapid reflex contraction in response to abdominal straining. The circularly arranged muscle fibres are striated and slow twitch in character. The positive pressure generated in the urethra during abdominal straining originates partly from direct transmission to the intra-abdominal urethra and partly from reflex sphincter contractions. The external sphincter is quite separate from the periurethral striated muscle of the pelvic sling which passes lateral to the urethra and inserts into the inferior pubic rami. It does not encircle the urethra as a sphincter would. This sling supports the bladder and proximal urethra posteriorly. Without this support the bladder neck becomes incompetent and abdominal pressure tranmission and associated reflex sphincter activity fails (Hald, 1984).

The prostate gland is present only in men, though there has been a fruitless search for a prostate analogue in women. The organ consists of a mixture of glandular tissue and smooth muscle. The muscle has a constant resting tone which can vary, and may influence the passage of urine through the prostatic urethra. Benign nodular hyperplasia of the prostate is universal over the age of 40, but only 10 per cent of men develop obstructive symptoms which are particularly common in Caucasians and American Negroes (McNeal, 1983).

In both sexes continence is usually maintained at the bladder neck because of the passive closure that the smooth muscle and elastic tissue promote, and because of its position in the abdominal cavity. The external sphincter plays a secondary role unless the bladder neck loses competence. Women, who have a short urethra and no prostate, have to augment the external sphincter function with the urethral elastic tissue, the pressure exerted by intramural arteriovenous sinuses, the smooth muscle of the urethral walls and the surface tension of the mucus. The position of the female urethra is also critical for the maintenance of continence (Hald, 1984).

The pharmacological anatomy

Most of the detrusor fibres carry muscarinic cholinergic receptors which are innervated by parasympathetic efferents originating in the intermediolateral columns of sacral segments two, three and four. Stimulation of these neurones results in a contraction. There are a number of other receptors within the detrusor but their clinical significance is limited (Malone-Lee, 1983).

The bladder neck and internal sphincter are richly supplied with excitatory alpha-1 receptors, some excitatory cholinergic receptors and a few inhibitory beta-2 receptors. The smooth muscle of the urethra has a similar receptor distribution (Gosling *et al.*, 1981). Cholinergic and alpha-adrenergic stimulation cause a rise in pressure at the membranous urethra.

The female urethra has oestrogen receptors throughout its length with maximum concentration in the distal two-thirds (Wilson *et al.*, 1981). Progesterone receptors have not been detected, though there is a sensitivity of the urethra to progesterone (Caine and Raz, 1973).

The afferent pathway function

The most important receptors in the bladder are tension receptors. The afferents which pass to the lumbar segments of the cord are concentrated in the muscle coats and submucosa of the bladder neck and urethra. Afferents going to the sacral cord are distributed throughout the bladder. The receptors respond, with varying thresholds, to tension produced by distension or contraction (Fletcher and Bradley, 1978).

The sacral afferents start responding at low bladder volumes and from about two-thirds of bladder capacity they activate a 'short reflex arc' which inhibits detrusor excitation, thereby permitting bladder fill without a related rise in pressure (Figure 29.3). This reflex fails in the presence of a sensory neuropathy and as a result a non-compliant bladder develops. The lumbar afferents respond to the extremes of distension and are stimulated at high bladder volumes. All tension afferents ascending to the brain do so in the lateral dorsal columns (Fletcher and Bradley, 1978).

Some sacral afferents are involved in a different reflex arc. The sensory neurones synapse with motor efferents either at sacral level or, more importantly, after traversing the spinal cord to the pontine reticular formation. This reflex, when activated, initiates micturition and is essential for

Figure 29.3: The sacral reflex mediating bladder relaxation during fill

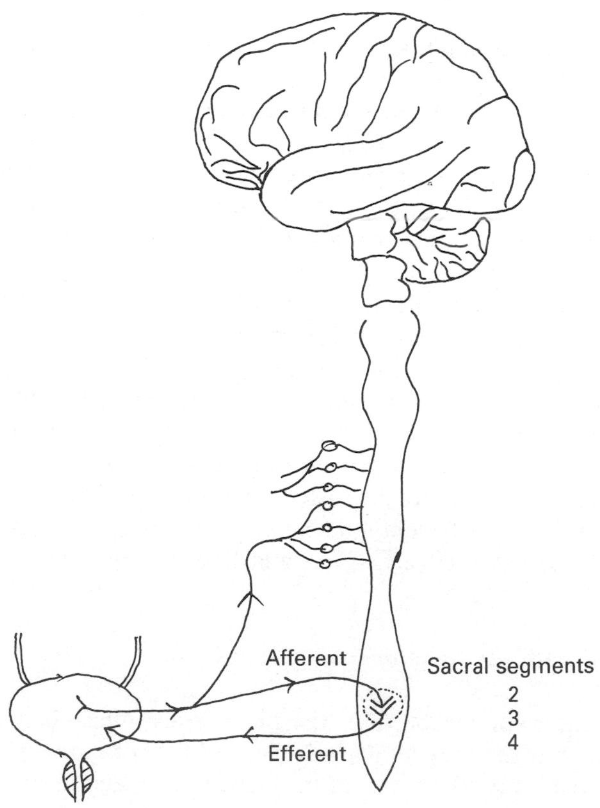

voiding. It is usually suppressed by the influence of neurones from higher cerebral centres (Figure 29.4).

The sensations of bladder fullness, touch and pain are conveyed from receptors in the submucosa via sacral and lumbar afferents up into the spinothalamic tracts with one-third crossing to the opposite side (Fletcher and Bradley, 1978).

Central nervous system control

The highest centres involved in the control of micturition are located on the superomedial aspect of both frontal lobes adjacent to the genu of the corpus callosum. They receive sensory fibres from the brainstem nuclei and the ascending tracts. Motor neurones arising at these centres pass to other parts of the cortex, cross the corpus callosum, or descend in the internal

Figure 29.4: The spinal reflex mediating the initiation of voiding

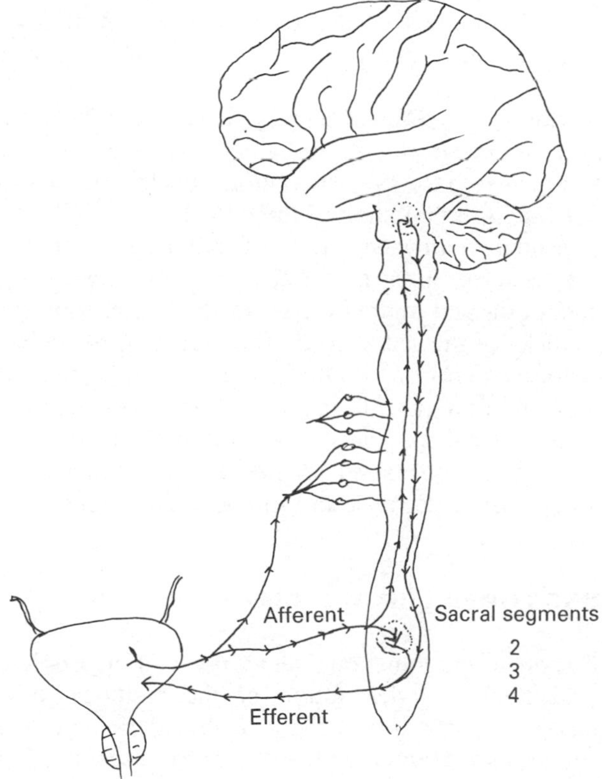

capsule to the brainstem nuclei and reticulospinal tracts. If these cortical centres are stimulated experimentally the detrusor becomes activated, but they also exert an inhibitory influence on the brainstem centres (Fletcher and Bradley, 1978).

The thalamus relays sensory signals from bladder, urethral and pelvic receptors to the cortical micturition centres. Some nuclei relay signals to other parts of the brain which mediate modifications of behaviour and autonomic function in response to bladder filling.

Motor efferents from the cortical centres synapse in the basal ganglia which send communications to the brainstem motor nuclei. Electrical stimulation of the basal ganglia in experimental animals leads to suppression of the detrusor and ablation results in detrusor hyperreflexia.

Distension of the bladder in experimental animals results in activity in the neurones of the posterior hypothalamus, and neurones from the anterior hypothalamus communicate with motor neurones travelling to the detrusor. We do not, however, know what influence the hypothalamus exerts on the lower urinary tract. In man the limbic system would seem to be unassociated with bladder function, as ablation of the temporal lobes is not associated with changes in bladder behaviour.

The main brainstem motor nuclei governing detrusor activity are situated in the pontine reticular formation. Stimulation of these nuclei results in precipitant detrusor activity, whereas ablation leads to detrusor inactivity.

The anterior vermis receives sensory signals from the lower urinary tract via the spinocerebellar tracts. From here neurones pass to the fastigial nucleus and thence to the brainstem motor nuclei. Stimulation of the fastigial nucleus results in inhibition of these nuclei.

The descending pathways from the brainstem motor nuclei become organised into three important tracts. Nerves originating in the pons, medulla oblongata and midbrain pass in the lateral spinoreticular tract to the motor nuclei of the sacral cord. They function to promote a sustained contraction of the detrusor with inhibition of the sphincters. Another group of fibres pass from the pons in the medial reticulospinal tract and function to inhibit the external sphincter. The third group of neurones arise in the medulla oblongata and travel in the anterior reticulospinal tract and function to inhibit the detrusor and stimulate the sphincters.

MEASURING LOWER URINARY TRACT FUNCTION

Having described the functional anatomy and neurophysiology of the bladder and urethra a description of the methods of assessing their performance is appropriate. A bladder should be able to store urine in volumes of around 500 ml without causing discomfort, and to empty efficiently and completely when appropriate. It should be capable of conveying accurate information about its state to the cerebral cortex. The bladder needs to remain free from infection.

The first-line methods of assessing bladder behaviour are examination. *The clinical history* must contain information about the following:

(a) the presence, pattern and frequency of incontinence;

(b) the daytime frequency of micturition;

(c) the presence of nocturia, urgency, stress incontinence, hesitancy, a poor stream, postmicturition dribbling, dysuria or haematuria;

(d) information on bowel habits and behaviour;

(e) sexual function and how incontinence affects it;

(f) a personal or family history of late bedwetting;

(g) information on parity and obstetric complications;

(h) information on previous disease of the genitourinary system, gastrointestinal system, or nervous system;

(i) details of current medication.

The clinical examination must include a proper vaginal examination and rectal examination. Women must be examined standing, on coughing, with a full bladder. Special attention should be paid to the neurological signs, the health of the genitalia and the genital reflexes. Assessments of mobility, dexterity and perceptual ability as well as cognitive function are relevant.

A postmicturition measure of residual bladder capacity should be made on all people with bladder problems. Passing a Jacques catheter is a simple and safe way of doing this. Urinalysis may be limited to a dip-stick test as urine culture is not always indicated. A plain abdominal X-ray should also be taken, as it is a good way of screening for bladder stones and an abdominal palpation and rectal examination do not always detect faecal impaction.

The application of the principles described above will lead to an accurate diagnosis of the cause of incontinence in an overwhelming majority of cases. In our unit we use the information obtained to treat many patients of all ages successfully. However, the measurement of the urine flow rate, while the patient is voiding prior to the estimation of residual capacity, is a very useful exercise. The equipment used for this measurement is called a 'mictiometer' and is not very expensive. The patient voids into a specially constructed commode and the mictiometer provides an analogue tracing of the flow rate throughout the micturition. A normal flow curve is illustrated in Figure 29.5. Note how maximum flow rate is greater than 15 ml/s and is

Figure 29.5: A normal flow curve from a woman aged 39. Voiding flow rate against time

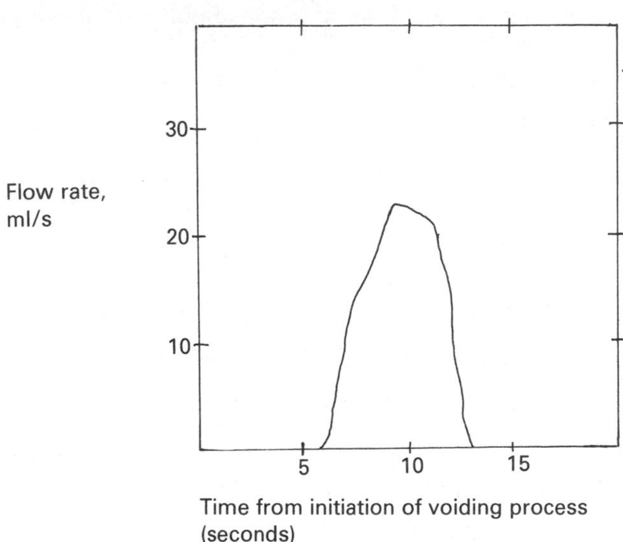

reached within the first third of the void. If the voided volume is less than 150 ml then the accuracy of the measured flow rate becomes doubtful. A typical flow curve from someone with an obstruction is shown in Figure 29.6. Note the prolonged void, the reduced rate of flow and the plateau shape of the curve.

The next stage in investigation is the urodynamic study. This should be employed in the following circumstances:

(1) whenever surgery is being considered;

(2) in the presence of a voiding problem;

(3) when first-line treatment has failed.

The basic urodynamic investigation using pressure-flow cystometry or video cystometry is illustrated in Figure 29.7 and has been described in a number of texts (Griffiths, 1980; Turner-Warwick and Whiteside, 1979). The bladder is emptied and two catheters are introduced through the urethra. One is used to fill the bladder with sterile water or saline. The other is used to measure the bladder pressure at an external transducer mounted at pubic level. A third catheter, capped with a latex balloon to avoid faecal plugging, is inserted into the rectum. This is used to measure

Figure 29.6: A flow curve from a 55 year old man with an obstruction. Voiding flow rate against time

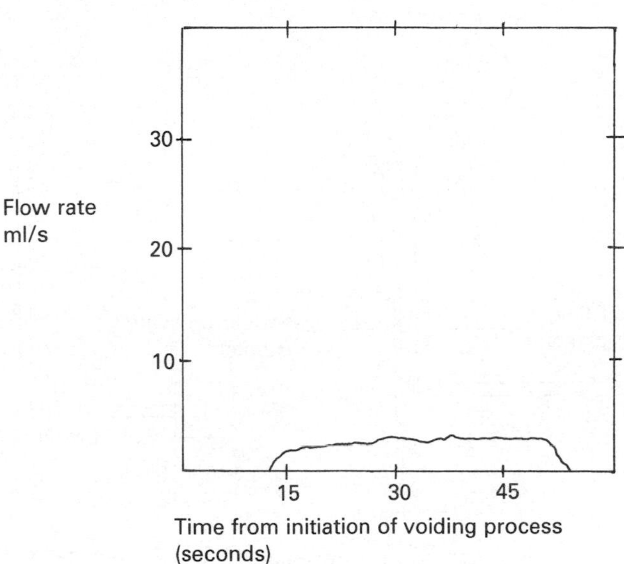

abdominal pressure at a transducer mounted next to the bladder transduccr. Thc truc intrinsic bladder pressure is calculated by subtracting the abdominal pressure from the bladder pressure. The bladder is filled at a rate of 60 ml/min to a volumc of 500 ml if possible. The pressures are recorded throughout fill on a chart recorder. At the end of fill the feeding catheter is removed from the bladder and the patient is asked to stand, cough, and to rock from heel to toe. Voiding occurs into a mictiometer with simultaneous recording of pressures. The investigation can be augmented by using a contrast medium to fill the bladder and screening with X-rays during parts of the investigation. The functional anatomy of the urethra can be checked by pulling a pressure measuring device down the length of the urethra and thus obtaining a urethral pressure profile. None of these techniques are easy to apply, requiring skill to perform and to interpret, but they can shed considerable light on the more difficult bladder problems.

THE INCONTINENCE SYNDROMES AND THEIR MANAGEMENT

Any breakdown in the normal physiology of the bladder and urethra may lead to urinary incontinence, which should be viewed as a symptom as

Figure 29.7: Diagrammatic representation of a urodynamic study

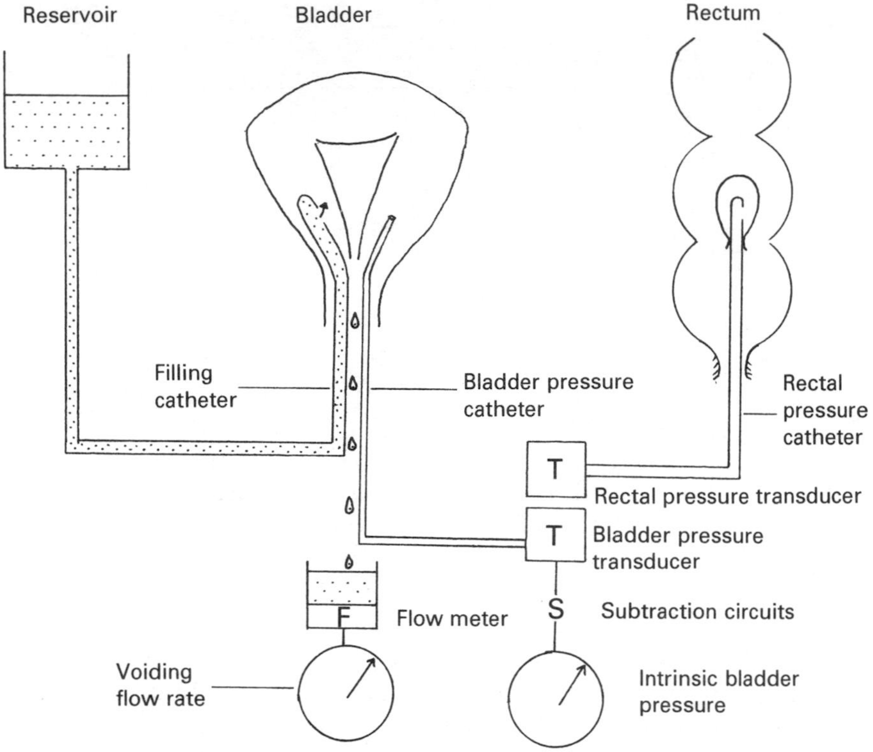

opposed to a specific pathological entity. Successful treatment depends on identifying the pathologies concerned, and remembering that frequently more than one precipitant may be involved.

Urinary tract infection

A significant bacteruria is defined by Kass and Brumfitt (1978) as at least 105 organisms per millilitre in three successive fresh, clean-catch, midstream specimens of urine. This provides a 95 per cent confidence level that there is a genuine infection. One specimen fulfilling the criteria gives an 80 per cent confidence level. More than half of the patients presenting with frequency and dysuria with or without fever or loin pain will be found to have sterile urine cultures on these criteria. The presence of more than ten white blood cells per millitre of urine indicates an inflammatory process. Asymptomatic bacteruria is a common finding. About 3 per cent of women aged 25 have bacteruria. The incidence increases by 1–2 per cent for each decade of age reaching 7 per cent at 65 and 9 per cent at 85 in ambulant women. Asymptomatic bacteruria has an incidence of 2–3 per cent in men aged 60–70, and 21–30 per cent in those over the age of 80. Any abnormality of the urinary tract will greatly increase the incidence of bacteruria (Dontas, 1984).

An acute urinary tract infection causing frequency and dysuria may well precipitate urge incontinence that resolves with treatment of the infection. The treatment of significant bacteruria in the absence of these symptoms is not likely to improve incontinence, and should only be pursued if other indications exist.

Detrusor instability

A detrusor instability or unstable bladder is the second most common cause of incontinence in women, and the most common cause in men. Its incidence increases with age. It can be caused by damage or failure of the pathways functioning to inhibit the long spinal voiding reflex; by failure of the third descending pathway in the anterior reticulospinal tract which functions to suppress the detrusor and stimulate the sphincters; by local disease of the bladder or urethra such as outlet obstruction. Consequently, a detrusor instability may be precipitated by virtually any neurological disease or trauma above the sacral cord. 'Idiopathic detrusor instability' describes the condition in the absence of a clear cause, though a history of late bed-wetting may exist.

The symptoms of detrusor instability involve frequency, nocturia, urgency, urge incontinence and nocturnal enuresis. The detrusor is inadequately suppressed and tends to contract inappropriately, resulting in expression of part of the bladder contents. Figure 29.8 shows a pressure recording taken during bladder filling from a patient with a detrusor instability. The inappropriate pressure rises are clearly shown.

An unstable detrusor is a spastic detrusor and the most important aspect of treatment involves stretching the muscle so as to encourage a reduction in tone. The bladder retraining regime is the simplest way of achieving this, as it results in the maintenance of progressively higher bladder capacities. The patient maintains a simple bladder diary chart recording, with a tick, each micturition or episode of incontinence, and works hard at increasing the intervals between micturitions. It is not logical to use fixed time intervals as normal micturition patterns have a circadian rhythm. We instruct the patient to delay voiding for as long as possible whenever a sense of urgency develops. We have found that once a minimum interval of four hours can be achieved the symptoms related to instability usually settle down. The most problematic times of the day are first thing in the morning ('kettle filling urgency') and in the evening ('homing urgency'). Retraining

Figure 29.8: The detrusor pressure during bladder filling from an unstable bladder

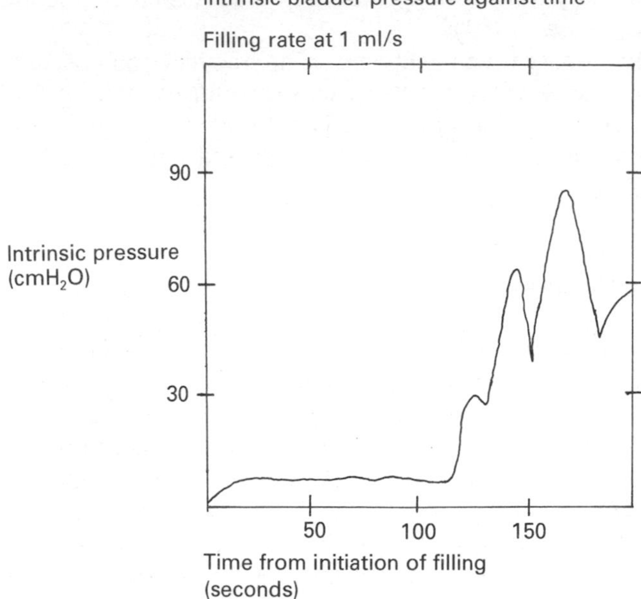

at night disrupts sleep and is inadvisable. Look after the day and the night will take care of itself. A good relationship with the patient and regular fortnightly follow-up, seem to be important for success.

The use of anticholinergic medication can be extremely helpful as an adjuvant to the retraining regime. Though many preparations have been advocated there are in fact few that have been shown to be genuinely effective. It is important to select a limited range and become familiar with each drug. In our unit we use two preparations: imipramine and oxybutinin.

The tricyclic antidepressant imipramine has anticholinergic, alpha-agonistic, antihistaminic and anti-5-HT properties. It has been shown to be effective for detrusor instability in a number of clinical trials. Most patients respond to a single daily dose of 10–20 mg at night. Some people with troublesome daytime symptoms require a morning dose as well. The dose–response varies among individuals and some people require high doses of 100 mg or more, but this is rare. Side-effects can be attributed to the anticholinergic properties, a dry mouth and constipation being common problems (Castleden *et al.*, 1981).

Oxybutinin is a tertiary amine with powerful anticholinergic and papaverine-like properties. This drug is well absorbed and highly effective at suppressing unstable detrusor activity but its use is limited by marked anticholinergic side-effects which make it difficult to tolerate. It is given in a dose ranging from 5 mg b.d. to 10 mg t.d.s. (Moisey *et al.*, 1980).

Propantheline, emmepronium bromide, flavoxate hydrochloride, non-steroidal anti-inflammatories and calcium ion antagonists have all been advocated for the unstable bladder, but responses have not proved very impressive. The first two are quaternary ammonium compounds which do not readily pass biological membranes; consequently their absorption is variable and high doses are often required.

The more troublesome unstable bladders which fail to respond to medical management may be helped by phenol injections into the pelvic plexuses (Mundy and Stephenson, 1984), an augmentation cystoplasty (Stephenson and Mundy, 1984), or by the Brindley nerve stimulator (Brindley *et al.*, 1984).

The voiding problems

The most common voiding problem encountered is that caused by prostatic obstruction. The prostate enlarges in all men over the age of 45 but symptoms requiring surgical treatment occur in only 10 per cent. The older a man is the more likelihood of a prostatic carcinoma which features in 80 per cent of resections performed on men of 80 and older (Karr and Murphy, 1984). Difficulty in initiating micturition, a poor stream, an intermittent stream, postmicturition dribbling and incomplete emptying are all symptoms of obstruction. Detrusor instability may accompany obstruction and give rise to appropriate symptoms. A significantly symptomatic prostatic hypertrophy requires surgical resection which will involve a transurethral approach 95 per cent of the time in most modern units. If the associated detrusor instability was provoked by the obstruction then it will be relieved as well; if it was a separate entity a troublesome incontinence is likely. An accurate preoperative diagnosis is important. Other urethral strictures produce similar symptoms and all require surgical treatment.

A hypotonic bladder may develop as a result of lesions of the sacral cord (as in spinal injuries involving the vertebrae below T11); in peripheral neuropathies (as in diabetes) and as a result of damage to the pelvic nerves (as after hysterectomy). The bladder will remain apparently hypotonic for variable periods after most spinal injuries. The stretching of the bladder that occurs in acute retention may cause hypotonia, which can be very persistent. The typical symptoms feature difficulties in initiating micturition, a poor urinary stream, an intermittent stream, incomplete emptying, stress incontinence and persistent dribbling incontinence. Recurrent infection is another important aspect and often involves serious septicaemia with the bacteria becoming increasingly resistant. Surgical procedures designed to reduce outflow resistance are used to treat this problem but often lead to incontinence afterwards. Using manual compression of the abdomen to promote voiding rarely leads to satisfactory emptying, and may damage already compromised bladder support mechanisms. Permanent indwelling catheters, though often used, ought to be avoided. Now the treatment of choice for a hypotonic bladder is the use of intermittent catheterisation, and this technique will be dealt with later in this chapter (Lapides, 1976).

If the central pathways controlling the coordination of the sphincters and detrusor fail to function then the sphincter mechanisms will not relax efficiently during voiding and a functional obstruction will result. This is called detrusor–sphincter dyssynergia and is a frequent feature of bladder problems associated with neurological disease, especially those affecting the spinal cord. It is usual for this problem to coexist with a detrusor instability. The symptoms are those of an obstruction, though difficulty in initiating voluntary micturition is more constant and postmicturition dribbling less common. Sphincterotomy is frequently used to treat this problem, but results are unpredictable if continence is sought, especially as the accompanying detrusor instability will be aggravated by a reduced urethral resistance. More gratifying results can be achieved by using intermittent catheterisation combined with an anticholinergic for the instability.

When describing the functional neuroanatomy we referred to an important descending spinal tract which bears neurones that function to sustain the micturition process once it has been initiated. If this tract fails voiding is incomplete and a persistent residual urine will result. This problem is usually accompanied by a detrusor instability and the incontinence that results will not resolve until the voiding problem has been corrected, despite energetic treatment of the detrusor instability.

In fact this condition often declares itself as an exacerbation of symptoms, or as a voiding difficulty developing after the introduction of anticholinergic medication. An unsustained detrusor is a feature of many diseases of the central nervous system, most notably multiple sclerosis, cerebrovascular disease, Alzheimer's disease and spinal injury. Recurrent infection and incontinence resistant to standard therapy are the usual presenting symptoms. The treatment of choice is intermittent catheterisation. Some patients, especially females, can often re-establish normal voiding after a short period on such a regime (Malone-Lee and Exton-Smith, 1985).

The development of the Brindley sacral nerve stimulator implant in recent years has proved an important advance. It is very effective for treating patients with spinal cord lesions that have resulted in a detrusor instability combined with a voiding problem. This procedure is becoming more available in specialist centres and offers an excellent alternative for suitable patients (Brindley *et al.*, 1984).

Urethral sphincter incompetence

The symptom of stress incontinence involves urinary leakage in association with coughing, laughing, running and other similar activities. It can be a feature of any of the bladder pathologies described in this section. For instance, a cough may precipitate an unstable detrusor contraction. However, it is most commonly associated with urethral incompetence. Failure of the urethral sphincter mechanisms is frequently related to childbirth but nevertheless occurs in 5–15 per cent of young nulliparous women (Hald, 1984). Epispadias and trauma contribute to some of the causes of the problem but many patients have no obvious abnormality. Lower motor neurone lesions of the sacral efferents to the urethra are more common causes of stress incontinence in rehabilitation units and are usually associated with hypotonic bladders.

Mild symptoms associated with minor anatomical defects will respond to pelvic floor exercises. The techniques used will depend on the preferences of the therapists concerned. Where this approach does not succeed then surgery should be adopted after thorough urodynamic assessment. Where the bladder neck has dropped a colposuspension or, if necessary, a sling procedure are appropriate (Stanton, 1984). When the urethral sphincters are failing in the absence of any descent of the bladder neck then an artificial sphincter should be considered. The Brantley Scott implantable artificial sphincter is the most successful prosthesis of its kind available at the moment (Scott, 1981). Though oestrogenisation is important for normal urethral function topical or system replacement therapy is not useful in treating incontinence.

NURSING ASSESSMENT AND MANAGEMENT

The assessment

A properly conducted nursing assessment should identify those factors, other than bladder dysfunction, which may be aggravating incontinence, and the problems that arise as a result of incontinence. It should complement the medical history and examination. Some of the most frequently identified factors include: immobility, impaired dexterity, poor eyesight, mental impairment and communication problems. Chronic constipation is almost invariable in the immobile and aggravates detrusor instability and any of the voiding problems. Diuretics and sedatives are notorious as precipitants of incontinence. The patient's environment also needs careful checking. What is the distance to the lavatory? Are there any obstacles in the way? Is the lavatory easy to identify? Is it well lit? Is it warm? Are the patient's bed and chairs suitable? A surprisingly common problem is the attitude of the caring staff and the use of unsuitable regimes and institutionalised settings.

The more usual complications of incontinence include: skin excoriation and maceration, and the use of fluid restriction in one way or another. Problems associated with odour must be identified, and it is important to enquire about laundry facilities and the financial consequences of the incontinence. The ability of the relatives or carers to manage the patient's incontinence is an important part of the social assessment as incontinence is often invoked as the precipitant of a crisis within the support system. Incontinence often causes some form of social isolation and problems with self-respect. The associated depression may compromise the ability to recover.

The assessment has to involve private interview with the patient and carers, together and alone. A structured questionnaire is an extremely useful way of aiding the assessment. Liaison with physiotherapists, occupational therapists, and social workers is recommended as their help is often invaluable. It is also important to observe the patient's toileting skills in the home environment.

MANAGEMENT TECHNIQUES

Bladder retraining regimes

The bladder retraining programme forms the cornerstone of treating detrusor instability. The principle is to increase the intervals between voiding until a normal frequency of micturition is achieved without urgency or incontinence. An explanation of the regime should be preceded by a description of normal bladder function and the nature of the abnormality involved. The programme adopted must be kept simple so as to encourage compliance, and the patient will require considerable support and regular review, a minimum of fortnightly. We ask patients to keep a basic daily chart marking with a tick for each micturition and each episode of incontinence. We instruct them to deliberately delay voiding whenever they get the urge, holding for as long as possible. This allows the new pattern of micturition to be developed on the normal circadian rhythm which is impossible with strictly clocked schedules.

If a patient is so dependent as to be unable to cooperate with a standard regime a personalised programme must be developed with the carers. This involves charting the patient's bladder behaviour over four to five days in a stable environment. The information obtained permits the designing of a toileting programme which anticipates the patient's needs. The programme is then redeveloped by trial and error. With careful designing this approach is remarkably helpful.

Pelvic floor exercises

Pelvic floor exercises are only likely to benefit women with mild stress incontinence associated with minimal descent of the bladder neck. They are also helpful to those women who present with a low-pressure detrusor instability in the presence of a low urethral resistance. The grosser forms of urethral sphincter incompetence require surgical solutions.

We teach the patients to identify accurately an effective contraction of the periurethral striated muscle. The therapist inserts a finger into the vagina and identifies the urethra. The patient is then encouraged to contract the periurethral muscles by mimicking the actions used to terminate micturition in midstream. An effective contraction can be detected by the instructor's palpating finger. Once this has been achieved the patient is asked to remember the actions and feelings associated with the contraction. She is advised to perform this contraction, in repetitions of five, regularly throughout the day every time she uses a tap. The use of a tap is usually associated with bladder awareness in those with an incontinence problem. If the exercises are performed adequately an ache is experienced in the perineum during the first two weeks. A response in the symptoms is usually noted over the ensuing two to three months.

Intermittent catheterisation

Intermittent catheterisation is an important method of managing the voiding problems described earlier in this chapter. The clean, non-sterile technique described by Lapides (1976) is the approach now widely adopted. We teach the patient or consort to pass a CH12 plastic Jacques catheter into the bladder during a single outpatient attendance. The technique is then practised at home daily for two weeks while using antibiotic cover and 1 per cent lignocaine jelly as lubricant. After two weeks catheterisatons can usually be achieved without difficulty and a personalised regime, best suited to the individual, is then developed. A bland lubricant jelly is used and catheters are passed with a frequency that keeps the patient continent, free from infection and the residual urine below 500 ml. The catheter is rinsed after each catheterisation and stored in a clean polythene container to be reused and then changed at weekly intervals.

Regular review of this type of management is essential, and the patient must have good access to nursing and medical help if problems, though rare, should occur.

Manual expression and suprapubic tapping

We do not advocate the Crede manoeuvre or other methods of manual expression. It is our experience that these techniques do not promote complete bladder emptying and the forces used may cause damage to the pelvic tissues. We do not use suprapubic tapping in order to promote detrusor contractions in patients with spinal lesions. Our approach hinges on suppressing the bladder using anticholinergics and promoting emptying by intermittent catheterisation. This facilitates the establishment of continence which cannot be achieved with an active detrusor instability.

The use of incontinence aids

A hand-held female urinal is of proven use to women with mobility problems and difficulty in getting out of bed to pass urine. It can be easily emptied into a bucket or commode placed by the bed. The function of a standard male bottle is improved by the use of the Raymed non-spill adaptor which prevents spillage if the bottle is knocked over. The disposable bottle, as made by Downs Surgical, used under a travel rug, is a discreet answer to problems on long journeys.

Very light male incontinence can be managed discreetly with a dribble pouch, an example is that made by 'L.I.C.'. The pouch is held in place with firm fitting stretch pants. The products currently available are expensive, but hopefully the future will see the development of cheaper versions.

Men are less likely to use incontinence pads, but they have a role for the elderly and for younger men who are toileting themselves normally. Kanga produce a pair of pants, modelled on the 'Y-front', which take a single pad in a special waterproof pouch, called the 'Kanga Male'. These are well accepted by men experiencing light incontinence.

Incontinence pads are an important method of management for women. Those that are mobile and independent are best served with a small pad which is easily stored and disposed of. The Kanga Lady or Kanga Bikini systems, or the Sandralux pants, are good examples of popular products. The immobile and less independent women usually require a larger pad, and the Molnlycke Tenaform Normal is a suitable choice of product. Special front-opening pants like the Brevet Sanitas range may prove more appropriate for wheelchair-bound patients who change their own pads.

The disposable bed pad is a time-honoured method of managing incontinence at night. Usually several are required to provide adequate protection, and there are usually problems with leakage and patient discomfort. Nowadays there are better alternatives to use during the night. There are a number of reusable bed covers which are proving to be effective, comfortable and cost-effective. They are all designed to have a high absorbency and to protect the rest of the bed from getting wet. The new Kylie absorbent bedsheet and the Domein 'Confidence' underpad are products worth considering. Molnlycke produce a larger body-worn pad that has also been shown to be effective for managing night-time incontinence. It is comfortable and well accepted and called the 'Tenaform Super'.

Younger men who are unable to toilet themselves are best managed by some form of sheath drainage system. The best products are those that incorporate an adhesive strip as the fixative for the sheath. The two most successful products available at the moment are the Coloplast 'Conveen' and the Squibb Surgicare 'Acuseal'. These are particularly effective when movement is restricted. Despite the advent of better adhesives the sheaths are still easily displaced. Good manual dexterity is required if a sheath is to be applied securely, but this can be achieved by a carer. The older latex urinal devices such as those produced by Downs Surgical are still useful for the heavily incontinent, mobile, male patients with limited manual dexterity. However, they are far from attractive and are often rejected because of this.

REFERENCES

Brindley, G.S., Polkey, C.E., Rushton, D.N. and Cardozo, L. (1984) Sacral anterior root stimulators for bladder control in paraplegia: the first 40 cases. XIV annual meeting of the International Continence Society, Innsbruck, Buch and Offsetdruck Plattner KG, pp. 53-4

Brocklehurst, J.C. (1978) The genitourinary system. In J.C. Brocklehurst (ed.), *Textbook of geriatric medicine and gerontology*, 2nd edn, Churchill Livingstone, Edinburgh, chapter 9, p. 306

Caine, M. and Raz, S. (1973) the effect of progesterone on the adrenergic receptors of the urethra. *Br. J. Urol.*, *45*, 131-5

Castleden, C.M., George, C.F., Renwick, A.G. and Asher, M.J. (1981) Imipramine — a possible alternative to current therapy for urinary incontinence in the elderly. *J. Urol.*, *125*, 318-20

Dontas, A.S. (1984) Urinary tract infections and their implications. In J.C. Brocklehurst (ed.), *Urology in the elderly*, Churchill Livingstone, London, pp. 162-92

Fletcher, T.F. and Bradley, W.E. (1978) Neuroanatomy of the bladder. *J. Urol.*, *119*, 153-60

Gosling, J.A., Dixon, J.S., Hilary, O.D., Critchley, O.H.D. and Thompson, S.A. (1981) A comparative study of the human external sphincter and periurethral levator ani muscles. *Br. J. Urol.*, *53*, 35-41

Griffiths, D.J. (1980) *Urodynamics*: Medical Physics Handbooks, Adam Hilger, Bristol

Hald, T. (1984) The mechanism of continence. In S. Stanton (ed.), *Clinical gynaecological urology*, C.V. Mosby, St Louis and Toronto, pp. 22-7

Karr, J.P. and Murphy, G.P. (1984) Carcinoma of the prostate and its management. In J.C. Brocklehurst (ed.), *Urology in the elderly*, Churchill Livingstone, London, pp. 203-29

Kass, E.H. and Brumfitt, W. (1978) *Infections of the urinary tract*, University of Chicago Press, Chicago

Lapides, J. (1976) Further observations on self catheterisation. *J. Urol., 116*, 109-71

McNeal, J.E. (1983) *The prostate gland: morphology and pathobiology.* Monographs in Urology 4: 3-33

Malone-Lee, J.G. (1983) The pharmacology of urinary incontinence. In G. Barbagallo-Sangiorgi, A.N. Exton-Smith (eds), *Ageing and drug therapy*, Plenum, New York, pp. 419-40

Malone-Lee J.G. and Exton-Smith, A.N. (1985) The disturbances of bladder and bowel. In M. Hildick-Smith (ed.), *Neurological problems of the elderly*, Baillière Tindall, London, pp. 183-98

Moisey, C.U., Stephenson, T.P. and Brendler, C.P. (1980) The urodynamic and subjective results of treatment of detrusor instability with oxybutinin chloride. *Br. J. Urol., 52*, 472

Mundy, A.R. and Stephenson, T.P. (1984) Transvesical injection of the pelvic plexus with phenol for the treatment of detrusor hyperreflexia/instability and bladder hypersensitivity. XIV annual meeting of the International Continence Society, Innsbruck, Buch and Offsetdruck Plattner KG, pp. 55-6

Scott, F.B. (1981) Current results with the AMS artificial sphincter. XI annual meeting of the International Continence Society, Lund. Skogs Trelleborg, pp. 93-4

Stanton, S. (1984) Urethral sphincter incompetence. In S. Stanton (ed.), *Clinical gynaeclogical urology*, C.V. Mosby, St Louis and Toronto, pp. 169-91

Stephenson, T.P. and Mundy, A.R. (1984) The treatment of the neuropathic bladder by enterocystoplasty with selective sphincterotomy, sphincter ablation and replacement or self intermittent catheterisation. XIV annual meeting of the International Continence Society, Innsbruck, Buch and Offsetdruck Plattner KG, pp. 57-8

Turner-Warwick, R. and Whiteside, C.G. (eds.) (1979) *Clinical Urodynamics, Urologic Clinics of North America*, Saunders, Philadelphia, Vol. 6, No 1

Wilson, P.O., Barker, G., Brown, A.O.G., Russel A. and Siddle, N. (1981) Steroid hormone receptors in the female lower urinary tract. XI annual meeting of the International Continence Society, Lund. Skogs Trelleborg, pp. 19-21

FURTHER READING

Incontinence. D. Mandelstam (1977) Heinemann/Disabled Living Foundation, London. (A practical book on aids to help maintain continence and manage incontinence. Second edition, due for publication in 1988 by Croom Helm/ Disabled Living Foundation, London)

30

Sexual Problems and Physical Disability

Mary Davies

Emotional and sexual relationships are highly significant in the lives of most people. This need for human relationships does not disappear with the onset of a physical disability. On the contrary, the person with a disability may need the comfort and security or the validation that a relationship can give, more than ever. People who have a congenital physical disability will have the same range of emotional and sexual needs and feelings as everyone else. Anyone can have problems fulfilling these. Most people do at one time or other in their lives, but a physical disability can be the cause of extra problems.

For staff to be able to help patients in this important area of their rehabilitation two things are necessary. First they need appropriate information on the problems which can arise as the result of a physical disability, as well as some ideas of how the problems can be resolved. Second, and of perhaps even greater importance, they need to feel comfortable with the subject of human sexuality in general, and in particular with the subject of sexuality and physical disability.

EXTENT OF THE PROBLEM

Problems can occur both as a direct and indirect result of physical disability. In a survey carried out by Stewart (1975) over 72 per cent of people with a physical disability experienced sexual and/or emotional problems often lasting a considerable time: 45 per cent were caused by physical factors, 15 per cent were due to psychological factors and 36 per cent were due to both. The greater the degree of disability the greater the problems.

EFFECTS OF PHYSICAL DISABILITY ON SEXUAL AND EMOTIONAL RELATIONSHIPS

Some disabilities have a very direct effect on sexual function, i.e. the usual sexual response does not take place even when the individual is sexually aroused. The man may be unable to get an erection or an ejaculation and the woman may not have the physiological response to sexual arousal which is an increase in vaginal blood flow and increased vaginal lubrication. Disabilities which can produce these effects include spinal injury, multiple sclerosis, diabetes mellitus and spina bifida. When a man gets an erection a nervous impulse passes down from the brain via the spinal cord and autonomic nervous system to the penis, causing a redistribution of blood flow and hence an erection. For both erection and ejaculation to occur the parasympathetic and sympathetic outflows need to be undamaged. When a spinal injury occurs the nervous pathway may be interrupted, so the man becomes impotent. In multiple sclerosis, impotence can occur due to effects of the disease on the autonomic nervous system, as can also occur in diabetes mellitus. An erection may also occur as a reflex — the reflexogenic erection. When this occurs the reflex arc operates, and is independent of the brain or the rest of the spinal cord. This means that, even after a spinal injury, a reflexogenic erection may still be possible, and some men have found this a source of great pleasure in their lovemaking. For many men, accepting impotence is not easy and can cause feelings of doubt about their 'manhood'.

The control system for sexual arousal in women is similar to that in men. Physical disabilities which interrupt the passage of the nerve impulse to the sex organs, such as spinal injury or multiple sclerosis, may have the effect of preventing the physiological changes of sexual arousal occurring. There are no measures we can take to produce the normal increased blood flow to the sex organs, but vaginal lubrication can be enhanced by the use of KY Jelly. Some disabilities make the attainment of an orgasm more difficult or impossible, a problem less easy to resolve.

Many physical disabilities do not produce such dramatic direct effects on sexual functioning, but can have profound effects on emotional and sexual relationships in indirect ways.

PAIN AND FEAR

Pain, particularly chronic pain, can be a source of problems. One very common example of this is in arthritis when the woman may find it too painful to lie with her legs spread apart, or the man may find it difficult to support himself on his elbows or to bend his knees. If sexual intercourse is associated with pain, as in these instances, then the person soon begins to avoid sexual contact. Pain affects the libido so that there is loss of interest in sex. If someone suspects that his/her partner may be pained by sexual intercourse, he/she may avoid close contact and sexual arousal. This can eventually damage the relationship.

Fear can also have this effect. Many patients leave hospital after an illness or an operation without any information on when and how to resume their sex lives. At the time of discharge from hospital many patients do not feel able to ask about this important aspect of their lives, and many couples — where a partner has had a stroke, or a heart attack, or cancer — postpone or give up altogether what could be a comforting part of their relationship.

LOSS OR LACK OF CONTROL OF BODY MOVEMENT

This can often lead to a loss of sexual relationships. After a stroke the patient may be left with partial paralysis, so that new positions for sexual activity may be necessary. Reassurance must be given that sex will not be harmful and cause further problems.

INCONTINENCE

Bladder or bowel incontinence is viewed with great distaste; it may be seen as a 'return to childhood', and for many it means an end to their sex lives. Some people feel ashamed to talk about incontinence, and would find it very difficult to raise this subject themselves, particularly when related to sexuality.

BODY IMAGE

Incontinence can cause individuals to feel quite negative about themselves and their body. One very important consideration in establishing and maintaining emotional and sexual relationships is that the person feels good about himself, and has a positive body image. If people's image of their own body is very different from their ideal of what they would like their body to be, a negative body image may result. This affects their response to others. There are many instances in which a physical disability can lead to a negative body image — a young athlete who becomes paralysed from a spinal injury and is confined to a wheelchair may see himself or herself as being far away from his/her ideal of a young attractive person.

Other examples of this include limb amputation, mastectomy, colostomy or a congenital physical disability, even if it only slightly affects the appearance. Such feelings can lead to a loss of libido or even impotence.

EFFECT OF DRUGS

Some prescribed drugs can lead to sexual problems, e.g. beta blockers can cause impotence. If patients are unaware that their impotence is due to the drug, then even if the drug is discontinued, impotence may remain — the cause then now being psychological. It is worth remembering that the most common cause of impotence is psychological. Some sedatives and antidepressents reduce libido, and monoamine oxidase inhibitors may make orgasm less attainable.

Many of the problems which people with a disability have to overcome can be summed up in one word — *attitudes* — of the society we live in, of members of the family, of professional workers.

THE MANAGEMENT OF PATIENTS

Lack of knowledge about the effect of the disability on sexual function can cause problems for patients, who can be helped by being given reassurance where appropriate, and information to enable him to get round the practical problems where these occur. Staff need to appreciate how much difficulty many patients find in raising the subject of sexuality. The staff may be embarrassed, not know what language is appropriate and be inhibited by other factors such as gender difference, age difference and cultural and/or religious differences. For staff the attitudes of their colleagues are of great importance. They need to feel that by raising the subject they are working within accepted practices and are supported rather than being undermined. The attitude of the patient's partner is crucial, for the partner may also be frightened and need information and reassurance. The timing of any information-giving may be critical. Unspoken anxieties can lead to a withdrawal from the partner; not just a sexual withdrawal but also a cessation of cuddling and kissing in case this may lead to more frightening sexual activity. Over the long term this can lead to a breakdown in the relationship.

In order to be able to provide this information, staff themselves need knowledge not only of the potential effect of the disability on sexual function but also of solutions to the problems. Even when they have this knowledge, unless they feel comfortable with the subject of sexuality they may well avoid it. If staff haven't had the opportunity to explore their own attitudes and feelings towards aspects of sexuality, such as homosexual or lesbian relationships or alternatives to sexual intercourse, then they may be unwittingly giving messages of hostility or disapproval to the patient.

Sexuality is something that belongs to every individual, whether severely disabled or old and infirm. We are all of us influenced by the media's presentation of sexuality as being the province of the young, fit and glamorous. This may cause distress to the patient, and may also affect how staff respond to the sexual rehabilitation needs of their patients. It is all too easy to look at the patient as a non-sexual person and deny him/her essential information.

It may happen that a particularly brave patient (brave for raising the subject) may ask a question which causes staff members to be taken aback because they don't know the answer. A positive way of responding is to say to the patient 'That's a good question for you to ask. I don't know the answer right now but I'll find out and then come back to you'. The attitude of staff towards the patient is of vital importance. They can respond positively, which reinforces the patient's dignity and sexuality, or laugh and make a joke about it which, although it helps them feel more comfortable, effectively denies the sexuality of the patient.

Many patients are far too embarrassed to raise the subject themselves even if they are very concerned about it. Ideally the subject should be raised by the staff in such a way that the patient can choose whether to continue the discussion or not.

CHANGES OF POSITION OR TECHNIQUE

In some instances, all that patients require is information on when it is safe to resume sexual activity, and reassurance that it will not harm them or their partner. Some of the problems require a practical approach, e.g. if a patient with severe arthritis finds sexual intercourse in one position uncomfortable, then other positions can be tried. Although the patient may be well aware that different positions can be tried, the fact that it has been suggested by the staff member can act as very helpful 'permission-giving'. Written advice in the form of leaflets can also be useful, since they can be used by patients to facilitate discussion with their partner. An example of an information sheet provided by SPOD is shown in Figure 30.1.

In some cases, when the patient has a partner who is not disabled, the partner may be able to take on the more active role in the lovemaking. After a man has had a stroke he may find lovemaking easier if his partner plays an active part and lies or sits on him if he is unable to support her weight. It *is* possible for patients to change their sexual practices of many years' standing. For some this can result in a renewed interest and enjoyment of sex.

COPING WITH INCONTINENCE

If bladder incontinence is the problem, patients require information that fresh urine is not harmful and that urine output can be temporarily reduced by restricting fluid intake for a few hours prior to sexual activity, emptying

Figure 30.1: Resuming sexual activity after a heart attack

The timing and manner of resumption of activity is important.

1. Patient can generally resume sexual activity when he is able to perform routine levels of physical activity (e.g. climbing two flights of stairs).
2. If palpitations or angina occur, he should stop immediately.
3. Advisable to have intercourse with the usual partner in the usual position.
4. The room should be at a comfortable temperature.
5. A hot bath, or eating or drinking too much prior to sexual activity, should be avoided.
6. A comfortable position for sexual intercourse should be used: partner could assume the active role.
7. There are alternatives to sexual intercourse as a way of giving and receiving sexual pleasure. See SPOD leaflets.
8. If erection is impaired due to beta blocking drugs, try sexual activity in the morning when male hormone levels are raised and the effect of the drug is at the lowest.
9. If there is persistent difficulty a doctor may be able to advise vasodilators to be taken prior to sexual activity.

the bladder before sexual intercourse. Patients with catheters do not always need to remove them. For the woman the catheter is taped to the abdomen. When the man has an erection the catheter can be taped into place along the penis or kept in place using a sheath. KY Jelly can assist comfort in both instances. Some couples will not be comfortable or confident in having sexual intercourse with a catheter in place, and may prefer to remove it, but discussion of the subject provides the opportunity for patients to air their anxieties, and may dispel some of the negative associations of incontinence.

Bowel incontinence can be best helped by encouraging the patient to improve management of his/her routine as much as possible, and to take care to be scrupulously hygienic. If the patient has a stoma, he/she may well need reassurance that sex will not harm it, and that with time management will improve. The bag or stoma can be covered during sex; sexy underwear is used by many people to enhance their lovemaking.

ALTERNATIVES TO SEXUAL INTERCOURSE

There are some patients for whom sexual intercourse is not possible. Either the man is unable to get an erection, or the woman is unable to experience penetration. Lovemaking can be carried out in other ways, by the use of the hands, or the mouth and tongue. Many couples get a great deal of enjoyment from mutual caressing and masturbation, and from orogenital sex. The whole of the skin is supplied with sense organs which can be a great source of delight when stroked or kissed. According to the Hite Report, many women find it easier to experience an orgasm via these techniques than by sexual intercourse, so lovemaking can go on in the absence of an erection. However, some couples prefer sexual intercourse to other methods of mutual stimulation. If the man is impotent a sex aid may enable the couple to continue to experience sexual intercourse.

SEX AIDS

These can range from everyday items like a pillow or cushion which supports parts of the body, or hold legs apart, to specially made appliances. Aids to getting and maintaining an erection are found to be extremely useful for some people. One such aid is an energising ring made of ebonite with copper and zinc electrodes set into either end. The ring is made in various sizes and needs to fit accurately in order to work well. It is worn around the scrotum and penis and encourages an erection due to a slight constrictive effect on the penile veins. The ring can often (not always) enhance an incomplete erection. The energising ring is not always effective, in which case an artificial penis may be useful. This is hollow at the end near the body; the man puts his flaccid penis inside it and holds it or straps it in position. Lubrication can be provided by KY Jelly. Another useful sex aid is the artificial vagina. It is lined with latex and contains a vibrator. It can be used when a woman is unable to have sexual intercourse, e.g. after surgery. The artificial vagina can be held between her thighs; for lubrication KY Jelly is necessary. The vagina can also be used to simulate masturbation for men who have no hand coordination or control. The sex aids just described are not designed specifically for people with a physical disability, which can be a point in their favour for some patients. If both partners feel happy and relaxed about using sex aids, they can provide much sexual satisfaction and pleasure. Professional staff giving information to patients must feel comfortable about showing them to patients.

During rehabilitation it is important that the subject of the resumption of sexual activity is raised. Whether patients are young or old they need to know:

(1) the effect that their medical condition has had on their body;
(2) which features of this, or of therapy, will continue to exert an effect;
(3) what can be done to reduce the disadvantages/disabilities ensuing in the sexual sphere;
(4) where to obtain helpful information and/or aids;
(5) the timing and intensity of resumption of sexual activity;
(6) the importance of close physical contact (of cuddling and kissing).

Most people see their sexuality as something that is extremely private, but patients need an opportunity to talk to a person who is sympathetic to the fact that they still have emotional and physical needs which may be increased by the insecurity of disability. They may need permission to rediscover how their body can be a source of pleasure to themselves and their partner. In some instances information and advice from the professional is not enough to enable patients to resolve their difficulties and they may need sex therapy or counselling. Further information is available from the agencies listed at the end of the chapter, and in Chapter 49.

For any of this to be helpful, the professional requires to have a positive attitude towards sexuality and physical disability, and to accept that there are many ways of giving and receiving sexual pleasure. Sexual intercourse is just one of these ways. To quote Don Smith, who became disabled at 19.

> I felt asexual for a long time because a man's sex is supposed to be in his penis — and I couldn't feel my penis — it didn't occur to me that it felt good to have the back of my neck licked or that it felt good to have my arms stroked lightly. I've taken the goals out of my lovemaking. I don't have to have intercourse or any kind of penetration if I'm going to have sex, I don't even have to do anything with the genitals. I can take my time. I feel less pressure and less performance anxiety.

Victoria Thornton has cerebral palsy:

> I walked around with my head in the clouds most of my early life because I was trying to avoid my body and I did not associate earthiness with sexuality at all. I did not associate sexuality with my body. I associated it with my emotions and with my spirit. I still have some wonderful platonic friendships. But it is through my sexual relationships that I find a greater acceptance of my whole person, body and mind.

FURTHER READING

Boiler, F. and Frank, E. (1982) *Sexual dysfunction in neurological disorders — diagnosis, management and rehabilitation*, Raven Press, New York

Brearley, G. and Birchley, P. (1986) *Introducing counselling skills and techniques — with particular application for the para-medical professions*, Faber & Faber, London

Bullard, D.G. and Knight, S.E. (1981) *Sexuality and physical disability — personal perspectives*, C.V. Mosby, St Louis

Comfort, A. (1978) *Sexual consequences of disability*, Stickley, London

Davies, M., Hasler, F., Holland, B., Dareborough, A. and Lowden, H. (1982) *Sexuality and the physically disabled*, SPOD, London

Dechesne, B.H.H. (1985) *Sexuality and handicap, problems of motor handicapped people*, Woodhead-Faulkner, Cambridge

Mooney, T.O., Cole, T.M. and Chilgren, R.A. (1975) *Sexual options for paraplegics and quadriplegics*, Little, Brown & Co., Boston

Stewart, W.F.R., (1975) *Sex and the physically handicapped*, The National Fund for Research into Crippling Diseases, London

Stewart, W.F.R. (1979) *The sexual side of handicap*, Woodhead-Faulkner, Cambridge

Advisory leaflets are available from SPOD (the Association to Aid the Sexual and Personal Relationships of People with a Disability)

HELPFUL AGENCIES

Disabled Living Centres
Multiple Sclerosis Society
Spastics Society
Spinal Injuries Association
} See Resources, Chapter 49

National Marriage Guidance Council
Herbert Gray College, Little Church Street, Rugby, Warwickshire CV21 3AP

SPOD
286 Camden Road, London N7 0BJ

31

The Skin, Tissue Viability and Rehabilitation

James Robertson, Michael Masser, Ian Swain, Christine Dowding, Simon Daunt and Ragai Shaban

The concept of tissue viability provides a framework for consideration of the care of skin and subcutaneous tissues. Failures of patient care may lead to loss of viability and the development of chronic open ulcers. These may be called pressure sores, chronic wounds or, on occasion, fistulae or sinuses. They are far too common. They can interfere with the rehabilitation of acute patients and may rob disabled patients of all ages of the quality of life, even if they do not shorten it. Sores also kill, and have profound effects on the health of patients.

Put simply, tissue viability is to the part as health is to the whole person. The term is to be preferred to 'tissue trauma' for the same reasons that the National Health Service is to be preferred to a National Sickness Service. To understand the disorders of tissue viability it is not enough to understand the underlying pathology, for the maintenance of tissue health is a more complex and a wider subject. To interpret abnormal values, the normal values have to be measured and understood (Robertson *et al.*, 1980). Unfortunately, we are only beginning to make the measurements of 'tissue viability parameters' and we do not yet have a consensus as to how to measure interface pressure, which is probably the most relevant parameter to study. Sampling of interface pressure during acute patient care throughout the 24 hours has proved useful.

Enough is known about tissue viability for most pressure sores to be prevented, and probably for many chronic open ulcers to be prevented also. The failure of our health care system to prevent sores is attributable equally to the lack of status of the subject, inadequate provision of physical facilities by the service, deficiency of patient self-care for a variety of social or personal reasons, and perhaps also lack of expertise on the part of professionals and carers. The limiting factors lie in the failure of care and caring systems to apply current knowledge. Even so, much more research remains to be done.

There is more to the concept of tissue viability than 'tissue health'. In the same way that the psychosomatic movement and its successor holistic medicine stress the necessity of diagnosis of, and care for, the whole patient in a family and work setting, so the concept of tissue viability underlines the importance of comprehensive and 24-hour care both internally, and especially externally, in the case of skin tissue viability disorders. This must be within the framework of a total approach to the whole patient. Similar principles apply to the part that is ulcerated. Putting it in another way, the process of rehabilitation must be applied to the whole patient as well as to the part. There are few short cuts; resources, including staff time, are limited; the need for care is infinite, and there is no end to learning, for the state of the art is advancing rapidly across the scientific territories of many disciplines. Teamwork is a necessity.

Study of skin tissue viability is repaid by the benefits resulting from better assessment of patients' problems. Traditionally pressure sore care was relegated to nursing staff, who were blamed for the very presence of the sores. The final common pathway of many illnesses, including those causing death, is through increasing disability, with its limitation of mobility. In the depressive there may be a lack of will to move; in the sensorily deficient, a lack of stimulus to move; in the respiratory or cardiac cripple, a lack of power to move, and in the stroke patient, a lack of control. Pressure sores result from lack of movement (Roaf, 1976). Movement affects the skin microclimate and determines the pattern of loading of skin and subcutaneous tissues. Thus the onset of a pressure sore indicates that disease is severe, or if the disease is not the main determinant of the sore then it marks a failure to provide adequate care. Indeed, pressure sores and other chronic open ulcers should be made notifiable, for they are good markers of morbidity and deprivation; they deserve to be part of the RAWP formula for determining care resources (Barton *et al.*, 1981). Pressure sores promote cross-infection in hospital and so may affect other patients who do not have sores. Wound exudate may contain viruses, and sores may provide a portal of entry for viruses. The AIDS virus is found in body fluids such as exudates from wounds and ulcers. Prevention of sores deserves the highest priority.

Pressure sores are the prime example of skin tissue viability disorders, but are only one of the dangers of recumbency or sitting, or of being too still for too long. Thrombosis, urinary stagnation, wasting of bones and muscles, and vasomotor instability are other dangers of immobility. Pressure sores are better markers of immobility than fatal pulmonary emboli, or osteoporotic fractures. Measures taken to prevent pressure sores, simultaneously prevent or minimise the other equally serious problems. Investment in care systems, especially patient handling systems, will benefit all patients, and has been proven to prevent pressure sores (Miller, 1984; O'Reilly *et al.*, 1981).

VIABILITY DISORDERS OF THE SKIN AND SUBCUTANEOUS TISSUES

These are listed in the form of a flow chart (Figure 31.1) which outlines what can happen to initially healthy skin when external factors affecting viability operate. Clearly the factors may also affect the compromised skin of patients with diabetes, peripheral vascular disease, loss of sensation, structural and locomotor problems. Good management will depend on the patient and the carer understanding the physical signs that differentiate a healthily adapted area of hypertrophied skin from a subcutaneous bruise or haematoma. Lesions indicating reversible compromise of viability due to recurrent application of abnormal forces need to be appreciated. They may indicate remediable causes of potential sores or necessitate the patient rationing the use of that part of his body. Such signs are the stock-in-trade of chiropodists, prosthetists and orthotists, and should be as well understood by nurses, therapists and doctors. Such experience needs to be shared widely. Hence the founding of multidisciplinary societies such as the Society for Research in Rehabilitation, and the Tissue Viability Society (Crow, 1985).

CLASSIFICATION

Pressure sores are classified as superficial (Type 1) or deep (Type 2) (Barton, 1981). Barton has cut through the complexity underlying many

Figure 31.1: Tissue viability disorders of skin and subcutaneous structures

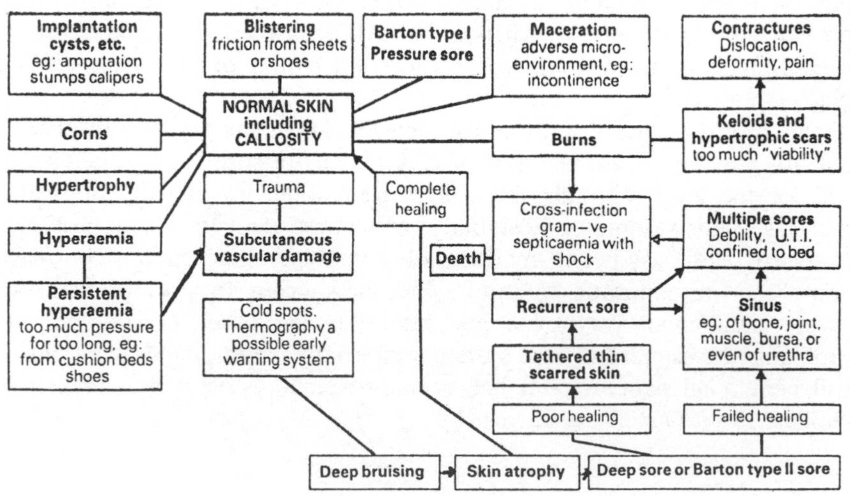

classifications and he is correct to consider that the two types are fundamentally different. The first is superficial and starts in the dermis and may progress inwards, whereas the second begins deep with vascular damage, and may progress both outwards and inwards. The types often coexist. For a full discussion on pressure sore classification and grading, readers should consult Lowthian's review (1985).

EPIDEMIOLOGY (Tables 31.1 and 31.2)

The Salisbury Health District's two-year survey of chronic open ulcers, or wounds not healing satisfactorily after two weeks, revealed a wide variety of associated diseases (Dowding, 1983). These included acute and chronic conditions, both life-threatening and disabling. The mortality of these mainly elderly patients was one in three. Wounds healed in only half the survivors. Table 31.3 lists the sources of patients, and indicates that all groups of health care workers are potentially involved.

Table 31.1: Two-year survey of chronic cutaneous ulcer patients in Salisbury Health District (population 160,000)

	Female	Male
314 patients	212	102
104 died	61	43
105 healed		
	1.6 ulcers per patient	

Table 31.2: Morbidity associated with chronic cutaneous ulcer patients

21%	osteoarthritis
14%	congestive cardiac failure
13%	cerebrovascular accident
12%	varicose disease
11%	fractured femur
9.5%	diabetes mellitus
8.5%	hypertension
7.3%	deep vein thrombosis
6.4%	rheumatoid arthritis
5.7%	myocardial infarction
5.4%	malignancy
5.4%	hiatus hernia
5.1%	depression
4.8%	dementia and/or Parkinsonism
4.5%	tetraplegics and paraplegics, half of whom were spinally injured

Note: There was an average of 1.4 diseases per patient.

Table 31.3: Sources of chronic ulcer patients

37%	found on acute wards
30%	on geriatric wards and day hospital
17%	domiciliary
10%	outpatients
4%	psychiatric wards
2%	chiropody

One-third of chronic ulcers are pressure sores, two-thirds of which are on the pelvic girdle and one-quarter on the legs. One in ten pressure sores involve the heels. The younger patients with pressure sores suffer from multiple sclerosis, spinal injury, spina bifida or diabetes. Sores are rare in disabled children, the usual association being with spina bifida.

Spinal injury patients are particularly at risk from pressure sores. In a patient questionnaire study 30 per cent of patients reported having a sore during their initial treatment, and 15 per cent had been readmitted (Lawes, 1984). In a study of 155 deaths occurring three months or more after spinal injury in patients attending the Stoke Mandeville Spinal Unit between 1964 and 1980, 61 died from renal amyloid. Of these, 50 were sufficiently well documented to permit further study. Forty-seven had pressure sores, 36 of whom had had them on admission to Stoke Mandeville after transfer from another hospital. Twenty patients had had sores for more than 66 per cent of their clinical lifetime. In these 20 the major or exclusive cause of the amyloid was pressure sore sepsis (Baker *et al.*, 1984).

A national survey of hospital patients showed a prevalence of 6.7 per cent pressure sores (David *et al.*, 1985). The 'sores' were graded into four groups. The first, the pre-sore grade, including scabbed areas and areas considered likely to break down, amounted to 19 per cent of all the 'sores' found. The second group had a superficial break in the skin (26 per cent). The third group was defined as a full skin thickness destruction (32 per cent). The fourth group consisted of deep ulcers (23 per cent). Groups two and three probably correspond with Barton Type 1, and group 4 with his Type 2. Despite the variation in the grading systems used in surveys the prevalence of sores (pre-sore grades excluded) lies between 3 per cent and 8.8 per cent of all hospital patients. In the community there are probably as many patients with pressure sores as there are in hospital, as well as those with other common chronic open ulcers, such as varicose ulcers. Perhaps for the population as a whole there is a prevalence of between one and five chronic open ulcer patients per 1,000 people.

FACTORS AFFECTING SKIN TISSUE VIABILITY

Several clinically important factors were demonstrated in the same national survey in which 885 hospital patients were found to have 1,506 pressure sores: 85 per cent of the patients were elderly, 50 per cent were immobile, and 31 per cent were incontinent. Forty-four per cent had been admitted urgently, most frequently for orthopaedic (18 per cent) or cerebrovascular (17 per cent) conditions; 77 per cent had chronic health problems, such as arthritis, paralysis, or diabetes, which also required treatment. Drugs thought to delay healing were being administered to 40 per cent of patients, and 41 per cent were taking sedatives. Simple clinical observations have proved reliable enough to form a risk scoring system, called after its originator Doreen Norton. This has been found to be reproducible between observers (Table 31.4) (Norton *et al.*, 1962). The emphasis on mental alertness, mobility in and out of bed, continence, and general health is clear.

LOCAL FACTORS: PRESSURES AND LOADS: distinguish/define pressure/load

Local factors may be influenced by local therapies, pressures, circulation, lack of skin ventilation, lack of skin sensation, and patterns of loading excess at certain points. *Sheer forces* (Figure 31.2) *are particularly dangerous and result in tension being applied to subcutaneous structures with distortion.* If extreme, larger cutaneous blood vessels may infarct and subsequently bleed. Failure to notice the resulting 'cold spot' may lead to repeated loading of the pressure point concerned, with eventual ulceration through the skin to cause a deep pressure sore. Such sores may 'surface' four to eight days after surgery (Petersen, 1976) especially after surgical treatment of a fractured femur (Dyson, 1978). The effect of ischaemia secondary to pressure on the capillary endothelium, and the subsequent inflammation and secondary damage, has been studied by Barton, who has also demonstrated the potential usefulness of ACTH in blocking the inflammatory reaction. A single injection of ACTH prior to hip surgery reduced the incidence of pressure sores from 16 per cent to 6 per cent (Barton and Barton, 1976). They believe that the inflammation induced by ischaemic capillary wall damage when the blood supply is restored, after the relief of pressure on the pressure point, is the cause of much secondary obstruction to blood flow. Inhibitors of inflammation may have a useful role in the prevention of sores. Similarities with small vein thrombosis will be apparent. Pressure continuously, unevenly or locally applied, especially if above skin arteriolar level, is the main cause of pressure sores. The relationship between the intensity of pressure applied locally and the length

Table 31.4: The Norton Score

A Physical condition		B Mental condition		C Activity		D Mobility		E Incontinent	
Good	4	Alert	4	Ambulant	4	Full	4	Not	4
Fair	3	Apathetic	3	Walk with help	3	Slightly limited	3	Occasionally	3
Poor	2	Confused	2	Chairbound	2	Very limited	2	Usually/urine	2
Very bad	1	Stuporous	1	Bedfast	1	Immobile	1	Doubly	1

Key: A total score of 14 or below means the patient is at risk.

Figure 31.2: Factors in the development of pressure sores: sheer, pressure and friction

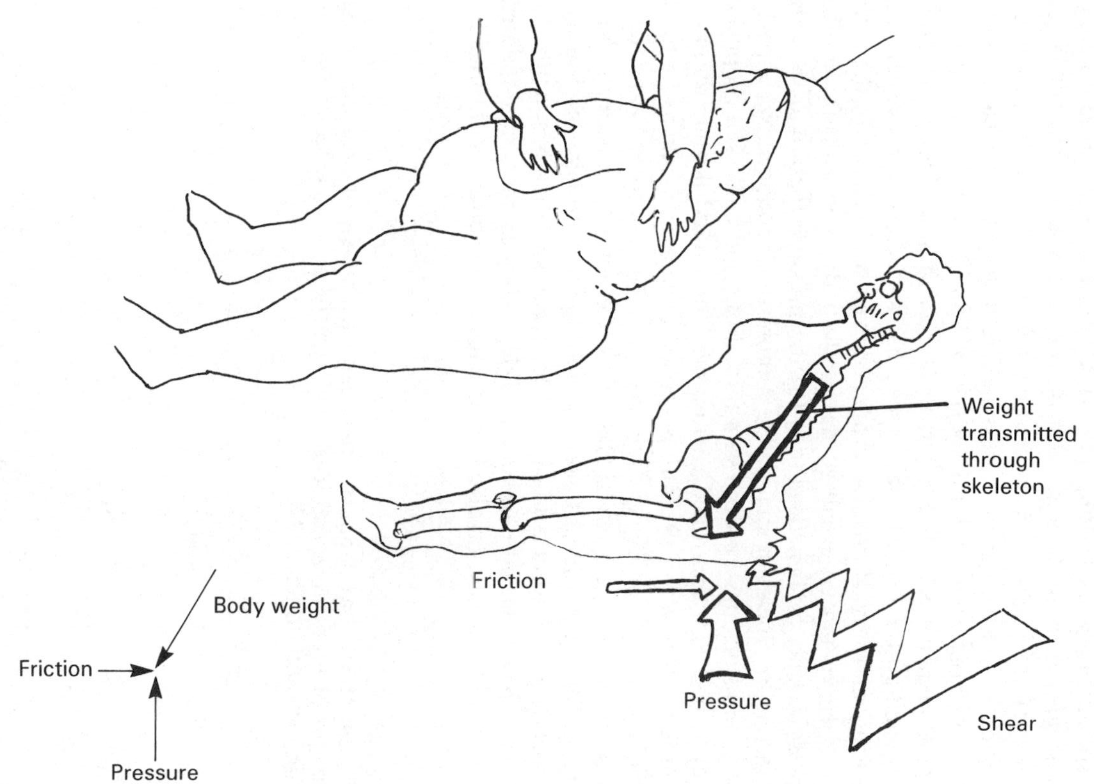

of time for which it is applied continuously without ill effect is shown in Figure 31.3 (Reswick and Rogers, 1976). This particular graph was obtained by medical engineers in a seating clinic, using the forerunner of the Talley 8 cm electropneumatic interface pressure sensor, which probably reads low. The same kind of time–pressure relationship is found in other experimental work (Brand, 1976a). Cycled pressure and repeated loading with an element of sheer, reduces the pressure bearable without damage, i.e. the curve in Figure 31.3 shifts to the left. That the pattern of loading may correlate with the patient's pressure sore history and clinical condition has been demonstrated by Bardsley *et al.* (1983) for young wheelchair-bound, spina bifida patients. The children who rocked from side to side rather than fore and aft on their wheelchair seats had suffered fewer sores and had less spinal deformity. If pressure is applied evenly to a region of the body such as a leg, or indeed evenly to the whole body as in a deep sea diver, the pressure may be beneficial, e.g. (a) the pressure therapy of hypertrophic scarring, (b) the even and graded compression produced by support stockings and stockings for deep vein thrombosis and embolism prophylaxis, or (c) as part of a controlled environment for wound healing on limbs after surgery. However, if pressure is applied circumferentially like a tourniquet (Johnson, 1972) or locally (Daly *et al.*, 1976) pressures as low as 10 mm/Hg may cause damage or affect blood flow. Certainly a pressure of 15 mm/Hg applied to the popliteal fossa can cause the appearances of obstruction on phlebography (Hosni *et al.*, 1968). Clearly pressure on skin and subcutaneous tissues may be harmful or beneficial depending on the amount, distribution and anatomical sites involved, or, in engineering terms, on the loading of the site.

Figure 31.3: The relationship between the intensity of local pressure and the length of time for which it is continuously applied *without ill-effect* (after Reswick and Rogers, 1976)

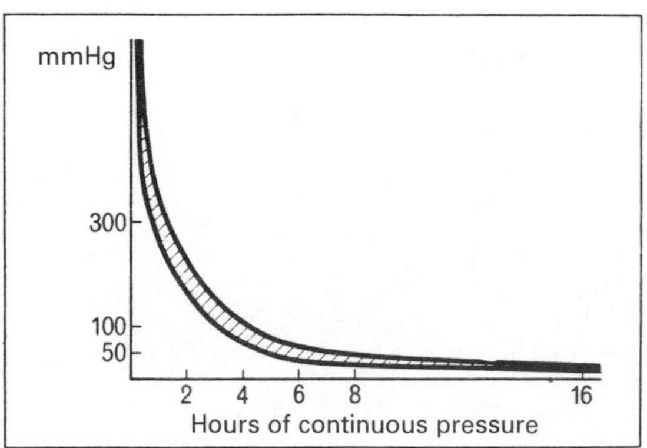

LOADING AND MOVEMENT

The *pattern* of loading is determined by movement. Only movement of the environment against the patient or vice-versa can alter the pressure, tension and shearing force at an anatomical pressure (or loading) point. Movement of resting patients lying on beds or in chairs has not been properly measured. It is thought to be inversely related to the plane or depth of sleep. Exton-Smith and Sherwin (1961) demonstrated that reduction in movement during sleep predisposed to bed sores. 'Relevant movement', that is movement that alters pressure at the so-called pressure points, has not been well studied, for there are many difficulties. One study suggested that small amplitude and high frequency may be prominent characteristics of the spontaneous movements occurring in the sleeper. Between 14 and 48 such weight-relieving movements per hour of sleep were recorded at the sacral prominence of a subject trained to lie on his back (Robertson *et al.*, 1980). It is unfortunate that Exton-Smith's machine cannot be applied to the modern hospital bed, for recording relevant movement, and indeed such simple parameters as 'time out of bed' are probably as important as recording the temperature, pulse and respiration rates.

Another elegant study (Clarke, 1974) showed that movement affected the microclimate in the pockets of air surrounding the recumbent patients covered by bedclothes. Movement of the patient affects the temperature, humidity, the rate of air interchange, and loading. If no movement occurs then the tissues are deformed by virtue of their viscoelastic properties (Wijn *et al.*, 1976). Lack of movement may raise the local temperature with metabolic consequences which enhance the ill-effects of pressure-induced ischaemia. Such an effect may be important for patients who spend their days sitting in wheelchairs, and especially when these patients are unable to perform regular pressure-relieving lifts, or to transfer off their chairs to standing or lying postures (Brattgard *et al.*, 1976) (Figure 31.4).

MEASUREMENT OF TISSUE VIABILITY PARAMETERS

Tissue viability parameters should be measured wherever possible. Perhaps interface pressure distribution is the most useful, supplemented by thermoscanning (Brand, 1976b). Other techniques are promising, and transcutaneous oxygen and photoplethysmography are used regularly as research techniques, and often as supplementary clinical investigations (Mani, 1985). Differential temperature measurement and radioactive uptake methods are seemingly in decline. Assessment of interface pressure is now easy using the Talley Scimedic 8 cm sensor for seating for near-flat interface condition or the Talley 28 mm sensor. More expensive techniques are available, and the Bader Oxford and Krouskop Texas methods are

Figure 31.4: Viscoelasticity of skin and subcutaneous tissues. (a) The buttocks of a paraplegic vegetarian patient with a non-progressive spinal tumour, showing deformity caused by the scars of plastic surgery for pressure sores. (b) View of buttocks shortly after the patient sat on transparent seat. The blackened areas represent air. (c) A quarter of an hour later the viscoelastic soft tissues have deformed under their own weight and trapped pockets of air in the hollows caused by the scarring

(a)

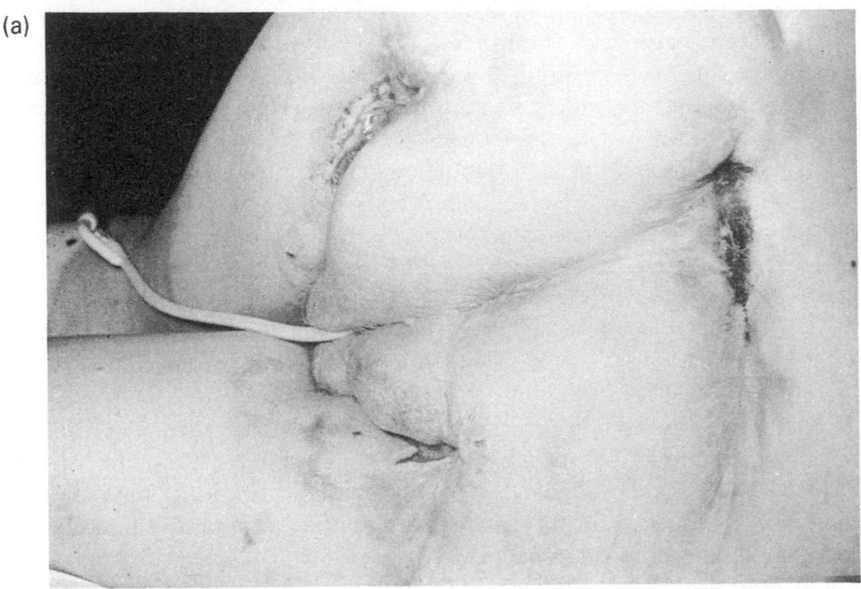

(b)

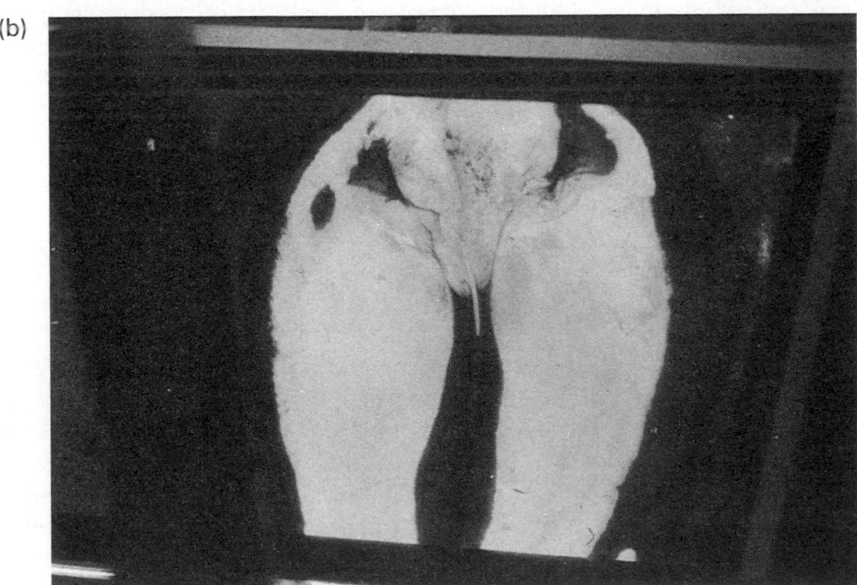

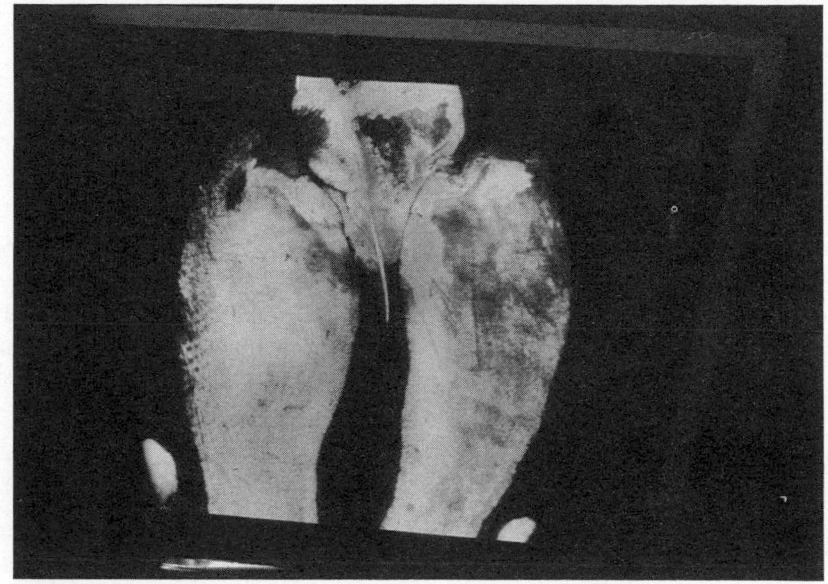

useful research tools, particularly where pressure distribution is of interest. The Talley 28 mm sensor developed at Roehampton and Odstock can be used with a baseline technique which makes it sufficiently accurate for research work, particularly on curved surfaces. It can be used continuously but is not without its difficulties as the sensors are not robust. Other techniques may become available, and researchers are strongly advised to consult experts such as the staff of district departments of medical physics and engineering (Grant, 1985).

Interface pressure measurement allows the assessment of fit between patients and their stockings, shoes, splints, callipers, sockets, or support systems. The fit can be too tight, too loose, or uneven. Such measured assessment can be used in outpatients, and should be a standard tool for arthritis, plaster technicians, occupational therapists and chiropodists.

CHRONIC WOUND HEALING — PRINCIPLES OF MANAGEMENT

Wounds are damaged areas of the body, involving the skin and often underlying tissues. If the wound is open and not showing signs of healing after two weeks it may be regarded as a chronic ulcer. Medical wounds are those which have to be managed without a surgeon's help, or do not need it. However, surgical opinions should be sought freely, particularly from those specialists concerned with repair; for example, plastic, spinal and vascular surgeons. The principles of managing chronic ulcers are:

(a) doing no harm to a lesion which ought to heal;

(b) reversing causative factors where possible;

(c) maintaining health (e.g. by keeping diabetes mellitus, anaemia, etc., under control);

(d) providing an effective, district-based, care system.

Choice of care will depend on the resources available. These include peer support from colleagues, and a district wound/ulcer policy and team for prevention and management as recommended in the Royal College of Physicians' Report (1986). The pressure sore team should include a nurse and consultant. Such a team should liaise with a similar incontinence team.

SERVICE PROVISION

It is our belief that every district should also have a multidisciplinary lower limb care clinic with immediate access to interface pressure measurement. Such clinics should be run with chiropodists, orthotists (appliance fitters), and interested doctors in association with the district appliance officer service and the medical physics and engineering service. Such clinics should have close liaison with limb-fitting surgeons, who, with their prosthetists and wheelchair technical officers, should be visiting the district regularly. Ideally wheelchairs and seating clinics should run concurrently, and all the clinics should have technical back-up to permit maintenance and minor alterations to be made during them. Purpose-built accommodation close to the main outpatients department of the District General Hospital is required. On the same site a home and hospital aids and equipment loan store could be operating as a source of supply, e.g. for walking aids, alternative wheelchairs, and cushions (Robertson and Haines, 1978). Patients should be able to stay over lunch, and patients attending regional centres at general hospitals may need hostel accommodation, as may their relatives. The above recommendations are supported by the findings of the McColl Report (1986).

INDIVIDUAL PATIENT MANAGEMENT: ASSESSMENT

The starting point for management of the individual patients is a *full assessment* of the whole patient and his situation. This must include a 24-hour consideration of both local and general factors which may affect healing, or which may precipitate further ulceration, perhaps of the other leg, or cause a relapse of the ulcer itself. *External local factors* include friction, uneven pressure, especially if applied continuously for long periods, excessive pressure and lack of movement. All of these may be associated with shear and with a less favourable microenvironment. Cold, heat, chemical, radiational and surgical trauma create wounds which can be further damaged by uneven dressings, infection or poor mechanical management. Internal local factors include peripheral vascular disease, arterial, venous or microvascular, paralysis, sensory loss, and local anatomy — *normal*, e.g. bone near skin or pressure points, and *abnormal*, e.g. a scar drawn tight over a greater trochanter.

HEALING

Local management

Having paid attention to general factors, external and internal, there are two further areas to consider. Both are local and both have to be managed over the whole 24 hours. They are: (a) dressings (*vide infra*), and (b) local external mechanical factors such as pressure.

Lowthian's 24-hour posture change 'clock' relates posture to 'daily living' function and distributes loading on the different pressure points, so coordinating prevention of sores and general care. Such a 'clock' will not be so easy to apply at home, but it provides a model for other wounds such as leg ulcers (Lowthian, 1979), and draws attention to many factors which might otherwise not have been thought to contribute to ulceration.

What happens to the leg ulcer at night? Does the medial malleolus of one ankle lie for hours across the tibial skin? Most patients lie on one side with their knees partially drawn up in flexion. What happens to the heels if patients lie on their backs and the bed sags? Is there a spring protruding through the mattress? What happens during the day when the patient falls asleep in a chair? Does the patient sit cross-legged or rest one calf, of perhaps the paralysed or arthritic leg, against the fender? Will the spastic leg suffer pressure from the heels or counter of the shoe, or from the straps of the calliper? No item can be taken for granted; certainly not wrap bandages and stockings, which are potentially dangerous in ischaemic and diabetic limbs.

Patient support systems should be reviewed. The lady with heart failure who is breathless, after getting up from a low chair, needs a high chair, high bed and high toilet seat, just as much as the patient with osteoarthritis of the knees or hips who may have oedematous legs or a varicose ulcer, or the stroke patient who could stand and walk given the right circumstances. Improving mobility enhances local healing factors by minimising oedema, increasing blood flow and ensuring that rest is taken in a better posture such as on a bed instead of a chair.

Remedial aspects

It can thus be seen that in the analysis of 'daily living' problems, OTs can contribute to management by the provision of aids and home alterations. Home aids and equipment schemes should be available on a 24-hour basis to nurses, particularly decubitus aids. The burden of supplying and training patients and relatives in the use of mobility, toiletry and incontinence aids should be shared between OTs, physiotherapists, and specialist nurse colleagues. A height-adjustable commode with removable arms may prevent incontinence, and pads, washable fleeces and pressure sore risk-reducing mattresses will either prevent chronic ulcers or enhance their healing. Prevention of, or healing of, chronic wounds is as important in the dying as it is in the younger disabled, and patient support systems must be promptly and conveniently available to nurses for both acute and chronic patients, whether in or out of hospital.

OTHER SOURCES OF HELP

Chiropodists can share the burden of care of patients with foot ulcers, especially those where local external factors play a part. NHS chiropodists can visit patients at home, and often undertake long-term follow-up, and may teach self-care effectively. Other sources of help may be available in particular districts, e.g. wound clinics, the ulcer nurse and clinic. While new dressings and other aids are helpful for the ulcer patient, too many changes of treatment may diminish confidence in nursing and medical expertise. Carers can get 'burnt out' and have to pace themselves. Referral to a supportive colleague, perhaps with a special interest in ulcers, may help enormously. Admittedly this may be far from easy in rural practice.

SURGICAL ASPECTS OF MANAGEMENT OF PRESSURE SORES AND OTHER CHRONIC WOUNDS

When soft tissue is compressed between a small area of bone such as the ischial tuberosity and a large area such as the surface of a chair, the highest pressures occur near to the bone and especially at its edges. This would correspond to muscle overlying the ischial tuberosity. Blood flow only ceases when pressure in excess of the arterial supply is applied to a vascular bed. Vessels close most readily in the most compliant tissue, which is muscle, less readily in the firmer dermis and not at all within rigid bone. At zero blood flow necrosis becomes certain as ischaemia times are exceeded. At 37 °C this may be approximately eight hours for skin but only five hours for muscle. At 20°C the corresponding figures may be 18 hours and twelve hours. When necrosis of muscle occurs a small zone may liquefy with survival of overlying skin, but a larger zone will deprive overlying skin of its fascial perforating blood supply. If dead muscle becomes infected whilst skin is intact, the resulting abscess may cause expanding tissue destruction. Pressure sores can also consist of cutaneous necrosis with preservation of deeper soft tissue. This can result from prolonged static contact if the temperature of the external surface is maintained in excess of core temperature (a danger with heated operating tables), and it can also result from repetitive cutaneous trauma or shearing forces.

The first phase in the evolution of an open wound is demarcation and separation of necrotic tissue. Sequestration of non-viable tendon, ligaments and bone may take many months. Final healing is never possible until this separation is complete. Surgical drainage of an abscess is obligatory, but early surgical debridement is highly desirable. All soft tissue and bone that does not bleed can be excised. If sensation is completely absent then, of course, a general anaesthetic is unnecessary. In a moist environment all newly exposed surfaces of viable tissue form a layer of granulation tissue over a period of a few days. The same surfaces exposed to dry air form a coagulum with a layer of secondary desiccation necrosis beneath it. The application of concentrated antiseptics may also induce additional necrosis. Over a period of weeks a dense layer of fibrous tissue forms deep to the granulations of a large open wound. During spontaneous healing this will contract through the action of myofibroblasts (Gabbiani *et al.*, 1971) unless the edges are rigidly bound to deep structures. In most other mammals, large granulating wounds heal almost entirely by contraction. In humans this mechanism plays a part, especially in defects around the pelvis, but much less in venous ulcers of the lower leg. When granulations with a sufficienty low tissue bacterial density and a moist oxygenated surface are in contact with an epidermal edge, a front of stimulated epidermal cells will advance at approximately one cell per hour, or 250 microns per day (Winter, 1964). When this second intention healing is complete the appearance is of a typical scar. The dermis and any other initially destroyed layers are permanently absent. The granulation tissue organises into a progressively maturing fibrous tissue bound to deep structures and covered by a flat and relatively unstable keratinised squamous epithelium. There is a positive relationship between the occurrence of spontaneous healing and the likely success of reconstructive surgery. The wound in which contraction has been observed is more likely to heal when excised and a flap inserted than is the static or enlarging defect. The shallow granulating wound over which edge epithelium is visibly advancing is usually capable of taking a split skin graft. It is most profitable to refer to a surgeon those patients with large but healing wounds, rather than only those for whom conservative measures have failed. A referral made as soon as any tissue necrosis is suspected will probably reduce total hospitalisation and systemic effect of the large open wound. When tissue loss has occurred treatment options may be summarised as follows.

TREATMENT OPTIONS

(1) Non-surgical.

(2) Primary debridement and then conservative treatment.

(3) Primary debridement with immediate reconstruction.

(4) Delayed wound excision and direct closure.

(5) Delayed excision and reconstruction by flap.

(6) Delayed skin grafting directly or following tangential excision.

Option 1 is usually unnecessarily slow. It may be acceptable for wounds of no more than 3 cm width when full exploration and radiographs have failed to detect dead tendon, ligament or bone. *Option 2* is a means of providing early diagnostic information and allowing second intention healing to start much earlier. The final scar will be similar. *Option 3* is particularly relevant to larger areas of shallow necrosis which, like thermal injuries, can greatly benefit from immediate excision and split skin grafting. Sound cover may be established, and the patient discharged only two weeks after injury. Immediate reconstruction, with a flap of vascularised soft tissue, must often be feasible for pressure sores but is, in practice, rarely performed. Option 3 allows the opportunity of primary wound healing without bacterial colonisation having taken place. *Option 4* is often used. The fibrous capsule of the established cavity is completely excised, together with 5–10 mm thickness of any bone in the base of the wound. Radical excision of normal bone in paraplegics as recommended over 30 years ago (Conway and Griffith, 1956) may prevent recurrence of an identical pressure sore, but it does, of course, result in new bony prominences upon which the weight of the body must rest. Excision of bone which shows radiological evidence of lysis, as well as sequestrum, is recommended. During wound excision blood loss may be in the region of 1 litre. Transfusion will certainly be required because these patients are anaemic and the wasted legs of the paraplegic contribute to a reduced total blood volume. When the defect is small, and the surrounding soft tissue can be mobilised, as is often the case over the ischial tuberosity and the sacrum, direct closure of all layers may be possible. Conversely, it may not be possible to close even a small ischial defect in a thin young patient with hip flexion contractures. Excision and direct closure of infected wounds with subsequent uncomplicated healing has been facilitated by appropriate perioperative prophylactic antibiotics, buried monofilament synthetic sutures and vacuum drains. With Option 4 the first three to four weeks delay allow recovery of the damaged vasculature in the wound edges. Further delay may be required for sufficient spontaneous contraction of the defect before direct closure is possible. *Option 5* relates to the treatment of large deep wounds in the region of the pelvis. Although flaps permanently change the local anatomy, they may be the only means of providing a full thickness of soft tissue cover. The flap, which may consist of a muscle with overlying skin (myocutaneous flap), deep fascia with overlying skin (fasciocutaneous flap), or merely superficial facia and skin (skin flap), retains its circulation from a defined pedicle. The secondary defect from which it is transferred may be closed directly or split skin grafted. The unnecessary use of flaps for small defects does preclude the future use of the same flap and often adjacent flaps, should the same sore recur with more extensive necrosis. Direct split skin grafting of deep defects around the pelvis has only a limited success rate and results in thin skin, rigidly bound to bone (Nuseibeh, 1974). It is not often used. *Option 6* is applicable to shallow ulcers in which the skeleton has retained some soft tissue cover. Thus, split skin grafting is almost always of some help in the treatment of lower limb venous ulcers, or in those over the heel.

Surgical measures so far mentioned are drainage, debridement, skin grafting and flap reconstructions. Venous and arterial surgery of the lower limb is outside the scope of this text. Following many years of chronic ulceration the sclerotic lower leg often benefits from compartment decompression by division of deep fascia. The most severely neglected decubitus ulcers with destruction of the entire sacral/ischial/posterior hip are, on occasions, best treated by disarticulation of the paralysed leg and closure of the defect by means of the quadriceps femoris as a myocutaneous flap.

DRESSING MATERIALS

For an open wound some type of solid fabric or compound is required as a dressing. This might be changed as frequently as two-hourly or as infrequently as every two days. It must be remembered that soiled dressing materials contain not only a wide range of bacterial flora, constituting a serious source of cross-infection, but also large quantities of any serum-borne viruses that the patient may be carrying.

Requirements for dressing materials:

(1) Easily and cheaply sterilised and replaced.

(2) Contour to wound surfaces without preventing contraction.

(3) Keep wound moist but avoid pooling of pus.

(4) Allow oxygen diffusion, when required.

(5) Avoid shedding particles or fibres which may act as non-absorbable foreign bodies.

Examples of materials

Woven cotton or cotton gauze has remained the most popular fabric dressing during the past century. It is a cellulose fibre, little affected by autoclaving or by bacterial enzymes. By rapid capillary action, dry cotton absorbs four times its weight without changing in volume. In deep cavities, multiple small swabs must be avoided. Tight packing is undesirable. Retained cotton causes continuing suppuration and failure to heal.

Debrisan is radiation-sterilised Sephadex G25. The dry beads, of diameter 80–250 microns, flow easily, and slowly hydrate to form a gel. Total exudate uptake is four times the initial weight, but with volume expansion. The material is usually flushed out of the wound with a stream of saline, but retained dextranomer is known to be harmless. From a controlled experiment with porcine wound chambers (Masser, 1982) it has been established that daily wound exudation is the same whether in contact with cotton gauze or with Debrisan. Certain bacteria may be reduced in the presence of Debrisan, but granulation and epithelial regeneration are quantitatively similar. Debrisan is most useful in deep cavities of small volume. Other gels can be applied to superficial as well as deeper wounds. They are sometimes more comfortable when pain is a problem. *Gelliperm* has a polyacrylamide structure. It may be applied dry as well as pre-hydrated. Less expensive *Granuflex* has an adhesive surface and a waterproof backing. *Comfeel Ulcus* is a comparable product. *Sorbsan* utilises an alginate gel which seems to be well accepted in contact with open wounds.

Silicone rubber foam (Wood *et al.*, 1977) is cast by pouring into a cavity. The soft casting so formed can be frequently removed, cleaned and replaced but wound contraction demands renewal.

Polyurethane foam is made in sheets (e.g. Lyofoam). It is applicable to flat wounds and provides a contact surface favourable to epidermal regeneration.

Placed over an advancing epithelial front, these membranes of polyethylene or polyurethane may be of value. *An oxygen-permeable polyethylene membrane* results in higher sub-epithelial oxygen tension (Silver, 1972) and more rapid epithelial regeneration (Winter, 1972), when compared with relatively impermeable polyester. This is relevant to split skin donor site or expanded meshed skin grafts rather than to large open wounds. In the presence of exudation such membranes should be perforated and backed by absorbent material.

Biological dressings include skin heterografts (usually processed porcine split skin), skin homografts and human amniotic membrane. Heterografts do not take. They appear to behave no differently from vegetable-derived and synthetic dressings. Homografted material is a potential carrier of viruses, and the donors must be screened in the same way as organ or blood product donors. Skin homografts take under the same conditions as autografts but subsequently reject. Amnion homograft does not take, but may be renewed. It is claimed to stimulate a more vascular granulating surface on which subsequent skin graft take is enhanced, but no results of controlled trials, nor of controlled experiments, are available.

DRESSING ADDITIVES

Countless substances have been applied to open wounds in the hope of promoting healing. Some change only the physical properties of the dressing material. Some diffuse into the wound and some remain in the dressing controlling its bacterial flora.

Requirements for additives:

(1) Minimal direct cytotoxic action in the wound.

(2) Hclp avoid cross-infection.

(3) No toxic effects from systemic absorption.

(4) Allergic sensitisation uncommon.

(5) No induction of antibiotic resistance.

Examples of additives

Paraffin is widely used to reduce adherence of fibre and textile dressing. In liquid emulsions and creams it helps retain moisture and it slows the release of water-soluble agents.

Polyethylene glycols are water-soluble alternatives to paraffins. Used with fibre or textile dressings there is some limitation of adherence and the hydrophilic action results in generally less oedematous wounds. Furacin contains 0.2 per cent nitrofurazone, which provides some bacterial control in the dressing. Plastics, iodine, silver and penicillins are incompatible with polyethylene glycols.

Eusol is an activated solution of calcium hypochlorite. Available chlorine is 0.25 per cent but shelf-life is only two weeks. With its wide action against vegetative organisms and viruses, chlorine remains the most valuable agent in the general prevention of cross-infection. Plain Eusol does have a brief cytotoxic action at the wound surface. Eusol and paraffin emulsions are very useful, but the activity and shelf-life vary widely according to the method of manufacture (Summers and McLaughlin, 1968).

Hydrogen peroxide has a brief, but aggressive, cytotoxic action. It does not reduce wound flora but can produce dramatic adverse effects when poured into wounds (Sleigh and Linter, 1985).

Povidone iodine is the only iodine preparation in current widespread use. A 10 per cent solution in water or further isotonic dilutions can safely be used to control the microbial flora of dressings (Barton, 1982). As it makes fibre dressings unduly adherent, povidone iodine may be more usefully combined with gels, plastic films and foams.

Chlorhexidine has superseded hexachlorophane as the most widely used hospital antiseptic for skin cleansing. A solution of 0.01 per cent can be safely applied directly to wounds if antibiotic-resistant staphylococci have been cultured. Bactigras is a tulle preparation containing 0.5 per cent chlorhexidine.

One per cent acetic acid is a useful temporary additive when wounds are heavily colonised with *Pseudomonas pyocyanea.*

One per cent zinc sulphate solution (lotio rubra) and zinc oxide pastes or ointments have long been applied to wounds, and there is some evidence for stimulation of granulation and epithelialisation. A therapeutic effect might be anticipated if the serum zinc level has been found low (Hussain, 1969).

A 0.5 per cent silver nitrate solution has been used for control of wound infection in burns, but absorption of silver and bacterial reduction of nitrate to nitrite (Strauch *et al.*, 1969) contraindicate its use in wounds of more than 5 per cent body area and for periods of more than four days. In small wounds, higher concentrations can be used to inhibit overgranulation.

A 1 per cent silver sulphadiazine cream (Flamazine) is currently in widespread use with burns dressings, but is equally applicable to all open wounds, especially when used for a limited period to inhibit a specific organism. The cream can be safely applied to large defects. It reduces dressing adhesion but often produces an oedematous wound.

Streptokinase streptodornase (Varidase topical) solutions may be expected to aid the proteolytic enzymes normally found in a wound during the phase of desloughing. Enzyme actions are very slow compared with even limited surgery.

Local antibiotics cannot be recommended for regular use in chronic open wounds because of the problems of allergic sensitisation and development of an antibiotic-resistant flora. These agents may be of value for one or two days in the preparation of a wound for reconstructive surgery. Absorption from large wounds may result in appreciable serum levels. Fucidic acid (Fucidin), framycetin (Sofra Tulle), and neomycin (Cicatrin) are examples of antibiotics applied locally.

Slow irrigation of wounds with nutrients or substances intended to enhance local metabolism, has been carried out for many years. Egg albumen, insulin and gaseous oxygen have been applied as well as the specially formulated parenteral nutrition mixtures. Such treatments remain controversial (Calver, 1983).

Activated charcoal, included as the outer layer of a dressing, is effective in reducing odour.

PHYSICAL CONSIDERATIONS IN THE LOWER LIMB

Outer coverings may be necessary to provide both physical and psychological support, and may include additional padding with mechanical and thermal protection (e.g. cotton gauze or wool). Shaped support bandages (or Tubigrip) may give better pressure conformity than elastic wrap bandage (Isherwood *et al.*, 1975) and so reduce oedema, hypergranulation and pain, encouraging mobility. Stockings discourage meddling with wounds and offer additional protection against shear. All forms of bandage which encircle limbs should be applied by experts, for bandaging ischaemic legs may precipitate gangrene. In a study of 100 patients with 188 ulcerated legs, there were 64 limbs with ulcers due to venous disease alone, 35 with abnormal superficial veins and 29 with deep vein incompetence. In 44 limbs, ischaemia was demonstrated by ultrasound and photoplethysmography. Arterial insufficiency may often be an unrecognised element is leg ulcers (Cornwall *et al.*, 1986).

Lower limb venous pressure (as well as contact pressure) may be relieved by elevation with bed rest, but this has its dangers. Rationing of time spent standing, combined with short, frequent periods of bed rest, may be as effective. Chiropodists are adept at relieving pressures on feet. The patient's footwear should be reviewed. If doubt remains, then a physicist may be able to advise on mechanical aspects after measuring parameters relevant to tissue viability.

Other physical treatments include multiaxial vibration, induced electromagnetic fields, ultrasound, massage and even light of various wavelengths. Some of these could become standard therapies, but their place in treatment has yet to be determined. A demonstrable placebo effect seems to be due to heightened interest of staff in their patients (Fernie and Dorman, 1976).

FOLLOW-UP, INSPECTION, AND PATIENT EDUCATION

These are interrelated items. In general, patients should know the danger signs and not be afraid to seek advice from any member of the team.

Ideally advice should be written. If anxiety exists then a named member of the team should inspect the wound at suitable intervals, such as the district nurse or occupational health nurse. Intelligent relatives may be briefed if the patient is unable to take responsibility for self-care. Prevention of pressure sores depends on the frequent inspection of pressure points by knowledgeable patients or relatives looking for persistent hyperaemia, i.e. redness lasting more than say ten minutes.

No chapter can do justice to the complex subjects of wound prevention and healing, which involve so many of the caring disciplines. Evaluation of new care systems and products must continue, but should not cloud the main issues, which are, on the one hand, a total approach to the individual patient, and, on the other hand, a determination by all concerned to improve the caring system. Only a collective approach to research and development will provide a better scientific basis to solve the tissue viability disorders, and only a consensus approach at district level will result in effective care policies and better management of individual patients.

REFERENCES

Baker, J.H.E., Silver, J.R. and Tudway, A.J.C. (1984) Late complications of pressure sores. *Care, Sci Pract.*, *3*(2), 56-9

Bardsley, G.I., Bell, F., Black, R.C. and Barbenel J.C. (1983) Movements during sitting and their relationship to pressure areas. In J.C. Barbanel, C.D. Forbes and G.D.O. Lowe (eds), *Pressure sores*, Macmillan, London, pp. 157-65

Barton, A.A. (1981) Pressure sores described. *Care, Sci Pract*, *1*(1), 7-9

Barton, A.A., Barton, M. and Crow, R. (1981) Mortality, morbidity and resource allocation. *Br. Med. J.* (letter), *282*, 484

Barton, A.A. and Barton M. (1976) Drug-based prevention of pressure sores. *Lancet*, *2*, 443-4

Barton, M. (1982) Pressure sores unit — our work. *Care, Sci. Pract.*, *1*(2), 7-8

Brand, P.W. (1976a) Pressure sores — the problem. In Kenedi *et al.* (1976), pp. 19-23

Brand, P.W. (1976b) Patient monitoring. In Kenedi *et al.* (1976), pp. 183-4

Brattgard, S.O., Carlson, S. and Severinson, K. (1976) Temperature and humidity in the sitting area. In Kenedi *et al.* (1976), pp. 185-8

Calver, R.F. (1983) Topical nutrition reviewed. *Care, Sci Pract.*, *2*(4), 20-3

Clarke, R.P. (1974) Microenvironmental air exchange rates in patient support systems. *Eng. Med.*, *3*, 6-7

Conway, H. and Griffith, B.H. (1956) Plastic surgery for closure of decubitus ulcers in patients with paraplegia. *Am. J. Surg.*, *91*, 946-75

Cornwall, J.V., Dore, C.J. and Lewis, J.D. (1986) Leg ulcers: epidemiology and aetiology. *Br. J. Surg.*, *73*, 695-6

Crow, R. (1985) The Society for Tissue Viability, shared knowledge, a new opportunity. *Care, Br. J. Rehabil. Tissue Viability*, *1*(1), 2

Daly, C.H. Chimoskey, J.E. Holloway, G.A. and Kennedy, D. (1976) The effect of pressure loading on the blood flow rate in human skin. In Kenedi *et al.* (1986) pp. 69-77

David, J.A., Chapman, E.J., Chapman, R.G. and Locket, B. (1985) A survey of prescribed nursing treatment for patients with established pressure sores. *Care, Br. J. Rehabil. Tissue Viability, 1*(1), 18-20

Dowding, C. (1983) Tissue viability nurse, a new post. *Nursing Times, 79*, June, pp. 61-4

Dyson, R. (1978) Bed sores, the injuries hospital staff inflict on patients. *Nursing Mirror, 146*, June, pp. 30-2

Exton-Smith, A.N. and Sherwin, R.W. (1961) Prevention of pressure sores, significance of spontaneous bodily movements. *Lancet, 2*, 1124-6

Fernie, G.R., and Dorman, J. (1976) The problems of clinical trials with new systems for preventing or healing decubiti. In Kenedi *et al.* (1976), pp. 315-20

Gabbiani, G., Ryan, G.B. and Majno, G. (1971) Presence of modified fibroblasts in granulation tissue and their possible role in wound contraction. *Experientia, 27*, 549-50

Grant, L.J. (1985) Interface pressure measurement between a patient and a support surface. *Care, Br. J. Rehabil. Tissue Viability, 1*(1), 7-9

Hosni, E.A., Ximenes, J.O. and Hamilton, F.G. (1968) Pressure bandaging of the lower extremity. *J. Am. Med. Assoc., 206*, 2715-18

Husain, S.L. (1969) Oral zinc sulphate in leg ulcers. *Lancet, 1*, 1069-71

Isherwood, P.A., Robertson, J.C. and Rossi, A. (1975) Pressure measurements beneath low knee amputation stump bandages. *Br. J. Surg., 62*, 982-6

Johnson, H.D. (1972) Mechanics of elastic bandaging. *Br. Med. J., 3*, 767-8

Kenedi, R.M., Cowden, J.M. and Scales, J.T. (eds) (1976) *Bed sore mechanics*, Macmillan, London

Lawes, C.J. (1984) Pressure sore readmission for spinal injured people. *Care, Sci Pract., 4*(2), 4-8

Lowthian, P.T. (1985) The classification and grading of pressure sores. *Care, Br. J. Rehabil. Tissue Viability, 1*(1), 21-3

Lowthian, P.T. (1979) Turning clock system to prevent pressure sores. *Nursing Mirror, 148*, May, pp. 30-1

Mani, R. (1985) Oxygen tension at wound sites. *Care Sci. Pract.*, Special ed, 22.26

Masser, M.R. (1982) An objective comparison of Debrisan with cotton gauze using a porcine model. *Care Sci. Pract., 1*(2), 27-33

Mccoll, I. (1986) *Review of artificial limb and appliance centre services*, HMSO, London

Miller, A.E. (1984) The nursing process. *Br. Med. J.* (letter), *288*, 719

Norton, D. McLaren, R. and Exton-Smith, A.N. (1962) *An investigation of geriatric nursing problems in hospital.* National Corporation for Care of Old People, London

Nuseibeh, I.M. (1974) Split skin graft and the treatment of pressure sores. *Paraplegia, 12*, 1-4

O'Reilly, J., Whyte, J. and Goldstone, L.A. (1981) A pressure sore survey. *Nursing Times*, Theatre Nursing Supplement, *77*, 7-19

Peterson, N.C. (1976) The development of pressure sores during hospitalisation. In Kenedi *et al.* (1976), pp. 219-24

Roaf, R. (1976) The causation and prevention of bed sores. In Kenedi *et al.* (1976), pp. 5-7

Reswick, J.B. and Rogers, J.E. (1976) Experience at Rancho Los Amigos hospital with devices and techniques to prevent pressure sores. In Kenedi *et al.* (1976), pp. 301-10

Robertson, J.C., Shah, J. and Amos, H. (1980) An interface pressure sensor for routine clinical use. *Eng. Med., 9*(3), 151-66

Robertson, J.C. and Haines, J.R. (1978) A community hospital home aids loan scheme. *Health Trends, 10*, 15-16

Royal College of Physicians, London, *Physical disability in 1986 and beyond.* *20*(3), 185

Silver, I.A. (1972) Oxygen tension and epithelialization. *Epidermal wound healing*, in H.I. Maibach and D.T. Rovee (eds), Year Book Medical Publishers, Chicago, Chap. 17

Sleigh, J.W. and Linter, S.P. (1985) Lesson of the week: hazards of hydrogen peroxide. *Br. Med. J.*, *291*, 1706

Strauch, B., Buch, W., Grey, W. and Lamb, D. (1969) Successful treatment of methemoglobinaemia secondary to silver nitrate therapy. *N. Engl. J. Med.*, 281, 257

Summers, F.H. and McLaughlin, C.R. (1968) Emulsifying eusol/liquid paraffin *Lancet*, *2*, 1299

Wijn, P.F.F., Brakkee, A.J.M., Stienen, G.J.M. and Vendri, K.A.J.H. (1976) Mechanical properties of the human skin in vivo for small deformations. In Kenedi *et al.* (1976), pp. 103-8

Winter, G.D. (1964) Movement of epidermal cells over the wound surface. In W. Montagna and R.E. Billingham (eds), *Advances of Biology in Skin*, vol. 5: *Wound Healing*, Pergamon Press, Oxford, Chap. 7

Winter, G.D. (1972) Epidermal regeneration in the domestic pig. In H.I. Maibach, and D.T. Rovee (eds), *Epidermal wound healing*, Year Book Medical Publishers, Chicago, Chap. 4

Wood, R.A.B., Williams R.H.P. and Hughes L.E. (1977) Foam elastomer dressings in the management of open granulating wounds: experience with 250 patients. *Br. J. Surg.*, *64*, 554-7

RECOMMENDED FURTHER READING

The management and prevention of pressure sores (1981) Anthony and Mary Barton, Faber, London

ADDRESS

Tissue Viability Society
c/o Mr John Gisby, Wessex Rehabilitation Association, Odstock Hospital, Salisbury, Wiltshire

32

Dental Care

Peter Hirschmann

The dental care of physically handicapped people has in the past been accorded a priority which is too low. Epidemiological studies have demonstrated that almost all such patients have more periodontal disease and poorer oral hygiene than the general population. The aims of dental care for the physically handicapped person should be no different from those for any other member of the community. These are:

(1) preventing pain and discomfort;

(2) improving (or maintaining) the patient's appearance;

(3) enhancing his/her ability to eat;

(4) assisting his/her speech;

(5) promoting a satisfactory standard (by the patient or the attendants) of oral hygiene.

In addition, and of particular relevance to the physically handicapped,

(6) maintaining the dentition for use as an accessory limb (O'Donnel *et al.*, 1985).

It should not be necessary to say that such dental care should be to the best possible standard, and of the same quality (as far as possible), as that offered to all other patients. It is also important to remember that dental treatment may be required early in, if not in some cases prior to, the rehabilitation process. For instance, professional oral hygiene, from a dental hygienist, should be available early in the management of patients with head injuries before chronic gingivitis becomes established. Patients may well complain of ill-fitting dentures shortly after a stroke: often this is due to loss of muscle tone and the consequent inability to control the lower denture in particular. 'Plumping' the surface of the lower denture to eliminate the buccal sulcus may prove helpful in both eating and speech. Intra-oral appliances have been described which are helpful in the speech therapy of acquired velopharyngeal disorders (Enderby *et al.* 1984).

ACCESS TO DENTAL TREATMENT

Dental treatment for the disabled is available either from a general dental practitioner (GDP, family dentist), working either within the NHS General Dental Service (GDS) or to private contract, the community dental service or the hospital dental service. It is the accepted policy that treatment for such patients should be provided, as far as possible, by the first of these three.

General Dental Service

Dentists' names are on the local dental list, which is available in libraries and main post offices. Alternatively, patients can telephone their local Family Practitioner Committee (FPC). Access to dentists' surgeries is often a problem, and the Dental Administrator of the FPC may have the names of those with ground-floor access, who are willing to undertake treatment for the handicapped.

Housebound patients may request a domiciliary visit from the dentist at no cost to themselves, and many practitioners are happy to provide such a service. The extent of the service varies: check-ups should present no problems; nor should the construction of dentures. Fillings and cleaning may be more difficult to provide, although some practitioners do have their own portable dental equipment to enable them to provide such treatment.

The ambulance service may also impose a further limitation on seeking treatment from a GDP: however, in some parts of the country the ambulance service appears willing to take patients to dentists' surgeries, but prior negotiation may be necessary before they will agree to convey personal wheelchairs. Most Social Services Departments will provide transport, and have suitable vans for transporting those confined to wheelchairs.

Community Dental Services (CDS)

The CDS can now provide treatment not only for children but also for adult handicapped. The extent of such provision may vary, but an inquiry to the District Dental Officer (DDO) (in Scotland and Wales the Chief Administrative Dental Officer), will establish the nature of local provision. Such officers can often negotiate with ambulance services.

Hospital Dental Services

Provision of dental care for the physically handicapped is as uneven between hospitals as in other areas of the dental services.

Most *dental teaching hospitals* have comprehensive adult handicapped services, whereas in *district general hospitals* the extent of the provision will depend on the attitudes and interests of the individual consultant oral surgeon. Some limit their service, consultation apart, to surgical treatment of those whose handicap is primarily medical. Others do have the staff and facilities to provide regular dental care. A telephone enquiry to the DDO should establish the extent of the service available. Finally, consultant oral surgeons may be willing to see patients for domiciliary assessments if not actual treatment, and dental hygienists may treat patients in their homes.

COST OF DENTAL TREATMENT

The rising costs of dental treatment may deter the physically handicapped from seeing a dentist. However,

(1) Dental examinations, including domiciliary visits, are free, as are repairs to NHS dentures.

(2) There are exemptions:
  (a) All treatment is free to those receiving any of the following: supplementary allowance, family income supplement, supplementary pension, housing benefit supplement, free prescriptions because of low income.
  (b) Those on low income (details in DHSS leaflet D11) may get some assistance. They should ask the dentist for Form F1D, which has then to be sent to the local Social Security Office. However, those in possession of a prescription charge exemption certificate do not need Form F1D in order to claim exemption.

Patients should always be advised to seek clarification about charges from their dentist *before* commencing treatment.

ORAL HYGIENE

The maintenance of an adequate dentition depends as much on the efficacy of the patient's own toothbrushing, and on the diet, as on the quality of professional care provided. There are increasing numbers of dental hygienists whose role as part of the dental team is to provide advice and active treatment in these areas. The need to maintain an adequate level of oral hygiene should not be overlooked in the management of the terminal stages of pseudobulbar palsy and motor neurone disease.

TOOTHBRUSHING

The toothbrush should be of a suitable size and design to reach all tooth surfaces and gum margins with ease and comfort. For those unable to grip a normal toothbrush there are now several readily available modifications, and if these prove unacceptable, then it is also possible for the dentist, and his dental technician, to construct a ‘made-to-measure’ handle.

Electric toothbrushes are particularly useful when manipulating a toothbrush (whether by the patient or the attendants) is difficult and, in some cases, may be obtained with financial assistance from the Social Service Departments of the local authority. The handle can be modified in the same way as conventional toothbrushes.

MOUTHWASHES

Although numerous mouthwashes are available, both on prescription and over the counter, only chlorhexidine gluconate (Corsodyl) has been shown to be efficacious in reducing plaque and maintaining oral hygiene. It is available either as a 0.2 per cent mouthwash or 1 per cent dental gel; the former can be applied with a swab, the latter on a soft toothbrush.

DIET

Dietary advice for the prevention of dental disease is just part of more general counselling: sugar-containing foods and drinks should be confined to mealtimes to minimise the risk of dental decay, and sucrose-based medicines given for chronic disease should be avoided wherever possible.

DENTURES

Dentures need to be cleaned as regularly as teeth, the simplest method being brushing wih soap and lukewarm, not hot, water. Dentures should not be worn at night, and should be soaked two or three nights a week in a proprietary denture cleanser such as 0.1 per cent hypochlorite (Dentural, Milton) to prevent the accumulation of plaque.

WHAT DENTISTS NEED TO KNOW

If access and cost are two of the barriers facing the disabled in their search for dental treatment, then apprehension is the third, not only for the patient but also for the dentist. Some GDPs are reluctant to treat patients who pose 'medical problems', due to the risk of sudden collapse in dental surgery or potentially hazardous drug interactions, and they may telephone requesting advice as to the suitability of your patient for treatment in their dental surgery: to which your reply should be, what treatment? There are few handicapped patients who cannot receive simple dental treatment, such as fillings and cleaning, if not single extractions, in the normal way under local anaesthetic. Patients should be advised to take their drugs in the customary fashion, and for those at risk from hypertension the use of prilocaine (Citanest), which contains octapressin, is thought to be safer than an adrenaline-containing local anaesthetic solution. Requests for advice as to the suitability of a patient for general anaesthesia in the dental chair should be referred to the appropriate consultant anaesthetist. Dentists should be

Figure 32.1: Clinical photograph showing the dental state of a 56-year-old lady with a 32 year history of rheumatoid arthritis. She last saw a dentist two years ago and can no longer clean her own teeth. There is widespread calculus and plaque, in particular on the upper right central incisor. Her gums are inflamed and there is much recession

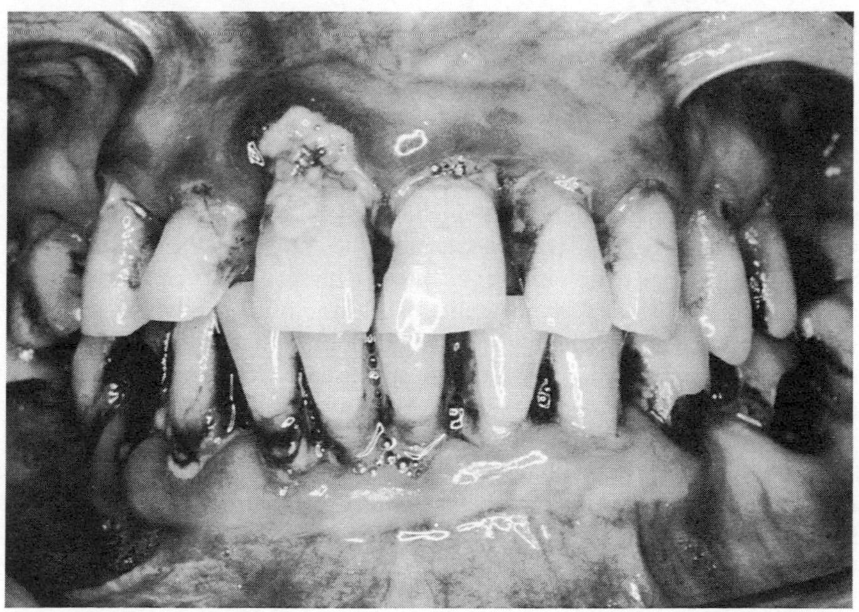

warned of the risk of atlanto-axial dislocation when treating patients with rheumatoid arthritis.

Some dentists may be able to offer the more apprehensive patients either intravenous sedation or relative analgesia. Nonetheless there will remain a small residue of patients who, because of their handicap, such as spasticity or behavioural problems, cannot receive comprehensive treatment in the dental chair. An endotracheal anaesthetic is needed for these patients, and this service is provided by either the Community or Hospital Dental Services. In case of difficulty, contact the DDO.

There are three other specific medical problems on which your advice will be sought:

(1) *Anticoagulant therapy.* Patients on anticoagulant therapy are at risk of excessive bleeding not only after extractions but also from scaling in the presence of either severe periodontal (gum) disease or marked gingivitis. In these cases the dentist would appreciate a prothrombin ratio in the region of 2.5 where this does not otherwise constitute a hazard to the patient's primary condition — for instance a prosthetic heart valve.

(2) *Corticosteroid therapy.* The relationship between the type of dental treatment and the degree of stress is impossible to quantify, and each patient must be judged on merit, but in general whereas a filling is not usually considered stressful, a single extraction under local anaesthesia is. In the latter instance the dentist should be advised to boost the steroid cover either by i.m. injection of 100 mg hydrocortisone hemisuccinate (or the equivalent oral dose) half-an-hour to one hour prior to the extraction. However, where more major dental procedures are involved the patient should be referred to the local consultant oral surgeon.

(3) *Antibiotic prophylaxis.* Antibiotic prophylaxis is essential for patients at risk from endocarditis when thir dental treatment, including fillings or gum treatment, produces a significant bacteraemia. The level of susceptibility varies: those with a heart valve replacement or a history of endocarditis are considered at higher risk compared to those with rheumatic heart disease, congenital anomalies and repairs or a previous valvotomy. Those with ischaemic heart disease or coronary artery autografts are considered at negligible risk. Antibiotic prophylaxis for those with a history of rheumatic fever alone may not be necessary if there is no evidence of consequent rheumatic heart disease. The antibiotic regime recommended by the British Society for Antimicrobial Chemotherapy is given in the *BNF* and should be adhered to.

Antibiotic prophylaxis may also be necessary when dental treatment is provided for patients with *prosthetic joint replacements*, whose mouths are less than healthy: if in doubt seek the advice of the local consultant orthopaedic surgeon. Finally, it is also indicated for patients, such as hydrocephalics, with *ventriculoatrial shunts.*

REFERENCES

Enderby, P., Hathorn, I.S. and Servant, S. (1984) The use of intra-oral appliances in the management of acquired velopharyngeal disorders. *Br. Dent. J.*, *157*, 157-9

O'Donnel, D., Yen, P.K.Y. and Robson, W. (1985) A mouth-controlled appliance for severely physically handicapped patients. *Br. Dent. J.*, *159*, 186-8

33

Psychological Assessment and Treatment

Helga Hanks and Carol Martin

INTRODUCTION

This chapter aims to discuss the nature of a clinical psychologist's contribution to the assessment of patients in the care of a rehabilitation team, concentrating particularly on the deficits shown by patients with brain damage. It contains sections on the patterns of neuropsychological dysfunction in common neurological conditions, neuropsychological testing including mention of the more useful tests and batteries, other types of assessment available to psychologists and a case history showing how these can be used in clinical practice.

For many years psychologists have worked with patients who have suffered brain damage. For much of this time they have focused on localising functions to a specific part of the brain. Over recent years, coinciding with progress made in psychological therapies, there has been an increasing interest in the more practical uses of psychology for patients disabled by neurological damage. For a history of the subject the interested reader may turn to Walsh (1978), and for a more comprehensive study of issues of localisation and assessment to Lezak (1976) and Hecaen and Albert (1978).

Some conditions have been examined and found to have specific patterns of change, e.g. memory impairment as a result of alcohol abuse severe enough to lead to Korsakoff's syndrome (Victor *et al.*, 1971). On the other hand conditions such as Alzheimer's disease result in global cortical cell loss and a more general loss of cognitive ability, although again with some evidence for patterning (Katzman *et al.*, 1978). A generalised condition such as hydrocephalus may eventually produce a breakdown of all complex behaviours regardless of localisation (Benson and Blumer, 1975). Elucidating the nature of the patterning is one of the ways in which assessment of functioning can assist diagnosis.

A list of conditions with their common psychological characteristics is given below.

Stroke

Deficits and recovery following stroke are variable, depending on the aetiology, extent and location of the cerebrovascular accident. Speech and language disorders are often seen in dominant-side stroke while spatial problems are more common in strokes on the non-dominant side. Each individual will show a different pattern of dysfunction, as described in Chapter 20.

Head injury

Again deficits observed will vary with the type, degree and site of the injury. Changes in memory, thought and concentration compatible with frontal lobe damage are commonly seen (Brooks, 1984) (Chapter 24).

Alcohol abuse

Organic complications often develop into a fairly specific pattern of a memory defect for current events, retrograde amnesia, disorientation and sometimes confabulation, named Korsakoff's syndrome (Victor *et al.*, 1971).

Dementia

Several common profiles are found in dementia, while conventional neuropsychological assessment is still possible. Early on most sufferers show a pattern of short-term memory loss and spatial/constructional problems with a relative sparing of language, reading and writing (Katzman *et al.*, 1978).

Degenerative diseases (e.g. multiple sclerosis, Parkinson's disease)

There is a growing body of evidence to suggest that such diseases produce idiosyncratic profiles of deficit (e.g. Albert *et al.*, 1974; Albert, 1978) who studied 'subcortical dementia' in patients suffering from supranuclear palsy. The pattern Albert described included apparent memory loss, personality change, slowness and difficulty manipulating previously acquired knowledge, such as problems with calculation.

There is still some call for assessments to localise dysfunction to areas of the brain. The correlation between behaviours and lobes of the brain seems to be the most reliable (Walsh, 1978). Further refinement becomes increasingly inaccurate because of individual variation.

More recently research in psychology has begun to influence the way the links between brain and behaviour are understood, for example in terms of functional systems (see Table 33.1).

Table 33.1: Neuropsychological functions and localisation

Area	Nature of dysfunction includes
Frontal	Abstract thought, planning and regulating activity
Temporal	Memory tasks, auditory perception
Parietal	Spatial tasks, constructional apraxia
Occipital	Colour naming and discrimination

It is uncommon for patients to suffer damage localised to one part of the brain. For this reason patients who suffer bullet wounds, or who have had brain operations (e.g. for epilepsy), have a special place in clinical research. Usually a patient will suffer more diffuse damage; for example, the deficits resulting from a head injury will be complicated by the effects of the contre-coup and by small tissue tears.

FUNCTIONS OF ASSESSMENT

The kind of psychological assessment needed by a rehabilitation team depends on the nature of the information required, and the form in which it is most useful. Below, we illustrate three common questions asked of neuropsychologists with case histories. For more information on this subject, and on some of the methods for treatment, the reader may turn to Brooks (1984) and Wilson and Moffat (1984).

Q.1: Is this patient capable of returning to work?
A teacher, Mr S., was referred after recovery from a stroke. He performed well on a standard test of intelligence, and on a memory test showed few difficulties. The tester paid particular attention to those aspects of the testing session which highlighted possible difficulties that the teacher would have to cope with at work. For example, it was noted that Mr S. was able to concentrate over a period of time equivalent to the length of a lesson, could effectively plan ahead, noted but was not easily disturbed by making errors, and was able to cope with frustration emotionally. Mr S. successfully returned to work as predicted.

Q.2: What is the nature of this patient's personality change?
A patient Mr F., was referred following complaints from his wife that he was difficult to live with and, in her words, was no longer the man she had married. Matters had come to a head about a year following an accident in which Mr F. had sustained a head injury which had necessitated several months of hospitalisation. Mrs F. commented that her husband was less affectionate and concerned about her and their children, that he had started to become increasingly bad-tempered and verbally aggressive, that he could not be trusted to collect the children after school and that he was handling his financial affairs badly. Testing showed difficulties consistent with frontal lobe damage. In particular, Mr F. had problems with 'forgetting to remember', planning and executing strategies and inhibiting behaviours. These deficits could explain most of the changes in Mr F's behaviour.

Q.3: Can this patient complete a particular test necessary to his everyday life?
Mr D. was referred for assessment following extensive neurological investigation which indicated a localised lesion. He was due to return to work as a driver, but the staff on the ward felt anxious about this without being able to explain their doubts, and an assessment was thought to be advisable. The assessment focused particularly on visuospatial skills. On a standard test of intelligence Mr D. performed well on most tasks but had difficulty with the Block Design and Object Assembly subtests. He was unable to draw a design. He also made errors on tasks requiring visuospatial analysis. It was felt that although Mr D. was able to cope in spite of these difficulties in many everyday settings, that driving was likely to put himself and others in danger.

USING THE RESULTS

It is important when analysing the test results to bear in mind that the scores cannot be taken in isolation. Below we have listed some of the factors that it is necessary to consider. One can think of the test situation as similar to an examination, and many of the factors which affect exam performance may be relevant. For example, concentration can be affected by fatigue, by anxiety, by preoccupation and by medication. Depression may result in lowered scores, particularly when the patient is discouraged by failure and sees no point in making an effort, or when a slow performance is penalised on items with a time limit. It is important to be aware of the beneficial effect that a good rapport between tester and patient can have. On the other hand anxiety over failure, or about authority figures, can contribute to a poor score. Educational difficulties need to be watched for — if a patient could not read or write before his or her illness or accident, the score may not reflect true ability. Where there is doubt, a glance at the overall pattern of scores may be helpful. These are some possible clues; poorer scores towards the end of each session (possibly fatigue); poorer scores in the first session (possibly anxiety); poorer scores on written items than items wih spoken or pictorial instructions (check premorbid literacy); variable scores from session to session regardless of content (check external variables, e.g. emotional events, medication change); poor arithmetic (check anxiety and schooling).

The three examples above illustrate how important it is for a rehabilitation team to have information that allows staff to predict the difficulties that a patient who shows impaired neuropsychological functioning will have in adapting to a normal life. This may necessitate a careful analysis of the tasks failed by the patient, to identify the nature of the dysfunction and its severity. This will not always be easy to do, as the effectiveness of tests varies; in particular, concentration and attention deficits are difficult to assess exactly in a clinical setting.

Let us consider failure to perform a simple motor task such as touching the nose with a finger of the right hand. Difficulties might occur at one of these points:

(a) understanding the instruction initially (aphasia);

(b) regulating motor behaviour, i.e. understanding the command but being unable to carry it out in spite of intact motor function (apraxia);

(c) difficulty initiating behaviour;

(d) coordination of one body part in relation to another, including disorders of body image and of sensory feedback and coordination;

(e) if the subject is asked to imitate a movement (asomatognosia) or read a written instruction, the ability to process visual information will be relevant.

To specify which of these processes is dysfunctional, several similar and related tasks have to be attempted. For example, if the subject can carry out the instruction when imitating, but not when requested to do it verbally, a difficulty in comprehending language might be suspected. Support for this hypothesis might be a failure to respond to a completely different request such as complying with an instruction to read a sentence out loud or to pick out an object from a display. An alternative train of thought might be: the subject can follow many verbal commands but cannot draw a simple design or put together bricks in a specified pattern. In this case a spatial difficulty, an apraxia, would be suspected. By a process of logical elimination of possible dysfunctions, sense can be made of a sometimes bewildering range of failures. Some problems may only be picked up by observing a patient's behaviour throughout a testing session, rather than assessing directly through a test; for example, problems with concentration or attention may appear more clearly after a period of testing, so that the most recently performed tests are done worse than the first, regardless of the nature of the functions necessary for correct completion of the tasks involved (Brooks, 1984; Hecaen and Albert, 1978).

Once the nature of the deficits observed has been clarified, it is necessary to predict the effects that these difficulties will have on an individual's attempt to resume activities and relationships. It is sometimes possible to enable someone to relearn old skills. Wilson and Moffat's work (1984) on memory retraining may be a good example. However, it is usually more successful to help modify the environment and to educate those involved with the patient as to what to expect and how to cope. We can require the environment to take over the function that our patient cannot do, as happens when the patient uses a diary to compensate for memory problems, or when someone prompts a patient who 'forgets to remember' when distracted, that he should go to turn off a boiling kettle. Alternatively, we can make it unnecessary that the patient has to use lost skills, so that a head-injured patient whose job involved the use of complex abstract thinking may return to work successfully in a job that requires different abilities.

BEHAVIOUR ANALYSIS

The use of behavioural techniques can be particularly helpful when dealing with patients whose neuropsychological difficulties have become confounded with behaviours which either disrupt their adaptation within social and family settings or which result in a loss of skills and independence out of proportion to the deficits as shown on testing. If it is easier and quicker for a relative to dress a patient than to allow him to do it himself, he may remain without those skills. If, in addition, the patient has difficulty tolerating frustration, as is common after head injury, the relative may be discouraged from letting him learn to dress again when this results in temper tantrums. In this way the relative may be punished in several ways if she encourages increased independence. The patient in his turn may be punished for his aggressive behaviour when his relative rejects or ignores him after an outburst; his frustration about this may lead to further violence. If the relative feels guilty and unkind letting the patient struggle, and then proceeds to complete the task for the patient, the patient may then learn that by showing distress or aggression he does not have to struggle with the tasks he finds frustrating. The same behavioural principles will hold in institutions (see the case history below). The principles used derive from learning theory. When analysing a patient's behaviour the assessor will be looking for those events which predictably presage or follow the behaviour which is of interest. An easy way of making sense of such observations is to construct a chart with three headings: A (antecedents), B (behaviour), C (consequences). For each behaviour selected, the antecedents and consequences can be listed and examined. In clinical settings a common example might be this: A patient causes concern to a member of the team. His mobility is not improving and he often seems unsteady in spite of practice with the physiotherapist. The behaviour (B) would be unsteady walking. In the team meeting it is mentioned that the staff on the opposite shift do not find this a problem, and that he seems to be able to walk well enough not to cause them concern (B′). Observations made over the next few days suggest that the patient does stumble more when the staff of one shift are on duty. The most important immediate antecedent (A) is therefore the presence of certain members of staff. The consequences (C) of unsteadiness when these staff are near include anxious attention, physical help and conversation. If the patient stumbles when these staff members are not present, there are no environmental consequences unless he loses his balance and falls. The patient therefore seems to discriminate between the presence and absence of particular staff, and is more cautious in their absence. Given that attention and help may be positive consequences for this patient (and at a premium generally on a busy ward) it might be possible for the attention to be given contingent on independent behaviours rather than linked to helpless or dependent behaviours. The analysis itself can be helpful in achieving this; if staff find that the patient can cope, their anxiety and vigilance for falls may be reduced, allowing them to encourage rather than caution. An assessment that includes not only the behaviour being evaluated, but also the stimuli which are thought to either increase or decrease the incidence of those behaviours, is called a functional analysis. For further information the reader may turn to Owens and Ashcroft (1982) or Mackrell and Toogood (1983). Common examples where this approach may be helpful might include: temper tantrums, especially when they occur in some settings and not others; sporadic antisocial or self-harming behaviour; learning difficulties.

WIDER ISSUES

It is important to bear in mind that interactions in families and in institutions are extremely complex. Emotional and developmental issues may affect prognosis (Brooks, 1984); for example, a young man was held back from optimal independence through his parents' fear of losing him and with him the focus of their lives — the empty nest syndrome. Relatives can also limit the patient out of concern and fear that he will not cope. These two factors can operate together, creating a situation which is self-perpetuating and ends up being distressing for everyone. (See the case history below for an example of problems arising in contrast in an institutional setting.) Return to work (or alternative forms of occupation) can be important milestones to consider.

TESTING

There are a number of tests which can be used to determine the functioning of a patient, and here we will only give a brief overview of major tests and what they might help us discover about the patient. Walsh (1978), Mittler (1970) and Lezak (1976) give a wide coverage of tests, and the reader is referred to these references for specific guidance. It seems that most clinicians select a battery of tests to assess patients and point out areas that need closer attention. Experienced clinicians often rely on a relatively limited range of tests with which they develop a set of internal norms to aid them when evaluating a patient's responses.

The following tests are commonly used (the tests are ordered so that psychometric tests appear at one end and qualitative assessments at the other).

Tests in common usage

Wechsler Adult Intelligence Scale — Revised (WAIS-R) — a battery made up of eleven subtests which give a verbal, performance and full-scale-score IQ. It is standardised on large numbers and is commonly used so that the results are meaningful to most clinicians. There is now a new version. Unfortunately the subtests themselves are not closely related to discrete psychological functions.

Wechsler Memory Scale — similarly made up of subtests which investigate different aspects of memory. Not as popular now because understanding of memory is more sophisticated, but again it has been well standardised.

Halstead–Reitan Battery — this is an influential battery of tests which examines a variety of psychological functions. It includes tests for abstraction, planning, auditory perception and constructional praxis. It has been well-used in research.

Luria–Nebraska Neuropsychological Battery — an American reworking of a Danish compilation of a Russian neurologist's clinical investigation which has all the problems arising from multiple translations of language and culture. The battery is comprehensive, with 14 scales covering, e.g., motor, language, memory, educational skills and intellectual attainment. The 267 items are short and simple, easily scored and related to neuropsychological functions. It is good as a training and research tool. However, the way the scales are constructed, and especially the concept behind the scoring, leaves much to be desired. Interpretation of the results is best done by an experienced practitioner.

Luria Neuropsychological Battery — this consists of an interview and testing instructions, a manual for interpreting results, cards and tapes. The items are taken from Luria's clinical assessment but, although roughly grouped, rely on the understanding of the interviewer when interpreting results. When used by an experienced clinician it is a sensitive tool for defining the nature of neuropsychological dysfunction. However, there is no way of quantifying the results so that it is difficult to measure severity or change.

In addition the following four tests provide a sample of material available:

Recognition Memory Test (RMT), Elizabeth K. Warrington — a new test for recognition of faces and words. Two well-designed simple tasks. The test has only recently become available and still has to find its place in common use.

Weigl–Goldstein–Scheerer (WGS) Colour Form Test — one of a battery of tests which evaluate abstract thought and concept formation. This takes the form of a clinical experiment. While at times too simple for intelligent patients, it preserves its place as an interesting and well-designed classic.

Williams Test of Delayed Recall — a short and simple memory test which provides a quick estimate of spontaneous recall, cued recall and recognition. It seems not particularly popular with clinicians but patients take well to it, and the delay recall is a useful and relatively uncommon feature.

National Adult Reading Test (NART) — this relatively recent reading test aims to provide a score that can be used as an estimate of premorbid ability. It is easy to administer and score — regional accents occasionally leave some responses in doubt.

Case history

Mr B is a single man in his 30s who, after a road traffic accident in which he sustained a serious head injury, was admitted for long-term care to a psychiatric hospital. There had been difficulties at home prior to admission and over a period of time he developed a reputation as an aggressive man following a series of violent incidents, both physical and verbal in nature. After one of these occurrences he was referred for assessment to the psychology department. At this time the ward staff and patients were feeling both anxious about, and hostile to, Mr B.

Neuropsychological assessment

Mr B was comprehensively assessed using a number of tests. Primarily the Luria–Nebraska was employed to give a global view of Mr B's functioning. The results showed a classical pattern of deficits common after head injury. He had difficulties with certain items in the motor scale and in the memory and intellectual scales.

On the WAIS-R Mr B gained an average IQ scoring only a little lower than would have been predicted from his educational background. This is a common result after head injury.

The WGS Colour–Form Test indicated difficulties with abstract thought, concept formation and ability to change set (from one way of thinking to another).

The Williams Delayed Recall showed difficulty remembering items spontaneously after distraction, but a reasonably good use of prompts. It is important to note that testing took place over many short sessions so that the effects of Mr B's problems, e.g. irritability and difficulty concentrating, were minimised. The tester also on occasion was willing to be distracted into conversation to make the sessions as easy-going as possible and ensure Mr B's continuing cooperation. The physical setting included choosing a quiet room to minimise his distractability, though it is relevant to point out here that it is important to remember to have another member of staff informed and standing by in case the patient develops disinhibited sexual or aggressive behaviour. Preparing assessment sessions in this way allows the tester to behave in a more relaxed and less anxious way. Mr B often responded to anxiety or pressure with an escalation of difficulties concentrating, frustration and eventually aggressive behaviours. On the other hand a secure and friendly situation enabled him to relax and consequently optimise his achievement on testing.

Day-to-day behaviour consistent with the test results included:

(a) difficulty using verbal instructions to modify his behaviour;

(b) inability to delay behaviour (waiting);

(c) difficulty inhibiting behaviour (not acting on his aggressive feelings);

(d) forgetfulness after distraction;

(e) difficulty working out problems (including explaining why he felt as he did).

Behavioural assessment

It became clear that on the ward Mr B was largely ignored or treated in a negative way by patients and even by staff, who were angry with him for what they felt was unprovoked aggression. He was expected to be able to behave in a 'reasonable' way, much as the other patients did, which, given the deficits described above, meant that Mr B was often left confused or unable to comply with others' expectations. An example of this might be when he lent money to another patient who told him he would pay it back to Mr B in a week's time. When Mr B needed some money the following day he became angry when his friend could not pay him back instantly. Because he would interpret situations like this as hostile acts, and respond accordingly, people avoided him. Eventually people only approached him when they felt angry with him.

A further complaint at this stage was Mr B's inappropriate sexual approaches to women.

Interventions

Mr B was transferred to a new ward for a new start. Staff were all involved in a discussion of Mr B's history and problems, including an explanation of the way an institutional setting and his own difficulties might have dovetailed to produce the disruptive behaviours. Further ways of helping Mr B to compensate for his difficulties on the ward were formulated: (a) repeating instructions in a straightforward way as often as necessary while showing as much patience as possible; (b) informing him of the most appropriate way to obtain appropriate goals; (c) interrupting inappropriate ways of behaving as soon as these could be recognised; and (d) supplying him with models and prompting to develop these.

Time for interesting and pleasant exchanges with staff and other patients was built into his routine, not dependent on his behaviour at other times. In addition a reward scheme was set up whereby Mr B could earn rewards for appropriate ways of behaviour. Further, he was given individual social skills training sessions using video and 'actors'.

Aggressive and inappropriate sexual behaviour diminished rapidly and Mr B built up warm and positive relationships with both staff members and other patients over a period of months. Mr B is, of course, left with the original deficits, but with some strategies for coping better, e.g. use of a diary for memory and planning. Part of Mr B's improvement can be seen as an educational process whereby he has begun to stop hitting people and start explaining to himself and others what has made him confused and angry. More important, the behavioural overlay has been reversed and Mr B can now hope to be returned to community living in, e.g. a hostel.

One other aspect the authors want to stress here is that it is recognised how demanding it is for the staff to help these patients. Training alone is not enough, and it must be understood that staff too have personal needs and difficulties. To handle situations like with the patient described above, staff need to be counselled and encouraged. Staff group support by appropriately trained psychologists or group therapists may be of great benefit.

SUMMARY

In this very brief chapter we have attempted to give the reader a flavour of some of the issues related to psychological assessment. Emphasis has been placed on the importance of a good fit between referral, assessment and real-life situations. A short list of tests and a case history have been included to show how the handling of a case might be conducted. The reader has been referred elsewhere for more detailed information.

REFERENCES

Albert, M.L. (1978) Subcortical dementia. In R. Katzman *et al.* (eds), *Alzheimer's disease; senile dementia and related disorders* (*Aging*, vol. 7), Raven Press, New York

Albert, M.L., Feldman, R.G. and Willis, A.L. (1974) The 'subcortical dementia' of progressive supranuclear palsy. *J. Neurol. Neurosurg. Psychiatry*, *37*, 121-30

Benson, D.F. and Blumer, D. (1975) *Psychological aspects of neurological disease*, Grune & Stratton, New York

Brooks, N. (ed.) (1984) *Closed head injury*, Oxford University Press, Oxford

Hecaen, H. and Albert, M.L. (1978) *Human neuropsychology*, John Wiley & Sons, New York

Katzman, R., Terry, R.D. and Bick, K.L. (eds) (1978) *Alzheimer's disease: senile dementia and related disorders* (*Aging*, vol. 7), Raven Press, New York

Lezak, M.D. (1976) *Neuropsychological assessment*, Oxford University Press, New York

Mackrell, K. and Toogood, R. (1983) Clinical application of principles derived from the experimental analysis of behaviour. *Behav. Anal.*, *4*(2), 11-20

Mittler, P. (1970) *The psychological assessment of mental and physical handicaps*, Tavistock Publications, London

Owens, R.G. and Ashcroft, J.B. (1982) Functional analysis in applied psychology *Br. J. Clin. Psychol.*, *21*, 181-9

Victor, M., Adams, R.D. and Collins, G.H. (1971) *The Wernicke–Korsakoff syndrome*, Davis, Philadelphia

Walsh, K.W. (1978) *Neuropsychology — a clinical approach*, Churchill Livingstone, Edinburgh

Wilson, B.A. and Moffat, N. (eds) (1984) *Clinical management of memory problems*, Croom Helm, London/Aspen Publishers, Rockville, MD

34

Occupational Therapy

Rosemary Curry and Helen March

DEFINITION

Occupational therapy (OT) is the treatment of physical and psychiatric conditions through specific selected activities in order to help people reach their maximum level of function in all aspects of daily life.

MAIN AIMS

(1) To assess the patient's difficulties in various daily activities.

(2) To facilitate maximum independence.

(3) To encourage maximum return of function.

(4) To help the patient, family and colleagues (e.g. at work) to adjust to his difficulty.

(5) To prevent deformity.

(6) To resettle the patient within the community and at work, where appropriate.

(7) In doing this, the OT will work with and reinforce the work of other members of the rehabilitation team (or other specialist treating team).

(8) To provide the necessary aids and appliances where appropriate, and thus encourage independence.

OTs treat patients with both physical and mental disorders. Many will acquire considerable specialist skills over the years and will work in a variety of specialties at basic grade level on rotational appointments commonly in geriatrics, neurology, orthopaedics and paediatrics, splint-making or other areas such as psychiatric fields before specialising.

ORGANISATION OF OT SERVICES

OTs are employed in many areas, including the Health Service, Social Services Departments (community OTs), the Prison Services and a variety of charitable organisations. The community OT sees the patient at home. She may come into the hospital to see the patients when needed to ensure smooth transition to their home. She may work in a day centre or in other areas administered by Social Services. When building alterations need to be done, and homes designed for the disabled, she may work with the architects' department on design and planning.

OT HELPERS AND OTHER NON-MEDICAL STAFF

OT helpers are found in many hospital departments; technicians with joinery skills or industrial experience usually work in OT workshops, others may help with certain aids and adaptations. The OT has much liaison work with referring doctors, with other remedial professionals including OTs in the community, with those responsible for employment, with Social Services and often with local authority housing departments, and, for some younger patients with educational departments. OTs need to go out to where the patient lives and works, i.e. to the home, school and workplace, not only to assess but to advise and train the carers and co-workers of disabled people.

REFERRAL TO HOSPITAL OT DEPARTMENTS

This usually requires the filling out of a referral form by the hospital doctor. Many departments are also open to direct access by the GP. Community OTs work on a similar referral system to their colleagues in the Health Service or via the local Social Services office which may be contacted by the GP, patient or carer.

It is important that full diagnostic information is given, as the therapist may not have access to the patient's notes. Such information should indicate whether the OT is to assess the patient, if so, to what end, and if the patient is to be treated, the goals which are sought.

The skills of the OT are used best when she is part of the rehabilitation team. In our hospital the OT is present at every rehabilitation outpatient clinic, so that decisions can be taken rapidly, e.g. as to whether the patient comes to the OT department, the OT does a home visit, liaises with the employer or Manpower Services, or education authorities.

ASSESSMENT

Assessment of a patient's disabilities will only be accurate when therapists have established some rapport with the patient who has relaxed sufficiently to allow the therapist to explore his difficulties. Specific counselling and relaxation techniques are also now being used more frequently by appropriately trained OTs. The OT needs accurate information to know what areas to explore. For instance, an older man, living alone in an area where support services are limited, may be unable to make himself a drink: until he can do so, he may be deemed unable to return home. A similarly affected man, with a fit wife, may need to do very little; the therapist may be more concerned with teaching the wife how to assist the man in dressing, using the toilet and other transfers. In both cases she would need a considerable amount of information about the domestic environment. In the case of a younger man at work, but temporarily in hospital, she might need to find out sufficient about the man's work and workplace, to ensure his effective and speedy return to it. It can thus be seen that several types of assessment may be undertaken, which will be of use to a variety of statutory, voluntary and private services.

Assessments include the following:

(1) activities of daily living;

(2) hand skills;

(3) mobility and access;

(4) social skills;

(5) numeracy and literacy; visuospatial skills;

(6) work skills;

(7) leisure skills and interests;

(8) other specific assessments (e.g. of chair and wheelchair requirements and splinting requirements).

Assessment may be repeated as the patient improves. The OT will be especially concerned with energy conservation (disabilities such as amputation or hemiparesis result in greater energy expenditure in walking, and many other tasks) and with safety, particularly in the kitchen and workplace. Goals should be reviewed and reset as the conditions alter (see Chapter 6, Functional Assessment Tests).

METHODS OF WORKING WITHIN HOSPITAL

Most hospital OT departments have within them several areas: domestic facilities (bedroom, kitchen, bathroom and toilet) will be found, as well as light and heavy workshops, quiet activity areas and those for general activities. Specialised areas such as a paediatric department, splint-making facilities, a head injuries workshop and, ideally, a garden, are found in some departments.

Specialist equipment is commonly found: a standing frame may be used in any area so that certain patients can stimulate the leg muscles or improve balance by standing to perform certain tasks.

THE HEAVY WORKSHOP

This is a most useful asset in an industrial city, even though the OT department may not be able to accommodate every type of equipment found in the industries around. Working conditions can often be simulated to some extent; it is possible to retrain patients on some of the equipment mentioned earlier sufficient to produce an assessment useful to the ERC or employers. Carpentry, metal work, brick and cement making, and work on various lathes are possible in many departments (Figure 34.1).

Figure 34.1: Making a rail in the workshop; one patient can help another

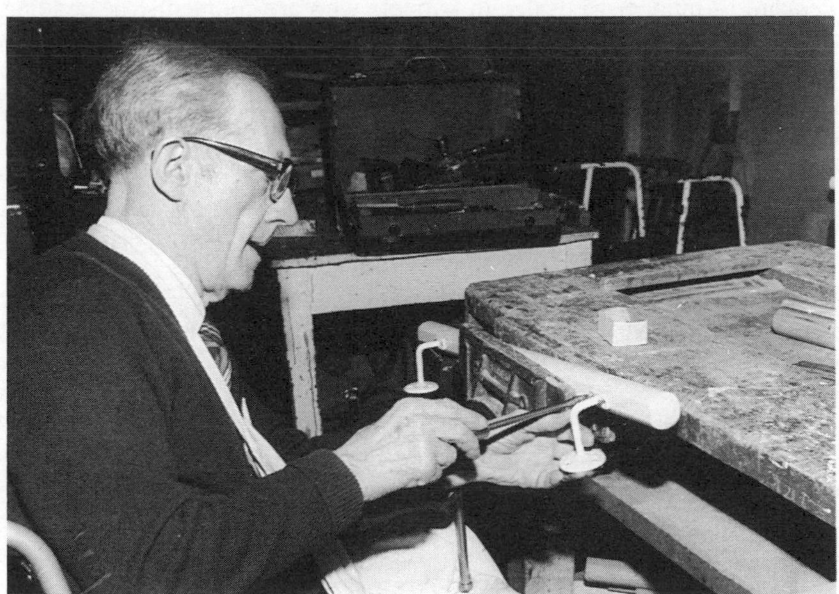

In the workshop a variety of manual and powered machinery (such as lathes, saws, woodwork or metalwork equipment) is found. Again, this may be modified as patients' requirements dictate, to build up muscle strength, or work tolerance, or to increase joint range, particularly after orthopaedic surgery and hand injuries, where the patient is aiming to progress to retraining or return to his own work. The machines can be used in different ways to achieve arm or leg exercise, to increase muscle strength or range of movement.

THE LIGHT WORKSHOP

The therapist must structure work to suit the individual's need and may simulate the working conditions. Here office duties, typing, packing, bookbinding, printing or engraving can be undertaken. Light work, machine sewing and machine knitting are possible in some departments. In others, enterprising OTs may seek the help of relevant departments of the hospital itself, or occasionally of friendly employers nearby. Alternatively, the patient's employers may allow the OT to bring work from the factory to the OT department, so that as early as a few weeks after a leg amputation (e.g.) the OT may be able to say that the patient retains job skills, and it only remains to work out the details of the journeys to and from work (turning to the MSC Fares to Work Scheme, perhaps).

A workshop is invaluable for head-injured patients provided that work is correctly structured for them, and that the experienced therapists are adequate in number to deal with patients who are frequently demanding, and who may need considerable help to regain social as well as other skills. It may be necessary to set this area apart from that used by other patients. It will also be useful to have a *quiet room* where patients' numeracy and literacy may be tested or trained (Figures 34.2 and 34.3).

GARDENING

The garden, including raised flower beds, and a wheelchair-accessible greenhouse are invaluable. They bring patients much pleasure; many enjoy being outside after weeks inside a hospital ward (Figure 34.4). Again, the therapist can assess the patient's ability to use old skills or to learn new activities. The patient may come to realise that some active leisure activities are still possible, such as growing indoor plants, gardening in a greenhouse, or from a wheelchair using adapted equipment on normal flower beds, or using raised beds. These can be bought or constructed from something as simple as car tyres or paving slabs fixed vertically in the ground to retain the earth. Many hobbies are possible from a wheelchair.

Figure 34.2: Perceptual testing, body image disorder

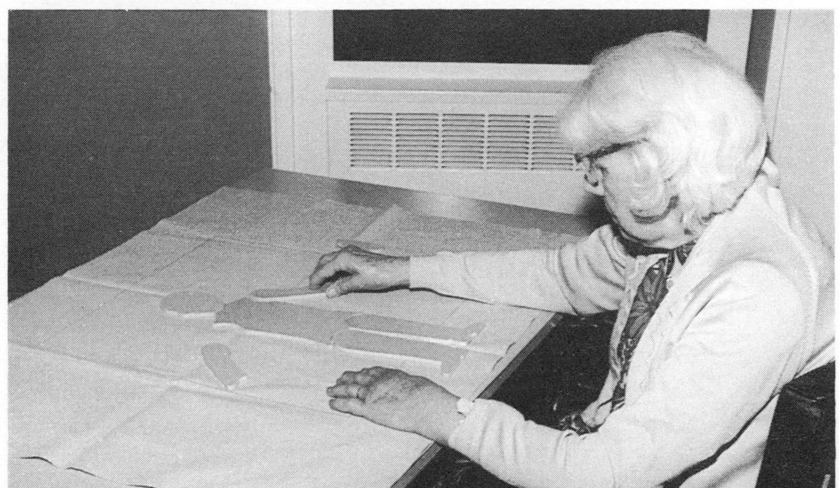

ACTIVITIES OF DAILY LIVING

Self-care activities

Eating and drinking

The patient's morale is considerably improved when he is able to eat and drink independently with as little mess as possible. Patients should be encouraged to dine at the dining room table in the ward: to this end the OT may bring the patient to the OT department and try out a range of equipment, such as non-spill cups, adapted cutlery, or plates with a raised edge or those with a reservoir of warm water under the food to keep it hot. A non-slip mat is often useful. Simple advice may be helpful: a cup may be only half-filled or a straw may be used by an ataxic patient. A patient who can use only one utensil may start with a spoon but progress to a fork if possible. Care should be taken to position the patient comfortably and correctly at the table.

Dressing

Again, a patient feels better if dressed in normal clothing rather than in nightclothes. As far as possible, practice in regaining this skill should be given at the correct time of day, although it may be easier to begin by

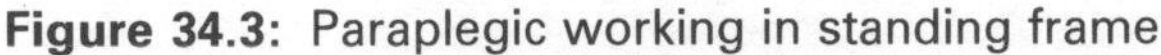

Figure 34.3: Paraplegic working in standing frame

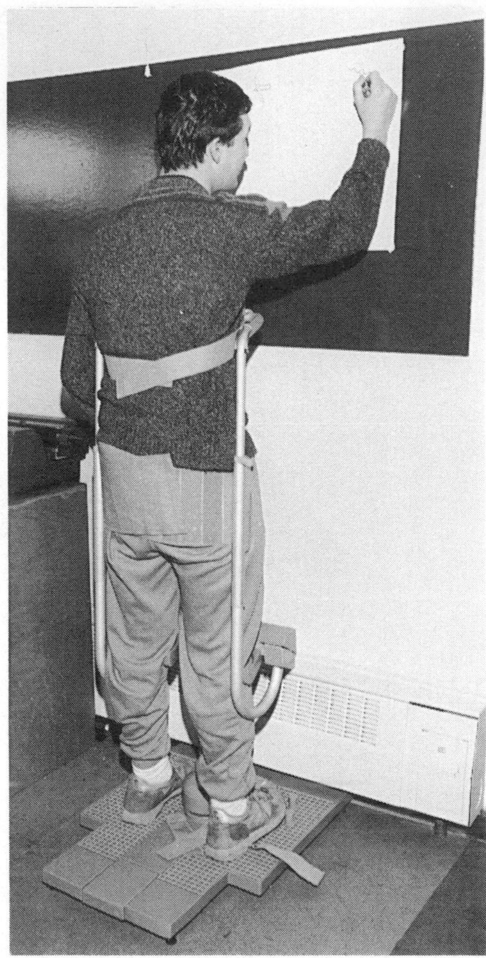

teaching the patient to undress, pulling the clothes over the head. The stroke patient takes clothes off the hemiplegic side last.

Clothing

Clothes should be simple, lightweight and loose. Front-fastening track suits are particularly useful, although some women manage better with full skirts. Waistbands may be elasticated, buttons replaced by velcro. Crutch-less knickers are available: indeed a wide range of beautifully produced and fashionable clothing is coming on to the market and should do much to make handicapped people feel more confident. There are even trousers and jeans which are shaped specifically for those who sit in wheelchairs all

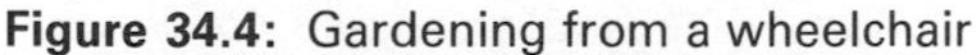
Figure 34.4: Gardening from a wheelchair

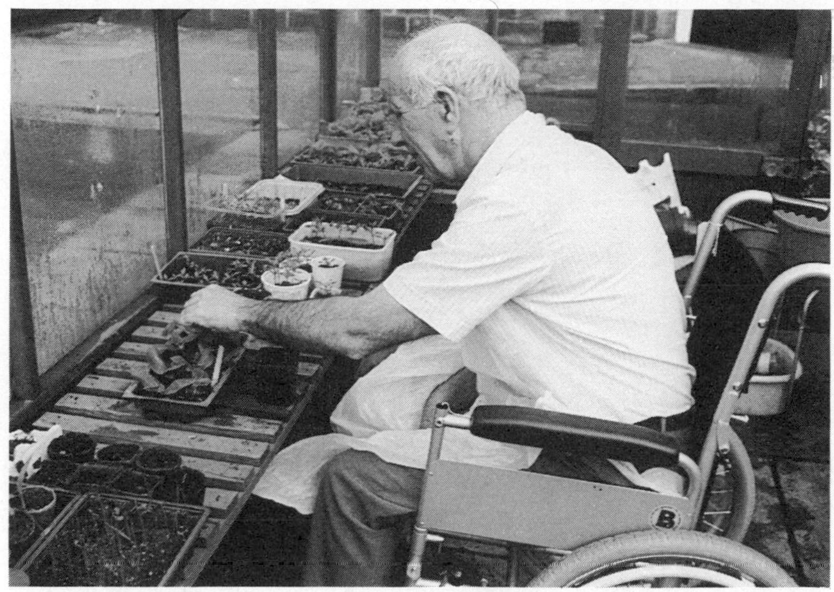

day, which can cffcctively disguise considerable trunk deformities. Shoes should be low-heeled and sturdy; trainers with velcro fastenings are often used (Figure 34.5).

For dressing the patient is seated *securely* on the chair or bed edge, with the feet firmly on the floor. The clothes are placed, in order, within reach and in a good light. If the patient is hemiplegic clothes may be placed on the hemiplegic side, which is inserted into the garment first. If there are perceptual problems (which frequently show up in dressing) the patient may have to be 'talked through' his dressing so that he learns the nature of his problems, and ways of overcoming them.

Balance is frequently impaired so that the patient cannot stand to put clothes on, or needs help with tights or trousers. Even when seated with legs crossed this may be a difficult activity which only improves with persistent training (in both physiotherapy and OT). Sometimes a patient finds it helpful to hold onto a fixed dressing bar fixed on a bedroom wall while donning trousers.

The patient may have to dress on the bed at first, and remain unable to put on socks and shoes for a long time. Orthoses (callipers) are often a persistently difficult problem.

Dressing aids

Dressing aids may be useful, as in arthritis, where a dressing stick helps to adjust clothes over the shoulders. Occasionally such things as a long-

Figure 34.5: Dressing — putting on a sock and shoe with one hand, supporting weak leg over the unaffected leg

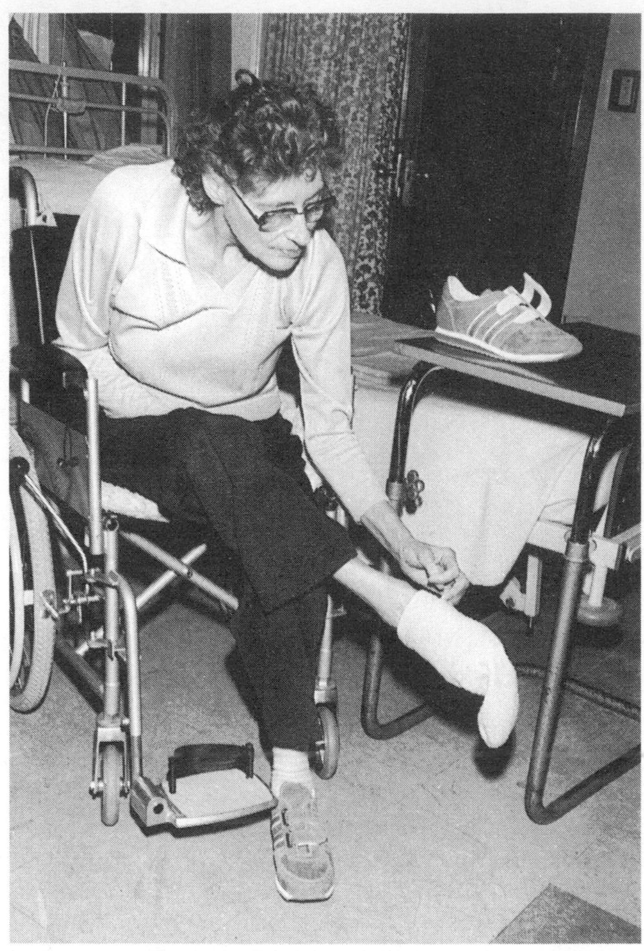

handled shoe horn, 'no bows' or elastic shoelaces or stockings aids are required.

Washing

Patients should be encouraged to be independent in washing and grooming. They normally need to sit to use a washbasin; there should be surfaces on either side for sponge bag, flannel and make-up. Good light and a large mirror are necessary. Those with arthritis may like lever taps. Men will need an accessible shaving point. A patient may take a long time to wash at first, so the bathroom should be warm and comfortable. As he becomes more confident and stronger, the patient will progress from washing only the face, to dealing with the top half of the body. Some remain unable to manage perineal washing and toileting with ease, but may do better using a bidet, or bathing or showering.

Just as some patients can stand for sufficient time to pull on trousers if given a dressing rail, so many find rails in the bathroom a great asset. These may need to be alongside the bath, toilet and washbasin.

Bathing

Bathing is a potentially hazardous procedure. Frail patients, or those with poor balance, should be encouraged to enter the bath from a seated position. A chair or stool is put beside the bath, or a bath board on top of the bath. The patient sits on this and swings the legs in, then lowers himself onto the bath seat and thence down into the bath. A grab-rail on the wall by the bath is often helpful.

A shower may be a better alternative, with a firmly placed plastic chair or stool for the patient to sit on. However, arthritic patients get relief from lying in hot water. They may need further bath aids such as a Manger bath seat or Ambulift bath hoist.

Simple aids such as a suction nailbrush, long-handled brushes and flannels are helpful. All these aids and adaptations are provided through Social Services Departments, but more sophisticated ones may take months to obtain (Figure 34.6).

Figure 34.6: Some aids to daily living: dressing stick, non-stick mat, egg whisk, spiked potato peeler/grater, rimmed plate, adapted cutlery, suction egg cup, bread buttering board

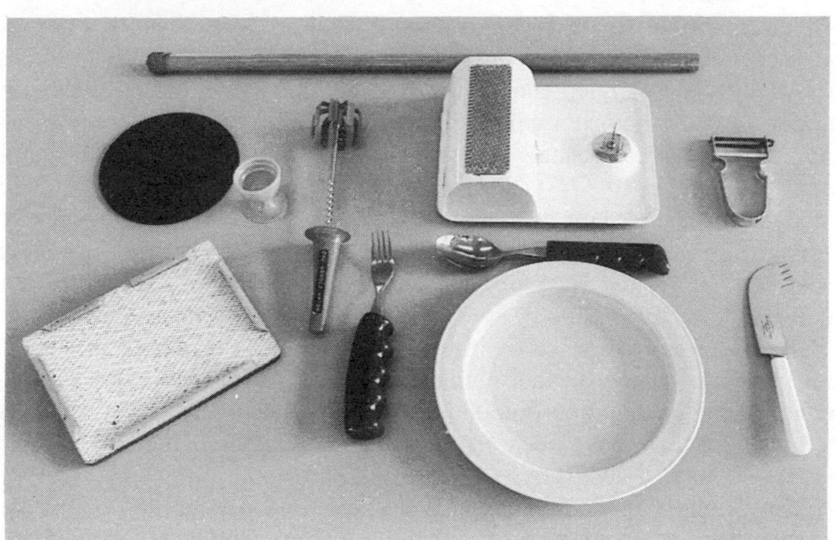

Toilet

It is important to most people that they can use the toilet independently and privately, even if they require help in getting there, or in transferring from a wheelchair to the toilet. The adjusting of one's clothes before and after urination or defaecation requires some dexterity and good sitting and standing balance. Rails alongside the lavatory may help the latter; toilet paper must be accessible; clothing has to be chosen with care; aids to perineal toilet may be necessary. Rarely a Closomat may be installed in a residential unit or a patient's home: this sophisticated lavatory cleanses the perineal area with hot water, then hot air, and is useful where the patient has no hand function and no helper.

Menstruation may be difficult to manage in women who have poor hand control, or lack of feeling in hands or perineum, particularly if they are obese. It may be worth putting them on the contraceptive pill as flow is then often sparse; occasionally the pill is given continuously for many months. Rarely hysterectomy or a radiation menopause is necessary.

Frequently the patient's toilet is small, and has a narrow doorway which will not admit a wheelchair. Many houses have no downstairs toilet. Although a commode may be used downstairs temporarily, a ground floor extension to accommodate a toilet, washbasin and perhaps a shower allows the disabled person to remain at home more comfortably and independently. Good access and room to manoeuvre is essential, and is easier to obtain if these are all in one room.

Domestic activities

An occupational therapy department kitchen is accessible to both the wheelchair-bound and the standing patient. A selection of aids for domestic activities is usually on hand. Most women (and some men) dislike being unable to run their households, and every effort should be made to preserve at least part of this central role. Most patients in hospital readily understand when the OT takes them to the department's kitchen to check on domestic skills. However, it may not be so readily appreciated that getting the patient to weigh out ingredients, count out and fill bun cases, make up recipes and wash up, assesses a whole range of skills (including reading, numeracy, ability to obey instructions, to sequence events, to time activities, to get on with other users of the kitchen). Training in all such skills can be given in further kitchen sessions. A patient may progress to menu planning, shopping (handling money) and using transport. At some point, where there have been profound changes in the patient's abilities, a home visit may be necessary.

Many kitchen appliances ease the physical work needed in food preparation, and are valuable to patients. In addition, non-slip mats, bread boards (on which a single slice of bread is placed for buttering), potato peelers, one-handed or electric tin-openers may be needed. Where grip is weak or poor the kettle or teapot may be placed on a specially designed tipper.

The microwave oven is simple and safe for most people, and valuable, particularly where sensation in the hands is poor. If the patient is ataxic he should be taught to half-fill larger containers. A simple drink can be heated in the microwave, or water for tea or coffee heated with a 'hot shot', which requires only the ability to press a button.

The amount a patient needs to do in the kitchen depends on the support he receives from carer, neighbours or statutory bodies. He may have a home help daily, and/or be provided with freezer meals or meals-on-wheels. Many patients have few resources, and their kitchens are often small and inconvenient. Some have never cooked before and live entirely from the fish and chip shop and the neighbouring pub. However, if living alone, meals bought frozen, ready prepared, and heated in a microwave may be helpful.

THE HOME VISIT

A home visit is beneficial when the patient's situation has changed considerably due to a new disability such as paraplegia or the death of a caring spouse; *the new problem may be medical or social.* The visit must be planned to ensure that neighbours or helpers are present, if wanted, or perhaps that the patient has the opportunity to use his kitchen, or to go upstairs. Such a visit may be invaluable in motivating him. Frequently the treating physiotherapist also comes on this visit. The journey itself can be informative: does the patient give directions to his home, does he recognise the immediate vicinity, and can he tell the therapists something about the area? Has he given any thought as to the difficulties he will encounter and solutions to overcome them?

Assessment will include access to the home (necessity for rails, ramps), transfers of patient into and within the house, accessibility of kitchen, of surfaces, equipment therein, of plugs, doors, cupboards and windows, means of heating, use of stairs (rails often required) and access to the toilet and bathroom.

Equipment, aids and alterations are then decided upon. Sometimes sophisticated environmental controls (to control entry to the house, the TV, heating, radio, telephone, curtains) may need to be ordered through the Regional Consultant Assessor (Chapter 48). Alternatively, a person living alone may benefit from an alarm system or merely a telephone.

Wheelchairs

The OT department should have a wide range of wheelchairs for assessment of disabled patients, enabling the OT to prepare a detailed presentation after discussion with the patient. She will ensure that the wheelchair is suitable for the situations in which the patient wishes to use it (usually the home, place of work and for travelling) — see Chapter 43.

PROGRESSIVE AND SEVERE DISEASE

Where patients are undergoing extensive rehabilitation a single home visit will need to be supplemented by 'trial' weekends (the first may be during the working week). The patient begins to cope with increasing success in his own home with necessary modifications *in situ*, and is gradually weaned to this. Carers also gradually become skilled at their new work, but may realise they need help or periodic relief.

With progressive illnesses, such as multiple sclerosis and motor neurone disease (MND), *positive thinking* and *long-term planning* are priorities. With care most patients can remain at home for a long time. Sometimes adaptations are necessary; sometimes a different approach to a task is all that is required. For instance, a stairlift might be dismissed as unsuitable for patients with MND simply because the patient is unable to get on or off its seat by standing to transfer (or it may take too long to fit). By the use of a simple sliding board this task can be accomplished with economic use of energy. In fact, *economy* is a key word in the management of many people with chronic illness: economy in the use of energy and resources. One must use available money for equipment in such a way that it is available for as many as possible. Similarly, the use of hospital beds for intermittent care makes good use of both hospital facilities and hard-pressed carers. The space at home can sometimes be better utilised, as by turning the upstairs over to teenagers, the downstairs to the disabled parent.

Games and crafts have many therapeutic applications. Individual activities may be undertaken in such positions as to encourage increased range of movement and greater muscle power. For instance, to encourage this at the shoulder, a stool could be placed at shoulder height on a wall for seat-weaving. The game of draughts is frequently played by hemiplegic patients, using both hands to move large pieces. Group activities are very often fun, and the element of competitiveness useful. Dressing practice may be disguised as a game that requires the patient to get a circle of webbing over the head, down the body and off the feet. Ball games encourage balance and coordination (Figure 34.7).

Figure 34.7: Playing skittles: trunk balance and coordination

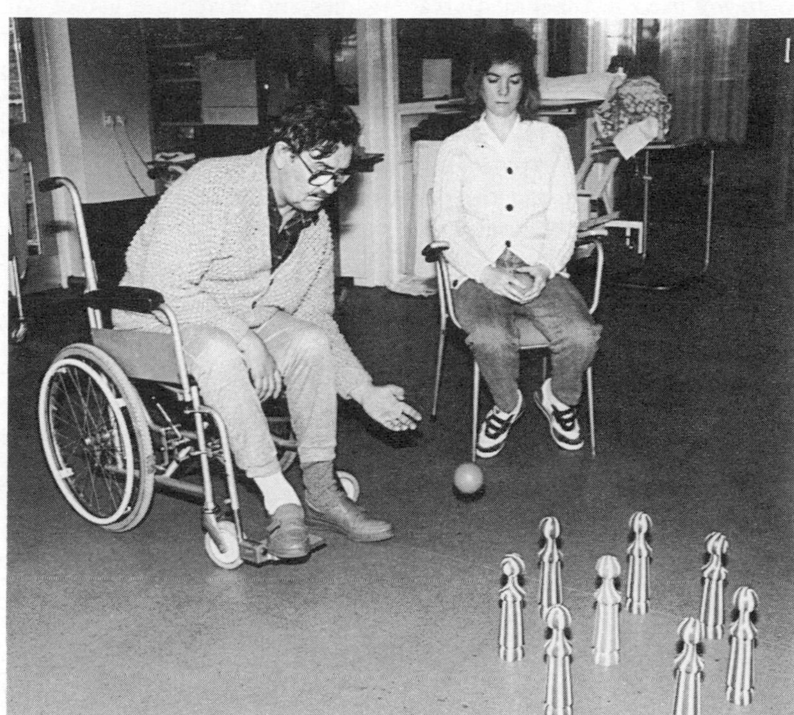

Microcomputers

Many OT departments have recently acquired microcomputers and are exploring their potential. They are especially relevant to younger patients, to those with head injury, or hand injury, and may be highly enjoyable ways of assessing and treating patients. Areas such as the following have been explored:

> concentration, motivation, reaction time, logical thought processes, perceptual skills, memory and communication, dexterity — other motor skills, educational ability, work tolerance — life skills can also be surveyed.

Where the patient has difficulty using conventional inputs, *modified inputs* may be used such as a keyguard, switches, joy sticks, the extended keyboard, concept keyboard, touch screen. A game may be slowed up using the slowmo. Two patients may operate the computer together. The computer can be activated by a two-switch input on finger, foot or suck–

blow control, if the patient is heavily disabled (Figure 34.8).

Software used has included arcade games and adventure games which demand decision-making, problem-solving and lateral thinking, traditional games such as chess and draughts, specific language programmes (e.g. written by speech therapists), and educational programmes including those written by local teachers, perhaps in special schools. There are also institutional programmes for typing and data management. Often liaison with local computer groups and the department of education is useful. Some patients may join local computer groups thereafter.

OCCUPATIONAL THERAPY OF THE STROKE PATIENT

The OT treatment of the man with a stroke, whose history and physiotherapy are detailed in Chapter 35, is given to show the use of progressive coordinated treatment in both OT and physiotherapy to a common aim, i.e. return home, alone.

On admission to the rehabilitation unit

Mr A required help to stand and don his trousers and shoes. His standing balance was poor. He was right-handed but learning to do domestic activit-

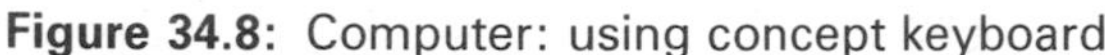
Figure 34.8: Computer: using concept keyboard

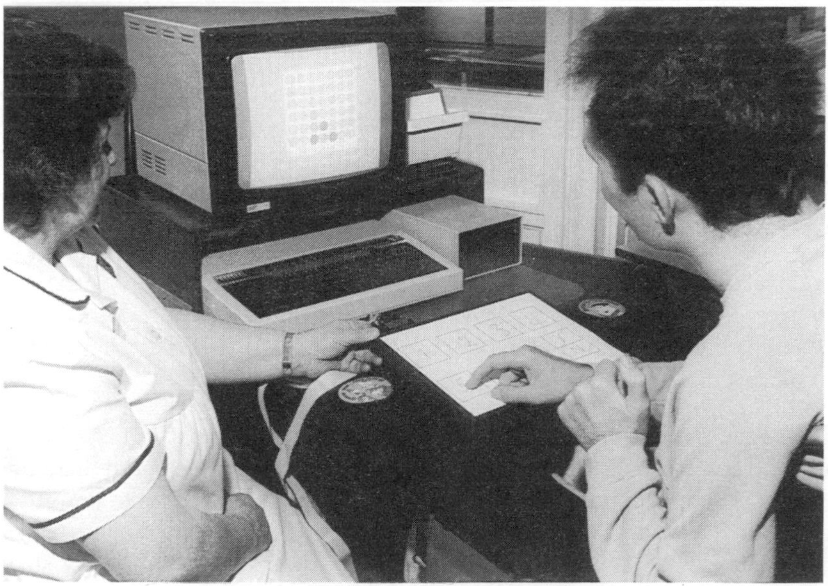

ies with his left hand and was well motivated to do this. He was independent in washing and shaving using his left hand. Because of his poor balance he needed help with the lavatory and used an Ambulift to bath.

Early treatment and progress

One week later, after intensive physiotherapy and occupational therapy, balance was much improved, so that Mr A had become independent in dressing and in use of the lavatory. As soon as he began to take steps he was able to practise bathing, use a bathboard, seat and non-slip mat. Mr A lived alone, was used to making his own meals and would still need to do this. He began to make tea and snacks from a wheelchair and then progressed to cooking full meals at a pace dictated by his understanding and his physical balance and endurance. After a further three weeks he was able to stand and walk round the kitchen. He could bend down to light the oven safely and was using his right hand to steady equipment.

Intermediate stage of treatment and progress

Mr A's first shopping trip occurred some six weeks after entry to the unit. It was felt that a supermarket was easier for him to use than a shop where language was needed. Mr A proved able to select the required goods, stand up from the wheelchair and place them in his basket, and pay for them at the checkout. Two successful trips were made to the pub. In spite of Mr A's jargon aphasia he was able to order a drink and pay for it.

A variety of occupational therapy activities had been used to gain these successes: some encouraged use of the hemiplegic limbs. For instance, Mr A had to find large objects placed in a pillowcase. The right hand had to find the objects, which had to be named. Gardening was tried but was not successful, and the patient did not like computer games. He was happy in the workshop, progressing from the wheelchair to standing, from varnishing to painting and sawing (again using both hands). He also worked in the kitchen and joined in group activities.

Later stages of treatment and progress

A home visit was made during the 12th week. Mr A lived in a modern bungalow which would be very suitable, but had trouble opening the front door which required the turning of two keys (now locked with one). Within the house he accomplished all necessary tasks; the rails he had varnished were installed by the workshop technician. Assessment for simple bath aids was completed, after which Mr A made tea for all. Because of the anticipated difficulties with communication, Mr A was sent on our experimental *family placement scheme.* A volunteer family looked after Mr A, at first in their home, later in his. They took him, and later sent him, on increasingly complex journeys, demanded more of him, liaised with the supervisory OT and employer's needs, and encouraged him to play his electric organ. On discharge Mr A was entirely independent in self-care and simple kitchen activities. Considerable work remained to be done to ensure re-employment.

FURTHER READING

The practice of occupational therapy: an introduction to the treatment of physical dysfunction, ed. Ann Turner (1981), Churchill Livingstone, London

Occupational therapy approaches to stroke, Anne Allert Wilcock (1986), Churchill Livingstone, London

Coping with disability, Peggy Jay (1984), Disabled Living Foundation, London

35

Physiotherapy

Mary Jackson, Jill Fisher and Philippa Perkins

INTRODUCTION

Physiotherapy is largely concerned with the improvement of function. A fuller definition is taken from the *Chartered Physiotherapists' Source Book*, 1985: 'A systematic method of assessing musculoskeletal and neurological disorders of function, including pain and those of psychological origin, and treating or preventing those problems by natural methods based essentially on manual practice and physical agencies'.

This definition should not be taken as restrictive; physiotherapeutic practice is evolving. Furthermore, physiotherapists are often asked to treat disorders of the chest, skin and circulation, i.e. those areas which are not primarily musculoskeletal or neurological.

Assessment

Assessment itself should not be viewed narrowly, but includes psychological, social and environmental factors related to the patient. Nor is assessment static. The physiotherapist will repeatedly evaluate the effectiveness of her programme, revising it as necessary.

Teamwork

Optimum results from physiotherapy are rarely achieved when the physiotherapist is isolated: good communication with other members of the rehabilitation team brings benefit to the patient. Easy access to the doctor is essential, and where possible the patient's progress should be reviewed regularly with all members of the team present.

Referral by doctors

Wherever possible, when doctors refer patients for physiotherapy they should give the patient's diagnosis (or diagnoses) and note specific details about the case which may contraindicate a particular form of treatment. They should indicate when they will see the patient again.

More general practitioners are now able to refer patients for physiotherapy assessment and treatment directly; in 1982 two-thirds of Health Districts were operating a direct referral system. This system is strongly recommended as being of great benefit to the patients, facilitating treatment in early and acute stages of conditions, avoiding, where possible, chronic developments and secondary complications. Direct referral may also shorten waiting lists for visits to consultants, who will then be able to devote more time for patients who are referred for their specific expertise.

There is an increasing emphasis on the advisory, preventive and health education role of physiotherapists. 'Clients may not always be patients'; for example, physiotherapists may work in Part III homes monitoring the general fitness of residents, and many physiotherapists use their expertise to teach others how to deal with problems such as lifting the elderly and handicapped.

Organisation of the District Physiotherapy Service

The Chartered Society of Physiotherapy recommends the appointment of a District Head of Services 'to create a cohesive physiotherapy service for the whole district and to maintain that service, coordinating and rationalising available resources and effecting change as appropriate'. Each hospital within the District is managed by a superintendent physiotherapist, and the larger hospital may be further subdivided into units with superintendents whose grade depends on the number of staff supervised.

Senior physiotherapists undertake 'highly skilled and specialised work requiring the exercise of particular expertise or ability'. The basic grade staff 'have acquired by their basic training and experience some degree of skill and expertise' (Whitley Councils for the Health Services (Great Britain) (1981).

The majority of Districts have now established a Community Physiotherapy Service to advise patients, their relatives and carers in the home and in residential homes and day centres. These physiotherapists work with the primary health care professionals and those in the paediatric field, and also visit schools and colleges.

'The Chartered Society of Physiotherapy (1985) believes that a comprehensive system of post-registration education for its members is essential.' This is organised on national, regional and local levels.

Provision is made for these four main areas of post-registration education and their development:

(1) clinical specialisms,

(2) management knowledge and skills,

(3) educational knowledge and skills,

(4) research knowledge and skills.

PHYSIOTHERAPY TREATMENT

Exercise

General principles

An exercise programme is planned following careful assessment of the patient's needs. Selection of exercises is based on an understanding of the mechanical principles involved with each type of exercise, and the physiological effects which are to be produced. Exercises may:

(1) strengthen muscle power and endurance;

(2) improve joint range;

(3) improve neuromuscular coordination;

(4) improve cardiovascular efficiency;

(5) re-educate functional activity.

A number of different techniques will often be combined in one treatment programme, and these will be altered according to the patient's progress and changing needs. For example, when treating a patient for osteoarthritis of the knees, one treatment session may include (1) free active exercise (no external resistance applied), (2) weight-resisted exercise, (3) gait re-education, (4) advice on activities of daily living and scheme of home exercises (Chapter 9).

Progress is largely dependent upon the patient's own efforts, not only when working with the physiotherapist but also when carrying out home exercises and putting into practice self-care advice, maintaining good postures and avoiding certain activities. Written exercises, where the patient has a planned future appointment with the physiotherapist, have proved to be an effective method of improving patient compliance (Chamberlain *et al.*, 1982).

Group treatment

When patients have some common disability or condition which will benefit from exercises and activities similar in character they may be treated in a group, e.g. frozen shoulder, Colles fracture, and cervical spondylosis classes. A variety of other classes will also take place, e.g. geriatric inpatient class and antenatal and postnatal classes. Two or more grades of class of the same type may exist, allowing for varying severity of disability, so that some patients may progress through the classes; others will be limited by age or some other factor. A major advantage of the group situation is the encouragement and support a patient receives from working with others in a similar situation.

Muscle strengthening techniques

To improve a muscle's performance a demand must be put upon it. The physiotherapist will seek to gain improvement in power by maximal loading and low repetition, and in endurance through lesser loading associated with frequent repetitions. There are various ways in which a muscle may be loaded.

(1) Weight loading. Weight loading may be done directly or indirectly: directly through use of a De Lorme boot, weighted straps (e.g. Portabell weights), sandbags, etc.; indirectly through the use of pulleys attached to weights. Pulley circuits facilitate alteration in the angle of pull through which the weight is applied to the body. Commercially produced weight-training apparatus such as the Multi-gym and Westminster pulleys use pulley systems offering weight resistance. There are three commonly used training regimes used with weight resistance to improve power: De Lorme and Watkins, McQueen and Zinovieff (Oxford). The main advantage of weight training is that a known weight is being moved; the patient may carry out much of the training alone, after initial instruction.

(2) Variable (spring) loading. When using a spring as resistance the load on the muscle increases as the spring is stretched. Springs are graded according to the weight which has to be applied to stretch them to a known length. The springs are attached to a fixed point, e.g. the head of the bed or fixed frame, and to the handle or strap on the patient's foot, and are also used in combination with sling suspension.

(3) Manual loading. In this method the therapist uses his own hands to give resistance. It has the advantage of an immediate and sensitive response to the patient's action (see Proprioceptive neuromuscular facilitation, PNF, p. 580).

(4) Self-loading. In this method the patient offers a self-resistance to his own muscle actions. This may be done where one part of the body resists the movement of another, e.g. crossing one ankle over the other and resisting knee extension or holding two ends of a pulley system resisting shoulder extension (this arrangement is commonly used to give assistance to the other arm). Movement of the body's weight itself may also be called self-loading, e.g. doing push-ups or standing up and then slowly lowering to a squat position. Self-loading is particularly useful as part of a home exercise programme, as small or large amounts of resistance may be produced without apparatus.

Sling suspension

In this treatment part (or occasionally all) of the patient's body is suspended by a number of ropes and slings. The suspension allows the body to move without friction and frees the physiotherapist's hands from supporting the weight of the limb. The position of the point of suspension determines the amount of resistance (or assistance) to movement when no other external resistance is applied.

Sling suspension is principally used for:

(1) improving range of movement;
(2) gaining relaxation (local and general);
(3) improving strength of musculature, power and endurance.

Suspension is a particularly appropriate mode of treatment for very weak musculature whether the weakness is due to a local condition, e.g. nerve lesion, or because the patient is generally frail.

Circuit training

In circuit training patients are given a series of different exercises to perform regularly. It is important to record performance to allow evaluation of improvement and appropriate progression of exercises. A circuit usually consists of about eight exercises, and these may vary from simple free exercises with no apparatus, to exercises with apparatus and weight resistance. The circuit may be arranged as a 'fixed time circuit' when a certain amount of time is spent at each exercise, or a 'fixed repetition circuit' where the patient carries out a specific number of repetitions of each exercise. Circuits may be arranged to improve general fitness or be directed towards a more specific aim, e.g. improving strength of lower limb musculature. This type of training is most often used for relatively fit patients in groups within a gymnasium.

Passive movements

Here the patient's joints are moved through anatomical range by an external force. These movements are normally carried out by a physiotherapist, but in certain circumstances are carried out by others, as when a patient carries out passive movements on the other hand following hand injuries, or when a carer carries out passive movements on a paralysed relative. The principal objectives of passive movements are:

(1) to improve or maintain joint range and muscle length, and the mobility of tissues in general;

(2) to assist venous and lymphatic return;

(3) to facilitate normalisation of muscle tone;

(4) to facilitate performance of controlled patterns of movement.

It is often appropriate to progress from passive to active assisted movements where the patient participates in the movement.

Relaxation

Techniques to gain improved relaxation are carried out in a variety of therapeutic situations for the treatment of physical and psychological conditions. Relaxation training is particularly beneficial in such areas as antenatal preparation, in asthmatic patients, and where a local muscular tension causes pain, as in some back and neck pain. A variety of methods may be used to help to achieve relaxation; a commonly used one is the Laura Mitchell method (1983), where the emphasis is on the patient becoming aware of the pattern of tension within the body. The patient then learns to reduce tension through relaxation of key muscle groups. Reversal of the position of tension and breathing control is important in this method of relaxation, and in many others. Relaxation is often first achieved in a favourable quiet environment and relaxed starting position, then progressed so that the patient is able to maintain relaxation in less favourable situations.

Hydrotherapy

The hydrotherapy pool water is warm (approximately 35°C) and hoists are available to assist less able patients; fixed supports and floating aids are used to assist the patient as necessary in the water. The psychological benefits from hydrotherapy are great; for example, the patient may be able to walk in water as it counteracts the gravitational forces which make this impossible in air.

Aims of treatment include decreasing pain, promotion of relaxation — local and general, increasing range of movement, muscle power and coordination. Various techniques are used, such as the Bad Ragaz Ring method (Boyle, 1981). Here the patient lies in the water, supported by a collar at the neck, a ring round the pelvis and a ring round one or both ankles. Active treatment in the form of resisted exercises are carried out in the PNF patterns.

Floats and paddles are used to influence the effects of buoyancy, turbulence and water resistance to provide assistance or resistance to movement. The physiotherapist in the water with the patient provides support (psychologically and physically) to the patient, as well as verbally and manually controlling the patient's actions.

Patients most commonly treated by hydrotherapy are suffering from rheumatic, orthopaedic or specific neurological conditions. Patients with ankylosing spondylitis, and with arthritis of the hips from whatever cause, usually find hydrotherapy of great benefit. Contraindications to pool therapy include severe cardiovascular conditions, some dermatological conditions, especially tinea pedis, which is a water-borne infection, patients with active febrile conditions and patients who are incontinent of faeces. Great fear of water may also preclude treatment. Patients with multiple sclerosis may fatigue easily.

Breathing exercises (Chapter 14)

The aims of breathing exercises are:

(1) to gain or maintain full expansion of the lungs;

(2) to control breathing and relaxation;

(3) to encourage expectoration.

The history is taken, X-rays checked, and the chest movements may be measured. The patient's colour, rate of breathing, breath sounds and any loss of full expansion, either local or general, are noted. Where movement is poor on one side it may be necessary to concentrate on the weaker side before proceeding to bilateral movements. Breathing exercises to expand the posterior basal segments, middle lobe area and apical segments may be given. Diaphragmatic breathing is taught, with accompanying relaxation of the upper chest and shoulders.

Postural drainage

Postural drainage is used to remove secretions from the chest. It may be useful to administer bronchodilators or humidification before treatment. The patient is positioned to drain the appropriate area or areas of the lung for up to half an hour, e.g. to drain the posterior basal segment, the patient lies prone, with a pillow under the hips and the foot of the bed raised 18 inches. However, because of breathlessness or other condition, e.g. presence of abdominal wound or age of the patient, it is often necessary to adopt a modified position. Percussion and shaking of the chest is given where necessary. The patient is advised how best to carry out postural drainage at home, and is taught self-percussion. Relatives may be instructed if this is more appropriate. During and after postural drainage, breathing exercises are carried out.

TRANSFERS (Figures 35.1 and 35.2)

Some patients are profoundly handicapped so that the physiotherapist is concerned not with general fitness, running or walking, but with teaching the patient merely to *transfer*: that is to move from bed to chair, from one chair to another (e.g. commode, lavatory or wheelchair) or between standing and sitting. After a severe stroke, paraplegia, or after amputation, it may take much practice to achieve transfers safely. Without the ability to transfer unaided few people can live safely alone; many have carers who can guide the patient in transferring, but cannot take his body weight. Carers will need to be taught how to help the patient most effectively, whilst conserving their own energy and backs.

Figure 35.1: Transfers: bed to chair, chair to standing, standing to sitting on toilet seat

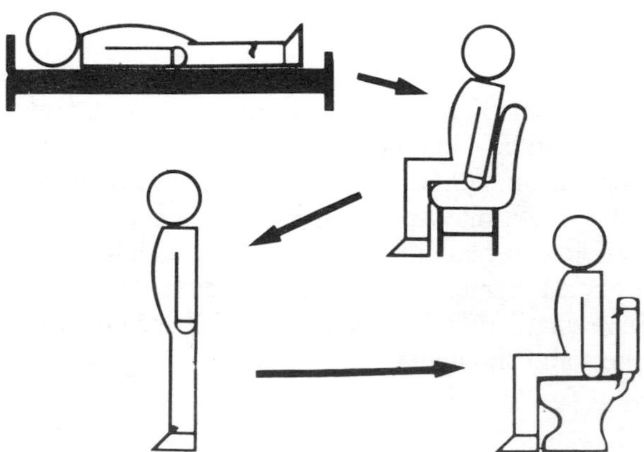

Figure 35.2: Stages in transfer: (a) patient taking weight on his hands; (b) physiotherapist bracing right knee as he rises to bear weight on right leg (continued over page)

(a)

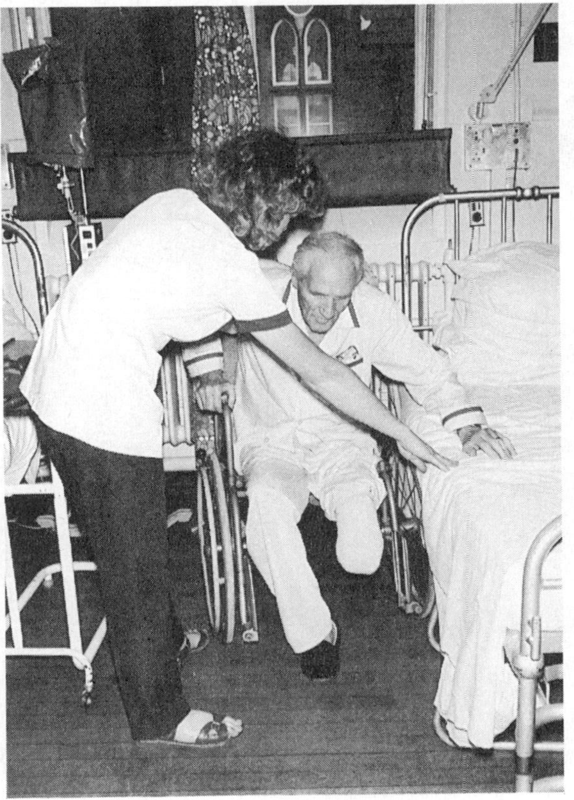

(b)

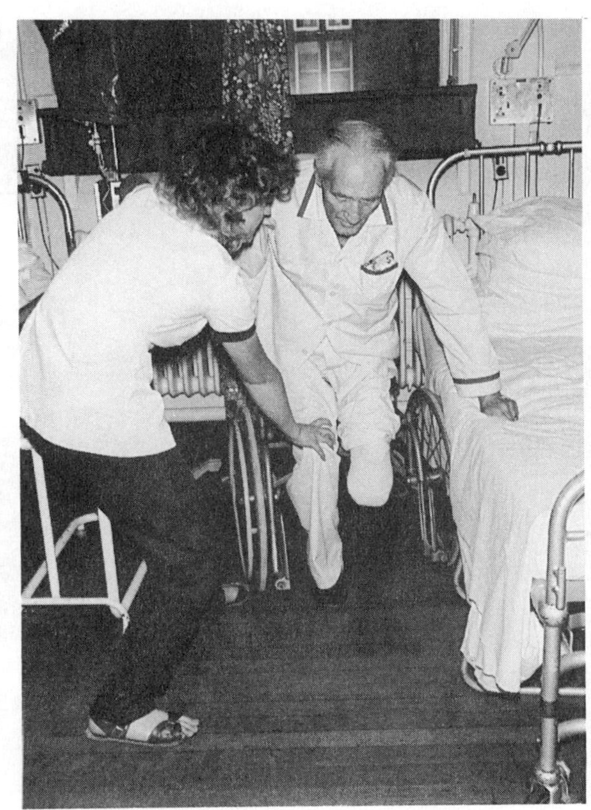

Figure 35.2: (c) arrived!

(c)

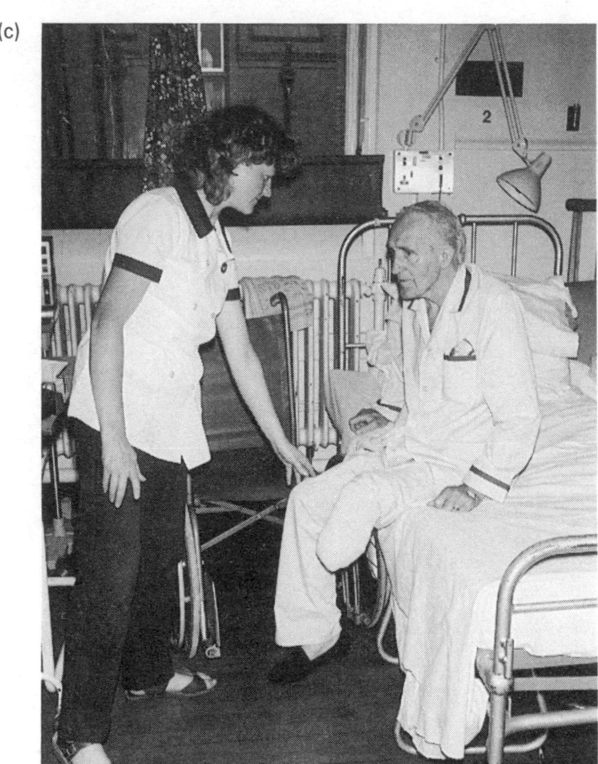

NEUROMUSCULAR RE-EDUCATION

Patients with brain and spinal cord lesions have a greater potential for recovery than was previously supposed. Recent work suggests that there is plasticity in the central nervous system, and if normal sensory-motor experience input is given to the patient so relearning is facilitated. In most therapeutic situations it is believed to be more appropriate for the physiotherapist to aim for re-educating to as near normal as possible functional movement, rather than to try to achieve rapid independence leaving the patient with abnormal patterns of movement. Various named approaches are used in the treatment of patients with neuromuscular problems, but as always these are combined with management of the person as a whole (Bobath, 1978).

Bobath

This is a system of evaluation and treatment of the hemiplegic patient based on inhibiting abnormal reflex activity, normalising postural tone and facilitating normal patterns of movement. The use of key points of control is emphasised, these being mainly proximal, e.g. neck, spine, shoulder, girdle and pelvis. Normalisation of tone in these areas is necessary for the patient to gain control of active movement throughout the body.

All movements are carried out without excess effort, which would itself cause increased tone. The importance of the patient learning the correct 'feel' of movement is emphasised. *The body is used as a whole, and an effort is made to avoid working only with the affected side.*

For the patient to receive maximum benefit the Bobath principles must be followed for 24 hours every day, not just during phyisotherapy sessions, which are of necessity limited. The importance of other members of the health care team, relatives, and particularly the patient, gaining understanding of the principles and applying them thus cannot be overemphasised.

Margaret Johnstone (1983)

This approach to the treatment of the hemiplegic patient is based upon teaching the patient to minimise developing spasticity, through inhibition of abnormal reflex activity, while regaining lost function. Orally inflatable pressure splints are applied for periods to upper and lower limbs to give deep, even pressure, to hold the limb in the 'recovery' antispasticity position and give support to the limb. In addition, weight-bearing through lower and upper limb is strongly advocated, as is the use of a rocking chair to help develop normal postural reactions. As the patient improves, activities are progressed in broadly the same sequence as a normally developing baby.

Conductive education (Cotton and Kinsman, 1983: Cottam and Sutton, 1985)

A system for the rehabilitation of patients with neurological conditions, where the patients repeat a series of specific tasks, leading to the acquisition of new skills. The patients are usually placed in matched groups led by a conductor. In Budapest, where the system was developed by Professor Peto, the conductors are specially trained. In this country, however, different members of the multidisciplinary team take the role of conductor. The patients are taught how to guide their movements using their own speech, first to describe the movement and then counting as it is carried out. Patients with speech difficulties may benefit greatly from the groups.

Conductive education aims to break up motor patterns, reduce spasticity and develop more selective movements, relying on the patient's own active participation, not on the handling of the therapist. Educational as well as neurophysiological principles form the basis of this approach.

Proprioceptive neuromuscular facilitation (Knott and Voss, 1968) (PNF)

PNF may be defined as 'methods of promoting or hastening the response of the neuromuscular mechanism through the stimulation of the proprioceptors'.

All coordinated movement is dependent upon an adequate feedback mechanism, including proprioception from muscles and joints, extraceptors from skin surface and from visual, auditory and equilibrium centres. Facilitation techniques aim to maximise the use of these pathways to stimulate and improve strength and coordination of movement. PNF techniques may also be used to reduce muscle spasm, and improve local mobility (joint range and muscle length).

A large number of specific patterns and techniques are incorporated with PNF. The exact position and pressure of the therapist's hands is most important, as is use of precise diagonal patterns of active and static muscle work. Facilitation is gained through pre-stretch of muscles, careful timing of activity, therapist's use of voice, and overflow where stronger muscles or groups facilitate contraction of weaker groups.

PNF techniques may be used with muscles at any point on the Oxford Scale Classification:

Oxford Scale Classification (classification of neuromuscular efficiency)

0 No contraction.

1 Flicker of contraction.

2 Small movement with gravity eliminated.

3 Movement against gravity.

4 Movement against gravity and some resistance.

5 Normal.

Frenkels exercises

This treatment approach is used for patients with ataxia in which the performance of precise rhythmical movements is accomplished with much repetition and intensive concentration. Initially the patient counts out aloud and selects his own natural rhythm. Progression is gained in various ways, e.g. changing rhythm, introducing halt, using more complex movements, using a less well-supported starting position.

The Frenkels scheme of exercises is used for exercising upper or lower segments of the body and for re-educating gross functional activities, e.g. walking.

Few controlled trials of any of these methods of neuromuscular education have been undertaken. Nevertheless, most of these principles are used in most physiotherapy departments.

Manipulation and mobilisation

Manipulation/mobilisation is practised widely by physiotherapists in the treatment of musculo-skeletal conditions. These skills were introduced into the training of physiotherapy students over 40 years ago at St Thomas's Hospital, London, by Cyriax (1978). Since then they have developed under the influence of Geoffrey Maitland, and are more widely used throughout the profession. The Manipulation Association of Chartered Physiotherapists was founded in 1968 to maintain a high standard of practice. It arranges and validates postgraduate courses. The principle of a thorough initial examination of the patient and a continuous assessment is essential to the skills of the manipulator. Treatment is given to spinal and peripheral joints. Manipulative physiotherapists have developed other skills, including McKenzie techniques and 'muscle energy' techniques, so that they are able to offer their patient a wide range of treatments. McKenzie advocates 'that the patient should be taught to be self-reliant and independent of therapists in the management of future low back pain'. 'Muscle energy' techniques are considered to be similar to PNF. Many hospitals have set up Back Schools to instruct patients on the basic anatomy of the back and the causes and prevention of back pain.

Traction

Traction to the lumbar or cervical spine may be given by a physiotherapist to relieve pain in the back or neck, and associated nerve root pain. It is usually given once or twice a day for short periods. For *cervical* traction the patient may be treated lying down or in sitting or half-lying position. A halter is placed round the neck with the pressure applied to the patient's chin and occiput. The halter is attached to a spreader and thence to a pulley system and weight. The trunk acts as counter-resistance.

Lumbar traction is normally given supine. It may be necessary for the patient's hips and knees to be flexed. A belt is placed round the thorax and another round the pelvis. The thoracic belt is then attached to a fixed point at the head of the bed, and the pelvic belt to a fixed point at the foot of the bed. The traction is then applied to the foot or head end of the apparatus. The position of the spine during traction, the length of treatment and the poundage of pressure should be carefully monitored as treatment progresses.

Massage

Massage is used comparatively rarely now in most physiotherapy departments. There are various techniques, e.g. effleurage, kneading, frictions, which may be selected as appropriate for the condition to be treated. The commonest used today are in the treatment of:

(a) Oedema. The arm or leg is placed in elevation to aid drainage during the massage.

(b) After skin grafting using lanolin to increase the circulation to the graft and soften the skin.

(c) Connective tissue massage where the connective tissue is stretched and mobilised.

(d) Friction to relieve pain in localised areas.

ELECTROTHERAPY; FORMS OF HEAT AND COLD THERAPY

Heating the tissues results in:

(1) increase in circulation;

(2) reduction of pain (usually);

(3) relaxation of muscles.

Heat treatments are not given to patients in whom there is a loss of skin sensation (e.g. some patients with multiple sclerosis or peripheral neuropathy), because of the danger of burning.

Short-wave diathermy provides a deep heating of the tissues of the body. The current commonly used for medical work has a frequency of 27.12 MHz and sets up waves with a wavelength of 11 m. This current is generated in a machine circuit, which is in turn coupled to a patient (resonator) circuit which is used to treat the patient' (Foster and Palastanga, 1985). Treatment can be given by using electrodes or by the cable method. In the former method a rapidly alternating electric field is set up within the area being treated. In the latter method an electrostatic and magnetic field is set up. Short-wave diathermy is a useful form of applying heat to the deep tissues, e.g. the hip joint. It should be used with caution in recent injuries and acute inflammation, as the increased blood flow can increase the tension in the tissue and may aggravate the symptoms. Metal implants also preclude its use. It may interfere with cardiac pacemakers.

Infrared radiation. Infrared rays are electromagnetic waves with a wavelength of 750–400,000 nm. Luminous and non-luminous lamps are used in physiotherapy departments. The depth of penetration depends on the wavelength. Infrared 1200 nm penetrates into the superficial epidermis, and short infrared through the deep epidermis and dermis.

Microwave diathermy is irradiation of the tissues with a wavelength between infrared and short-wave diathermy. The effective depth seems to be about 3 cm, and only one aspect of the body can be treated on any one occasion. It is therefore most useful in the treatment of small areas and more superficial tissues and joints. There is a danger of injury to the lens with exposure to the eye to microwave diathermy, it is therefore not used near the eyes, and patients and staff are advised to wear protective goggles. Other effects and dangers are similar to shortwave diathermy.

Electric heating pads are like small electric blankets. The heating is by conduction. They are available commercially and are safe to use as long as they are kept in good order and protected from damp.

Hot packs are used increasingly in physiotherapy departments to produce superficial heating. The packs are steeped in hot water and then wrapped in dry towels before being applied.

Wax baths are the most convenient method of applying conducted heat to the hands and feet. In physiotherapy departments the wax is kept at a temperature of 40–44°C. The foot or hand is dipped in and out of the bath, producing layer on layer of a wax glove or sock, until a good covering adheres to the part. It is then wrapped in a plastic bag and towels, or blanket for a short time, usually 20 minutes. At this time the wax has cooled off and easily peels off.

Cold therapy

Cold therapy is used to relieve pain, reduce oedema and effusion, depress spasm and facilitate motor activity. Cold packs or ice packs may be used. It is commonly used in the treatment of recent injuries, particularly sports injuries where the application of cold therapy limits the oedema and effusion and reduces pain. Ice packs may also be applied to muscles to reduce the spasm. Ice cubes may be stroked briskly over the skin to stimulate muscle contraction.

Faradic-type current is a short-duration interrupted direct current with a pulse duration of 0.1-1 ms, and a frequency of 50-100 Hz. Faradic stimulation is used to obtain a contraction of muscles when there is a weak response to voluntary contraction. It is most often used to re-educate the intrinsic muscles of the foot, and in re-education of the patient with quadriceps muscle weakness. The patient is encouraged to carry out voluntary movement at the same time as the muscles are stimulated electrically. In this way the patient learns to perform movements which previously had been difficult or impossible. Faradic stimulation also relieves pain, probably in the same way as transcutaneous nerve stimulation.

Transcutaneous nerve stimulation (TCNS)

TCNS is used to stimulate large-diameter afferent nerve fibres to achieve analgesia in cases of chronic pain. It is thought to reduce pain by 'closing the gate' to pain and by stimulating the release of endogenous opiates (Chapter 7).

Biofeedback

Biofeedback refers to procedures whereby information about an aspect of bodily function is fed back to the brain following an auditory, visual or other signal, giving the patient the means of controlling aspects of bodily function which are normally independent of direct control and awareness. It may be used to aid relaxation when electrodes are placed over a key muscle, e.g. frontalis. The machine indicates when there is tension in the muscle and the patient is made aware of the failure to relax this muscle. Another common use is to encourage weight-bearing through the affected leg after a stroke. The patient stands on a pad which is connected to the machine, and a positive signal is given when weight is carried through the affected leg.

Intermittent compression

This treatment is given to reduce oedema and increase circulation in the limbs. A double sleeve or legging of plastic material is applied to the arm or leg. This is attached to a compressor which alternatively inflates and deflates the sleeve to a predetermined pressure. This can safely be used by patients at home.

Pulsed high-frequency energy

Within the past few years pulsed high frequency electromagnetic energy has been used to accelerate healing and increase circulation. The machines most commonly used for this treatment are the Diapulse, Megapulse and Curapulse. They operate on a frequency of 27.12 MHz in common with most short-wave diathermy machines, but the output is pulsed so that there is a relatively short 'on' period followed by a relatively long 'off' period before the next 'on' phase. This high-frequency energy is thought to affect the electrical potential across the cell membrane and the permeability of the cell membrane to Na^+. It is believed that the magnetic field produced by the machine restores to normal cell potential and the K and Na^+ balance which have been disturbed as a result of injury or inflammation. It is used to promote healing and repair of tissues, for dispersal of oedema, absorption of haematoma and reduction of inflammation.

Ultrasonic therapy

Therapeutic ultrasound uses frequencies in the region of 1–3 MHz. It may be used in a continuous or pulsed mode and its intensity varied. The intensity of the ultrasonic beam is reduced the deeper it passes into the tissues, which are heated. The mechanical or micromassage effect is used to reduce oedema and help reduce pain.

Care must be taken not to produce standing waves during the treatment, by keeping the treatment head moving. These standing waves produce blood cell statis and if this is prolonged it can damage the walls of the blood vessels. Ultrasound is used to reduce pain, soften and stretch scar tissue, remove traumatic exudate and reduce oedema.

Interferential therapy

In interferential therapy two medium-frequency currents are used to produce a low-frequency effect in the patient's tissues. One of the currents is kept at a constant frequency of 4000 Hz and the other can be varied between 3900 and 4000 Hz. The effects of the therapy are produced in the deep tissues where the two medium-frequency currents cross without unnecessary skin stimulation.

The physiological effects are the relief of pain, reduction of oedema and motor stimulation. Muscle contraction is produced with little sensory stimulation, and can be of deeply placed muscles, e.g. pelvic floor. It is frequently used therefore in the treatment of stress incontinence, and for pain relief and the absorption of exudate in the treatment of sports injuries.

Care must be taken in the covering and positioning of electrodes to prevent electrical burns.

PHYSIOTHERAPY FOR THE STROKE PATIENT: A CASE HISTORY

Physiotherapy aims to increase the functional ability of the stroke patient (see Chapter 20) by re-educating normal bilateral control of movement.

This is achieved by approaching the patient's symptoms directly rather than circumventing them by teaching compensatory techniques. It is complemented by occupational therapy (Chapter 34).

Each patient presents with a different combination of deficits, so it is not possible to describe a single series of techniques which can be universally employed. The basis of the treatment is always set on a thorough understanding of normal movement patterns.

The patient is assessed to discover where his/her attempts to achieve functional movements differ from normal patterns of movement.

The treatment of the patient is based on the belief that external sensory input can influence the plasticity of the CNS sufficiently to affect and re-educate normal control of movement (Figures 35.3-35.6).

Case report (the OT management is detailed in Chapter 34)

A 44-year-old male, Mr A, presented following collapse at work, with a

Figure 35.3: Untreated stroke patient with contractures

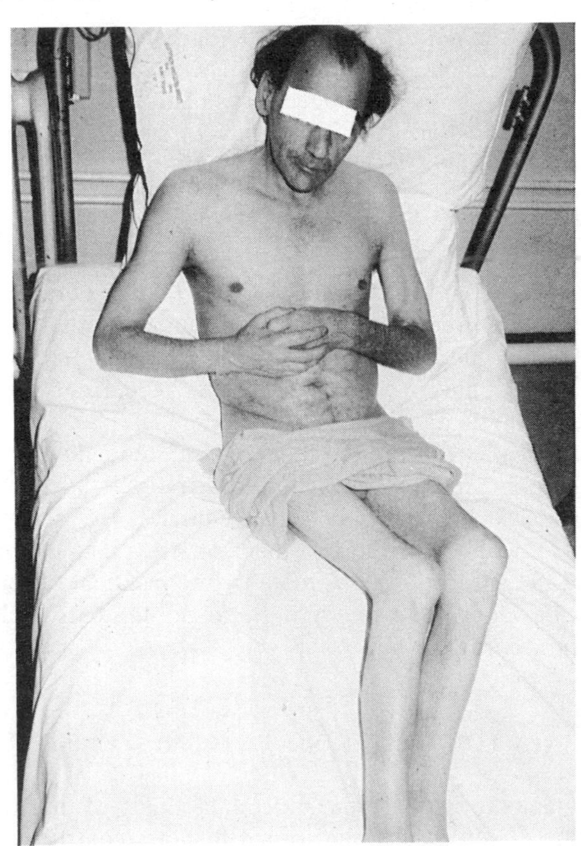

Figure 35.4: Good bed position for patient with right hemiplegia

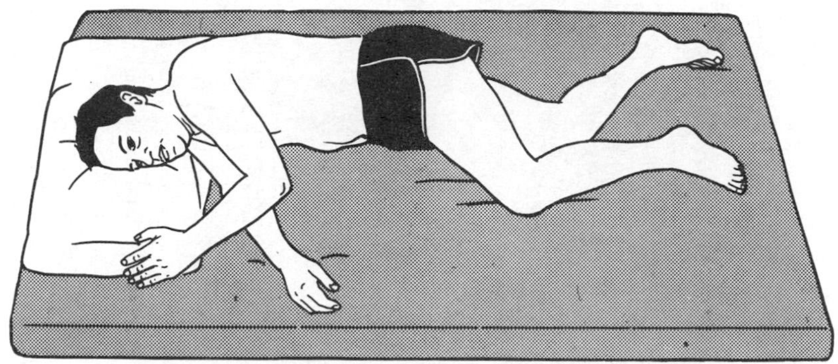

two-week history of temporal headache. He had a right-sided weakness and a fluent dysphasia. CT scan revealed an extensive intracerebral haematoma which was evacuated. Passive movements of the right side were carried out twice daily to normalise muscle tone and to maintain full range of movements, particularly of the shoulder, wrist, fingers, ankles and toes. The patient was positioned carefully in bed to prevent overstimulation of abnormal reflex activity of the right side.

At one week the patient was alert but only able to make inappropriate noises. He exhibited no active movement of his right side. Angiography revealed a large left middle cerebral artery aneurysm with some spasm and a small left posterior communicating artery aneurysm. These were clipped two days later. When he was stable medically and fully alert the patient was transferred to the rehabilitation unit. Mr A's performance on admission to the rehabilition unit was assessed using the checklist in Tables 35.1. and 35.2.

The treatment plan was to

(1) *Teach* the patient awareness of his difficulties and the reasons for these.

(2) *Re-educate* normal movement control, using *functional activities* designed to: increase sensory input, normalise muscle tone, whilst using existing movement correctly and facilitating more movement control.

Progress

Treatment was carried out in lying, sitting, kneeling and standing positions. He was helped to move between these positions correctly.

The physiotherapist aimed to enable the patient to achieve a function

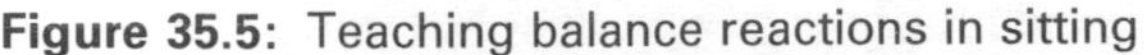

Figure 35.5: Teaching balance reactions in sitting

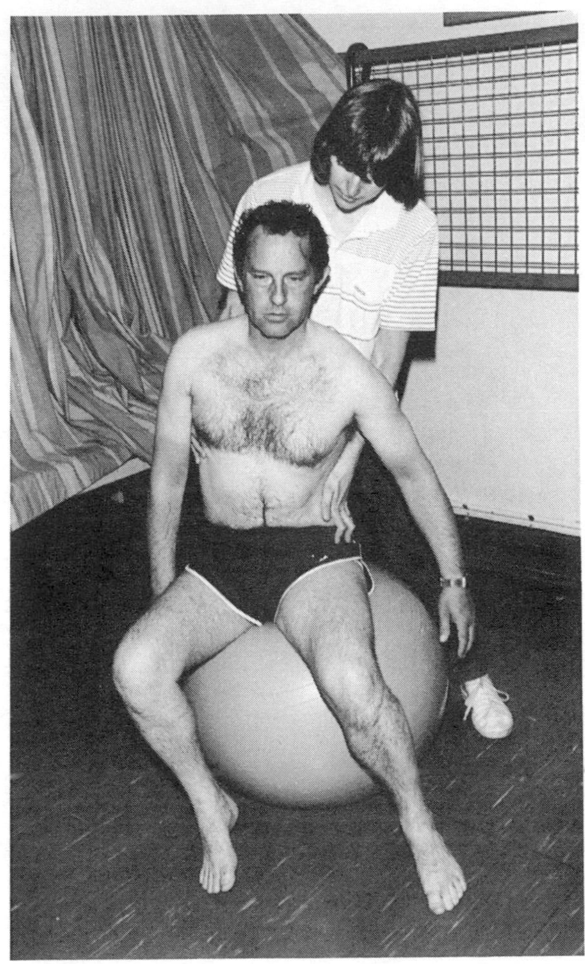

which lay just outside his present capability, by handling and supporting Mr A at key points, such as the shoulder or pelvis, thus controlling and normalising his movement, particularly fine ones. To decrease muscle tone, weight-bearing through the right leg/arm was encouraged. Many normal movements involve rotation of the shoulder girdle on the pelvis, and this ability had to be restored to improve trunk control and decrease abnormal tone.

Progressive activities

When Mr A could move from sitting to standing with his weight distributed

Figure 35.6: Balance reactions in standing. Mr A in stride position using affected right arm to support himself and taking weight through the right leg

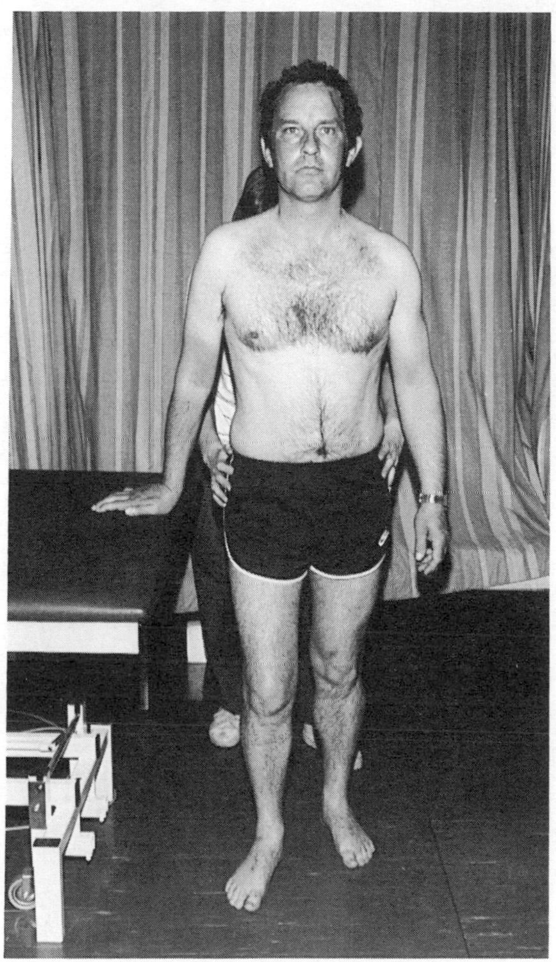

correctly, increased extensor tone in the right leg was found only when he attempted to step with the left leg. The right hip remained retracted. The patient had to be taught to recognise and correct this, so that the right leg could bear weight correctly.

Activities in standing and kneeling were always carried out with the right arm in a supported, weight-bearing position to encourage hip protraction.

Elbow control began to return some weeks after the incident. The combination of active shoulder movement and elbow control now allowed

Table 35.1: Results of initial assessment of Mr A (pertinent features only)

A	*Social:* lives alone in own bungalow; has several supportive friends.
B	*Perception of situation:* not fully aware of the extent of his physical disability; unaware of fluent dysphasia; highly motivated.
C	*Communication skills:* receptive dysphasia and fluent jargon, expressive dysphasia.
D	*Visual disabilities:* diplopia.
F	*Posture:* poor in standing, weight being borne mainly through the left leg.
G	*Muscle tone:* increased through the right side, particularly in his trunk and leg in an extensor synergy; increased tone in elbow extension and wrist flexors.
H	*Movement control:* gross movement patterns present, i.e. the patient moved his leg from total extension to total flexion but was unable to select a movement from within these patterns (e.g. he could not extend the knee keeping the hip flexed). Mr A had minimal control of the arm, with some shoulder protraction and some elbow extension being the only active movements he could undertake. Movement control decreased as he moved into upright positions.
I	*Sensation:* diminished superficial sensation in the right arm and trunk. Proprioception was absent.
J	*Functional activities:* see Table 35.2.

Table 35.2: Functional abilities (an initial assessment and on discharge from inpatient physiotherapy)

	On admission	On discharge
Transfers	***	***
Sitting balance	***	***
Shoes and socks	*	***
Sitting to lying	***	***
Rolling to left	**	***
Rolling to right	***	***
Lying to sitting	***	***
Sitting to standing	*	***
Standing balance	*	***
Stepping with left leg	*	***
Stepping with right leg	*	***
Walking	*	***
Stairs	*	**
Getting up from floor	*	**
Balance reactions		
In sitting	Fair	Good
In standing	Poor	Fair

Code: independent, ***; with aid, **; with physical help, *.

the patient to move his arm along the supporting surface whilst practising stepping.

Walking backwards proved to be a useful activity to improve control of hip and knee extension whilst protracting the hip, dorsiflexing eccentrically and maintaining good arm support.

At *three months* post-onset Mr A could move normally from lying to sitting and from sitting to kneeling on the floor, given some facilitation at the shoulder girdle. He could kneel correctly and also move in kneeling. In standing he was able to bear weight equally through both legs. The right arm was used automatically to support him when standing, and Mr A was able to pick up large objects (see Figure 35.6). He still had difficulty when moving from kneeling to standing, and when walking, as he found it hard to control dorsiflexion of the right foot.

Treatment at this stage had changed considerably: the physiotherapist worked to facilitate balance reactions both in sitting and standing. She aimed to allow him to be able to reach and grasp and perform a variety of activities from these positions, and thus worked with Mr A to encourage automatic trunk and arm control. At the same time they also aimed to improve the control of dorsiflexion of the foot, with the same aim of increasing stability in a variety of maneouvres.

The final assessment of Mr A, after considerable inpatient treatment gave the results shown in Table 35.2.

Conclusion

This patient became safely independent in all normal activities required for mobility in the home and its immediate environment, and was discharged there to live alone. He was referred to his local physiotherapy department for follow-up treatment. Mobility was no longer a dominant problem and the possibility of return to work was to be explored.

REFERENCES AND FURTHER READING

Bobath, B. (1978) *The evaluation and treatment of adult hemiplegia*, 2nd edn, Heinemann, London

Boyle, A.M. (1981) The Bad Ragaz ring method. *Physiotherapy*, *67*, 265-8

Caudrey, D. and Seegar, B. (1981) Biofeedback devices as an adjunct to physiotherapy. *Physiotherapy*, *67*, 371-6

Chamberlain, M.A., Care, G. and Harfield, B. (1982) Physiotherapy in osteoarthrosis of the knees: a controlled trial of hospital versus home exercises. *Int. Rehabil. Med.*, *4*, 101-6

Chartered Physiotherapists Source Book (1985) Parke Sutton Publishing, in association with the Chartered Society of Physiotherapy

Cottam, P. and Sutton, A. (1985) *Conductive education: a system for overcoming motor disorder*, Croom Helm, London

Cotton, E. and Kinsman, R. (1983) *Conductive education for adult hemiplegia*, Churchill Livingstone, Edinburgh

Cyriax, J. (1978) *Textbook of orthopaedic medicine*, vols. I and II, 7th edn, Baillière Tindall, London

Davies, P.M. (1985) *Steps to follow*, Springer, Germany

DHSS Health Circular H.C.(77)33. Health Services Development Relationship between the Medical and Remedial Professions

DHSS Health Notice H.N.(78)68. Physiotherapy in the Community

Downie, P.A. (1986) *Cash's textbook of neurology for physiotherapists*, 4th edn., Faber & Faber, London

Forster, A. and Palastanga, N. (1985) *Clayton's electrotherapy*, 9th edn, Baillière Tindall, London

Gardiner, M.D. (1981) *The principles of exercise therapy*, 4th edn, Bell & Hyman, London

Gaskell, D.V. and Webber, B.A. (1985) *The Brompton Hospital guide to chest physiotherapy*, 4th edn, Blackwell Scientific Publications, Oxford

Gloag, D. (1985) Need and opportunities in rehabilition. Introduction and a look at some short term orthopaedic rehabilitation. *Br. Med. J.*, *290*, 43-6

Grieve, G.P. (1985) *Common vertebral problems*, Churchill Livingstone, London

Hollis, M. (1981) *Practical exercise therapy*, 2nd edn, Blackwell Scientific Publications, Oxford

Johnstone, M. (1983) *Restoration of motor function in the stroke patient*, 2nd edn, Churchill Livingstone, Edinburgh

Knott, M.B.S. and Voss, D.E. (1968) *Proprioceptive neuromuscular facilitation patterns and techniques*, 2nd edn, Harper and Row, London

Licht, E.D. (1961) *Therapeutic exercise*, 2nd edn, Elisabeth Licht

Lunderberg, T. (1984) Electrical stimulation for the relief of pain, *Physiotherapy*, *70*, 98-100

Maitland, G.D. (1986) *Peripheral manipulation*, 2nd edn, Butterworths, London

Maitland, G.D. (1986) *Vertebral manipulation*, 5th edn, Butterworths, London

McKenzie, R.A. (1985) *Treat your own back*, 3rd edn, Spinal Publications Ltd, New Zealand

McKenzie, R.A. (1983) *Treat your own neck*, Spinal Publications Ltd, New Zealand

McKenzie, R.A. (1981) *The lumbar spine: mechanical diagnosis and therapy*, Spinal Publications Ltd, New Zealand

Mitchell, L. (1983) *Simple relaxation*, J. Murray, London

Musa, I.M. (1986) The role of afferent input in the reduction of spasticity: an hypothesis. *Physiotherapy*, *72*, 179-82

Nichols, P.J.R. (1980) *Rehabilitation medicine: the management of physical disabilities*, 2nd edn, Butterworth, London

Skinner, A.T. (1983) *Duffield's exercise in water*, 3rd edn, Ballière Tindall, London

Smith, C.R., Lewith, G.T., and Machin, D. (1983) TNS and osteo-arthritic pain, *Physiotherapy*, *69*, 266-8

Weerdt, W. and Harrison, M. (1985) The use of biofeedback in physiotherapy. *Physiotherapy*, *71*, 9-12

Whitley Council for the Health Services (Great Britain) (1981) Professional and Technical Council A, Pay and Conditions of Service

Williams, S.I. (1985) Management in physiotherapy. *Physiotherapy*, *71*, 43-5

36

Bioengineering in Rehabilitation

Colin Roberts and David Porter

INTRODUCTION

The past decade has seen the emergence, within the health care team, of a new professional — the rehabilitation engineer. Presenting in a variety of forms the rehabilitation engineer brings together and integrates the skills of the bioengineer, the electronics engineer, the biomechanic and the materials scientist in the assessment and rehabilitation of the disabled. This chapter will give some indication of the breadth of activities of this field and, by concentrating on one area, the rehabilitation of locomotor disability, give some idea of its depth. Certain areas such as orthotics and environmental controls are dealt with elsewhere in this book (Chapters 45 and 48). The management of any disability and the rehabilitation engineer's role fall into two distinct classes of activity: firstly the assessment of dysfunction, and secondly the design and use of aids. Clearly functional assessment also plays a role in the evaluation of prescriptions.

ASSESSMENT OF FUNCTION

Motor function

Goniometry

One of the earliest fundamental measurements to be made in functional assessment is the range of joint movement, both under passive and active control. The earliest device for the measurement of the range of joint movement, the goniometer, remains largely unchanged since its invention. Essentially a protractor, the two arms of which are attached or passively held against a limb, it can be read directly for static measurements. Where dynamic measurements are required (for example, during walking) the two limbs of the device are attached to some displacement or rotation transducer which can be used to drive a display/recorder or be fed to a computer for analysis.

Though ostensibly simple devices, the problems which beset goniometry face all methods which are intended for joint mobility assessment. The most obvious is the difficulty of defining *precisely* the axis of rotation of a joint — this is rarely uniaxial. The second is related to the superimposed force required to move the joint. Whether this is applied passively by the investigator or actively by the subject, large variations can be expected — not only between observers, but within the same subject from hour to hour. Typical variations in excess of 10 per cent may be found, and the effectiveness of any therapy must be viewed in the light of these variations (see Wright, 1982). Fatigue may be a further factor to be considered in assessing the variability of muscular action (Helliwell *et al.*, 1987).

Though effective for 'static' assessment of joint movement, goniometers are far from ideal for dynamic assessment, during walking for example. The need for non-contacting techniques for kinesiology has led to the worldwide creation of gait laboratories. These are concerned with locomotion, but many are equipped with instrumentation which can equally well be used for the assessment of upper arm motor disorders.

The modern gait laboratory relies on three independent activities: qualitative observation, quantitative measurement and biomechanical analysis (Saleh and Murdoch, 1985). Although a skilled clinician will be able to recognise the major improvements in a patients' walk — as he/she becomes accustomed to a prosthesis or an orthosis, minor changes will be much more difficult to detect. Asymmetrical gait, for example, following amputation or stroke, further complicates the task, making objective measurement mandatory if comparisons are required over time or between patients.

A recent study of amputee gait by Saleh and Murdoch (1985) revealed that a quantitative measurement system was able to pick up three times as many deviations as did the skilled observers. Such quantitative methods, formulated within the framework of biomechanics, can be used effectively for prosthetic and orthotic design and prescription. The principal parameters on which gait assessments are based fall into three major classes: temporal and spatial, kinematic, and finally kinetic. Metabolic assessments have also been made.

Temporal and spatial investigation of gait

In the study of temporal and spatial parameters of gait, stride time, swing time, stride length, velocity and cadence are the most obvious parameters to measure. Measurement techniques have included the study of footprints (Kirby *et al.*, 1985) using cellophane-covered carbon paper, and instrumented pressure-sensitive mats (Laughman *et al.*, 1984). This latter technique uses a series of switches embedded in a substrate, which are scanned by a microprocessor. Such a method can yield both the temporal and spatial gait parameters. A review of many of these will be found in Porter and Roberts (1987).

Kinematic data

The kinematic variables of locomotion describe movement in terms of linear and angular displacement, velocities and accelerations, but with no reference to the forces producing the motion. Most of these variables are obtainable using one of the many dynamic imaging techniques. These range from standard cinematography (Golbranson, 1980), which is subsequently analysed frame by frame, to the more complex optoelectronic and TV–computer systems. These latter techniques, where the motion of a body is viewed simultaneously from at least two positions (Hicks *et al.*, 1985) (see Figure 36.1) can provide a very powerful tool whose real clinical potential is only just being realised. Other workers have obtained

Figure 36.1: System used for collection and analysis of kinematic data on gait. The distribution of the cameras and subject is viewed from above. A footswitch is used for event timing

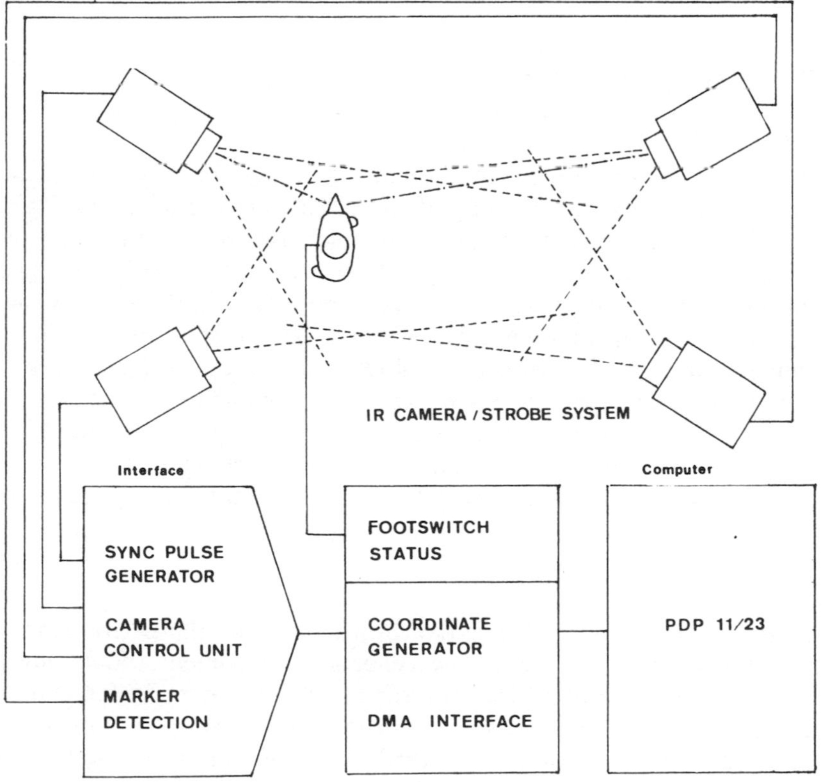

kinematic data with the aid of electrogoniometers (Chad and Hoffman, 1978) and accelerometers (Gage, 1964).

Kinetic data

Human gait involves the creation of a complex system of intrinsic and extrinsic forces. The dominant extrinsic force is the ground reaction which occurs during foot/floor contact. This may be measured using a force plate which is usually incorporated into some form of walkway. Because the ground reaction is three-dimensional, force plates must be able to resolve the vertical, anterior–posterior and the mediolateral components. A less expensive alternative which can be used to measure only the maximum vertical pressure and its point of application is the pedobarograph (Lord *et al.*, 1986).

In the most extensive biomechanical analyses the combination of kinematic data (obtained using TV systems) with kinetic data (obtained from force plate and EMG signals) provides the database. Such integrated systems cost around £100,000 and as a consequence are not widely found. The simplest goniometers and footstep devices cost only £100s and as a result are much more often used.

The assessment of sensory function

Auditory function

Hearing defects are surprisingly common, resulting not only from disease and physical accident, but most often as a natural effect of ageing. In providing communication aids for the disabled assessment of hearing must form a first stage in the management of the patient. Standard audiological techniques, in which a patient is exposed to pure tones at different frequencies and intensities, may be used to assess the extent of hearing loss in relation to the patient's own perception. A less subjective, though more complex, assessment can be made using the technique of evoked response audiometry in which changes in the EEG signal in response to stimuli such as clicks or tone bursts can be monitored. Such techniques are clearly of more value when making assessments of young children or in patients with speech defects (Chapter 17).

Visual function

Visual feedback is of vital importance in monitoring the performance of assist devices, and as a consequence patient assessment should *always* include visual evaluation. The assessment of vision can, as for auditory assessment, rest on patient testimony or may also be supported by the use of evoked response methods in which EEG changes in response to visual stimulation are monitored. However, whatever assessment is made it must be carried out in the context of the disability and of the probable assistive devices — be it a TV screen or a row of red-light-emitting diodes. A good description of methods of visual screening in assistive devices may be found in Coleman *et al.* (1980). (See also Chapter 16.)

Tactile function

In the case of tactile function, assessments need to be made in response to various stimuli such as pressure and temperature. In some cases, however, evoked response techniques are used in which the EEG response to topical electrical stimulation can be used to map the sensory nerve supply to patient's skin — the somatosensory evoked response. This evaluation is best carried out in conjunction with an evaluation of motor skills, since the two are intrinsically related.

DESIGN OF AIDS

Nye and Bliss (1970) have encapsulated the major components of all assist devices. Figure 36.2 shows the general form of sensory aids and communication or control aids. The structure applies equally well to orthotic or prosthetic devices.

Locomotor aids — passive

The area in which biomechanics has played a major role is in the design of locomotor aids. These may range from simple orthoses through complete artificial limbs to wheelchairs and general mobility aids.

In the design and optimisation of lower limb prostheses, for example, gait analysis has been found to be of very considerable value. In particular, several workers have used gait analysis to optimise the alignment of prostheses. The work of Hannah *et al.* (1984) showed that optimal alignment of prostheses tended to minimise asymmetry of the pattern of rotation of the hip and knee. Furthermore, they also found that small alignment changes to the prosthetic foot affect gait to a greater extent than do alignment changes.

In current practice the alignment of prostheses is usually carried out subjectively by an experienced prosthetist. However, with the growth of gait laboratories and the dissatisfaction with current limbs, this process is starting to become more quantitative.

Gait analysis has been used to assess the effects of prosthetic knee friction. Hicks *et al.* (1985), using a three-channel video system to collect three-dimensional kinematic data from juvenile above-knee amputees, showed that knee friction could be used to match the heel rise of the prosthetic limb to the sound limb, and that this could provide a more

Figure 36.2: The essential components of assistive devices. The loops are completed by the modification of the environment by the communication/control aid and by the provision of an environmental stimulus for the sensory aid

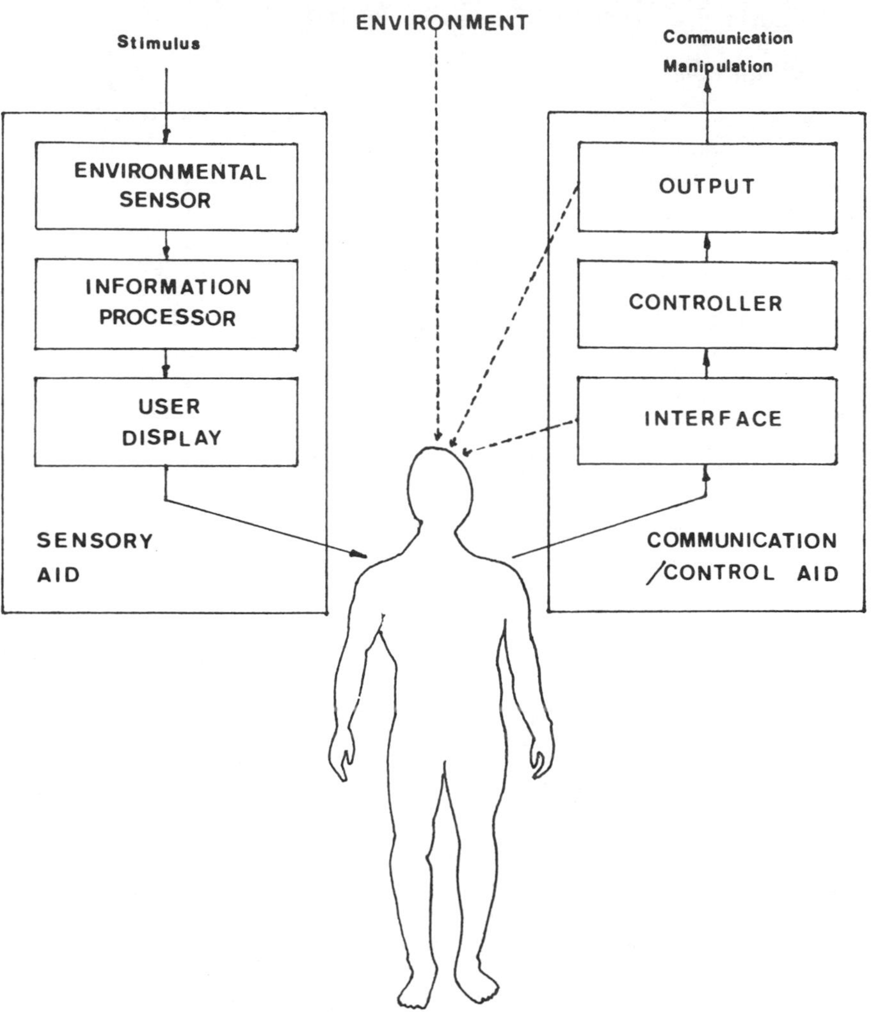

symmetrical gait pattern. Others have used similar techniques to optimise the hydraulic dampers used in prostheses.

Instrumented pylons have been used to collect data on forces and moments encountered during the stance phase of gait in below-knee amputees. Jones and Paul (1978) used this information to optimise prosthetic alignment. Others (Ishai *et al.*, 1983) have developed computer-based techniques for alignment correction based on the minimisation of axial torque at the thigh. Instrumented pylons have also been used to investigate the relationship between the shape of the patellar tendon insertion in the socket and the dynamic load transmitted through it. Such studies (Mizrahi *et al.*, 1985) are helping to better define the optimal shape of prosthetic sockets.

Prosthetic weight and its effect on gait has been studied by several workers. Lower mass means lower inertial forces, which can lead to less expenditure of energy — an important requirement for the elderly amputee.

Work with most of these systems is, however, difficult to use on a routine basis, and latterly attention is being focused on the development of techniques which can easily be used in the routine treatment of patients. Noteworthy is the work of Seliktar and Mizrahi (1986), who have explored the possibility of representing locomotor abnormalities solely by their reflection on the ground reaction forces. In this work the ratio of the anterior–posterior impulse was found to be very sensitive to the quality of gait. Perturbations of the AP force curve were also found to reflect stump/socket interfacial incongruity — effectively stump/socket fit (Chapter 11).

Locomotor aids — active

Active locomotor aids which incorporate functional electrical stimulation (FES) of the muscular system have been pioneered particularly in Yugoslavia. The first successful efforts in FES were directed towards the correction of the drop foot. Conventional treatment is the provision of a spring-loaded orthosis which prevents the foot dropping as the heel leaves the ground. The FES version incorporates some means of stimulating the peroneal nerve. A heel switch is used to trigger the stimulation for a (usually adjustable) period at heel lift-off (Gracanin, 1971). Nerve stimulation can be achieved with a fully implanted nerve stimulator, coupled transcutaneously to control circuity (see Figure 36.3). Patients with drop foot often exhibit other gait abnormalities and multiple muscle stimulation may prove necessary.

Paraplegic patients present an altogether different challenge. In these patients multiple activation of several muscle groups is required if locomotion is to be assisted. Again, the work of the Lubljana team has been at the forefront of solving this problem (Kralj *et al.*, 1983) and considerable progress has been made towards effective ambulation (Mizrahi *et al.*, 1985). Mention must also be made of the work of Petrofsky *et al.* (1984), who have done much to improve the applicability of FES techniques by the addition of complex computer feedback techniques, in which the patient's movement is used to control the degree of electrical stimulation applied.

Feedback techniques have also been widely applied to the prosthetic arm. In this area the combination of electromyography, providing the control signal for the prosthesis, together with some form of sensory

Figure 36.3: Implanted peroneal foot-drop brace. The electrode/receiver are implanted close to the peroneal nerve and are activated transcutaneously from a waist band transmitter/power supply

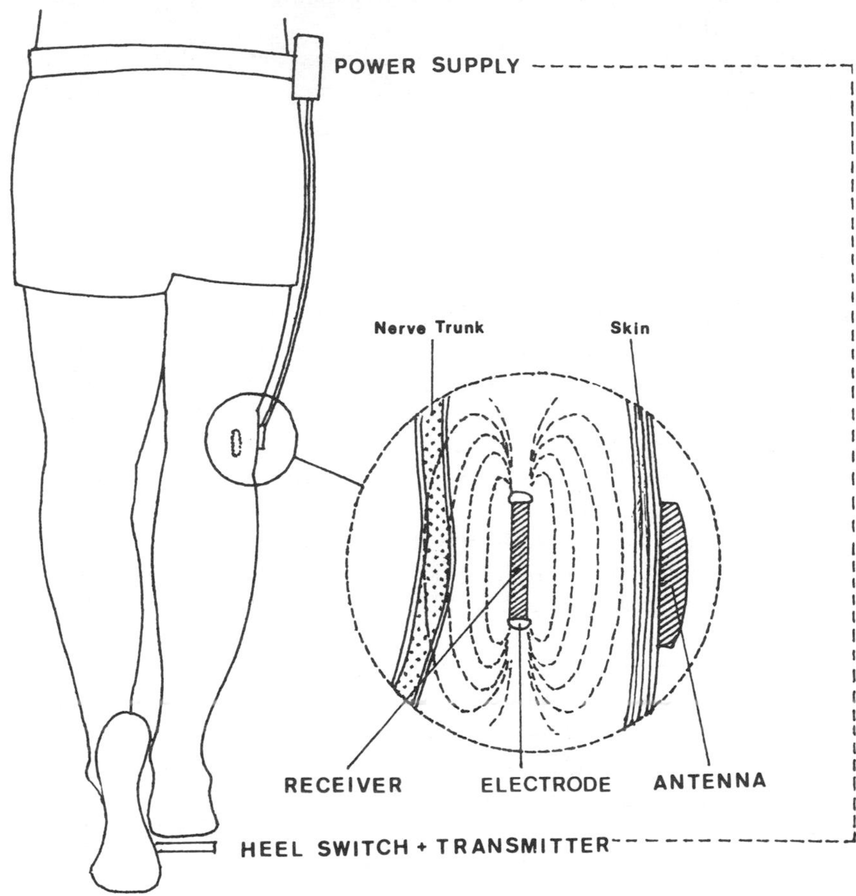

feedback, is necessary for good closed-loop control of function. In this area the work of Childress (1973) and his colleagues in the late 1960s and early 1970s was germinal to much of the development which has gone on since. Latterly, work on the artificial arm, particularly for the young, has been most evident from Sweden.

Mobility aids — wheelchairs

For some patients artificial limbs or the application of FES techniques are not suitable for the rehabilitation of movement or locomotion. For many the wheelchair must remain the sole means of effective transportation. For these patients the interface between user and machine is critical. The design of the chair must take into account seating and body support, as well as aspects of control. In the latter area the control of the powered chair is most often achieved using some form of joy-stick, though other methods which use residual motor function in the head, shoulder, finger, etc., can be used, as may the mouth (blow–suck) or in extreme cases even EMG signals. In the application of any of these control activations, sensory (usually visual) feedback is critical. In any event, however, controllers often employ electronic circuitry which deliberately limits either velocity, acceleration or both.

A number of wheelchairs have been designed to give the user omnidirectional capability. Although these have for the most part been experimental, and designed to complement people's existing mobility, they have been successfully used by patients with such disabilities as muscular dystrophy, multiple sclerosis and cerebral palsy. Most of these chairs have been bulky, but recent designs for unicycle-based chairs (see Figure 36.4) have shown that versatility can successfully be integrated with performance (Roy *et al.*, 1985). Roy's chair is based on a single central driving wheel which carries the patient's full weight. Stability is achieved with four peripheral castors placed at the extremity of the circular base of the chair. Designed for use in the home, such a chair has been found to confer considerably increased mobility to many groups of patients, and in addition permits easier eye-to-eye contact between the user and someone who is standing (Chapter 43).

Communication aids

Communication aids fall broadly into hearing, seeing and speaking aids, and excellent reviews of work in this area is to be found in Copeland (1975) and Webster *et al.* (1985).

Hearing aids

This group of aids is aimed to assist the deaf. At their simplest the aids consist of systems to amplify sounds and feed them to the ear, either directly or by bone conduction. The response of a typical 'behind-the-ear' aid peaks at around 2 kHz, with a maximum gain of around 120 db (amplification of 1,000,000). Such high gains can give rise to unpleasant acoustic feedback, a problem which is still awaiting a good solution. The total performance of the aid is very much determined by the microphone characteristics. Miniature aids consequently have a far inferior performance to portable systems which may be carried on the belt or in the pocket, and make use of a better-quality microphone. Accoustic feedback, leading to howling, can, however, still be a problem.

Recent work has concentrated on the development of a cochlear

Figure 36.4: Five-wheel unicycle showing the basic components. The steering loop is coupled to a ground reference point through an adjustable vertical post. (Reproduced by permission of the International Federation for Medical and Biological Engineering)

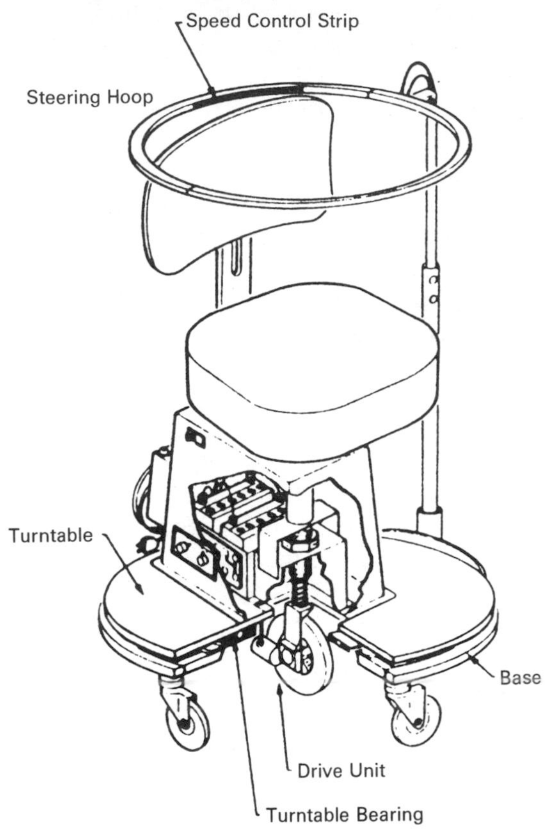

prosthesis which can be used to stimulate electrically the viable parts of the auditory system. Several groups have been developing such devices, most of which are implanted (White, 1982). Coupling from the external microphone/amplifier is achieved by frequency modulation of a radiofrequency signal which can be transmitted transcutaneously (see Figure 36.5). (See also Chapter 17.)

Aids for the visually impaired

Aids for the visually impaired appear in many forms. At their simplest, where the disability is slight, they take the form of small reading aids such as magnifiers. More technological devices include enlarged-print books, high-intensity lighting, through to closed-circuit TV systems. The latter,

Figure 36.5: In the cochlear implant the transmitter system is coupled inductively through the skin to the fully implanted receiver/stimulator. The stimulating electrode is positioned in the scala tympani

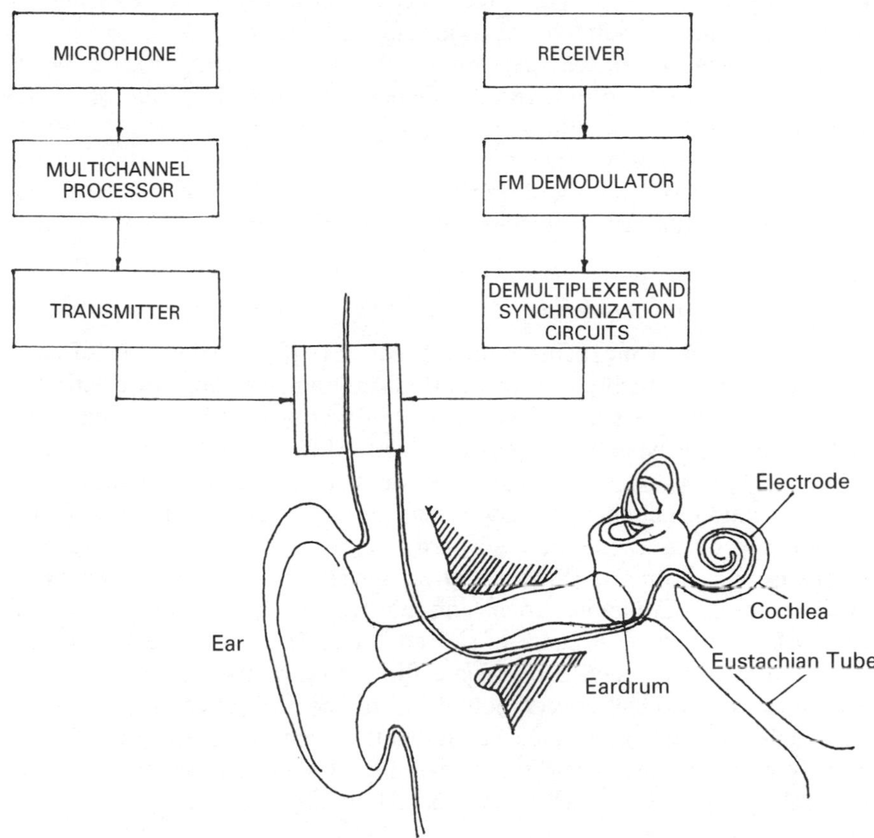

which are essentially electronic aids, confer the possibility of image manipulation and enhancement. Control of image contrast, an important variable for partially sighted people, is easily achieved with such technology. The disadvantage of these systems is, however, their cost and often their lack of portability. However, some devices are compact enough to be used for work or study in a classroom.

Braille has for long been the most established of reading aids relying on tactile acuity. The production of braille books has, until recently, been a time-consuming and expensive exercise. However, recent developments have harnessed computer technology, and portable braille readers have been constructed in which, for example, a row of 12 braille cells can be activated electromechanically to form lines of text. Activation may be achieved from signals derived from a cassette or floppy disc, thus condensing dramatically the physical storage space needed.

Other systems have recently been developed in which the microcomputer is coupled to a braille typewriter, voice synthesiser and braille reader — in effect a complete bidirectional communication device.

At the other end of the spectrum of vision loss, much work has been done on the generation of a visual prosthesis in which the visual cortex is stimulated directly. Donaldson (1983) has presented an excellent review of work in this area which has had to overcome enormous technological problems. However, despite the progress made in this area, it now seems unlikely that a full visual prosthesis will become a practical reality in the near future.

Aids for the vocally impaired

With the advent of inexpensive microprocessors the development of aids for the vocally impaired have centred around the use of electronic keyboards with some form of display or vocal encoding. Several commercial devices are available which are dealt with elsewhere in this book (Chapter 15). Many of the devices, however, are slow as a means of communication; patients with additional motor handicap being unable to achieve speeds in excess of five words per minute. The use of speech synthesisers has done much to improve this situation, but most currently available devices are limited to around 200 words. Greater capacity would be possible, but at the expense of size and cost. The most recent developments which look likely to overcome these constraints are based on the generation of artificial speech sounds from the fundamental phonemes. Although communication aids based on this technology will initially be more difficult to use, their total flexibility should remove most of the vocabulary and speech constraints imposed by other devices.

CONCLUSION

This chapter has attempted to bring together some ideas of areas in which bioengineering is contributing to the rehabilitation of the handicapped. In the space of the chapter it has only been possible to touch briefly on a few areas. Indeed whole books have been written on the subject (Copeland, 1975; Webster *et al.*, 1985) and the reader is directed to these for more extensive discussions. Much has come and gone in the development of technology for rehabilitation. Sometimes work in one area finds application in another. The work on the development of neurological prostheses, for example, has now been very successfully reapplied to the problem of bladder control in paraplegics (Brindley *et al.*, 1986).

It is clear, however, that with the increasing availability of relatively inexpensive technology, particularly in the computing field, the incorporation of the rehabilitation engineer into the clinical team is necessary for the proper management of the handicapped patient. The multidisciplinary skills that such engineers can bring to bear on the complex problems of handicap, give encouragement and hope for a greatly improved quality of life in future.

REFERENCES

Brindley, G.S., Polkey, C.E. Rushton, D.D. and Cardozo, L. (1986) Sacral anterior root stimulators for bladder control in paraplegics: the first 50 cases. *J. Neurol. Neurosurg. Psychiatry*, *49*, 1104-14

Chad, E.Y. and Hoffman, R.R. (1978) Instrumented measurement of human joint motion. *ISA Trans.*, *17*(1), 13-19

Childress, D.S. (1973) Powered limb prostheses: their clinical significance. *IEEE Trans. Biomed. Engng.*, *BME-20*, 200-7

Coleman, C.L., Cook, A.M. and Meyers, L.S. (1980) Assessing non-oral clients for assistive communication systems. *J. Speech Hear. Disord.*, *45*, 515-26

Copeland, K. (ed.) (1975) *Aids for the severely handicapped*, Grune & Stratton, New York

Donaldson, P.E.K. (1983) Engineering visual prostheses. *Eng. Med. Biol. Mag.*, *2*, 14-18

Gage, H. (1964) Accelerographic analysis of human gait. ASME Paper no. 64-Wa/ NUF 8

Golbranson, F.L. (1980) The use of gait analysis to study gait patterns of the lower limb amputee. *Bull Pros. Res.*, 10-34 *17*(2), 96-7

Gracanin, F. (1971) *Instruction manual for the Ljubljana functional electronic peroneal brace.* ZRI, Ljublyana and TIRR, Houston

Hannah R.E., Morrison, J.B. and Chapman, A.E. (1984) Prosthesis alignment: effect on gait of persons with below knee amputations. *Arch. Phys. Med. Rehabil.*, *65*(4), 159-62

Helliwell, P., Howe, A. and Wright, V. (1987) Functional assessment of the hand: reproducibility, acceptability, and utility of a new system for measuring strength. *Ann. Rheum. Dis.*, *46*, 203-8

Hicks, R., Tashman, S., Cary, J.M., Altman, R.F. and Gage, J.R. (1985) Swing phase control with knee function in juvenile amputees. *J. Orthop. Res.*, *3*(2), 198-201

Ishai, G., Bar, A. and Susak, Z. (1983) Effects of alignment variables on thigh axial torque during swing phase in AK amputee gait. *Prosthet. Orthot. Int.*, *7*(1), 41-7

Jones, D.P. and Paul, J.P. (1978) Analysis of variability in pylon transducer signals. *Prosthet. Orthot. Int.*, *2*, 161-6

Kirby, R.L., Stewart-Gray, J.F. and Creaser, G.A. (1985) Usefulness of footprint sequence analysis in lower limb amputees. *Phys. Ther.*, *65*(1), 31-4

Kralj, A., Bajd, T., Turk, R., Krajnik, J. and Benko, H. (1983) Gait restoration in paraplegic patients: a feasibility demonstration using multichannel surface electrode FES. *J. Rehabil. R & D*, *20*, 3-20

Laughman, R.K., Asken, L.J., Bleimeyer, R.R. and Chao, E.Y. (1984) Objective clinical evaluation of function. Gait analysis. *Phys. Ther.*, *64*(12), 1839-45

Lord, M., Reynolds, D.P. and Hughes, J.R. (1986) Foot pressure measurement: a review of clinical findings. *J. Biomed. Engng.*, *8*, 283-94

Mizrahi, J., Susak, Z., Bahar, A., Seliktar, R. and Najenson, T. (1985) Biomechanical evaluation of an adjustable patellar tendon bearing prosthetis. *Scand. J. Rehabil. Med.* (Suppl), *12*, 117-23

Mizrahi, J., Braun Z., Najenson, T. and Graupe, D. (1985) Quantitative weightbearing and gait evaluation in paraplegics using FES. *Med. Biol. Engng. Comput.*, *23*, 101-7

Nye, P.W. and Bliss, J.C. (1970) Sensory aids for the blind: a challenging problem with lessons for the future. *Proc. IEEE*, *581*, 1878-98

Petrofsky, J.S., Heaton, H.H. and Phillips, C.A. (1984) Leg exerciser for training of paralysed muscle by closed loop control. *Med. Biol. Engng. Comput.*, *22*, 298-303

Porter, D. and Roberts, V.C. (1987) Gait assessment in the lower limb amputee — a review. *J. Biomed. Engng.* (in press)

Roy, O.Z., Duries, N.D., Farley, R.L., Perkins, G., Tierney, K. and Skrypnyk, R. (1985) Five wheel unicycle system. *Med. Biol. Engng. Comput.*, *23*, 593-6

Saleh, M. and Murdoch, G. (1985) In defence of gait analysis. Observation and measurement in gait assessment. *J. Bone Joint Surg., (Br)*, *67*(2), 237-41

Seliktar, R. and Mizrahi, J. (1986) Some gait characteristics of below knee amputees and their reflection on the ground reaction forces. *Eng. Med.*, *15*(1), 27-34

Webster, J.G., Cook, A.M., Tompkins, W.J. and Vanderheiden, G.C. (1985) *Electronic devices for rehabilitation*, Chapman & Hall, London

White, R.L. (1982) The Stanford artificial ear project. *The Stanford Engineer*, Spring/Summer, pp. 3-10

Wright, V. (ed.) (1982) Measurement of joint movement. *Clin. Rheum. Dis.*, *8*(3)

37

Social Services and Benefits

Brian Meredith Davies

GOVERNMENT-BASED SERVICES

In the United Kingdom the main government department which has central responsibility for social services, and which also controls the various financial benefits and pensions, is the *Department of Health and Social Services (DHSS)* — the same which administers the health services. From time to time the DHSS issues helpful free pamphlets including *Help for handicapped people* (pamphlet H.B.1) which not only summarises various social services but indicates how they may be obtained. The DHSS also promotes various research projects and makes grants to voluntary bodies working with disabled people (mainly for specific projects). The Artificial Limb and Appliance Service (ALAS) is a specialised part of the National Health Service which works directly with the DHSS. It is responsible for supply of artificial limbs and wheelchairs (Chapters 11 and 43). The DHSS is not the only government department concerned with the needs of disabled persons. The Register of Disabled Persons under the Disabled Persons (Employment) Acts of 1944 and 1958 is kept by the Employment Services Division of the Manpower Services Commission, which is set up by the Department of Employment. The Department of Education and Science is responsible for the education of handicapped children and the further education of adult persons.

LOCALLY BASED SOCIAL SERVICES

The Social Services Departments (SSDs) of major local authorities (county councils, metropolitan district councils and London boroughs) are the main suppliers of community-based social services for disabled persons. There are now 120 such departments compared with 194 health authorities, so that each usually covers a larger area than the local health services. Each has an elected Social Services Committee (to which at least one disabled person is coopted) and their chief officer is the *Director of Social Services.* Each SSD divides its geographical area into a number of Areas (or Districts) each with about 30,000–50,000 population under the control of an Area (or District) Social Services Officer (Meredith Davies, 1983)

TYPES OF SOCIAL SERVICES PROVIDED BY SSDs

Information

Each SSD must ensure that (a) it is adequately informed of the numbers and needs of handicapped persons so that it may plan and develop appropriate services — each department maintains a *Register of Disabled Persons*; (b) all disabled persons and their families know what help is avaiable locally.

Provision of services

These are divided into eight groups, and the SSD provides:

(1) practical assistance in the homes of disabled people, using social workers, occupational therapists and home helps;

(2) radio, library and similar facilities in the home;

(3) recreational facilities outside the home (these include arranging access to sports centres, day centres and clubs);

(4) help with travelling facilities for disabled persons — the SSD provides group transport, and the DHSS help with individual transport through the Mobility Allowance;

(5) assistance in carrying out adaptations within the home of disabled persons — the SSD also provides personal aids to disabled persons;

(6) assistance for a disabled person to take a holiday;

(7) meals service at home and elsewhere;

(8) a telephone and any extra equipment needed for its use.

Most of the legal powers to provide such services are in the Chronically Sick and Disabled Persons Act 1970. However these powers are general and mainly permissive; therefore levels of service vary considerably throughout the country. In conjuction with the local Education Authority and national organisations such as the Open University, SSD can give assistance to disabled persons wanting to take advantage of educational facilities.

In addition, this Act gives special duties to each local housing authority (in the county areas this is the smaller district local authority) to plan and provide special housing accommodation for handicapped persons. The Act also lays down a number of requirements for *public buildings* including:

(1) Means of *access* to and within the building, and in *parking facilities* and provision of *sanitary conveniences suitable for use by disabled persons. Such services must be considered before planning permission is granted.*

(2) Requirements for local authorities to provide public conveniences suitable for disabled persons.

(3) Requirement for anyone providing sanitary conveniences in premises open to the public for accomodation, refreshment or entertainment to make provision, *as far as is practicable*, for disabled people and for adequate signposting. The term 'as far as practicable' has resulted in a number of premises being excluded.

COMMUNITY SERVICES PROVIDED BY SOCIAL SERVICES DEPARTMENTS

Practical assistance in the home

This mainly covers help and advice given by social workers, occupational therapists or home helps within the home of the disabled person. *Social workers* normally work in small teams based at Area or District. Some of these will have a specialised knowledge of disabled people, and some will be specially trained to work with the blind or deaf. In addition, there are specialised senior social workers who can act as the liaison personnel with the health and education services.

Most SSDs have community based fully trained *occupational therapists.* These staff work in two main ways: (a) in visiting, assessing and helping individual disabled persons in their own homes; (b) in day centres. Most occupational therapists concentrate on practical ways in which disabled people can learn to live a more normal life at home. They are particularly concerned with the provision of various aids or adaptations and with active rehabilitation of disabled persons early in their disability whilst they are attending day centres.

Home helps are provided by all SSDs. Their main task is to help in the individual's home when, because of age, acute or chronic illness or disability, the person cannot adequately look after the home himself. Eighty-eight per cent of persons receiving such help are elderly, and many will have some chronic disability. About 6 per cent of home helps look after younger disabled persons. The duties of a home help include the usual tasks carried out by any housewife — cleaning rooms, preparing food and meals, cooking, shopping and lighting fires. Home help is usually provided on a part-time basis so as to encourage the disabled person to remain as active as possible, but in an emergency can be provided full-time. A usual arrangement would be for a home help to provide two or three sessions of three hours to a disabled person each week.

Each home help, especially in long-standing cases, gets to know the individual she is attending very well, and this can be helpful in watching over the disabled person and acting as a source of information, especially in the case of an elderly person living alone. By sensible use of the home help service, together with the meals services, it is often possible to keep an elderly disabled person at home for some years longer than would otherwise be possible. Charges are made for home help services, but if the disabled person lives solely on a pension, etc., no charge is made. In others a sliding scale of charges applies.

In addition there are various *good neighbour schemes* in operation, whereby arrangement are made through SSDs to provide regular visitors to disabled persons. Some authorities, such as Liverpool, have developed a special *home care programme* in which elderly persons at special risk, including those living alone, are provided with free home help for four hours a day for at least four weeks after being discharged from hospital. Such a service is organised *before discharge*, so that the home help is at the person's own home to welcome the patient on discharge.

Radio, television and similar recreational facilities in the home

Many *radios* are provided for blind persons and other bedfast or housebound patients through national voluntary bodies and SSDs. There is legal power for an SSD to provide televisions, but very few have given this service a high priority, although more authorities help with payments towards the television licence.

Library facilities

These include specially printed books such as the large-print series stocked by all public libraries, which are invaluable for those with low vision. Another useful service for the blind and partially sighted is the library of tape-recorded books maintained by the Royal National Institute for the

Blind which is financied by contributions from SSDs. A tape recorder is lent to each person and a changing supply of recorded readings of books is available through the post. There are no postal charges for this and other services for the blind. For those who have learnt braille a library of such books is kept nationally, and is also supplied on demand through the post.

Recreational facilities within the home include a wide range of interests, hobbies and cultural pursuits. The main object is to provide disabled people, many of whom cannot work, with an increased sense of purpose so that each may look forward to tomorrow in a new and purposeful way. Occupational therapists from the SSD will advise, and in many instances, will call in colleagues from the library and educational services.

Recreational facilities outside the home and assistance in taking advantage of educational facilities

Physical recreation of all kinds now plays an increasingly important part in the life of many disabled adults. This movement started after the 1939–45 war for those disabled with paraplegia. People paralysed from the waist down must rely on shoulder, arm and chest muscles to lift themselves, and therefore recreational pursuits which strengthen these muscles are very valuable in rehabilitation and in maintaining mobility, which is so essential if the disabled person is to continue to lead an active and independent life. A wide range of sports are recognised as being very suitable, and SSDs arrange (a) access to swimming pools and sports centres, (b) group transport to help disabled people to attend such facilities. Special sessions at swimming pools and sports centres are arranged, and these are particularly useful for newly handicapped persons, many of whom are reticent and embarrassed initially and require quiet conditions if they are to be persuaded to participate. Later a number will happily join in public sessions with their families and friends.

Adult educational facilities can be of particular value to many disabled persons, especially if they have much time on their hands. Each SSD will advise and arrange, if need be, for the local education authority to make special arrangements (i.e. to find a suitable course which is held on the ground floor of a convenient building with suitable WCs nearby). The SSD will arrange transport.

The *Open University* welcomes disabled students, and makes special arrangements for those wishing to enrol on courses. Such applicants are exempt from the 'first come, first served' principle, and are given priority of admission. There is also no lower age limit (usually 21) for disabled students and this can be very useful for disabled school-leavers wishing to enrol on such courses. Each SSD can advise on the facilities available, or the disabled person can write direct to the Open University at Walton Hall,

Milton Keynes, Bucks. A special senior counsellor is employed by the Open University to help and advise disabled students.

Travelling facilities for disabled persons

Group transport (minibuses and specially equipped vehicles with lifts) are provided by all SSDs to help disabled persons. Individual transport is a government responsibility and is discharged via the Mobility Allowance and Motability (see later). Group transport can either arrange to pick up the disabled person directly from home or at a convenient pick-up point. Such transport is used to take disabled people to day centres and to various club activities; such transport is free.

Assistance in carrying out adaptations in the home and the provision of aids to daily living

This is an important service provided by all SSDs, for the ability of any disabled person to continue to lead a reasonably normal life depends on being able to move freely around the home and to remain independent for as long as possible. Occupational therapists (Chapter 34) are the professionals who are specially trained to advise on and coordinate the various complicated procedures, and many now work in SSDs as well as in hospitals. An increasing number of excellent *aids centres* (Disabled Living Centres) are now in existence, some funded by SSDs and some voluntary bodies. Most are located in major cities, and local enquiry will indicate the most convenient. Many SSDs will be able to arrange for the disabled person to purchase aids on a wholesale or discount basis; indeed some SSDs make generous contributions towards the cost of larger aids (Chapter 49). Sophisticated electronic aids such as Possum are provided by government through the national health service (Chapter 48) with SSDs also helping with the alterations within the home, i.e. electrical fittings and extra tables or shelves needed.

Most SSDs assist with the cost of major adaptations *provided they have agreed before the adaptations have been started.* In such cases it is usual for the SSD to insist on a contract being signed so that if, within a reasonable period (usually five years), the home is resold at a profit a proportion of the costs of the grant has to be repaid.

Holidays

SSDs can help disabled people in four ways with holidays:

(1) By providing the fullest information about various types of holiday accommodation. Excellent guides are now published for all parts of the UK giving full details of hotels, boarding houses, farms, etc., and these particularly record where downstairs bedrooms, bathrooms and WCs can be found. This helps disabled people and their families to plan their own holidays in the normal way, and the majority choose to do this.

(2) By arranging special holidays – these are usually of two kinds: (a) for the blind who may need to go to some modified accommodation, especially if they are on their own; or (b) for groups of young disabled persons to whom the adventure type of holiday is often very attractive (i.e. camping, etc.). Careful planning is essential, and it is always necessary to take an equal number of able-bodied helpers. These usually include some permanent staff and some volunteers, who are often students on holiday.

(3) By assisting with group transport. Some SSDs send vehicles equipped with lifts which are based in various holiday resorts (including some abroad) in the peak summer months to help those disabled in wheelchairs, who can then go on package holidays with their families knowing that they will still be able to get about in the resort using special transport.

(4) By making small monetary grants (in the region of £25) to help with the more expensive arrangements often essential for those who are disabled (i.e. it may be important to choose a hotel with an adequate-size lift and private bathroom).

Meals services

There are two types of meals services provided by SSDs: (a) *meals-on-wheels*, where a two-course hot meal is delivered to the disabled person at home; and (b) a *similar meal is provided at a day centre or luncheon club.* Both are useful. In practice the first is more commonly used for elderly persons living alone, and the second for the younger disabled person, most of whom attend some day centre or workshop. A small subsidised charge is usually made for the meals-on-wheels, but some SSDs provide meals at day centres free.

Provision of a telephone or other special equipment

This was a new discretionary power given to SSDs by the Chronically Sick and Disabled Persons Act 1970, and can be a most valuable service especially for physically disabled people who live alone and find it impossible to leave their home without help. The usual criteria which must be satisfied for anyone to qualify for a telephone are:

(a) he/she must not be able to leave their home in normal weather without help.

(b) he/she must either be living alone or be left alone for long periods of the day or night.

The usual arrangement is for the SSD to pay the rental charges and, if necessary, the installation charges leaving the disabled person to pay the cost of any calls. SSDs have responded in varying ways to this service, and unfortunately there is wide variation throughout the country in the level of such telephone provision. The best SSDs provide telephones for about 20–25 per cent of all their registered disabled people; the worst about 1–2 per cent.

For more details about social, educational and employment services for disabled persons, the reader is referred to the book *The disabled child and adult*, written by myself (Meredith Davies 1982). This book was written from a different angle, being mainly aimed at a wider group of professionals in the health and social services, and may be of value to readers and the staff who work with them.

COMMUNITY-BASED DAY CARE SERVICES FOR DISABLED PERSONS (DAY CENTRES)

One of the most valuable groups of services which SSDs provide for disabled people is *community-based day care in special day centres.* Many of these are purpose-built and can provide a wide range of services including workshops. In most days centres two types of service are available:

Rehabilitation for those recently disabled

Most of this rehabilitation is under the control of an occupational therapist, and it is usual for a wide range of equipment to be available. Much of this service concentrates on teaching the disabled person how to live more normally even though he/she may now have to face life with some permanent disability. There may be a large number of special personal aids provided at the centre, and it is here that many disabled people can learn which aids are most suitable, and how to use them properly. It is always important for any disabled person to try out any such equipment at such a centre, at home or in a hospital department before it is installed in the home, to make sure that the individual understands the aid and will be able to manage it. This is especially important with hoists and lifting equipment of various types.

Most day centres have special bathroom and WC equipment, and access to private sessions in a swimming pool. Many who are struggling to become mobile again after a disabling condition find rehabilitation sessions in a warm swimming pool particularly helpful, as the effect of gravity is reduced, allowing weaker muscles to be more effective.

For the more chronically disabled person in whom rehabilitation is limited

Attendance at an SSD day centre can be most useful for this group, as it gives the disabled person an opportunity to get out of the home and to meet other people, and thus lead a more normal life. It also combats any tendency towards isolation, which in certain individuals can become a major problem

AIMS OF DAY CARE

Day care has four aims:

(1) To encourage self-help and independence. Although disabled people are often initially taken to the day centre by special transport (private bus or minibus) every effort is later made to encourage them to use public transport (free bus or rail tickets being provided).

(2) To continue with training and some education. The best day centres concentrate upon this aspect of care, and local education authority staff will also visit and work at the centre.

(3) To increase communication with others. This is always important if the tendency towards self-pity is to be avoided. It is often helpful for the disabled person to meet others who have worse problems to face, for then it is difficult to feel sorry for oneself.

(4) To improve 'socialisation'. Another problem, particularly for the younger adult who has to cope with a serious permanent disability, is that he/she probably will have very little opportunity to learn how to live within a group and to play a useful part in developing that community (this is especially so for those who have never been able to go to work, because of their disability). Any day centre helps young disabled adults to learn how to live and function happily together, especially if arrangements can be made for them to play a part in the organisation of the centre through the management committee. This can be a particularly useful lesson if later the disabled person has to live in a residential home.

RESIDENTIAL HOMES FOR DISABLED PERSONS

Residential homes for disabled persons are provided by both local authorities through their SSDs and voluntary bodies. In England and Wales there are approximately 4,000 disabled people under the age of 65 who live in such homes run by SSDs and 4,500 by voluntary bodies. *Provided the SSD has agreed to the admission beforehand*, the local authority may contribute towards the cost of keeping the person in the voluntary home, although increasingly DHSS benefits are used for this. In all such arrangements, if the individual cannot afford to pay the charges out of income, any capital owned by the disabled person in excess of £3,000 must be taken into account. This usually means that the individual has to pay the full cost until the capital has been reduced to £3,000.

Many disabled people who are elderly do well in ordinary old persons' home and settle down very happily there, especially if they have been living alone and only managing with difficulty. But many studies have shown that this is not the case with younger disabled people, who often are in serious danger of becoming institutionalised when they have to live permanently in a residential home. The reasons for this are complex, and often depend on the lack of a sense of purpose which follows, rather than on the treatment received within the home, although if this is restrictive and authoritarian the effect will be worse.

From studies carried out by the DHSS in 1970 it appears that nearly half the disabled persons under the age of 65 who at present are living in homes are in the 'minimally dependent' category, being continent, mobile without assistance, able to feed themselves and mentally alert. There is little doubt that such people would be better off living in some form of independent sheltered accommodation.

In this respect much can be learnt from other countries. For instance, the 'collective home' in Denmark, which was developed many years ago for frail elderly persons, can be ideal. This scheme consists of purpose-built accommodation (usually flats) into which the elderly person can move any time after retirement. Essentially a centrally heated flat (the cost of the heating being included in the rent) is provided where the elderly person receives a three-course lunch which is taken in a central dining room. Also contained within the unit is a small old person's home. Any disabled persons who can no longer stay in the flat because they have become too frail to look after themselves, even with the help provided, have priority to enter the attached home, where they now can be fully cared for by the same staff. This means that the disabled person never needs to leave the district and their friends, and know that if they do eventually have to be admitted to a home with full care, they will be spared a complete change of environment, which in many elderly frail people can be traumatic and damaging. Such a scheme certainly encourages independence as well as enabling an unobtrusive surveillance to be carried out. If the disabled person does not turn up for lunch, staff can make an immediate enquiry to ensure that the resident is all right (Chapter 38).

VOLUNTARY BODIES

Voluntary bodies also play an important role in providing social services. Many specialised services for blind and deaf people are mainly provided by the Royal Institute for the Blind, Royal Institute for the Deaf or by the British Deaf Association. In many instances these act as agents for SSDs who reimburse their costs. There are many other specialised voluntary bodies working both nationally and locally with other groups of physically disabled people: examples include the National Spastics Society, British Epilepsy Association, Arthritis Care and the British Sports Association for the Disabled (Chapter 49).

ADULT FOSTERING

Adult fostering of disabled persons has been tried out by some SSDs. It can be successful but needs careful planning, particularly if the disabled person suffers from a progressive condition such as multiple sclerosis. Although fostering can be ideal at an early stage, sudden deterioration can produce a crisis and, before any scheme is finally arranged, full discussions should take place between staff from the local SSD, the doctors involved, the patient and family so that some agreed contingency plan is on hand if and when fostering is no longer practicable. Failure to do this has produced serious difficulties in the past, and has resulted in the disabled person having to be admitted in an emergency to some unsuitable hospital ward.

FINANCIAL PROBLEMS AND THEIR SOLUTIONS

There are a number of specialised financial benefits available to disabled persons and their families, but in this chapter all that is attempted is to introduce the range of such help and describe a few special benefits and allowances. Such financial benefits are provided by the DHSS, and one of the best ways to understand the scope of them is to read a copy of the free DHSS booklet *Which Benefit?*, which can be obtained from local DHSS offices or main post offices. It will be noted that the range of benefits is complicated, and many are continuously changing. Some are contributory, others non-contributory; some tax free, others taxed as income. The study of welfare rights has become so complex in recent years that many SSDs now employ a specialist welfare rights officer to advise social workers, clients and their families as to which benefits they may be entitled. It is therefore important for disabled persons and their families to realise that, unless they are prepared to seek expert help, it is quite likely they will not manage to obtain all the benefits to which they are entitled. DHSS staff are helpful, but many decisions about benefits can and ought to be challenged; for experience has repeatedly shown that where a claim for a benefit such as an Attendence Allowance has been turned down, a request for a review supported by expert help has reversed that decision.

There is a particularly useful national voluntary body — the *Disability Alliance*, 5 Netherhall Gardens, London NW3 — whose main aim is to introduce a comprehensive approach to financial disability. It publishes an extremely helpful booklet each year, the *Disability Rights Handbook*, which gives an up-to-date account of significant changes in welfare rights for disabled people and their families; it also highlights recent decisions regarding successful appeals which can be most helpful. Certainly no hospital department or SSD, or other professional group concerned with advising and helping disabled persons, should be without an up-to-date copy of this booklet.

Attendance allowance

This is an allowance for a person who, because of serious physical or mental disability, has needed frequent help from another person for six months or more. It is tax-free and usually does not affect other income (exceptions include a disabled person already receiving a constant attendance allowance or an industrial, war or service pension, or extra money for attendance needs from supplementary benefit).

There are two rates of attendance allowance. If the individual needs attendance during both day *and* night, he/she qualifies for the *higher rate*. If the disabled person needs attendance by day *or* night he/she should get the *lower rate*.

To qualify, the disabled person must be so severely disabled that for six months he/she has needed;

By day: frequent attention throughout the day in connection with his/her bodily functions, *or* continuous supervision throughout the day in order to avoid substantial danger to himself/herself or others.

By night: prolonged or repeated attention during the night in connection with his/her bodily functions, *or* continual supervision throughout the night in order to avoid substantial danger to himself/herself or others.

In practice this means that any disabled person should be able to obtain an attendance allowance if, for example, he/she needs much help to walk and get around or to eat and drink, use the toilet, wash, dress, shave, or has to use a kidney machine at home. *Because the allowance cannot be paid for any period before a claim has been made* (even if the person would clearly have qualified) it is most important for the doctor, nurse or other professional caring for any newly disabled patient (say someone who has suffered from a severe stroke) to recommend a claim be made six months after the start of the disabling condition. When in doubt a claim should always be made (studies have shown that many severely disabled persons fail to make a claim, or do so after an unnecessarily long period). Claims are made by completing the form attached to the attendance allowance leaflet. A medical examination will be arranged. All claims are decided by an Attendance Allowance Board at Norcross House, Blackpool. *If a claim is turned down, or the disabled person is granted the lower rate when the higher rate would seem to be more appropriate, the disabled person should ask for a review.* More than half those asking for a review have been successful.

Mobility allowance

The Mobility Allowance is a weekly cash benefit paid to any disabled person between the ages of five and 75 years who is unable, or virtually unable, to walk. However, the individual has to qualify before the age of 65, and the claim must be made before the individual is aged 66. The allowance is tax-free and does not make any difference to the amount of any other benefits; the individual becomes exempt from paying vehicle excise duty (the car licence) and also qualifies for the orange badge scheme for parking, and for help from the Motability Scheme.

To qualify, the disabled person must be able to make use of the allowance; a person in a coma, or who for medical reasons cannot be moved, would not qualify. The disabled person must also be living in the UK (Isle of Man qualifies and there is a parallel scheme in Northern Ireland), and must have lived there for at least 12 months in the preceding 18 months from the date on which a claim is made.

The allowance is intended to be spent on outdoor mobility, but may be spent in any way, towards a vehicle even if owned by someone else, to pay for taxis for hire, a car, or to pay for holiday transport. *The decision is entirely at the discretion of the severely disabled person.* The mobility allowance can be paid to more than one person in the same household or family, which is extremely useful for those rare cases of familial disability where they may be a number of persons eligible in the same family.

Any person who at present has a car provided by the DHSS, or has a DHSS three-wheeler car or had such a car before November 1976, can, if they are still medically eligible, switch to the Mobility Allowance *without further medical examination and without age limit.*

Vehicle excise duty (car licence) exemption

Anyone receiving the Mobility Allowance no longer has to pay the vehicle excise duty on a vehicle used by the disabled person. It is also important to note that *if a person is no longer able to claim the Mobility Allowance because he/she is over the age limit, he/she can still qualify for vehicle excise duty exemption if the disability is severe enough to qualify for the Mobility Allowance had they been younger.* This can be very helpful to an elderly disabled person finding it increasingly difficult to afford the expense of running a car.

Motability

This is a voluntary organisation formed on the initiative of the government to help disabled people with a Mobility Allowance to obtain a car or wheelchair. It has negotiated excellent discounts with motor manufacturers, wheelchair manufacturers, insurance brokers and others. In addition the banks have agreed to provide finance for Motability's hire, and hire purchase, schemes on favourable terms through a finance company specially set up. Motability receives a government grant annually towards part of its administrative costs. It offers four types of schemes: (1) a new car on hire (a leasing scheme), (2) a new car on hire purchase, (3) a used car on hire purchase, (4) an electric wheelchair on hire purchase (for full details of the wheelchair scheme an application should be made direct to Motability).

New car on hire

This is available to holders of a Mobility Allowance, who will continue to be eligible to receive it for at least a further three years. Anyone who is less than three years from the top age limit cannot use the scheme. The whole of the mobility allowance is paid over to Motability for the period, together with any annual increases.

In return, Motability provides the new car chosen by the disabled person. For the smallest cars available, such as most Austin Minis and some Metros, there is no extra payment, but if a larger car is chosen there is an additional single payment to be made at the start of the hire. No further hire charges are due unless the car exceeds 12,000 miles a year (averaged over three years). The arrangement covers full costs of maintenance and repairs for the three-year hire period with the exception of new tyres for some larger cars. A block insurance scheme has been arranged with the Zurich Insurance Company, and this forms an integral part of the scheme. The disabled person must arrange comprehensive insurance with this company. The cost of any adaptations will be an additional expense. If large-scale adaptations are needed they can only be fitted to cars supplied on hire purchase (see below), as all cars have to be returned in their original form and the cost of removing large-scale adaptations would be too great.

The disabled person has to pay for running costs (petrol and oil) and at the end of the hire the car must be returned in a proper state of repair and in good serviceable condition. The hire scheme has been a great success, and has enabled severely disabled people without capital to obtain a new car. One advantage is that the scheme covers the cost of all maintenance and repairs, which is an expense often overlooked and allows the disabled person to calculate exactly what the costs are likely to be.

At the end of the hire the car has to be returned, but the disabled person can reapply to take out a lease on another new car exactly as before.

Hire purchase scheme for new cars

The cost of buying a new car outright on a special hire purchase scheme can also be covered with the help of Motability.

The disabled person must be the holder of the Mobility Allowance for the whole of the period (four years) and disabled persons are allowed to cover part or all of the cost by paying over their Mobility Allowance to Motability. In addition, the disabled person usually has to pay a deposit for all but the smallest cars. The disabled person is responsible for paying repairs, maintenance and fully comprehensive insurance. Further details, and a list of insurance brokers offering special rates, can be obtained from Motability.

Hire purchase scheme for used cars

If the disabled person wishes to use the hire purchase scheme for used cars, the car must be under four years old, have done less than 40,000 miles and have been inspected by the Automobile Association. The dealer supplying the car must be a member of the Motor Agents Association (or Scottish Motor Traders Association) or hold a franchise from a motor manufacturer). Full details are available from Motability at Boundary House, 91-93 Charterhouse St, London EC1 6BT.

ORANGE BADGE PARKING SCHEME

If a disabled person has considerable difficulty in walking, or is blind, there is a special parking scheme to help. An orange badge can be obtained from the local council, which will enable the handicapped person to park free without time limit at parking meters, limited waiting areas, and to park for up to two hours on single yellow lines. It does not apply to parts of central London, but is of considerable help to those with walking difficulties. More details can be obtained from social service department or transport departments of local authorities.

OTHER BENEFITS AVAILABLE

A wide range of financial benefits is available to help disabled people and their families. The best way to understand them is to obtain a copy of the free booklet *Help for handicapped people*, HB1 from DHSS offices or Citizens' Advice Bureaux. If the person is disabled following an illness and has been contributing to the national insurance scheme at work, he/she may claim *invalidity benefit*, and if the disability started before age 60 for men and 55 for women *an additional invalidity allowance* can be obtained (see DHSS leaflet N.I. 16A).

The more important non-contributory benefits (available to everyone) include:

Non-contributory invalidity pension (NCIP)

This is available to people of working age who have not been able to work for at least 28 weeks and who do not have enough National Insurance contributions to get sickness or invalidity benefit. Married women can claim only if they are also unable to do normal household duties (see DHSS leaflet N.I.210).

Housewives' non-contributory invalidity pension (HNCIP)

This is a benefit paid to a married woman who had not been able to work and carry out normal duties for six months because of illness or disablement (see DHSS leaflet N.I.214).

Invalid care allowance

If a man or woman of working age has been unable to work because of having to stay at home to look after a severely disabled person who is getting an attendance allowance or a constant attendance allowance, he/she can get an invalid care allowance (see DHSS leaflet N.I.212).

Rent rebates and rate relief for disabled persons

These means-tested benefits are available both to council and private tenants and, in the case of rate relief, additionally to owner-occupiers. Full details are given in DHSS leaflet BR1, or can be obtained from local council offices or Citizens' Advice Bureaux.

Assistance with fares to work

Help is available to severely disabled people who, because of their disability, are unable to use public transport for all or part of their journey to work — leaflet DPL13 from Job Centres gives further details.

REFERENCES

Assistance with fares to work. Leaflet DPL13 from Job Centres
Meredith Davies, B. (1982) *The disabled child and adult*, Baillière Tindall, London
Meredith Davies, B. (1983) *Community health, preventive medicine and social services*, 5th edn, Baillière Tindall, London
Disability Rights Handbook, published annually by Disability Alliance, 5 Netherhall Gardens, London NW3
Help for handicapped people, DHSS booklet HB1
Motability free booklet on new cars and hire purchase schemes for handicapped persons, from Motability, Boundary House, 91-93 Charterhouse St, London EC1 6BT
Non-contributory invalidity pensions, DHSS leaflet N.I.210
Rent and Rate relief, leaflet BR1
Which benefit?, DHSS free booklet FB2

(See Chapter 49, Resources Available)

38

Housing and Residential Care

John Harrison

Whenever long-term admission to a residential home or hospital is being considered, or a move to specialised housing, the issues are essentially those of *relocation*: helping or causing a disabled person to live in a new environment. Relocation is often wrongly believed to be necessary because of particular kinds or degrees of dependency, or because other options have either not been given serious thought, or are reckoned not to be available even though they could be. It is genuinely necessary when all the resources available in the existing environment are demonstrably inadequate to match the dependency in an individual case. People with disabilities, or the others with whom they share their households, may of course themselves seek somewhere else to live, for many different reasons: in such circumstances a move may not be strictly essential but it can undoubtedly be desirable.

Any disability can be catered for in a private household when the personal help and motivation to provide it are there, unless the disability is very unstable or is associated with disturbed behaviour of a kind which could be dangerous. The three factors most likely to be associated with requests for relocation are mental inadequacy, including not only disturbed behaviour but also any other kind of childlike dependency, loss of use of both upper as well as both lower limbs, and incontinence. The desirability of a move also, however, depends on the prevailing climate of opinion: whether in some general way a person 'ought' to be somewhere else, or whether a family or the available services or a particular establishment 'ought' to be able to cope.

Against this background is general agreement that disabled people have every right to choose their style of living, but sadly the opportunities for unprompted, carefully considered and well-informed choice are all too limited. Usually the options are few, or the disabled person is apprehensive and bewildered and not ready to decide, or the wishes and prejudices of others are allowed to prevail. Moreover, even when choices are very clearly stated they cannot always be allowed to override other priorities, in particular the needs and wishes of people whose predicaments may be more extreme.

Although the physical environment is important, and can often reduce the severity of dependency, the essential components of support and care are people. In private households the usual situation is that most or all of the personal help is unpaid, and this is why community care is cheaper than a hospital or residential home where most or all of the help is paid for. Overwhelmingly, paid help is provided through public funds: even the numerous voluntary and private homes and hospitals depend on public subsidy for their labour. The economic and planning arguments are therefore about the most effective ways of using public money.

During the 1970s and 1980s there has been a big shift of emphasis from residential care to care in private households. By its very existence, investment in residential care generates demand for it, together with diversion of resources from community services, and is a strong influence on the climate of opinion. Long-term residential care is also inflexible: residents' security of tenure conflicts with the ability of the institutions to respond quickly to the need of others, a conflict which can lead to ever-increasing numbers of residential homes unless it is resolved in different ways. In contrast, besides incorporating and supporting informal, unpaid care, community services can be flexible, deployed according to individual requirements rather than the staffing regimes of institutions. It so happens that many, perhaps most, disabled people do not want to live away from their own homes, and that many people in residential units regret being there. Consumer choice therefore becomes an additional argument in support of the sound economic and administrative reasons for preferring community care.

Clinicians and other professionals have to make decisions within whatever system they find themselves, but the system is itself partly determined by the succession of decisions they make.

The financial and legal framework for housing and residential care in the United Kingdom

(a) *True voluntary and private enterprise*, with services given freely or entirely paid for by charitable endowment or by charges to the consumer, contributes to a significant proportion of the specialised housing stock, but a very small proportion of residential care. The reason is that capital schemes are relatively easy to fund privately, but ongoing programmes of support and care which last for more than a few weeks, let alone many years, are beyond the financial means of most charities and private individuals. Charities also find it much easier to appeal for capital projects than for wages and salaries, even when those salaries are spent on personal care.

(b) *State-subsidised voluntary and private enterprise*: for residential homes and hospitals this usually takes the form of discretionary fee-for-service support for individual residents, from one of three possible sources.

(1) Health authorities, by direct payment to the institution: a few authorities pay for beds on a contractual basis rather than individual residents.

(2) Local authorities, by direct payment to the institution in support of individual residents, empowered by the National Assistance Act 1948.

(3) Social Security benefit offices, by payment to the resident or a person acting on his/her behalf, empowered by Supplementary Benefit regulations. There are four ceiling rates which depend on whether a resident is in a nursing home or residential home and over or under the age of 65, but the total budget is open-ended.

Tenants and owner-occupiers of *specialised housing* are eligible for Social Security and housing benefits on the same basis as anyone outside a residential home or hospital, but the total payments cannot match those payable to or on behalf of the institutional residents. Capital for housing schemes is awarded to non-profit-making housing associations through the Housing Corporation.

(c) *Direct provision by local authorities*: residential homes and private houses managed by social services departments and housing departments respectively. The sources of funds are local rates and the rate-support grant from central government. Provision is restricted by budgetary limits and competing priorities. Fees or rents are charged according to residents'/tenants' ability to pay.

(d) *Direct provision by central government*, through regional and district health authorities, to hospitals and other units managed by the National Health Service. As with local authority services, budgetary limits and competing priorities limit the quantity and quality of what is provided. No charges are made to the consumers.

According to the National Health Service Act 1946, a hospital is an institution for the reception and treatment of persons suffering from illness or mental defectiveness, or who require convalescence or medical rehabilitation. The National Assistance Act 1948 states that local authorities are obliged to provide residential accommodation for persons who, by reason of age, infirmity or any other circumstances, are in need of care which is not otherwise available to them. Voluntary and private residential institutions must register and be inspected by the public authorities, according to the provisions of the Nursing Homes Act 1975, the Residential Homes Act 1980 and the registered Homes Act 1984. Nursing homes have to register with health authorities, and residential homes with local authority social services departments, thus extending the ill-defined concept of two kinds of institution into the voluntary and private sector. Establishments which are incorporated by Royal charter are exempt from registration.

Section 17 of the Chronically Sick and Disabled Persons Act 1970 states that, so far as practicable, persons under 65 who are suffering from chronic illness or disability, and who are in hospital for long-term care, should not be cared for in any part of the hospital which is normally used wholly or mainly for the care of elderly persons 'unless he is himself ... suffering from the effects of premature ageing'. A Ministry of Health memorandum in the same year tried to clarify this concept by describing it as deterioration to such a degree that the environment of an old people's ward would be just as appropriate. Sections 17 and 18 of the Act required that information about all persons under the age of 65 who are living in hospital wards, nursing homes and residential homes which are primarily intended for old people, should be placed annually before Parliament.

Patterns of housing for disabled people

Physical modifications to the domestic environment may be required because of obligatory wheelchair use, or inability for other reasons (such as arthritis or cardiorespiratory failure) to negotiate steps and stairs, or limited reach for other reasons (such as arthritis, paralysis or inability to stoop), or inability/limited ability to use the hands. The majority of these modifications can be and are provided by adaptations to existing dwellings, and are outside the scope of this chapter. They therefore do not require specially built housing and the consequent relocation, unless the required adaptations would be impossible or uneconomic in existing property; in practice this applies only to wheelchair living. Moreover, rehousing should not be confused with the need for intensive programmes of support and care; it may even hinder such programmes, if for example a person moves away from a neighbourhood where people are willing for personal reasons to contribute informal support. Nevertheless some special housing schemes do have special care programmes incorporated in them, and at least one is even registered as a residential home.

Another motive for rehousing may be a perceived element of risk requiring occasional but unpredictable outside help. People who live alone are obviously vulnerable in this way, and disabilities which increase the risk of falling are one obvious reason why they might be. Both these predicaments are especially likely in old age, and help to explain the popularity of sheltered housing schemes for the elderly. All that is really necessary, however, is some form of alarm, telephone link, or surveillance system, the exact nature of which should depend on the nature of the likely risk and the likely ability of the person(s) at risk to operate any equipment. Communication technology now makes almost any system practicable in any household, and reduces the need for relocation on these grounds alone (Chapter 48).

A newly built dwelling may, of course, be specially commissioned by or on behalf of a disabled person, but most 'purpose-built' housing for disabled people is provided in a range of off-the-peg schemes which may be classified in the following ways. Only the first three are at all common in the United Kingdom.

(1) Isolated wheelchair units in ordinary neighbourhoods.

(2) Similar units which are, however, grouped within the neighbourhood but have no special arrangements for support and care.

(3) Similar groupings with the services of one or more attendants who are often called wardens; this is the category most often referred to as 'sheltered housing'.

(4) Units which form part of a community of households which undertakes, as a condition of tenancy, to provide mutual help.

(5) Units with personal care services as an integral part of the tenancy.

(6) Units attached to a residential home or hospital, from which services are available as required.

(7) A separate village community.

Eligibility for special housing belonging to local authorities is the same as for any other prospective tenant, and usually demands prior residence in an authority's area. In most cases applications are made to housing departments, but assessments of need are usually made by occupational therapists attached to the corresponding social services departments; some authorities require medical assessments too. Methods of establishing priority for allocation vary from one authority to another. Tenancy agreements often state that when a property is no longer required for a disabled person the remaining occupants will be offered another suitable home. Comprehensive information about property belonging to housing associations can at present only be obtained by a round of enquiries: the allocation systems vary from one association to another and all too often success is largely a matter of chance.

Residential care

Some of the indications for relocation have already been discussed. It is important to recognise that residential care should not be recommended too soon in the course of a progressive illness or a deteriorating household situation, or become too easy an option when, two or three months after the acquisition of a severe disability, further rehabilitation is evidently going to be difficult. It only becomes essential when every option for rehabilitation and household support has been fully exploited, or if a household is so fractious that the care, contentment and especially the safety of the dependent disabled person is manifestly at risk. On the other hand some residential homes argue that, with progressive diseases such as multiple sclerosis, they prefer to admit their residents relatively early so that the staff can get to know them before the diseases take their toll of personality as well as physical capability.

Essentially there are two patterns of residential care, which can be described as the medical and the alternative or ('social') models (Table 38.1). The medical model is almost always inappropriate as a long-term way of living, both for residents and for staff, and there is much confusion about the disabilities which are considered to require it. Because nursing skills are so obviously relevant to the care of severely disabled people it is often believed that trained nurses are always necessary, and that the health services should assume administrative responsibility where they are. Yet experience in homes where the alternative model is operated, not to mention experience of care in private household, shows that neither proposition is correct: when disabilities are unchanging, and carers have close

Table 38.1: The medical model and the alternative model of residential care: some distinguishing features

	Medical model	Alternative model
Customer		
title	Patient	Client or resident
status	Recipient of care	Participatory recipient of care
Environment		
general layout	Emphasis on service given (nursing)	Emphasis on domesticity
bedrooms	Emphasis on ease of observation	Emphasis on privacy and personal choice
Decision-making		
management	Divided between medicine, administration and nursing	Delegated to person in charge
clinical/casework	Medical prerogative	Emphasis on social work and client's consent
Staff		
qualifications	Strong emphasis on nursing	Variety of special training or none
clothing	Uniforms	No uniforms
Occupying the customer's time	Centred on remedial therapy	Centred on diversional or workshop activity

Source: Royal College of Physicians Report (1986) (reproduced with permission).

and regular acquaintance with the people they care for, whatever their previous experience, they can learn the necessary skills. Very often the medical model is adopted more for reasons of history and convenience than because of any fundamental need.

Given that medical, surgical and diagnostic procedures, especially in the management of acute illness or injury, are not recognised functions of residential homes and units, there are nevertheless *five distinct tasks* with which these institutions may be involved: *rehabilitation, planned short stay, the ability to respond to certain kinds of emergency, terminal care of people with disabling disease, and committed long-term care.* This last is the function which is most often expected, and which requires the provision of a home and an acceptable way of life. In some instances *a sixth function, day care,* may also be included, although it is strictly a contradiction in terms. The five or six tasks do not have to be performed in the same place, although they all may be: the first four are commonly associated with the medical model but none of the six has to be. It is therefore not surprising that policies and practice vary according to the managing agency, the availability of resources elsewhere in the locality, and in many cases decisions made by the residential units themselves.

Residential and nursing homes in the *voluntary and private sectors* occupy a variety of premises in a variety of environments, from remotely situated country houses to unobtrusive suburban dwellings or modern purpose-built complexes. The management style varies too, adopting either the medical or the alternative model but frequently a hybrid of both. Most homes take pride in offering residents a home for life, and partly for that reason they usually reserve the right to choose for themselves the people they admit, often involving their existing residents in the choice. Some homes specialise in particular diseases, usually because of their ownership and management (The Spastics Society and the Multiple Sclerosis Society, for example) but also because a particular commitment may simply have seemed appropriate to them. The Cheshire Homes have made such a big contribution to the residential care of younger disabled people that in some parts of the country they are regarded as the principal provider of that service (Table 38.2).

Local authority homes almost universally avoid the medical model. Although at first many of them occupied old or adapted buildings the policy has been for these to be closed, so that the majority are now purpose-built. Nearly all are therefore in situations where the authority happened to have land, which means that they are usually part of a housing development. Architecturally they are rather stereotyped, with single bedrooms opening off corridors, a large communal dining area and several sitting rooms. More recent designs have tended to group the bedrooms round smaller communal facilities which give an opportunity for self-catering. The staff are often apprehensive about accepting responsibility for

Table 38.2: Organisation of institutional residential care in the United Kingdom (RCP Report, 1986)

Type of institution	Accountable to	Financed by
National Health Service	District and Regional Health Authorities Central Government (Secretary of State for Health and Social Security)	National taxation
Local authority	Social Services Committees	Means-tested fee-for-service Local rates National taxation
Voluntary: registered charity	Charities Commission Local registering authority (District Health Authority and/or Social Services Department* of the local authority)	Means-tested fee-for-service Board and lodging payments (Social Security)
Voluntary with Royal Charter	The Crown	Fee-for-service grants from District Health Authorities and/or Social Services*
Private	Local registering authority (District Health Authority and/or Social Services Department* of the local authority)	

* Known as Departments of Social Work in Scotland. In Northern Ireland the responsibilities of local health and social services departments are combined.

people who might require nursing care, although these fears may have more to do with low staffing levels than a real need for technical expertise. For this reason the local authorities tend to refuse admission when levels of dependency are high.

National Health Service wards and units almost always follow the medical model, as might be expected; although a few units have tried to escape it their efforts have not been very successful. Even the newest buildings have failed to provide an environment which could realistically be called domestic, and the routines of hospital administration and conventional nursing are usually very prominent: dormitory bedrooms and large communal day areas are the rule. Partly no doubt to escape from these rather dismal ways of providing committed long-term care, many have diverted their emphasis to the other possible functions of a residential unit, although they may also have had these functions thrust upon them. The units can and do refuse residence to people whom they consider inappropriate, but they are nevertheless very vulnerable to pressures to admit, especially from other hospital departments. Decisions about admission are traditionally assumed by hospital consultants, whose discretion it is whether to involve staff or residents in the process.

Financially, the three different systems within which residential care is provided have different consequences for the residents. People who live in voluntary or private homes are not eligible for supplementary benefit until each person's own capital has fallen to £3,000 (in 1986). For residents supported by local authorities the arrangement is similar except that most authorities allow personal disposable capital to fall to £1,250 before they take over full financial responsibility. The National Health Service is unable to make any board-and-lodging charges, even for residents who have received injury compensation awards in the courts. Personal disposable income in residential care of course includes income from private sources and certain non-taxable State benefits, especially the Mobility Allowance which is payable if the disability which justifies it began before the age of 65. Otherwise, 'pocket money' payments are reduced to £7.65 per week for residents financed by local authorities and in National Health Service care. The legislation, and the precise way in which it is implemented, are constantly changing, so the figures quoted in this paragraph are soon likely to be out of date.

To some degree conflicts are inevitable between the desire to construct and preserve a harmonious residential community and the need to provide asylum for any person who may require it, and between the guarantee of a secure place in which to live and the ability to respond quickly to requests for admission. Waiting lists can be very long, indeed so long as sometimes to be meaningless: few homes or units admit people simply because of the length of time they have been waiting, and in recognition of that fact many prefer simpy to accept or reject without establishing waiting lists at all. In principle, if more places were available the conflicts might be reduced, but resources and attention would then be diverted further away from community care, and requests for admission would almost certainly increase, as experience in countries such as Canada, Australia, the Netherlands and Sweden has shown.

As with specialised housing, there is no standardised way of seeking admission. In the voluntary/private sector applications are usually made direct to individual homes, but some have to be routed through a national agency. Local authority homes commonly restrict their help to the populations of their own districts, and nearly always require a social-work assessment: social workers therefore usually process the applications, which often involve much paperwork. Hospital and hospital units in most cases also work to catchment areas but require little more than a consultant's acceptance. There is, however, an increasing tendency for local authorities to ask for specialist medical assessment, and for hospitals to request social work help before final decisions are made. Arrangements differ in detail from one locality to another.

Whatever the precise reasons why individual people enter residential care, there is a remarkably uniform pattern of disabling diseases and injuries among the residents, as follows:

80 per cent are conditions which involve or potentially involve the brain;
10 per cent are disorders of the spinal cord or peripheral nervous system;
10 per cent are other disabling conditions.

The disabilities may also be classified according to whether they are:

stable, such as cerebral palsy, head injury, spinal injury and some cases of stroke;
unstable, such as many cases of stroke and multiple sclerosis;
progressive, such as muscular dystrophy, motor neurone disease, and again many cases of multiple sclerosis.

More than half the residents in homes and units for younger disabled people have either multiple sclerosis or cerebral palsy: in hospital units for old people the equivalent conditions are stroke and senile dementia. Disabilities which are congenital or date from childhood are much more likely to be found in residential homes than in hospital units, but acquired disabilities are catered for in all kinds of residential care.

Principal deficiencies of existing resources

A major problem is that although genuine consumer choice exists for a tiny minority of disabled people, hardly any district has a comprehensive set of resources catering adequately for all kinds of disabling predicament. Collaborative planning and opertional policies involving the different agencies remain exceptional: health services, social services and the various voluntary organisations usually pursue their own objectives, all spending public money yet relatively unconcerned about deficiences and lack of choice, which they do not regard as their particular responsibilities. Difficulties are notably troublesome for younger physically disabled people, for whom an absence of clear commitment within the hospital service adds further confusion.

Boundaries of responsibility give plenty of scope for disagreement, even geographical boundaries which, although easily defined, are rarely coterminous for the different agencies. Four important issues regularly recur: the discontinuity and withdrawal of services when people pass school-leaving age; the distinction between medical/nursing and non-medical responsibilities to which reference has already been made; the problems of physically disabled people who have brain impairment and (especially) disturbed behaviour, and of mentally ill or mentally handicapped people who have physical disabilities; and the difficulty or impossibility of drawing a line between young or 'younger' people and 'the elderly'. These last two issues require a little more comment.

The failure to provide more than a tiny handful of services which cater for the behavioural consequences of acquired brain impairment, and are based on sound practice and understanding, is a major source of unhappiness. The people who have the disabilities all too often can feel, and in fact are, socially rejected, not just by their close partner and families but by otherwise caring institutions too. Those who stay in private households are often the cause of tremendous tensions, if only because supporting services are so commonly unhelpful or unsympathetic. The staff of the institutions which do accept them are often bewildered by the behaviour patterns they are presented with, for which their education and training has given no relevant preparation. The whole area of responsibility urgently needs new initiatives.

Despite the undoubted frustrations of young disabled people, severe disability in late middle age and early pensionable age is not only much more prevalent but also less sensitively catered for. Neither very old nor very young, most disabled people in this age range are expected to put up with residential services which are orientated principally towards 'the elderly', and severely disabled stroke victims often get a particularly bad deal. Social Security benefits payable because of disability also diminish after retirement age. The issue of ageing and disability can indeed be hopelessly confused, to the extent that ageing is often equated with brain injury. More sympathetic provision for this group of people and their carers is another urgent need.

While it is easy to point out deficiencies, it is less easy to make definite statements about the resources that every district should possess. Between the ages of 16 and 65 there are about 36 physically disabled people in residential care for each 100,000 total population in the United Kingdom as a whole, but the geographical distribution is uneven and more than half are in ordinary hospital wards or old people's homes. Evidence is also accumulating that many of them could just as well be in private households. The equivalent number of people over the age of 65 is many times greater, by a factor somewhere in the region of 10. Outside residential care there are almost 100 people aged 16–65 whose physical disabilities are severe enough to justify possible relocations, again for each 100,000 total population: only a quarter of them are likely to be under 45, whereas half are over the age of 55. The equivalent number of people over 65 is nearly three times as great.

Clearly the 'necessary' provisions depend on many factors besides numbers: they include the expectations and living standards of the local community and the availability of domiciliary support and care. Equally important is the perceived division of responsibilities between the various services for the main dependent groups: people with mental illness and mental handicap, old people, and the younger physically disabled. There is sketchy evidence that Health Service units for this last group may need no more than five beds per 100,000 total population; since in management terms an effective unit may well require the resources which are likely to go with 20 beds or more, each one would therefore need to serve a population of at least 400,000. Any such conclusion depends, however, not only on the factors already mentioned but also on the resources provided by the voluntary/private and local-authority sectors of residential care, and the extent to which the special units might take over the existing functions of some general hospital wards.

SUMMARY AND CONCLUSIONS

Housing and residential care must not be considered in isolation, but as integral parts of a full service to dependent disabled people and their careers. Services in the United Kingdom have developed in a tripartite fashion, according to whether they are managed by voluntary or private agencies (almost always subsidised by public funds), local authorities, or the National Health Service. The diversity has produced a wide range of resources but it has also produced uncoordinated developments, so that real choice is a rarity and inappropriate responses are frequent. The demands for special housing arise chiefly from obligatory wheelchair use; demands for residential care overwhelmingly relate to diseases and injuries which involve or potentially involve the brain, and to a relatively small number of other people with severe impairment of all four limbs. The most urgent priority for development is better-judged targeting of resources to the realities of dependent disability and the reasonable aspirations of severely disabled people.

SUGGESTIONS FOR FURTHER READING

Brattgard, S.O. (1972) Fokus: a way of life for living. In D. Lancaster-Gaye (ed.), *Personal relationships, the handicapped and the community: some European thoughts and solutions: Sweden*, Routledge & Kegan Paul, London, pp. 25-40
(Describes a pioneer scheme with a personal care service as an integral part of the tenancy)

Clough, R. (1982) *Residential Work*, Macmillian, London
(An admirable account of the principles of managing residential units: well worth reading)

Dartington, T., Miller, E. and Gwynne, G. (1981) *A life together*, Tavistock Publications, London
(Includes descriptions of a housing scheme of the Fokus type, and of an innovative system of residential care)

Davis, K. (1981) 28-38 Grove Road: accommodation and care in a community setting. In A. Brechin, P. Liddiard and J. Swain (eds), *Handicap in a social world*, Hodder and Stoughton, London, pp. 322-7

(Describes a pioneer housing scheme in which able-bodied tenants help to support tenants who are disabled)

The Disability Alliance (1985) *Disability rights handbook*, 10th edn, section L8, pp. 118-30.
(Sets out the financial rights and obligations of people in residential care: new editions published at regular intervals)

Goldsmith, S. (1976) *Designing for the disabled.* 3rd edn, RIBA, London
(A compendium volume, full of information about housing)

Harrison, J. (1986) *The young disabled adult*, Royal College of Physicians, London

Harrison, J. (1987) Severe physical disability: responses to the challenge of care. Cassell, London (two complementary accounts based on tenure of a research fellowship of The Royal College of Physicians of London)

Home life: a code of practice for residential care (1984) Report of a working party sponsored by the Department of Health and Social Security and convened by the Centre for Policy on Ageing. Centre for Policy on Ageing, London
(Important because it sets national standards, but only for residential homes: it makes the assumption that nursing homes are necessarily different)

Inskip, P.H. (1981) *Leonard Cheshire Foundation Handbook of Care (1). Residential homes for the physically handicapped*, Bedford Square Press, London
(Similar to *Home life*, but shorter and without the residential home/nursing home distinction)

King, R.D., Ranes, N.V. and Tizard, J. (1971) *Patterns of residential care: sociological studies in institutions for handicapped children*, Routledge & Kegan Paul, London
(A classic study highlighting the deficiencies of hospital care)

McCoy, L. (1978) *Policy issues in residential care: a discussion document*, Personal Social Services Council, London
(An excellent review of history and legislation)

Martin, J.P. (1984) *Hospitals in trouble*, Basil Blackwell, Oxford
(Reviews recent enquiries into standards of care in mental handicap hospitals: relevant because of its conclusions about management responsibility)

Miller, E.J. and Gwynne, G.V. (1972) *A life apart: a pilot study of residential institutions for the physically handicapped and the young chronic sick*, Tavistock Publications, London
(Another classic study in the context of the younger physically disabled)

The Prince of Wales' Advisory Group on Disability (1985) *Living Options*, London
(A checklist of requirements, which helps to set housing and residential care into perspective)

Spath, F. (1977) *How the Cheshire Homes started*, Leonard Cheshire Foundation, London
(An instructive piece of history)

39

Housing Modifications

David Hughes

INTRODUCTION

Life can be a great struggle for many, particularly if the person's home is damp, inconvenient or inhospitable. Poor home circumstances may make it quite impossible for a disabled person to remain there, or for someone newly disabled to return home from hospital. On the other hand, severely handicapped adults such as quadriplegics can live comfortably and happily in their home for many years, even without a companion if the home environment is right for the individual. This is not always a costly exercise but usually depends on the installation of aids and adaptations to the person's needs, and such help should be obtained as soon as possible.

AIDS AND ADAPTATIONS

Help available

Finding help can be difficult both for the disabled person and the professional. The key people in providing help in the first instance are the hospital consultant or GP, so that it is essential they have an understanding of what statutory provision is available, and which professional person to refer to in order that the patient receives maximum help and support. Leaflet HB I, *Help for handicapped people,* which is available from the local Social Security office or by post from the DHSS Leaflets Unit, explains what help is available and the method of referral. If more details are required the *Disability rights handbook* is a valuable asset.

District Health Authority

We are here assuming that medical and nursing loans are obtained from the Health Service and aids to daily living from Social Services. Arrangements may differ from place to place and local provision should be ascertained. Some health authorities and social services operate a joint loans system with a common store accessible to professionals from both sources, e.g. Leicester supply home nursing aids on loan through their Community Loans Service via local health centres. Common items include incontinence products, commodes and hospital beds. Contact local health centre, health visitor, district nurse, GP.

Hospital

Aids can be supplied direct from the local hospital (usually by the occupational therapist or physiotherapist) where the patient can be fully assessed. The occupational therapist can provide aids to daily living and advice on home adaptations, the physiotherapist advising on appropriate walking aids and appliances. Communication aids are usually supplied through the speech therapist (Chapter 15). Environmental controls are supplied after assessment by a consultant medical assessor (Chapter 48).

Local authority

The local authority is responsible for housing, social services and education. Each authority will allocate its resources differently, and requests for assistance should be directed through the appropriate department.

The Department of Social Services usually provides aids to daily living, e.g. bathing, toileting, eating, dressing and feeding. For both these and home adaptations contact the relevant occupational therapist or Area Manager in Social Services. *The Housing Department* provides suitable housing or adaptations to *council* property. Many provide improvement grants. Contact the local Housing Manager or Social Service OT. *Environmental health* — improvement and intermediate grants (for privately owned housing) are usually administered by environmental health officers, although some authorities use the Housing Department. *Improvement grants* are discretionary and are used to provide improved facilities for a disabled person and include help towards extensions. *Intermediate grants* are mandatory, and are used for providing standard amenities like a bath or WC, if the existing facilities are inaccessible to the disabled person.

Circular 59/78, *Adaptations for people who are physically handicapped*, lists items which can be considered for grant purposes (see Appendix). Since the Departments of Social Services arrange for adaptations to be carried out, they may be involved in contributing towards the outstanding cost after the grants have been paid. Privately rented accommodation may also be eligible for grants, and the environmental health officer will advise accordingly.

SIMPLE HOUSING ADAPTATIONS

Adapting a house can involve many agencies and be a complicated and time-consuming task. It is important to contact the Social Services Department where the community occupational therapist will coordinate the services and, more importantly, liaise and keep the client informed of progress.

With any adaptation the client's prognosis and long-term needs have to be clearly established from the outset. With the more severely handicapped the needs of the carer(s) take equal priority when determining appropriate adaptations. Usually a decision has to be made whether to adapt the existing house or move to more suitable accommodation. In either case it is imperative that the family consult the community occupational therapist who will liaise with the consultant, GP, housing manager and possibly environmental health officer when making the decision to adapt or rehouse. Consideration should be given to the considerable support often given by neighbours and family, vicinity of shops and local resources; the amount of space inside the house allowing adequate wheelchair circulation; the width of the hallway and staircase and its style. Can a stairlift or through-floor lift be installed? Can an extension be built on to the property? No house is likely to be ideal, and the positive and negative aspects of each potential solution have to be considered before a decision is reached. The house must at least be suitable for adapting. Furthermore, there is a temptation for the family to accept alternative accommodation only to find, after a short period of time, that the property is unsuitable, leading to more frustration.

The following section briefly outlines the most common areas to consider when adapting the disabled person's home. Each case has to be individually assessed according to the person's needs and the accommodation available. For those planning accommodation intended for the disabled the bibliography lists those texts and organisations able to provide help and advice in this field.

ACCESS

If a car is essential then garage facilities or a hard standing near the house should be available allowing enough space for a wheelchair transfer if required. The kerb outside the house may need to be dropped. The garden should afford an area to allow the person to sit out, and the pathways be wide enough to allow wheelchair access (100–120 cm). Either the front or rear door should provide suitable level access; hand-rails and grab-rails can be provided for the ambulant disabled or alternatively ramped for wheelchair access, if possible.

RAMPS

The preferred ramp gradient is 1:20 for the wheelchair user who can propel himself independently. The maximum gradient is 1:12. A level platform should be constructed outside the entrance door, and with a long ramp a rest platform should be provided at a maximum of 10 metres. Surfaces should be non-slip, edged and with hand-rails on the outside. Temporary ramps can be constructed in timber, or alternatively metal channels can be provided.

DOORS

The minimum clear opening width should be 75 cm for wheelchair use. All doors should be checked and widened if necessary to offer maximum circulation space (this is expensive). Raised thresholds can be overcome with an internal wooden ramp. Door handles should be of the lever type. When space is limited consideration should be given to sliding or folding doors, or re-hanging so that the door swings in the reverse direction.

WC (Figure 39.1)

Simple aids can be provided to allow a person to get up and down from the lavatory: these include raised toilet seats, toilet frames and rails secured to the adjacent wall at the height to meet the needs of the individual. When adapting for wheelchair use there should be sufficient space to allow wheelchair access, usually assuming a sideways transfer. It is important to note the method of transfer, and whether the person requires the assistance of a carer, to provide adequate space when planning for future needs. If an over-toilet chair is to be used then there should be no obstruction. Hardwear can include toilet-paper holder for one-handed operation, low mirror, lever taps on shallow hand basin, etc., to suit the individual needs.

BATHING

This is the most common area of concern since most elderly and physically handicapped people seek help when they are unable to bathe independently. The occupational therapist can assess needs. Most people are helped by simple aids, a non-slip mat, a bath board and seat and a grab-rail secured to the wall are provided, and the person is instructed in their use, the aim being to enable the person to enter and leave the bath safely, preferably from a seated position. when conventional aids are unsuitable then consideration should be given to bath hoists (Chapter 44).

Figure 39.1: WC layout: (a) plan view; (b) side view. Ideal dimensions for lavatory for a disabled person in a wheelchair (dimensions in millimetres)

Key: C coat hook at 1500 mm
F flushing handle on transfer side
G fixed grab-rails
G1 hinged support rail at 700 mm height
L lever handle with inside bolt and outside quick release at 1040 mm height
M mirror 400 mm wide × 900 mm high, fixed at 900 mm from floor
P toilet paper holder for single-handed use
S soap dispenser
T towel dispenser
W waste towel receptacle
Basin: shallow hand-rinse fitting with lever spray mixer tap.
Light switch: near door on opening side at height of 1040 mm.
Alarm bell pull cord with ring, near WC and basin.

(a)

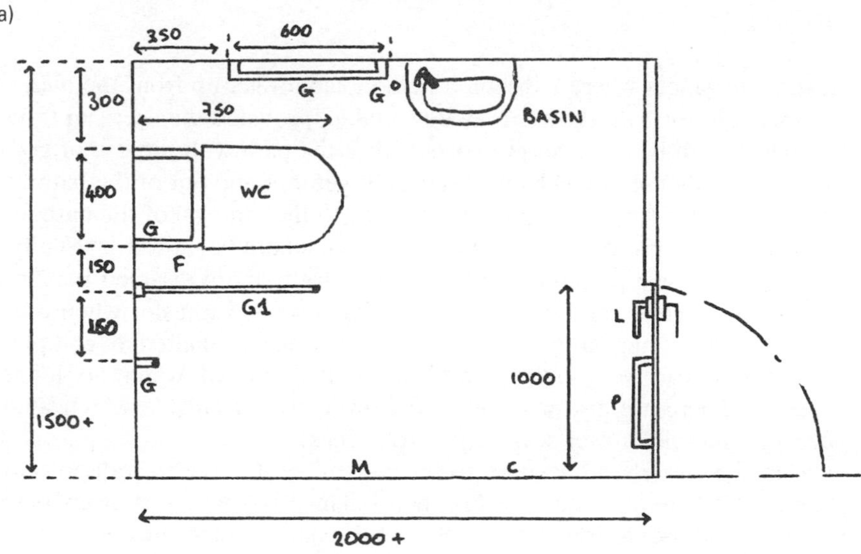

Figure 39.1: continued

(b)

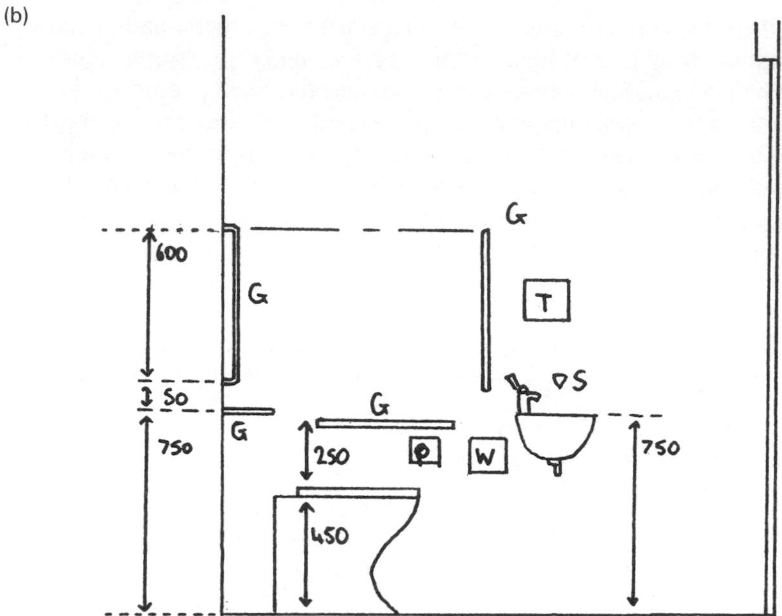

(Figures 39.1a and 39.1b are taken from publications of the Centre on Environment for the Handicapped, by kind permission of the Access Committee for England)

SHOWER

In some instances where a disabled person cannot get up from the bath or bath seat an overbath shower may be suitable, provided the user can transfer onto a bath board to shower or stand in the bath with the use of grabrails. When the use of mechanical hoists to get into and out of the bath has been discounted, then thought can be given to the removal of the bath and installation of a shower. The decision between a bath or shower is usually a matter of personal preference. However, with the more disabled person a toilet/shower chair can be used, eliminating a second transfer when using the WC and giving good support. Where space is limited a complete shower unit can be provided, and is easily removed when no longer required. There are also a variety of shower bases available which allow access for mobile shower seats, e.g. Ambi-deck.

Folding shower seats secured to the wall allow the user to walk into the shower and take a seated shower when balance is poor. A shower bench will allow the user to transfer from his wheelchair into the shower.

Tiled shower floors which have a slight incline to drain water away allow the use of over-toilet/shower chairs which give easy access to the WC and shower. The floor should slope approximately 76 mm to the drain outlet, and the tiles should be non-slip. The shower must be thermostatically controlled and non-conductive grab-rails should be used.

Plumbed-in units are usually more suitable than the instant-heat types, provided the cold water tank is in the correct position to given an adequate water pressure. Appropriate controls to allow, for example, a rheumatoid sufferer to operate the shower independently, or the carer to remain outside the shower, should be provided. Shower chairs can be easily operated by the carer, or can be self-propelled by the user, giving greater independence and privacy.

KITCHEN

The design of the wheelchair kitchen

As described in the 'Pilot study of disabled housewives', the work sequence of the disabled person is similar to that of the able-bodied, although the disabled person will take longer to carry out tasks. Therefore the design should be carefully chosen in order to cut down the number of journeys and amount of energy expenditure each task entails. There are various texts covering this subject: *Design for the disabled*; *An introduction to domestic design for the disabled*; *Spaces in the home*; *Kitchen sense for disabled or elderly people* (see Refs). Many books give recommended heights for kitchen design, but ideally the kitchen should be tailored to the individual's needs where possible. BSI standards for height apply only to people of average height. Several kitchen units are manufactured specifically for disabled people: contact local Disabled Living Centre for information.

STAIRLIFTS (see also Chapter 44)

Contact the Department of Social Services: they will advise on whether the house is suitable for a lift and which type will be most satisfactory. In most cases consideration will have to be given to rehousing, or a possible ground floor extension, depending upon the nature of the disability and in particular the prognosis. It is important to determine as accurately as possible the disabled person's future needs, especially if the disability is progressive and there is any likelihood of the person requiring a wheelchair in the future.

A lift should only be considered if the disabled person will use the upstairs facilities, and where the bathroom and WC are adequate or can be adapted for present and future needs. Before installing a lift the occupational therapist and client must be convinced that such an expensive solution is the only sensible answer to the problem (Figure 39.2).

GROUND FLOOR EXTENSION

When both rehousing and the provision of adaptations to the present property are found to be unsatisfactory, then application for an extension should be made. An extension will provide additional ground floor space to incorporate the facilities required by the disabled person, and thus allow full independence and privacy without encroaching on the often limited space used by other members of the family.

It is not easy to get an extension built to high standards; the process of planning and of grant provision may be lengthy and involved, and the patient needs the help of the occupational therapist who will liaise with the

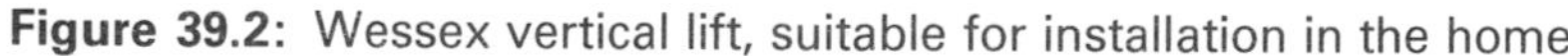

Figure 39.2: Wessex vertical lift, suitable for installation in the home

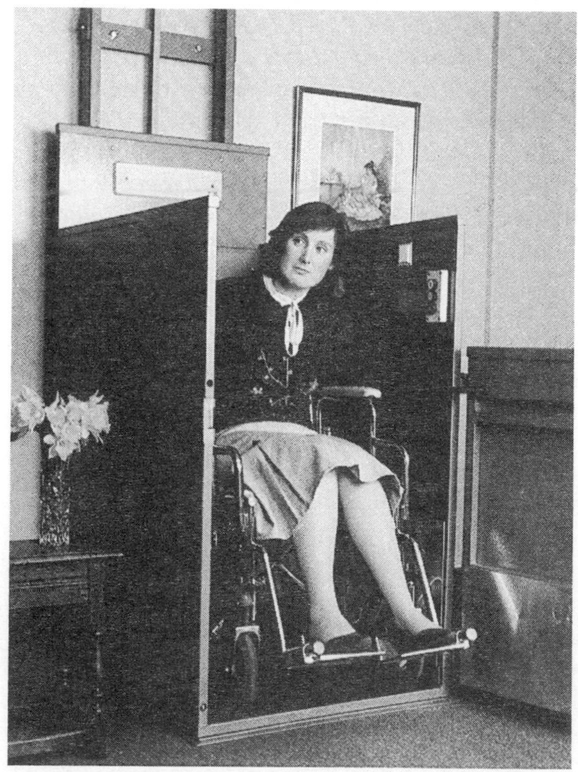

Department of Environmental Health and others. Equally important, the architect involved must be given as much relevant information as possible on the client's projected needs and, in turn, the detailed specifications should be adhered to by the builder. The occupational therapist should scrutinise the architect's plans before work commences.

It must be remembered that extensions are expensive, especially when a bedroom is incorporated and all financial aspects of the grant and topping up (i.e. the balance between the total cost and grant awarded) must be determined before starting the work. Extensions fully adapted for a disabled person do not necessarily increase the value of the property, and in some cases may actually make the sale of the house more difficult.

DISABLED LIVING CENTRES (AIDS CENTRES)

Disabled Living Centres provide a resource for professionals, disabled people and their friends to look at a vast array of equipment of potential use to the disabled person. The centres are manned by professionals who are able to provide advice and reference material on many of the possible solutions to the problems discussed in this chapter (and to many other related matters) (Chapter 49).

APPENDIX/BIBLIOGRAPHY

Designing for Disability. CEH Sheets:
(1) *Entrances*; (2) *Windows*; (3) *Bathrooms*; (4) *Kitchens*; (5) *Floor finishes*; (6) *Bedrooms*; (7) *Lifts*; (8) *Controls*; (9) *Safety.* Centre on Environment for the Handicapped, 126 Albert Street, London NW1 7NF (Publish information on the subject)

British Standards Institution (1979) *Code of Practice for Access for the Disabled to Buildings BS5810: 1979*, BS1, London

Goldsmith, Selwyn (1976) *Designing for the disabled*, 3rd edn, fully revised, RIBA Publications, London (Standard book on the subject)

Royal Association for Disability and Rehabilitation Access Data Sheets: (1) *Approach to buildings*; (2) *Doors*; (3) *Internal circulation areas*; (4) *Lifts*; (5) *Internal staircases*; (6) *Lavatories*; (7) *Auditoria*; (8) *Induction loop systems*, RADAR, London

Thorpe, Stephen (1981) *Access in the High Street: advice on how to make shopping more manageable for disabled people*, Centre on Environment for the Handicapped, London

'Disabled housewives in their kitchens': a series of one-day conferences, June 1969, Disabled Living Foundation

Made to measure — domestic extensions and adaptations for physically handicapped people, Cheshire County Council, 1980.

Foott, Sydney (1977) *Handicapped at home* (A Design Centre Book), Design Council, 28 Haymarket, London SW1

Boswell, D.M. and Wingrove, J.M. (eds), (1974) *The Handicapped person in the community*, Open University

Conacher, Gwen (ed.) (1986) *Kitchen sense for disabled people*, Croom Helm, London, for the Disabled Living Foundation,

Mobility housing. DOE/HDD Occasional Paper 2/74. DOE, 2 Masham Street, London SW1D 3EB

Housing for special needs — the physically handicapped. Scottish Local Authorities Special Housing Group, 53 Melville Street, Edinburgh

Access for disabled people: design guidance notes for developers. CEH, March 1985.

Hunt, J. (1980) *Housing the disabled*, Torfaen Book Co., Cwmbran, Wales

Adaptations of housing for people who are physically handicapped, HMSO, London; Department of Environment Circular 59/78, 1978 15 BN 0 117513369

Penton, J. and Barlow, A (1980) *A Handbook of Housing for Disabled People*, 2nd edn, London Housing Consortium West Group

Tarling, C. (1980) *Hoists and their users*, Disabled Living Foundation

Houine, P.M. (1968) *A pilot study of disabled housewives in their kitchens*, Disabled Living Foundatiopn

Walter, F. (1970) *An introduction to domestic design for the disabled*. Disabled Living Foundation

Spaces in the Home — DOE Design Bulletin 24, Pt 2., HMSO, London

BS 3705: 1972 BSI Recommendations for provision of space for domestic kitchen equipment, HMSO, London

Selected legislation — housing and environment

Practitioners in this field should be aware of the following:

Local Authority Social Services Act 1970

National Assistance Act 1948 — Section 29

Chronically Sick and Disabled Persons Act 1970 — Sections 1, 2, 3-8

Disabled Persons Act 1981 — Sections 1, 2, 3, 4, 5, 6, 7

Disabled Persons (Employment) Act 1944 — Section 1

Public Sector Housing Act 1957

DOE Circular 59/78 (WO 104/78), Adaptations of Housing for people who are physically handicapped

Private Sector Housing

Housing Act 1980

DOE Circular 36/81 (WO 56/81) Housing Acts 1974 and 1980. House Renovation Grants for the Disabled.

Designing for the disabled, by Selwyn Goldsmith, is internationally acclaimed as the foremost in its field and should be consulted by architects, planners and others when designing adaptations for the disabled.

Manufacturers of equipment

Autolift, Mecanaids Ltd., St Catherine Street, Gloucester GL1 2BX

Mangar Bath Lift, Mangar Aids Ltd, Presteigne Industrial Estate, Presteigne, Powys

Aqua-jac Bath Lift, Llewellyn & Co Ltd, Carlton Works, Carlton Street, Liverpool, Merseyside, L3 7ED

Commodore Hoist, SML Ltd, Bath Place, High Street, Barnet, Herts EN5 5XE
Wessex Hoist, Wessex Medical Equipment Co Ltd, Unit 2, Budds Lane Industrial Estate, Romsey, Hants SO5 0HA
Chiltern Shower Unit, Chiltern Medical Developments Ltd, Chiltern House, Wedgewood Road, Bicester, Oxon OX6 7UL
Ambi-deck Shower Tray, J.W. Swain (Plastics) Ltd, Byron Street, Buxton, Derbyshire SK17 6LY

40

Further Education for the Young Adult with a Physical Disability

Alastair Kent

INTRODUCTION

Consider the situation facing a young person with a significant congenital disability as he or she approaches the end of the statutory period of schooling. There is a wide range of options (Figure 40.1) potentially available for an individual to choose from when planning the next stage. If anything, the choice for the young disabled person is theoretically greater than for his able-bodied counterpart, although in practice it may be severely limited by a number of factors, both educational and non-educational in nature.

For the able-bodied school-leaver at 16+ the options are initially restricted to the choice between remaining in full-time education, either by staying on at school or transferring to the local college of further education, or by leaving education and seeking work. This can be either a job, or more usually through one or other of the programmes provided by the Manpower Services Commission as part of the Youth Training Scheme. For the able-bodied school-leaver the option of sheltered employment, day care, specialised colleges of further education or long-term care do not even exist in theory, much less in reality.

Of course for the school-leaver with a physical disability some of these options may not exist either — the severity of the impairment may preclude open or sheltered employment, or Local Authority facilities may not be developed to the point where real choice exists. Despite this, disabled school-leavers have the same range of aspirations as anyone else, and the apparent complexity of the system of provision can be very confusing.

Consider also the typical young person leaving a special school or unit for physically handicapped children. In so far as it is possible to generalise, he or she is likely, in addition to a significant degree of impairment, to have spatial and perceptual problems, be immature socially and emotionally (although probably not physically) and present a jagged and unpredictable pattern of academic attainments, either as a result of missed learning, perhaps due to extended periods of hospitalisation during childhood, or as

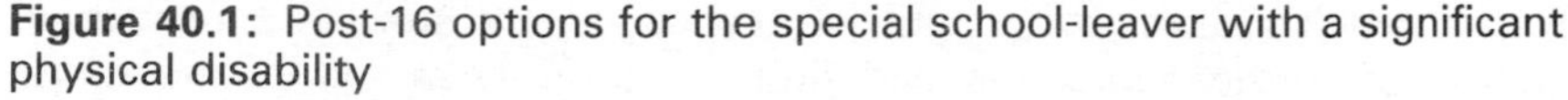

Figure 40.1: Post-16 options for the special school-leaver with a significant physical disability

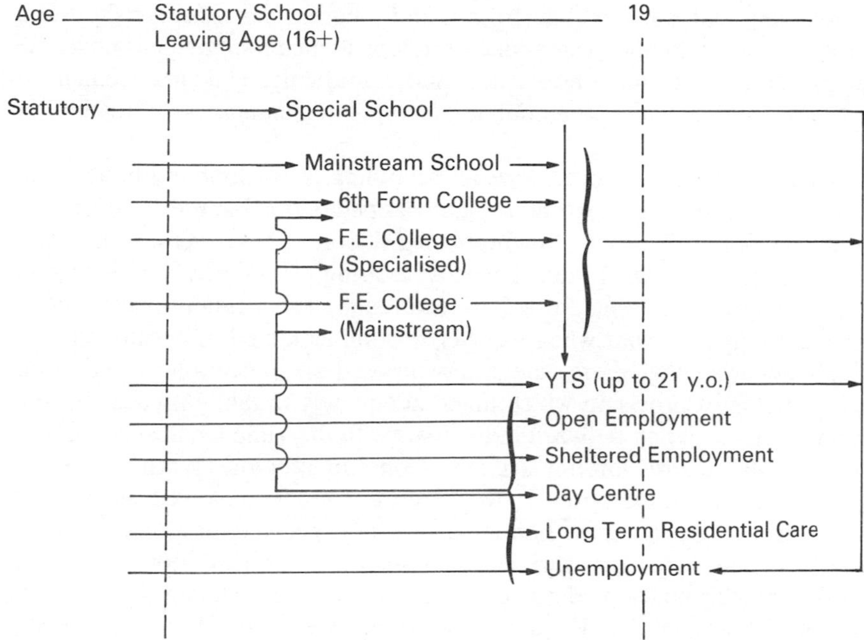

a direct consequence of neurological damage resulting from the handicapping condition. Furthermore this child is likely to have a more restricted experience of everyday life than his or her able-bodied peers as a direct result of increased dependence on others (usually parents).

For able-bodied young people the years leading up to school-leaving age are usually a time of increasing independence as greater mobility and relaxing parental control open up possibilities for new experiences and trial of adult modes of conduct and behaviour. For those who depend on others to open up social situations the opportunity to exercise choice and try new behaviours is necessarily limited by the physical presence of those others, be they carers, parents or other professionals. One has only to think of the activities of able-bodied teenagers that would be curtailed or rendered impossible by the presence of adults to appreciate the restriction of opportunities for the acquisition of adult social competences afforded to young people with severe physical disabilities. As a direct consequence of this, information about adult life, opportunity to make decisions about careers, further education or whatever, based on an accurate understanding of the issues involved and the consequences of each of the possible outcomes, is very restricted. Take, for example, the case of Simon, a 17-year-old boy with cerebellar ataxia who until he started on a course at a residential college of further education had literally never been out of the house without his mother. She had taken him to the taxi which took him to school, and had collected him from it and escorted him wherever he went. Following a systematic programme of independence training he is now able to go out into the community safely and confidently. The enhancement to his quality of life and potential for future independence can readily be imagined.

Until relatively recently special schooling was disability-based and derived from the ten categories of handicapped defined in the 1944 Education Act and subsequent amending legislation. These were: Blind and Partially sighted, Deaf and Partially hearing, Physically handicapped, Delicate, Epileptic, Maladjusted, Educationally subnormal, Speech defective. Although relevant when the Act was implemented, it became increasingly apparent that these categories imposed an unnecessary rigidity on the planning of provision which failed adequately to take into account the tremendous variation between individuals with the same medical condition, or a similar degree of impairment. Consequently the Warnock report (1978) recommended a move away from this model as a basis for special schooling towards one based on the concept of special educational needs — a concept subsequently enshrined in legislation as the 1981 Education Act.

Among the many recommendations of the Warnock report was that: 'A pupil's special needs should be re-assessed with future prospects in mind at least two years before he is due to leave school' (para. 10.7). This has been retained in the 1981 Education Act as a statutory re-assessment between the ages of 13½ and 14½. This assessment is in itself not without controversy. Much research and development has gone into devising tests for the normative evaluation of readily quantifiable skills in a school-based setting, e.g. literacy and numeracy. In these cases it is possible to reach a consensus view of the attainment of the skills being measured — a person can or cannot read or perform a certain mathematical procedure. In others areas not only are the criteria much more subjective, but also the validity and reliability of the methods for measuring them are much less well established.

Further, we have not yet established norms for success in the sufficiency skills of everyday life — those skills which a person must have if he or she is to be able to cope with the demands that will be made by independent adulthood. A satisfactory methodology for the assessment of the majority of school-leavers is still to be established. How much more difficult will it be to achieve for those with significant disabilities?

It is possible to devise a programme which will provide a systematic opportunity for school-leavers with physical disabilities to experience everyday living situations within a supportive and structured environment, thereby enabling progression to be one of the main aims of specialised further educational provision for this group of school-leavers and opening up possibilities for progression into a variety of options for adult life.

AIMS OF POST-16 EDUCATION FOR THE YOUNG ADULT WITH A PHYSICAL DISABILITY

Until comparatively recently the primary option for school-leavers with a physical disability has been to seek work. This has been in direct contrast to their able-bodied peers, who have traditionally seen a period of further education as a necessary precursor to employment. Only as unemployment has risen and formal employment become virtually unavailable to school-leavers with disabilities has active consideration been given to further education for this group of young people.

Traditionally the aim of post-school education has been to provide a skills- and knowledge-based curriculum leading to the acquisition of academic or vocationally relevant qualifications. Some school-leavers with disabilities may be able to transfer directly to mainstream further education courses without difficulty, but many more will have special educational needs which will preclude direct progression onto mainstream courses.

This group of students need a curriculum which will enhance their independence, and which will ensure that — given the limitations imposed by physical disability, by intellectual ability, emotional maturity and by social competence — students' sense of personal autonomy and control over their lives is enhanced. Only if this is the case will it be possible for individuals to make decisions about their future which are based on a realistic self-assessment, an understanding of the demands and responsibilities of an adult lifestyle and how these two components interrelate. It should not be forgotten that the concept of independence for students with physical disabilities is of necessity a very broad one, encompassing mental attitude as well as practical skills. Those young people who are totally dependent by virtue of their physical disability must be given the opportunity to understand and accept responsibility for the management of their own lives in order that they may assume responsibility for the direction of their careers, rather than being the passive recipient of externally directed care. For this to happen there will have to be a considerable attitude shift on the part of many professionals, so that the subordinate role of the disabled person in many relationships (e.g. doctor/patient, teacher/pupil, parent/child) is altered to that of an adult member of an adult group with a purpose.

This general aim for post-school education can be interpreted in terms of a number of different areas of activity, all of which interrelate and have a direct bearing on course content for students with special educational needs.

The key issue in course planning, and for determining an individual's special educational needs which prevent him or her from making a direct progression to a mainstream course of further education, is assessment.

ASSESSMENT

The process of assessment is discussed elsewhere in this volume (Chapter 18). In this section it is necessary only to emphasise certain features associated with the nature of assessment which must be considered by those responsible for the development and administration of procedures to ascertain special educational needs.

Perhaps the most important of these is the need to know whether one is measuring an individual's standard of performance in a given area against that of others (i.e. the assessment is *norm-referenced*) or whether one is measuring the individual's performance against a given task (*criterion*-referenced). In the latter case the yardstick for progress is the student's own level of development. It is important to make the distinction in order to identify discrepancies between the individual's performance in a given area and that of those around him, and to be able to measure change — either from a baseline level or towards the achievement of a set goal.

Secondly it is necessary to be confident that the measurement procedure adopted measures that which it is intended to measure, and not some other factor or trait; i.e. that the procedure has *validity*, and that the measurement process repeated by the same person on different occasions, or by different people, gives comparable results, i.e. the procedure has *reliability*.

The importance of validity is highlighted by the case of Christopher, who did not know where his hands were when he could not see them. As a consequence he was unable to clean himself after defaecation. This was interpreted as attention-seeking behaviour, and was a major factor in the decision to educate him in a school for the behaviourally disturbed. It was not until the real reason for his actions was diagnosed that appropriate action could be taken. This did not happen until he was in a specialised centre for assessment and further education of school-leavers with physical disabilities.

Assessment procedures must also be sensitive to the dynamic nature of human learning. The process of assessment is conducted by people who bring with them their own attitudes and prejudices, and who vary from day to day. This inevitably introduces an element of unpredictability into procedures for the measurement of human behaviour by other humans and which are, for the reasons given in the introduction to this chapter, not sufficiently well established to resist the pressure without constant vigilance on the part of the assessors.

Traditional assessment procedures, such as examinations or tests, are of relatively little use in establishing special educational needs. For this reason a system of *profiling* (for an example of a profile record sheet see Table 40.1) has emerged in many centres accepting students with special needs on to post-school courses. This allows a formative assessment of progress to be made by means of continuous review, culminating in a summative assessment, or statement of progress, and needs at a given point to be made for the benefit of both the student and those working with him or her, enabling an agreed plan for the future to be developed.

The profile that emerges should also give an indication as to whether a student has a generalised learning difficulty which operates in all areas of the curriculum, or has a specific loss which may either mark or be marked by relatively higher levels of attainment in other areas.

Deficits thus identified may arise either as a result of limited ability or due to gaps in education because of prolonged periods of hospitalisation or time spent away from lessons for therapy or other treatments.

Assuming that it is possible to design a satisfactory assessment procedure, the information that emerges as a result of its application will be relevant to the student's education in a variety of curriculum areas (see Figure 40.2).

Figure 40.2: A basic teaching model

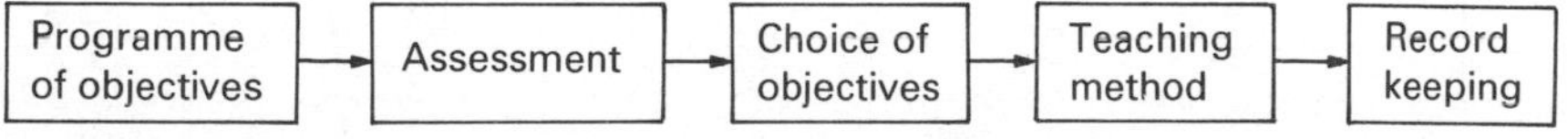

ACADEMIC EDUCATION

Consequent on the outcome of the assessment process, the nature of academic input to a student's programme or course will vary, and should be geared towards helping the students to make progress in terms of:

(a) Basic skills of literacy, communication and numeracy

Basic teaching skills can be seen either as a continuation of schooling or as a remedial process designed to ensure that the individual is able to cope confidently with the demands of everyday adult life. In order to do this effectively he or she must be able to read reasonably fluently, to count, measure and handle money accurately and communicate orally — in writing, or by means of some intermediary device (e.g. Bliss symbolics or a

Table 40.1: Workshop assessment

Student's name: ....

	7	6	5	4	3	2	1	
Hardly ever makes mistakes								Often makes mistakes
Excellent standard of work								Poor standard
Good work rate								Poor work rate
Steady performance from day to day								Inconsistent from day to day
Grasps instruction quickly								Slow to grasp instruction
Works continuously								Works for short periods only
Eager to work								Avoids work
Shows initiative								Shows no initiative
Retains what he has learned								Quickly forgets what he has learned
Willing to change jobs								Very unwilling to change jobs
Good attitude to authority								Poor attitude to authority
Realistic about own limitations								Unrealistic, overconfident, under confident
Aware of personal safety								Careless of personal safety
Accurate use of measurement and drawing aids								Unable to use measurement or drawing aids
Able to use hand tools								Unable to use hand tools
Able to use machinery								Unable to use machinery
Punctual								Unpunctual
Would benefit from further training								Would not benefit from further training
Able to work without supervision								Requires continual supervision

7 is equivalent to acceptance into sheltered employment; 4-5 implies good standard for training to sheltered work level; 1 implies very poor.

portable communication aid) — his or her needs and wishes to those in the community with whom some form of interaction is desired.

(b) Coping skills

For those unable to achieve sufficient proficiency in basic skills to function independently it will be necessary to devise strategies to enable them to 'get round' problems. For example, a person who is unable to read may be able to learn a social 'sight vocabulary' of words in everyday life, such as 'bus stop', 'ladies' or 'pay here'. For those unable to manage money learning always to tender a five pound note may facilitate independence. There is no set list of skills, but there is a great need for the involved professional to be perceptive and inventive when helping students to overcome specific difficulties.

(c) Preparation for progression to the next stage

For some students with special needs it will be possible to identify clear career or educational goals which are within reach but require specific preparation if they are to be attained. Many courses or careers have educational gatekeepers in the form of prerequisite qualifications; and it will often be necessary to incorporate these into the programme. In this context access to accurate information by all concerned is crucial if these are not to be overlooked. Even when formal qualifications are not essential there is often a requirement for a certain standard of literacy or numeracy in order to cope with the demands that will be made. This is particularly important where open or sheltered employment has been identified as the goal. It is also necessary to plan non-urgent medical intervention to take into account educational implications of any decisions, liaising with other involved professionals in order to ensure that actions taken in one sphere do not cut across those in another.

(d) Knowledge of rights, benefits, duties and entitlements

For the able-bodied person the introduction to citizenship is usually by a process of modelling on parents, teachers and other members of society. Knowledge of the 'way of the world' is transmitted to children by their own experiences. For young adults with a disability this is often inadequate, in that the world they are entering will be significantly more complex than that of most of their able-bodied peers. They will need to be able to understand the workings of statutory health and social services, the DHSS, housing and perhaps voluntary bodies as well.

SOCIAL EDUCATION

For a young adult with a physical disability and limited experience of everyday life the acquisition of social competence cannot be assumed to occur by a process akin to osmosis. The able-bodied adolescent, often by means of trial and error, is able to identify the limits of socially acceptable behaviour which must usually be taught to his or her disabled peers. This is in part due to the restricted opportunities for social interaction for many young disabled people, and in part due to the generally heightened reaction of the general public to any social gaffe on the part of a disabled person. Programmes of social education should be designed which will enable the disabled young adult to identify social norms, and pick up verbal and non-verbal cues which will help to ensure the individual is able to cope with a wide range of social situations.

A social education programme for the adult with a physical disability should have a number of distinct elements if it is to be comprehensive. These include:

(a) Understanding the social consequences of disability

This includes public perceptions of disability, stereotyping ('all deaf people are mentally handicapped', 'epilepsy is contagious', etc.), fears and myths and the publicly acceptable face of disabled people. If a person understands why people behave as they do in the face of disability, then he or she can come to terms with it and react appropriately as situations arise.

(b) Getting on with other adults on a peer group basis

As has been stated, young disabled adults are more often accustomed to being treated as 'junior partners' in relationships. If they are to become contributing adult members of any group then they must understand the social processes by which groups operate, and be able to act in a way which facilitates acceptance rather than rejection. This applies to social and recreational groups and also to work and employment settings, where incorrect interpretation of social cues may result in dismissal.

(c) Response to authority

Because the reaction of many people to those in authority is often one of acceptance of what is offered, failure to take full advantage of opportunities and facilities available is widespread. Disabled young adults should be encouraged to develop the skills which will ensure that they get what they need — that they are assertive without being aggressive and yet can also accept direction from those legitimately wishing to exert it over them. The relationship between an employer and employee is significantly different from that of doctor and patient, or claimant and DHSS visiting officer. All three will require different management skills on the part of the disabled individual if a productive encounter is to ensue.

Social education is not something which can be confined to one particular corner of an individual programme. It is not something that only happens at 3.30 p.m. on a Thursday, but should spread into all aspects and be undertaken by all disciplines working with an individual at any given time. For this reason communication and cooperation is essential if a consistent message is to be conveyed to the individual, and he or she is to be left more rather than less clear about appropriate behaviour in everyday social encounters.

A CAREER

For able-bodied young adults choosing a career is one of the most significant and difficult decisions that has to be made. It does not often happen at one discrete time, but more often emerges gradually as the young person matures and understands more about himself or herself and the world of work. In terms of their vocational maturity many young people leaving special schools are at the level of wanting to do something totally unrealistic based on a false picture of themselves and the demands of the job they aspire to — for example the young person with spina bifida who goes riding at a Riding for the Disabled Centre, enjoys it, and decides that he will be a jockey. Under these circumstances the first task is to make the individual aware of the range of opporunities that exist, and to begin the process of narrowing down to those career areas which are realistic and attainable, and yet which provide the individual with a sense of self-worth and fulfilment.

Vocational education has two distinct components. Firstly there are those skills and aspects of knowledge directly related to achieving the central task of the chosen job, be it typing, welding or whatever. Usually the job-specific component of any necessary training will be provided by the employer. The role of further education is to provide the individual with the general skills necessary in a form whereby they can be transferred to the specific situation required by the employer. Thus further education will teach word processing, and the employer may train the individual in the use of an IBM word processor. This applies across the board, and is not restricted to young adults with a disability. In this latter case the further education course should also aim to identify the job-specific implications of the disability and devise methods of overcoming them so that the disability does not become a handicap. Secondly, vocational education includes the teaching of non-task-related skills and knowledge. This includes building up individuals' stamina so they can cope with the physical and mental demands of the workplace — particularly important if previous experience has been restricted to the special school with its relatively short day, and the development of understanding of working to a standard every time. In school a score of eight out of ten represents a creditable achievement. At work the same level of performance signifies a 20 per cent failure rate, and is not normally acceptable.

Even for those so disabled as to make open or sheltered employment an unattainable goal, it is important to experience the demands of a work environment in order to develop understanding of the norms and pressures of everyday life.

Vocational education should also consider preparation for unemployment. This is a disproportionately common experience among young disabled people compared with their able-bodied peers, and unless disabled young people are given the skills to cope with the experience in a positive way there is a real risk of regression to higher level of dependence than is necessary or desirable.

ACTIVITIES OF DAILY LIVING (ADL)

Programmes for the development of independence in young adults with a physical disability must take account of the skills necessary for domestic and personal survival. Once again this involves not only the acquisition of basic skills, but also instillation of an attitude of mind in the young adult whereby he or she is motivated to take responsibility for these aspects of everyday life. For this to happen the curriculum must be firmly grounded in reality, and must provide the opportunity for students to undertake tasks 'for real' rather than as mere simulation exercises.

A curriculum to develop competence in this area should include the following topics:

(a) hygiene — bathing, toileting, dressing and eating;

(b) domestic skills — cleaning and home care;

(c) laundry — hand and machine washing, ironing, using a launderette;

(d) food preparation and cookery — including the use of convenience foods and 'bed-sit' cooking skills;

(e) nutrition — planning a balanced diet;

(f) shopping — what to buy, where and how much will it cost?

(g) Care and maintenance of clothing.

The amount of effort that has to be put into the development of any given individual will vary enormously according to the degree of disability, social and emotional maturity, intellectual ability and previous experience. Even the most severely disabled young adult, who is and always will be totally dependent, should be given the opportunity to participate in such a programme, in order that he or she will at least gain an understanding of what is involved in everyday life, and thereby be better able to, for example, form the link between the food on the supermarket shelf and the meal on the table.

It is only with the development of understanding that the opportunity for real choice comes, and with it the acceptance of responsibility for the consequences of that choice. Without this understanding the disabled person can unwittingly make unreasonable demands on carers, or feel that his or her individual freedom is being unduly restricted. The acquisition of daily living skills is a gradual process, and opportunity for individuals to increase the level of performance in all the areas listed above should be linked to a gradual shift in control from staff to the student.

It should not be overlooked that the aims of daily living skills programmes should be to develop individuals to a level which they are able to sustain, rather than to bring them to a peak of performance which it is unrealistic to expect will be adhered to day after day. There are, for example, those physically capable of dressing and undressing completely without assistance, but for whom the time and effort required is such that it would preclude any other form of activity. Much better to use an ADL programme to identify where help is necessary, and provide it, thereby enabling individuals to use their abilities in other areas with consequent enhancement of quality of life.

TRANSITION

The period of adolescence is a time of uncertainty during which childhood is left behind and the role of an adult in society is assumed. For the young person with a physical disability the successful management of this difficult period is of crucial importance. The involvement of the health, education and social services, and the statutory requirements of the 1981 Education Act, have tended to institutionalise this transition process for disabled individuals as compared to the experience of their able-bodied peers, with the resultant possibility of a loss of flexibility to respond to individual need.

During this transition the disabled individual will be gaining knowledge and experiencing the increasing demands of adult life. For any young person this will involve trying out new roles, and reacting to new situations. A period of further education is important in that it allows the individual to escape from the child-centred environment of the school and grow up while still within the ambit of education, and where he or she can be introduced to adult behaviour in an environment where this is the norm. Under these circumstances systematic guidance and counselling should be provided, to enable the person to cope with and assimilate the changes that he or she is experiencing, and also to allow the family to recognise and accept these, so that the necessary alteration in their perception of their disabled son or daughter can occur. In this way the disabled young person can become an adult within the family in the same way as his or her sibling, and without undue strain on relationships.

There is a further role for guidance and counselling in helping individuals to come to terms with the realities of their situation. For congenitally disabled young people it may be necessary systematically to strip away years of conditioning so that they no longer see themselves automatically as dependent on others, and subject to external control, but are enabled to make real choices about their lives and formulate realistic and attainable plans for the future. For those with an acquired disability there is a process of mourning which individuals and their families must go through, during which time they can grieve for the loss of the able-bodied person who is no more, and be helped to accept the new situation, and see the possibilities that are now attainable. Unless this is done there will almost inevitably be resentment and frustration which will prevent adjustment and hinder progress, resulting in unfulfilled potential and a lifestyle of greater dependence than otherwise might be the case.

LEARNING ABILITY

For the reasons outlined in the introduction many disabled young people reach school-leaving age with a very erratic profile of experiences and attainments. In some areas of their development they may be contemporary with their peers, but in others will lag behind by several years or more. Everyone needs a good learning environment if they are to maximise their potential, and in all cases there are a number of factors which may influence an individual's ability to learn. These include:

(1) *Reasoning ability*: many students have limited reasoning ability. When trying to teach a student, the task to be tackled should be at an appropriate level. A student cannot learn with understanding if the task is too complex for him or her.

(2) *Attention and concentration*: as concentration can often be a problem for students, it is essential that the student is paying attention to you or the task in hand if he or she is to learn. Choose short, quickly completed tasks for those who can only concentrate for a limited period.

(3) *Memory*: poor memory is often the result of poor learning (or poor teaching), although some students will have memory problems due to brain damage. In order to minimise this problem, teach small steps at a time and monitor progress continuously. Check whether students are better at remembering what you *tell* them or what you *show* them or demonstrate, and concentrate on the way they learn best.

(4) *Motivation* : a person learns best if he or she is interested in the task in hand; allow the student to choose from a range of activities.

(5) *Environmental factors*: outside noise, a stormy day, etc., can affect a person's capacity to learn. Those with certain disabilities may find that they work or learn best at particular times in the day. Check on this if you are introducing a new activity. If it is a 'bad' day or time of day for a student, it may be better to go over tasks already learnt and leave the new tasks for a better time.

(6) *Emotional status*: a person who is temporarily upset, or who shows a more long-term emotional disturbance, is unlikely to learn efficiently. Learning may in such instances fluctuate and this will need to be allowed for.

(7) *Perceptual difficulties*: perception is the ability to understand and interpret the information that our senses are presenting to us, and to organise this information in the light of past experience. Those students with perceptual difficulties may have a distorted view of the world which is likely to affect their learning ability in certain areas.

BANSTEAD PLACE ASSESSMENT AND FURTHER EDUCATION CENTRE

Much of the foregoing has been learned as a result of experience at Banstead Place, a centre for school-leavers and other young people with physical disabilities, operated by Queen Elizabeth's Foundation for the Disabled in Surrey.

Like any other young person whose local college of further education does not provide the particular courses or facilities he or she requires, students with special needs must sometimes look further afield for their post-school education. As a residential centre, Banstead Place provides a useful step towards adult life. The student has an opportunity to experience life away from home and to make a gradual move towards greater independence. Specialised staff are always on hand to provide support, tuition and guidance as necessary.

The main criterion for entry is the student's ability to participate in his or her own programme and to benefit from it. People with all types of physical handicaps, including multiple handicaps and sensory impairments, are accepted, but those with severe or uncontrolled behaviour disorders cannot be considered. Banstead Place and Hethersett College operate a joint programme for students who, in addition to having a severe physical disability, are registered as blind or partially sighted.

Students must have attained the minimum statutory school-leaving age before the commencement of their course. There is no upper age limit, but in practice most students are under the age of 25.

An individual programme is arranged for each student, based on the need for him/her to accept increasing personal responsibility and understand the demands of normal everyday life. The programme includes further or remedial education, training in independence and mobility, vocational assessment, work experience, social activities and the use of leisure and, where possible, learning to drive and use public transport. The programme is regularly reviewed with the student, and much of it is carried out away from Banstead Place with the help of local facilities of every kind.

Students may also attend further education colleges when relevant to their educational, emotional and/or social development. In such instance support is provided for students while they are at college by the staff at Banstead Place. Use is made of a wide range of academic, vocational and recreational courses as appropriate.

Amongst the facilities at Banstead Place are a shared bed-sitter and a single flat. These provide a variety of opportunities for students to live independently to a greater or lesser extent, and to demonstrate their mastery of the relevant skills and knowledge.

Individuals with little or no speech, or an impaired ability to communicate, are assessed for special aids or other items of equipment including micro-electronic and computer-linked systems.

SOURCES OF HELP AND INFORMATION

Many different professional disciplines are involved with young adults having physical disabilities. These include hospital consultants with a wide range of specialisms, GPs, nursing and paramedical staff, teachers, psychologists, careers officers, social workers and others. Each will approach the resolution of the individual's difficulties from the standpoint of their own professional discipline, and if anything like a coherent policy is to be adopted then a team, rather than a fragmented, approach must be employed. For this to happen each member of the team should have an understanding of the role of the other members, and also the constraints under which they operate. Ideally planning should evolve collectively rather than being a collection of decisions each taken in isolation. In addition residing within the team there should be the information about help available from statutory bodies like the MSC, and from voluntary organisations.

The specialist careers officer is an employee of the Local Education Authority Careers Service with a specific brief to provide guidance and counselling for school-leavers with all forms of special educational needs. As such these officers have a key role in planning and managing the transition from pupil to adult status by means of further education, YTS or other MSC schemes or whatever else is appropriate. Although there is no formal upper age limit to the specialist careers officer's work, by the time their clients reach their early 20s they tend to hand over primary responsibility to the disablement resettlement officer (DRO). This is an officer of the MSC whose primary role is placement in employment (either open or sheltered) of adults with disabilities. In order to secure this aim the DRO can call on the schemes to assist disabled workers outlined below. These schemes are also available for use by specialist careers officers, and the two professionals often work closely together to try and ensure continuity for their clients. In the first instance school-leavers with disabilities should normally be referred to the specialist careers officer, who can be contacted through the local careers office (in the telephone directory under Careers Service or the name of the local education authority).

For the resolution of particularly complex issues regarding employability, or vocational guidance or training, it is possible for either the specialist careers officer or DRO to refer an individual for assessment at an Employment Rehabilitation Centre. Here the opportunity is provided to try a range of different types of work — clerical, electronic, practical — the range varies from centre to centre, with a view to determining aptitude and ability and providing guidance. The instructional staff are supported by social workers and occupational psychologists. Medical advice is also available when required. Some of the services available are listed briefly below:

Manpower services commission

Employment

(1) Job introduction scheme — a wage subsidy for a disabled person during the first few weeks employment.

(2) Adaptations to premises and equipment (up to £6,000 is available to employers).

(3) Fares to work — for those unable to use public transport because of their disability.

(4) Special aids to employment — tools or equipment provided free to individuals.

(5) Sheltered employment.

Training

(1) On the job — to enable a disabled person to perform a particular task.
(2) Off the job — at a Skill Centre or local college of further education, or at one of the residential training colleges run by voluntary organisations but funded by the MSC. These are Queen Elizabeth's Training College, Leatherhead; Portland Training College, Mansfield; St Loyes Training College, Exeter; and Finchale Training College, Durham.
(3) Assessment of employment potential and suitability of particular career areas is available at Employment Rehabilitation Centres.

More information on any MSC scheme is available from the disablement resettlement officer (DRO) at local Job Centres, or from the Manpower Services Commission, Moorfoot, Sheffield.

Voluntary organisations

Many voluntary organisations provide a wide range of services to disabled people. Some of these are specific to a particular condition or group of conditions — e.g. the Muscular Dystrophy Group of GB — while others range over the whole field of disability — e.g. the Royal Association for Disability and Rehabilitation (RADAR). Addresses of voluntary organisations are contained in the *Directory of voluntary organisation*, published by NCVO, 26 Bedford Square, London WC1 and regularly revised (see Resources, Chapter 49).

These services exist over and above those provided by statutory health education and social services. The priority given to the needs of the young adult with a disability will vary according to where he or she lives and the degree of priority afforded to disability by the statutory authorities of that area.

Some aspects of provision are (nominally at least) guaranteed by statute — for example full-time education up to the age of 19. Others are not mandatory duties but discretionary powers, and access to services may depend on a sound knowledge base and forceful advocacy by those committed to meeting the needs of the young adult with a disability.

CONCLUSION

For the young adult with a significant physical disability the transition to adulthood is a time of uncertainty. The possibilities are legion, but plotting a course which is logical and progressive, and will ensure that potential is realised, is beset by difficulties. For many young people in this position a period of further education will be an essential part of their development into autonomous adulthood and a fulfilled life, however that may be defined. For those without significant disabilities this is difficult enough, but at least there is generally the possibility of learning from mistakes and trying again. Disabled young people not only have more adverse factors to contend with, but are also under a significantly greater pressure not to fail. If the exercise of a particular option has involved much preparatory work from a range of different professionals, then the chances of repeating the attempt in the event of failure for whatever reasons, are slight. Hence there is an overriding need for planning and interprofessional cooperation to ensure that the opportunities presented by further education in the life of the young adult with a physical disability form part of a seamless robe, which takes the young adults from where they are on leaving school to where they want to be as functioning adult members of the community.

REFERENCES

Dee, Lesley (1984) *Routes to Coping*, Further Education Unit, London

Education Act 1981, HMSO London

Special Educational Needs (1978) Report of the Committee of Enquiry into the Education of Handicapped Children and Young People (The Warnock Report), HMSO, London

FURTHER READING

Bradley, J and Hagerty, S. (1981) *Students with Special Needs in F. E.*, Further Education Unit

Evans, C.D. (ed.) (1981) *Rehabilitation after Severe Head Injury*, Churchill Livingstone, London

McCarthy, G.T. (ed.) (1984) *The physically handicapped child: an interdisciplinary approach to management*, Faber & Faber, London

Gregg, T.M. (1981) 'Vocational assessment, training and placement', Report from National Rehabilitation Board, 25 Clyde Road, Dublin, Ireland

Holgate, L. (1982) *The effects of hydrocephalus on vocational and non-vocational training*, ASBAH, London

Hutchinson, D. (1982) *Work preparation for the handicapped*, Croom Helm, Beckenham

Male, J. and Thompson, C. (1985) *The educational implications of disability: a guide for teachers*, RADAR, London

Pankhurst, J. and McAllister, A.G. (1980) *An approach to the further education of the physically handicapped*, NFER, Slough

Sousa, J.C., Gordon, L.H. and Shutleff, D.B. (1976) Assessing the development of daily living skills in patients with spina bifida. *Dev. Med. Child Neurol.*, *18* (Suppl. 37), 134-41

Tizard, J. and Anderson, E. (1979) *Alternative to work for severely handicapped people*, OECD, Paris

Willoughby, R.H. and Hoffman, R.G. (1979) Cognitive and perceptual impairments in children with spina bifida — a look at the evidence, *Spina Bifida Ther.*, no. 2. (October)

41

Employment

Mary Moore

INTRODUCTION

Everyone who requires medical intervention over a prolonged period is at a significant disadvantage in the current employment market. To facilitate full integration back into the community consideration must be given to overcoming the barriers preventing such integration. This chapter defines clearly what these barriers are, how they can be overcome and the various services available to help overcome them.

EMPLOYMENT

The common element of all 39 *Oxford English Dictionary* definitions of 'work' refers to action for a purpose, which includes, though is not restricted to, employment. Employment is more aptly described as work under contractual agreement involving material reward. The International Labour Office has for decades attempted unsuccessfully to establish an internationally acceptable definition of unemployment, but the legal definitions still vary from one country to another. In the UK the basis for establishing official rates of unemployment is registrations at local benefit offices. There is continuous debate about the degree of over and/or under-representation of the number of unemployed, arising from certain inherent weaknesses in the accuracy of official unemployment statistics due to (a) unemployed people not registering at local benefit offices as they receive no financial gain (due to a spouse earning or independent means of some kind, or they are unaware of their entitlement or simply do not wish to claim it); and (b) people registering for benefits who are in fact working and not entitled to them: the so-called hidden economy.

STATISTICS OF DISABLED PEOPLE IN THE LABOUR MARKET

In considering the problems that disabled people face in the labour market it is important to define disability. The definition used in relation to employment is that given in the Disabled Person's (Employment) Acts 1944 and 1958, which define those eligible to register as disabled as 'those people who because of illness, disease or congenital deformity are substantially handicapped in obtaining or keeping employment of a kind that would otherwise be suited to their age, experience and qualifications'. As registration under the Act is voluntary, the Manpower Services Commission (MSC) classifies people as disabled on the grounds of their eligibility to register, and not on their actual registration. Under the Act disabled people are classified as suitable for *open employment (section I)* or as most unlikely to gain employment except under *sheltered conditions (section II).*

Registration as disabled should not be confused with registration for employment. In October 1982 compulsory registration for employment in order to receive unemployment benefit was dropped. As a result there was a reduction in the number of people using the Jobcentre services generally, and a consequent drop in registrations of disabled people. As registration had previously been the source of official statistics for the disabled unemployed there was a consequent loss of statistics in this field.

Statistics from 1981 revealed certain trends that are true today: disabled unemployed people tend to be older than their able-bodied counterparts, as Table 41.1 shows. They also have a markedly different occupational profile (Table 41.2). Lack of skill is a major characteristic of the unemployed generally, but it is overwhelmingly the case for disabled unemployed people (Table 41.2).

The 1981 statistics revealed very significant evidence that disabled people, once unemployed, are likely to experience greater problems regaining work than the unemployed generally. At that time the proportion of disabled people who had been out of work for over 52 weeks (49 per cent) was twice the equivalent of the able-bodied (24 per cent). We do not have

Table 41.1: Age distribution of unemployment (%)

Age	Disabled	Able-bodied
Under 20	6.7	21.3
21–24	8.3	20.1
25–44	33.0	33.9
45–54	24.6	10.6
55 and over	27.3	14.1
	100	100

Table 41.2: Occupations in which employment is sought (%)

Occupation	Disabled	Able-bodied
Clerical and related	10.1	14.8
Other non-manual	3.0	7.0
Craft and similar	6.4	17.1
Other manual	20.6	29.1
General labourers	59.9	32.0
	100	100

statistics for the disabled unemployed in 1986, but as the percentage of long-term unemployed has generally increased the discrepancy is likely to remain high.

The initial results of the Labour Force Survey, 1984, indicate that poor health and disability problems were reported more frequently by the economically inactive and unemployed than those in employment. For all age groups the economic activity rate of people reporting a limiting health problem or disability was much lower than the average for persons of that age, and unemployment rates were higher (*Employment Gazette*, May 1985).

THE EMPLOYMENT MARKET, JOB ANALYSIS AND ASSESSMENT

The employment market is undergoing rapid change in the redistribution of skills. There is a general shift away from heavy manufacturing industries towards service industries; from 'blue-collar' to 'white-collar' jobs and from unskilled to semi-skilled, and semi-skilled to skilled employment. New technology is a significant causal factor in this redistribution of skill, and is revolutionising industry in terms of both number and types of jobs available.

This shift in the employment market affects the unskilled, the old and the disabled most hard; the competitiveness of the labour market means that anyone returning to employment after a period of unemployment finds it more difficult to get a job. This obviously has major implications for rehabilitation of the disabled back into employment even after good recovery from illness or injury, and is more severe for those with residual disability or handicap.

There are three stages in the return to employment of an individual who has had illness, injury or handicap as a result of longstanding disability:

(1) *analysis of the labour market* exploring what jobs are available, the skills they require, the physical, educational and experiential requirements;

(2) *assessment of the individual*, to assess all those attributes important for matching to an appropriate job;
(3) *rehabilitation*, to enhance the assessed individual attributes to a level matching that required in the employment market.

Job analysis identifies and specifies in detail all the key skills required to perform a particular job or task; the skills are categorised into groups and, depending on the type of task-analytic technique used and its aim, the group labels refer to essential components of tasks with reference to training, selection or transferability. There are many different task-analytic techniques of varying quality and usefulness; this is a growth area of research and development in both the USA and Britain. The Basic Skills Checklist is one example of such techniques; in this technique a checklist is used which itemises the basic skills employed in a task under 400 skill labels, these are then classified into six groups: calculation, measurement and drawing, listening and talking, reading and writing, planning and problem-solving, and practical skills. From such an analysis it is possible to draw up a skill hierarchy of combinations of skills required to perform higher-level tasks, skills essential at the recruitment stage, skills that can be taught on the job and skills that are advantageous but not essential to the job. From this kind of information it is hoped that more effective comparisons can be made of skills required in different jobs and their transferability from one job to another.

The skills matrix in Table 41.3 is an example of another checklist method used in the Job Components Inventory. This adaptation is taken from a checklist of several hundred core skills and is designed to demonstrate the way in which certain core skills occur in several different jobs, whereas others are unique to a particular job. This type of skill analysis has major implications for the stucture and method of providing training for the employed and unemployed in a changing labour market. It is also an important tool in matching individuals with appropriate jobs, but in order to do this a detailed analysis of the specific attributes of the job applicant is required.

MSC SERVICES

The Manpower Services Commission (MSC) is the branch of the Department of Employment which deals with recruitment, retention, rehabilitation, training and special services to facilitate the return to work for the unemployed such as Community Programme, Youth Training Schemes and other less well known schemes.

The MSC is responsible for policy and practice in employment and training; the Employment and Enterprise Group controls the Employment

Table 41.3: Skills matrix

			Skill/profession					
			Professional/ technical	Clerical with figures	Food preparation and services	Hairdressing	Sewing machinist	Plumbing
Physical and perceptual	B1	Finger dexterity	**	***	***	***	***	***
	B5	Arm/leg coordination	—	*	—	***	***	*
	B16	Close-up work	**	**	*	*	***	*
	B21	Good sense of smell	—	—	**	*	—	**
Mathematical	C50	Use whole number	***	***	***	***	***	***
	C26	24-hour clock	*	—	*	—	—	*
	C33	Use screw sizes	—	—	—	—	—	—
	C106	Read plumbing diagram	—	—	—	—	—	*
Communication and interpersonal	D3	Record written information	***	***	**	—	—	**
	D1	Complete standard form	***	***	**	—	—	**
	D15	Instruct others	—	—	**	**	—	—
	D16	Interview people (formal)	—	—	—	—	—	—
Decision-making and responsibility	E1	Decide about work order	**	*	*	*	*	*
	E6	Responsible for death/injury	**	—	**	*	**	**
	E5	Decide about standards	*	*	*	—	—	*
	E7	Responsible for damage to tools	**	*	**	*	**	**

*** *Very frequent:* more than 50 per cent of job holders use the skill very often; more than 75 per cent of job holders use the skill quite often. Equivalent combinations.

** *Frequent:* More than 35 per cent of job holders use the skill very often; more than 50 per cent of job holders use the skill quite often. Equivalent combinations.

* *Less frequent:* more than 25 per cent of job holders use the skill quite often; 30 per cent use the skill occasionally. Equivalent combination.

— *Blank:* Skill is extremely rare or never occurs.

(Adapted from: *MSC training studies, a skills compendium,* MSC, 1983).

Rehabilitation Centres (ERC), Jobcentres, and the Disablement Advisory Service (DAS) which provides advice and material support to employers in recruitment and retention of disabled employees and markets the MSC services for the disabled to employers generally; the Vocational, Educational and Training Group deals with policy in training provision within the MSC, in the Skillcentre Training Agency, and externally with employers, trade organisations and in colleges.

Jobcentre services

Disabled people may approach the Jobcentre of their own accord, or be referred by the GP, specialist or a DHSS doctor. Every Jobcentre has the services of a disablement resettlement officer (DRO) who deals personally with clients with significant functional handicaps and who arranges appropriate assessment, rehabilitation, training or employment according to their need. The DRO has a specialist knowledge and training in the effects of various disabilities and the services available to help disabled individuals back to work. Clients who have disabilities that cause only a minor handicap for employment are usually dealt with by the employment advisers and not by the DRO, as a specialist help is not usually required in these cases.

The DRO has available to him (or her) a number of special MSC resettlement schemes designed to remove or overcome obstacles to employment for disabled people. These are:

(a) Job Introduction Scheme

Under this scheme if the DRO considers that an unemployed disabled person is well suited to a particular vacancy, but the employer has doubts about his ability to perform the job to the standard required, the DRO can offer a grant of £45 per week toward the cost of employing the person, who is then paid the normal wage. This is payable for a trial period of six weeks, extendable to 13 weeks if necessary. There is no compulsion for the employer to retain the employee, although approximately 60–70 per cent are so retained.

(b) Job rehearsal

This may be offered by the DRO or an ERC but is solely for current ERC clients or those who have recently left ERC. Under this scheme the MSC pays the client the ERC allowance for the first two weeks of a new job to give the employer the opportunity to try out the client before offering employment. This scheme can also be used solely to give a client work experience where there may not be a permanent job vacancy to be filled. The time period can be extended if considered necessary.

(c) Adaptations to premises and equipment

The MSC will give grants to employers who need to make essential adaptations to premises or equipment in order to recruit or retain an existing employee. A maximum of £6,000 can be paid, and a contribution from the employer is required if the business will benefit materially from the adaptation.

(d) Fares to work

Disabled people, who are registered under the Act, who cannot use public transport to travel to work due to their disabilities, may be eligible for a contribution of up to 75 per cent of their travelling costs up to a maximum of £49.50 per week. For those in receipt of a Mobility Allowance from the DHSS a third of this allowance is offset against the MSC contribution.

(e) Business on own account

Under this scheme capital grants are available for the initial outlay involved in setting up a business. Only severely disabled people who have been classified as fit for sheltered employment are eligible for this grant, and then only if other avenues of resettlement have proved unsuccessful. These grants are only for setting up costs and not for continuing support.

DISABLEMENT ADVISORY SERVICE (DAS)

In addition to the DRO service in Jobcentres, a further specialist team, the DAS, exists primarily to advise employers on policies of recruitment and retention of disabled people. There is one DAS team per MSC area which usually comprises one large town or city and two or three smaller towns and countryside around. Each DAS team consists of three or four personnel who have commonly had experience as DROs in Jobcentres. They visit employers, help in their liaison with jobcentres and in the recruitment of disabled people; they assess and advise whether aids and adaptations might be suitable, and generally try to foster a positive employment policy for disabled people. The team also helps employers with employees who become disabled, and with the ongoing support of disabled employees recruited by employers; they also provide a link between employers and ERCs who help in assessment of the employee's current potential and likely aids or adaptations they require.

EMPLOYMENT REHABILITATION (Figure 41.1)

There are 27 ERCs in Britain; three of these are residential, designed for the more severely disabled who would have mobility problems travelling

Figure 41.1: Elements of an employment rehabilitation course

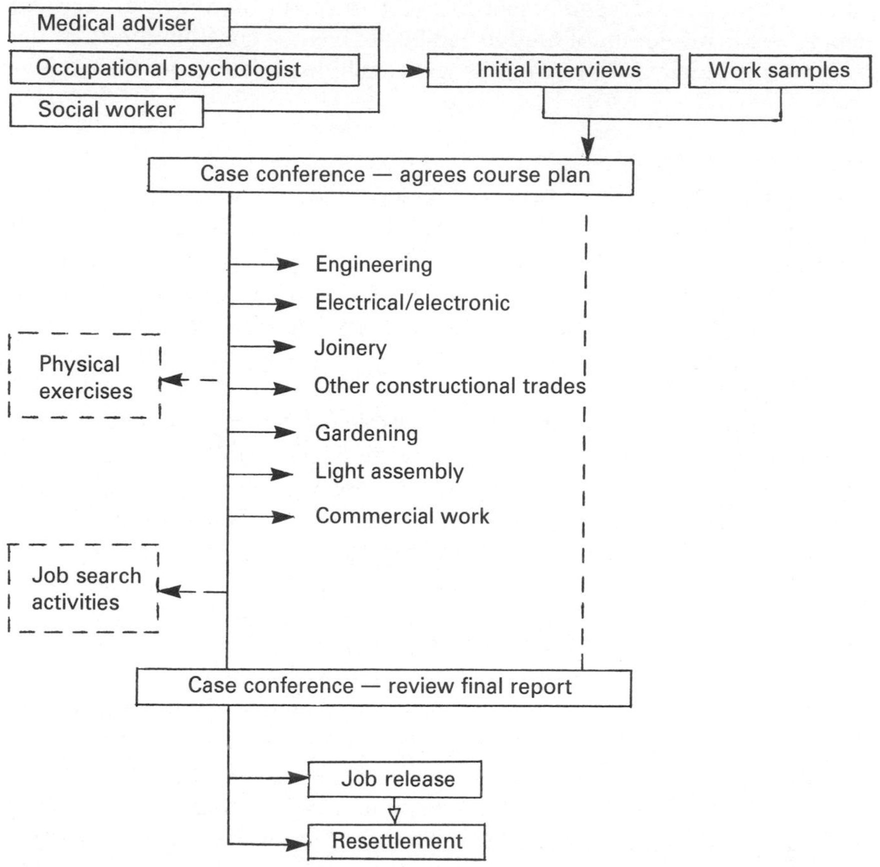

daily to an ERC, and for those who do not have ERCs within daily travelling distance. The centres vary in size, offering 60–175 places, but all offer a similar service.

Referrals are made to ERCs by doctors (GPs, specialist and DHSS) directly, by Jobcentres, when a disabled client goes to them seeking work, and a minority by employers whose employees have been ill or injured and wish to return to work. There are in addition referrals from other authorities such as Adult Training Centres, the Probation Service and local authority social workers. Most ERCs also run special courses for a small number of disabled school-leavers who are referred by the local authority Careers Service for the purpose of introducing disabled young people to the world of work and to assess their suitability for specific Youth Training Schemes

(YTS) or employment. In addition to these schemes there are several different schemes to help the unemployed generally for which disabled persons are eligible and in some cases may get preferential treatment.

Clients need not be registered as disabled but must be considered as having a significant degree of handicap which affects their employment potential, but which does not render them totally unfit for employment. If the referring body is unsure of the employability of a client the ERC runs a short course to investigate this prior to accepting the client on a longer rehabilitation course if they are considered able to work.

The ERC staff consist of a multidisciplinary team of a social worker, a nurse, an occupational psychologist, technical staff, administrative staff and the services of a doctor part-time from the Employment Medical Advisory Service, a branch of the Health and Safety Executive.

Courses are individually designed by the psychologist in conjunction with the client who agrees with the goals set and is actively involved in the evaluation, change of goals and feedback during the course. The course involves a preliminary assessment, consisting of interviews with the social worker, the occupational psychologist and the doctor, paper-and-pencil tests where required, and short standardised practical exercises called work samples. A client who requires rehabilitation and/or further assessment will then proceed onto a further period of assessment and rehabilitation which is goal-orientated, while clients who only required assessment leave their course and return to the Jobcentre for placing action.

Assessment of a disabled person's readiness to return or enter the employment market after illness, injury or long-standing disability can be broken down into six planes.

(a) *The medical plane* involves the professional assessment by a doctor of the degree to which a medical condition confers a disability. The doctor then needs to consider how far this disability constitutes a handicap for specified work; for instance aphasia may be of little relevance to a gardener but may bar future employment as a barrister. Those responsible for helping a client to find work also need to know whether the handicap is likely to continue, to resolve, to progress or to fluctuate, and whether it brings in train secondary disabilities relevant to employment. The doctor decides on his/her level of supervision of the patient and the degree of medical rehabilitation required in order to render the patient fit enough for referral to employment rehabilitation. It is sadly common for the gap between the fitness required to cease medical intervention and that required for the return to demanding employment to be unrecognised or negotiated.

(b) *The physical plane* involves an assessment of both current physical capacity and potential. In about half of the ERCs an occupational therapist is responsible for this assessment, but in the others there is no specialist professional input on this plane. An employment-oriented assessment is required involving a job specification analysis of the capacity to perform certain types of activity as revealed by skill analysis of the relevant jobs. The occupational therapist working in an ERC environment has the advantage of working as part of a multidisciplinary team with other specialists who have skills in task analysis, trainability testing and placing individuals into employment.

(c) *The psychological plane* is extremely complex. A client who has suffered some sort of psychiatric illness will usually receive a skilled analysis of his/her ability to adjust to daily life with varying degrees of support, during the psychiatric rehabilitation. Specialists involved in this assessment vary greatly in their degree of knowledge of the skills required in the employment market, and in their ability to make an accurate predictive assessment of their client's potential to carry out a specific job effectively; this of course is a feature of prognostic evaluation in the psychiatric field due to the complexity of such disabilities.

Those who have suffered short or long-term handicaps due to other types of disability also require assessment as to their psychological adjustment to the lives they will be leading. This is often carried out initially by medical staff, and subsequently by family and friends who make a limited assessment of whether the individual is coping with daily life adequately. It is only when the individual's behaviour or attitude is markedly aberrant that a professional assessment by a psychologist or psychiatrist is called for. The majority of medical and related staff in Britain receive sufficient basic training in psychology to help them detect overt problems of this nature. The major stumbling block in the return of disabled people to the employment market is frequently not the severity of their disability (for the physically handicapped) but the inadequacy of their psychological adjustment in employment terms: their overprotective attitude to their health, their feeling of inadequacy as a result of the change in physical and psychological capacity, their changed role in personal relationships, their lack of awareness of what other jobs they may be able to do if they cannot return to their former employment, their lack of knowledge about their current state of health and prognosis — these are just a few of the more common reasons for inability to take up a successful role in employment.

(d) *The psychometric plane* involves educational testing or exploration, intelligence testing, investigation of the client's ability to undergo various forms of training and where their particular intellectual skills lie: spatial, numeric, written, etc. When matching an individual to a job it is important to know that he has the education required to do the job, be it to read safety signs, use imperial or metric measurement, do statistical analysis, etc. It is also of importance to know whether the client can absorb training, and at what level if this is to be provided in the job. This is particularly relevant to disabled people who are frequently attempting to transfer skills to new fields of employment or enter jobs of which they have little or no experience (Chapter 33).

Educational testing is not simply a case of giving an individual a short test. A disabled client who left school many years before will have forgotten much and need to revise; he may also be unused to tests and therefore perform at a level lower than his true potential; one also finds occasionally that an individual may have left school early, or not made the best use of their time at school, and have an unexploited ability to acquire a higher level of education; a decision has to be made whether it is worth undergoing further education or training. In order to do this, psychometric testing is required to give an indication of the individual's potential to absorb training (to what extent and in what areas). Tests most commonly used include intelligence tests, reasoning tests, tests of mechanical insight; but the range is large depending on the nature and level of job being sought. There are also many psychological tests looking at the effects of specific types of disability such as concentration, attention span and various other cognitive abilities, for example in the brain-damaged. Many of these tests are clinical in nature but have important implications for occupational potential.

(e) *The social skills plane* is another area which is crucial for resettlement into employment, but too often inadequately assessed. All jobs have some minimum acceptable level of social skill but they differ greatly in the degree to which it is required. It is common to recommend that a shy, nervous person work alone or in a small group, but even the individual who operates a machine all day has to achieve an acceptable degree of communication with colleagues at break time and at arrival and departure from work. A salesman has to be able to get on with anybody, be adaptable and enjoy meeting people; similarly a retail manager requires different social skills from an accountant. This dimension is usually assessed at the minimum acceptable level; consequently inadequate attention is given to accurate assessment of the social skills required in a work situation and appropriate matching of the client to a job on this dimension.

Social skill assessment is relevant not only to clients with psychiatric problems or effects of head injury; it is also important for the client disabled by a heart attack, the loss of a limb or an eye. Most disabilities have secondary effects which can crucially affect a person's social skills: problems manifested in belligerence, sullenness, shyness, under- or over-confidence, etc. The effects must be assessed and matched to the social skills required in specific jobs. A specific area of social skills training which is being developed in Employment Rehabilitation Centres (ERCs) and in the Manpower Services Commission (MSC) employment and training services generally is job search training. This involves selecting and applying for jobs, telephone and interview techniques and social skills required in the work situation. Research in psychology, education and training has provided the database for development of job search training packages which have the most valuable information base and effective methodology for improving clients' skills in this direction.

(f) *The practical skills plane* (see Figure 41.2) is designed to assess the core skills a client possesses in practical tasks, and how these combine to match the higher-order skills required for specific jobs. As some skills are transferable or component skills of several jobs it is not always necessary to assess an individual on the specific task that he/she will be doing in a job, but the component skills that make up a job must be assessed; e.g. when testing for the potential to be a car mechanic a set level of mechanical insight, educational ability, physical ability, tool use, theory and ability to absorb training are required; all of which can be assessed without actually putting the individual to work on a car engine.

These six planes of assessment are required for every individual and type of job, though the extent and balance of assessment in different planes will vary widely according to the individual and the type of job being sought. The ERC is able to assess and rehabilitate on all six planes to provide an effective means for facilitating the return to work of disabled people who retain a desire and potential for employment, either in the sheltered or open employment market. Clients continuing onto a rehabilitation course, after their preliminary assessment, will typically work on sections supervised by an instructor, where their specific job skills, social skills and ability to follow instructions will be further developed. Each ERC has between five and seven sections, each reflecting a type of work available in the local employment market. These commonly include some of the following: commerical work, electrical/electronic work, engineering, light manufacturing and assembly, construction trades and horticulture. The specialist staff have differential roles in the rehabilitation process dictated by the individual needs and wishes of the client. This orientation towards the individual needs in the ERCs results in considerable flexibility in course length; a course can run from one day to six months, although the majority of clients pursue a course between two and seven weeks.

Recent developments in ERCs have resulted in them taking a much more active part in getting their clients jobs. This involves providing in-depth training in telephone techniques, writing application forms and letters, interview techniques; and in submitting their clients directly to job vacancies notified to them on a computerised system from all Jobcentres that refer clients to the ERC.

A further new development in employment rehabilitation is the setting up of ASSET centres in areas not adequately covered by the existing ERC network. These centres have a similar function to ERCs but they concentrate on assessment and job search training in the ASSET premises, followed by placements in local firms for rehabilitation and work experience; many of the clients attend part-time, or full-time for a short period; there are approximately nine staff with less technical and medical staff than ERCs,

Figure 41.2: Clients assessing manual dexterity and the ability to follow instructions using standardised work samples

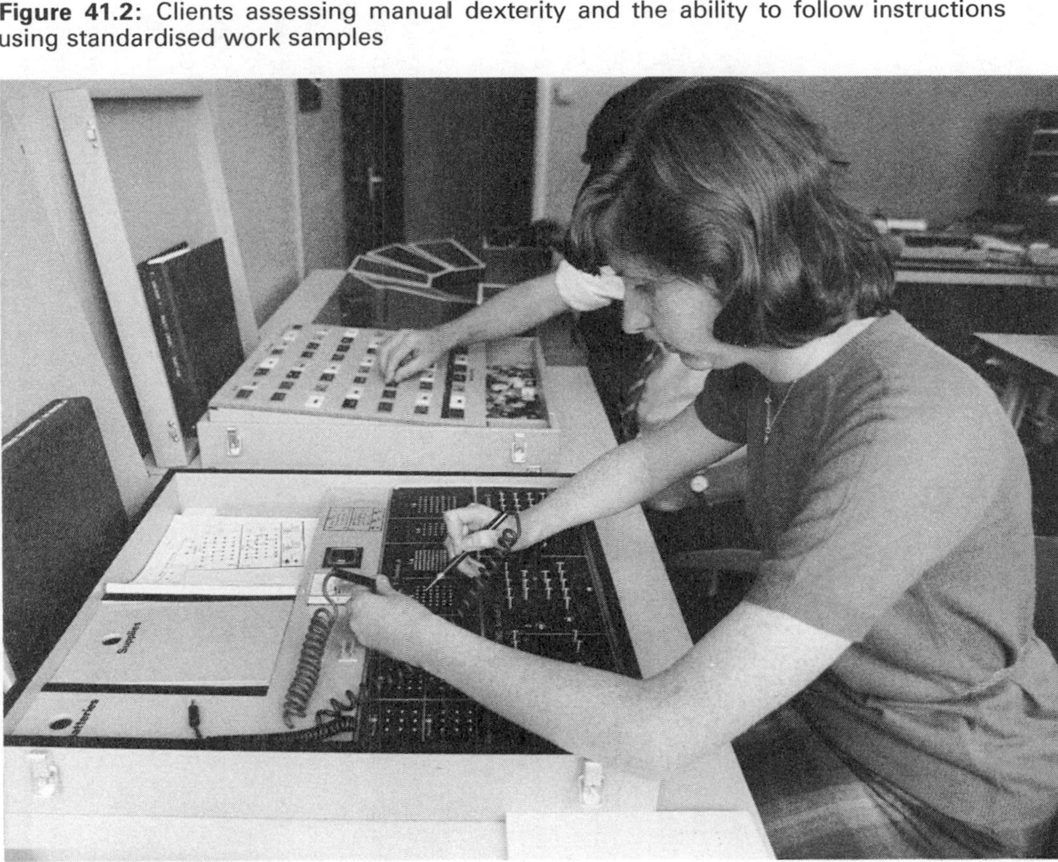

but the same specialists in occupational psychology, social work and placing.

VOCATIONAL TRAINING

Vocational training has undergone major change over recent years, largely due to the changing requirements of industry for new skills. During the 1970s there was a visible reduction in apprenticeship training by employers, and this was coincident with a reduction in the traditional 'trades' generally. The short skill training of MSC Skillcentres was then producing a labour force trained in skills for which there was a declining demand.

These sweeping changes in the employment market have prompted major changes in policy and practice in vocational training provided by MSC. The current adult training strategy of the MSC has shifted emphasis away from traditional trade training to that required in order to supply the employment market with the skills it needs in order to maintain and develop British Industry. The strategy relies largely on employers to provide the impetus and to fund training in industry itself, and on its trade organisations to provide training of the type required by the firms themselves or by local colleges in collaboration with industry. MSC Skillcentres will continue to provide some training, but on a reduced scale and with a different emphasis. They will concentrate more on short courses introducing industry to new skills and technology, trainees being in the main employees sponsored by their firms. Skillcentres will continue to give training in basic skills for the unskilled and semi-skilled to try and provide them with greater flexibility, and for the unemployed a variety of skills to make them more competitive in the job market. In general there will be less skill training available to the unemployed, but a higher standard of training provided by industry itself in firms and colleges to train new recruits in appropriate skills and upgrade the skills of the existing workforce.

Training courses for the unemployed do give special consideration to the disabled by putting them to the top of waiting lists, and allowing applications to continue for the disabled when waiting lists would otherwise be closed.

In addition many Skillcentres will adapt courses to suit the individual needs of the disabled, provided these adaptations still enable the individual to get sufficient benefit from the course to be able to enter employment. There are also four residential training centres specifically for training people whose disabilities preclude them from attending other training courses and therefore require training specifically adapted to their needs. These centres are independent, but largely funded by MSC and are situated in Nottingham, Durham, Surrey and Cornwall.

Disabled people can apply for all these courses at their local Jobcentres, who arrange for them to sit appropriate pre-entry tests if required. If there are doubts about a client's suitability the Jobcentre may recommend preliminary attendance on a short ERC course to assess suitability for a particular course.

A further method of training is available to disabled clients called ITTWE — Industrial Training Throughout with Employer. Under this scheme the DRO in the Jobcentre or ERC seeks out an employer who is prepared to offer specialist training to a particular disabled client which conforms to training standards set by MSC; the trainee then receives a training allowance, similar to that they would receive on a Skillcentre course, for the period of training agreed between the employer and MSC. Adaptations and tools required by the trainee are paid for by MSC up to an agreed financial limit. The quality and nature of the training given is supervised by a technical officer from MSC's Training Division. Understandably employers willing to provide such training are rare, and finding them is a time-consuming exercise, but this sort of training is receiving increased emphasis by the MSC.

In discussing the provision of the MSC for the disabled in the employment market, I have made reference largely to open employment, but for those whose disabilities are such as to enable them to be classified under section II of the Act, the MSC provides additional guidance and financial support.

SHELTERED EMPLOYMENT

The DRO is usually the person responsible for classifying a client as section II; in order to do this they seek medical evidence from the client's GP or hospital doctor and if necessary seek further advice from the Employment Medical Adviser. Classification as section II entitles the client to special provisions from the MSC, in the form of sheltered employment.

Sheltered employment is subsidised by the MSC to facilitate employment of disabled people in a productive capacity in a viable business. The majority of sheltered employment is in REMPLOY factories. REMPLOY is an independent national company which has factories all over the country specialising in different types of work relevant to the local employment markets. MSC sponsors REMPLOY for 40 minutes of every hour worked, on condition that it employs section II disabled people; this means that it can employ people who can work at only a third of the rate of an employee in open employment doing a similar job. REMPLOY is an independent company and has to be profitable to pay its workers and survive; it thus requires its workers to achieve these minimum standards, and pays a bonus scheme and promotes employees to chargehand and foreman, etc., if they show the relevant skill required. REMPLOY selects its own employees from a pool of appropriate section II applicants referred by the DRO. If, after a trial period, the applicant is unable to achieve the required standard he or she is not recruited. Most local authorities own one or more sheltered workshops with their own funds and grants from MSC and/or the European Social Fund.

MSC also funds the Sheltered Placement Scheme, where a sponsoring organisation, usually a local authority or charity, finds an employer who is prepared to consider a severely disabled person (section II) for a job within a normal working environment. The sponsor and employer do a detailed study of the rate of work that the person can do, and the sponsor agrees to fund the employer for the difference between that rate and the normal worker standard, in a familiar fashion to REMPLOY. The sponsoring body then claims that percentage of the finance back from MSC. The DAS team is usually the MSC contact in this arrangement, and frequently is the moving force in finding sponsors and employers for this scheme; in addition DAS may organise the funding, the aids and adaptations that might be required and are available to help resolve the problems that may arise after the apointment.

ALTERNATIVE TO EMPLOYMENT

For those disabled people who cannot achieve even the standards required in sheltered employment there are some alternatives. Both the quality and variety of these are insufficient to meet the needs of all disabled people. Adult Training Centres (ATC) run by local authorities primarily take clients who are mentally retarded but, depending on the local authority, they have admitted also a variety of other clients (with respect to age, disability and intelligence levels); places are usually in great demand and there are insufficient places to go round. ATCs have workshops and technical staff, and often produce a variety of goods and production work for sale.

Many local authorities have extensive day-care provision to cater for people who would otherwise be confined to their homes, but there are rarely sufficient places to cater for all those who might benefit, and frequently a priority system of those most in need has to be applied. These centres vary in the quality of provision from constructive, satisfying work with good supervision to facilities that are little more than holding centres where the people sit around with little stimulation or individual attention that goes beyond basic health care.

In addition to the above-mentioned facilities there are a few charity organisations which run rehabilitation centres, residential centres and day centres, typically for specific disability groups, but these are few and far between. A feature that all these provisions have in common is their focus on a disabled client group of low intellectual ability making them generally unsuitable for the more intelligent, severely disabled client; provision for this category is very poor.

CONCLUSION

Rehabilitation of the disabled individual into the employment market may require considerable skills; rarely is medical intervention alone sufficient. Prolonged unemployment produces barriers of its own to the return to work, which are superimposed on residual handicap from illness, injury or long-standing disability. This makes it essential that medical intervention is followed as soon as is feasible by further help to facilitate entrance to the employment market and enable the individual to live as full and satisfying a life as possible.

The MSC range of facilities and expertise helps the disabled person back into the employment market via its Jobcentres, ERC's advisory bodies, training provision and various special schemes giving incentives to employers and potential employees alike.

It is not easy to prevent a patient from becoming unemployed long-term, living a diminished existence on benefits. For intervention to be successful it is essential that doctors are aware, early, of the threat that ill-health and disability pose to employment. It requires considerable awareness and management skills to ensure that a patient is given every chance to return to work, and it is usually necessary to seek the help and continued involvement of professionals in MSC.

RECOMMENDED READING

MSC Publications:

Employment Gazette (monthly)

Employment Rehabilitation Research Centre Information, Papers 1-13

MSC Training Studies Paper

Employment Rehabilitation: Proposals for the Development of MSC Rehabilitation Service, 1984.

Available from MSC Head Office, Moorfoot, Sheffield, S1 4PQ

Jahoda, Marie (1982) *Employment and unemployment: a social psychological analysis* Cambridge University Press, Cambridge

Sinfield, Adrian (1981) *What employment means*, Martin Robertson, Oxford

Topliss, Ena (1979) *Provision for the Disabled*, 2nd edn, Basil Blackwell, Oxford

Walsh, Kenneth, and Pearson, Richard (1982) *U.K. Labour Market Guide*, 5, Institute of Manpower Studies, Brighton

Part 7

Equipment

42

Seating and Support Systems

Peggy Jay

INTRODUCTION

A suitable chair may be the most important piece of equipment used by a disabled person. It is likely to be in use for many hours a day, during which time it should provide a comfortable base for a variety of activities. A chair should not imprison the patient but be designed to facilitate rising and sitting down, so helping the patient to remain mobile. Patients with arthritis of weight-bearing joints, or with paralysis, spasticity or rigidity of the lower limbs — for example due to Parkinson's Disease, hemiplegia or spinal cord disease — are likely to have seating problems. Weakness or pain in the upper limbs will make rising from a chair more difficult.

Seating must be compatible with the patient's needs, and patients should be consulted about what these are. Too often people are trapped in chairs from which they cannot stand up, or are expected to eat while leaning backwards in easy chairs so that they spill food down their clothes. Good seating will maximise function. Good sitting posture should be combined with freedom to shift position. Similarly, armrests should not prevent arm movements. If a table is needed it must be at a suitable height. The chair needs to be well positioned within the patient's environment, whether facing the television so as to prevent neck strain, or with the best view of any stimulating action, which may be looking onto the street.

Appropriate seating should encourage patients to walk around. This will depend not only on the design of the chair but also, particularly for elderly patients, on relearning the techniques of getting up from a chair with least effort. When rising from a chair is easier, reaching the lavatory is less of a problem, and this may prevent or cure incontinence. Moving from an easy chair to the dining table will make eating easier. The ability to move about will encourage exercise that may help to improve circulation, prevent oedema, sustain muscle tone, prevent contractures, increase independence and go some way to overcoming social isolation. Sitting immobile in a comfortable chair all day is not good rehabilitation.

ASSESSMENT

It is very important to assess patients before advising them on the most suitable form of seating. This assessment will usually be carried out by an occupational therapist, a physiotherapist or a rehabilitation engineer. It will entail identifying both their medical condition, with the help of the referring doctor, and also what functions they want to carry out from the chair. The assessment will include body size and shape, posture, balance, oedema, perceptual dysfunction, confusion, continence, risk of tissue ischaemia, prognosis of deterioration, joint stiffness, muscle weakness, coordination, and the ability to get out of a chair. Sitting in a better position with a more upright posture can prevent contractures, and reduce the likelihood of tissue ischaemia caused either by unequal sideways pressure or sheer forces generated by sliding down in the chair. But sitting someone with a fixed deformity, such as a scoliosis, in a more upright position can result in an increase of pressure under one ischial tuberosity which may need special cushioning.

CRITERIA FOR CHAIR SELECTION (Figures 42.1 and 42.2; Table 42.1)

Easy or fireside chairs are often used by disabled and elderly people. Many of the criteria for selecting these chairs will apply to other types of chair. Easy chairs can be bought as standard furniture; some are sold with extra-high seats and others are designated 'geriatric' or 'orthopaedic' chairs (DLF, 1985). Although guidelines of choice may be given, the shape and dimensions of a 'comfortable' chair are very individual, (ICE, 1983). Lumbar support in different chairs, even the best chair, will only minimise discomfort. It is advisable to spend at least 15 minutes sitting in a chair before deciding it is the right one. Better still, some manufacturers will supply a chair on a trial basis. Disabled Living Centres usually have a selection of chairs which can be tried out during a visit. The following points should be considered when selecting a chair:

(a) *Seat height.* The feet should rest flat on the floor when the knees are at right angles, allowing the legs to move easily. There should be only nominal resistance when sliding the flat hand between the thigh and seat just behind the knee. A higher seat may be easier for rising and safer for sitting down. When a comfortable seat height is too low for rising unaided, the compromise may be a footstool, but only if this can be positioned and removed safely and easily.

(b) *Seat depth.* The sacrum should be touching the backrest to prevent slumping in the chair, and there should be a gap between the front of the seat and the lower leg to prevent calf pressure. A deep seat may look more

Figure 42.1: An unsuitable chair for a disabled person (courtesy of Mr A. Chesters, of Hangman Backdrops)

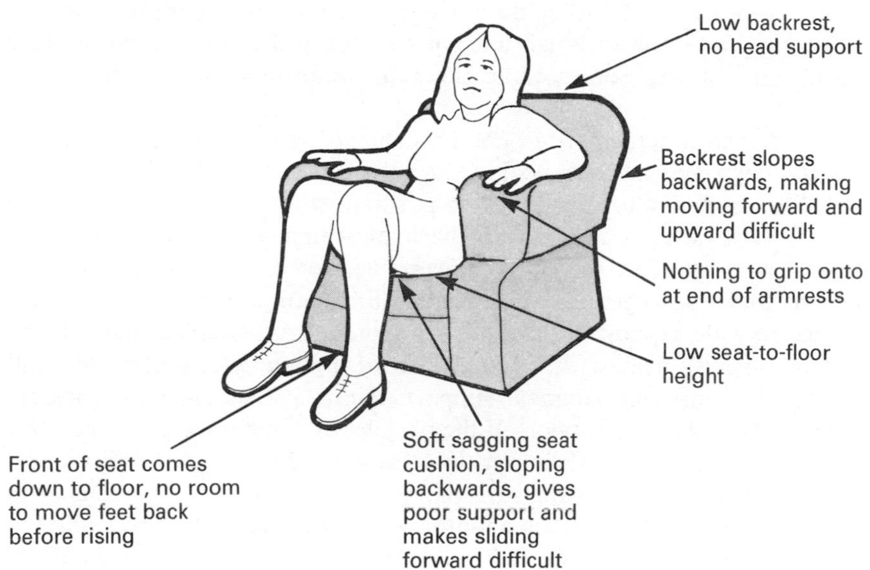

Figure 42.2: A suitable chair for a disabled person (courtesy of Mr A. Chesters, of Hangman Backdrops)

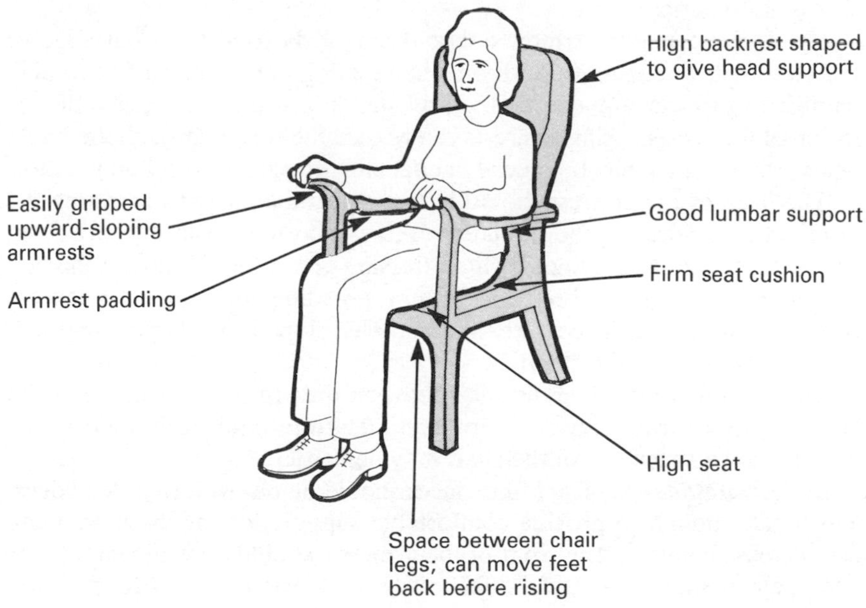

comfortable but back pain is often aggravated by sitting too far forwards in the chair, and then either slouching backwards or leaning forwards with a rounded back.

(c) *Seat width.* This should be wider than the sitter, both to allow for changing position in the chair and for sitting down clumsily (and possibly hitting an armrest). Some people like extra width to store belongings near to hand.

(d) *Backrest height and width.* This should be high enough to support the shoulders and for most people also the head. It should be broader than shoulder width to allow for changing position.

(e) *Backrest slope and shape.* A backrest with a gentle, backwards slope from seat to shoulder height is comfortable, but if the slope is too great, leaning forwards to get up from a chair will be more difficult. The backrest should provide support in the lumbar region but if the lumbar bulge is too low it will push against the sacrum instead. People with long trunks will need higher and longer lumbar support. Above the shoulder the backrest needs to provide head support. If the backwards slope is too great the sitter will use excessive neck flexion to look straight ahead or downwards. If it is too upright it may restrict neck movement. People need to be able to turn their heads freely to look about, and also to lean back to rest with the head supported. An adjustable head or neck rest can be positioned at the correct height and will allow neck movement. It should support the base of the skull, not the back of the head.

Wings on the chair are popular as head rests with people who sleep in chairs, but leaning the head so far sideways results in poor sleeping posture. Wings also restrict vision.

(f) *Armrest height.* Armrests should extend beyond the front edge of the seat, be low enough to push on when getting out of the chair and high enough to provide support until nearly standing without excessive dorsiflexion of the wrists. Using armrests can reduce the forces through the knees when rising, which may be crucial in enabling the patient to get up unaided.

The back of the armrest should be a comfortable height for resting the arms without elevating the shoulders, and should not get in the way when carrying out chosen activities such as dressing or knitting. Armrests that are the optimum height at both the front for getting up, and the back for comfort and convenience, are likely to be sloped or shaped upwards towards the front of the chair.

(g) *Armrest width.* The distance between the armrests (as much as the height) may restrict activities. However, if armrests are too wide apart, pushing down to get out of the chair may be harder.

(h) *Armrest design.* The top surfaces should be flat with rounded edges, and broad enough to provide comfortable support for the arms. Padding can increase comfort. The front of the armrests should be wide enough for good palmar support and of a thickness that allows the fingers to grasp the underside. Many people prefer filled-in armrests because these reduce draughts and make it easy to keep belongings within reach, but there are contraindications. Anything spilled will get trapped, a dropped lighted cigarette will be a fire hazard and unsupported vinyl sides may stretch and look unsightly. Belongings may end up beneath the seating area creating high-pressure points. Filled-in armrests, which leave a gap between sides and cushion, reduce draughts and make cleaning the chair easier.

(i) *Chair leg design.* To get out of a chair easily it must be possible to position the feet almost under the front of the chair, so bringing them below the body's centre of gravity. A low front rail or too deep a seat frame makes this impossible. Chairs should remain stable even when used by an unstable or atonic person, who may grab at the armrest or backrest for support. Chair legs that extend forward under the armrests, backwards under the backrest or are slightly splayed out sideways increase stability. If they project too far they could cause a fall.

(j) *Upholstery and coverings.* The seat and backrest should provide firm but well-padded support. Softer padding in the shoulder area may be needed to accommodate bony prominences and spinal curvature. Any armrest padding should be supportive and should not 'bottom out'.

When there is insufficient support in the seat the patient may slide into a hollow. This will make getting out of the chair difficult, prevent moving in the chair and induce a dorsal kyphosis. It may mean that the thighs are resting on the front edge of the frame.

Many chairs have foam upholstery and this can burn. Flame-retardant foam burns less fiercely but may produce more smoke and toxic fumes, so foam is often covered in a flame-retardant material. Flammability is a risk for a disabled person who smokes, but for others comfort and pressure relief are more important. After all, clothes and much else in the home will be flammable. BS5852 and DOE/PSA Flame Retardant Specifications Nos. 3 and 6 cover upholstered furniture. All chairs purchased for hospital use should be flame-retardant.

Chairs are often covered with vinyl because this is hardwearing, impervious to liquids, easy to clean and flame-retardant. However, some vinyls harden after prolonged contact with urine or with body oils from scalp or hands. Many people dislike sitting on vinyl because its impermeability pools perspirations, so it feels hot and clammy. If skin and clothing stick to vinyl, movement can produce sheer forces. For comfort, chair coverings should be absorbent to dissipate perspiration. Natural fabrics absorb moisture better than man-made fabrics. Vinyl can be covered by a loose cover of cotton or other natural fibre or one of the stretch fabric covers which can be bought to fit most shapes of chair.

Table 42.1: Check list for selecting a chair

Getting into the chair	
The sitter should not drop uncontrolled into the chair	armrest height (from floor at front) seat height upholstery/suspension
The sitter should not impact with hard areas	upholstery/suspension width of chair
The chair should not tip	stability splayed/curved legs
Sitting in the chair	
The sitter should be able to reach and lean against the backrest	seat depth seat slope backrest slope backrest shape
The sitter's feet should be supported	seat height/footrest seat depth
There should be no pressure on the calves and minimal pressure under the thighs	seat depth seat height upholstery/suspension
The sitter's back should be supported in the lower and upper regions	upholstery/suspension backrest shape backrest slope backrest height
The sitter's head should be in a comfortable position when leaning on the backrest but should not be restricted when not fully reclined	backrest slope backrest shape backrest height headrest
The sitter's arms should be comfortable, supported and free for activities	armrest height (to seat at rear) armrest width armrest shape
The sitter should not slide forward in the chair	upholstery/suspension seat slope
The sitter should be able to change position as required	upholstery/suspension seat slope armrest width armrest height (to seat at rear)
Getting out of the chair	
The sitter should not have to struggle forward to the edge of the chair	upholstery/suspension seat slope seat height backrest slope
The sitter should be able to place the feet beneath the front of the chair prior to rising	stretchers/legs seat height
The sitter should be able to give the initial push on the front of the armrest	armrest height (from floor at front) armrest width grip area
The sitter should be able to rise without unnecessary exertion or struggling	armrest height (from floor at front) seat height seat slope

The sitter should be able to gain support from the chair until almost standing	armrest height (from floor at front) grip area extending armrests
The chair should not tip or slip	stability curved/splayed legs

Adapted from *Seating for elderly and disabled people*, Report No. 9, by kind permission of the Institute for Consumer Ergonomics and the DHSS.

High-seat chairs

To get out of a chair a patient will normally lean forward and move the buttocks towards the front of the seat. He will then bring the feet back under the front edge of the chair, grasp the armrests and push himself forwards and upwards. A patient with limited knee flexion will need a higher seat in order to bring the feet closer to the front of the chair, and a patient with quadriceps weakness will need a higher seat to increase the mechanical advantage at the knee joint. Frail elderly patients are more likely to be able to get up from a high seat.

There are many high-seat chairs on the market. Wooden frames look more 'normal' and come in a variety of seat heights; some metal frames adjust in height. Backs may be contoured or straight and some are more upright to facilitate rising. Arms may be open, side-panelled, upholstered or removable. Upholstery may be cloth, which may be fire-retardant, or vinyl. These chairs are more expensive than standard chairs.

Some manufacturers will alter chairs to suit individual needs. These options range from merely adjusting seat height to made-to-measure seating systems which can include optional lifting and reclining seats (DLF, 1987).

Some patients raise the height of an existing chair by using an extra cushion, but this makes the armrests relatively lower and adversely affects the position of the curve of a shaped backrest. Chairs can be raised. Chair-raising sleeves are safer than raising blocks because sleeves become an integral part of the chair leg and will not be dislodged when the chair is moved.

Self-lift chairs

These actively assist patients to rise, and may be indicated for someone with painful joints or generalised weakness. They are not suitable for someone with poor balance or a limited range of hip or knee movement.

Self-lift seat units and self-lift mechanical chairs are hinged at the front and have either a strong spring or a hydraulic mechanism which lifts the seat from the horizontal to an angle of about 45°. Self-lift units fit into existing chairs and work best on a chair with a firm base.

Self-lift chairs lift higher than the seat units. The spring or the hydraulic system must be matched to the weight of the patient. As the patient leans forward and takes weight over the feet he or she will be pushed into the three-quarter standing position, and will need good quadriceps to straighten up into standing. Patients will need an assessment of lower limb function, followed by teaching and practice to use these seats safely and effectively. Some springs are noisy.

Electrically operated self-lift chairs are not affected by the patient's weight. Some systems raise the seat, others raise the seat and arms, and yet others raise the whole chair and tilt it forward. There are also variations in the height of raise and angle of tilt between chairs. Those with armrests that rise and tilt far enough to provide support right up to the standing position are best. These electrical chairs are easier to use but are much more expensive.

Rocking chairs

These can help a patient change position, relieve pressure, encourage gentle leg exercise and relieve backache. They are unlikely to give help in rising unless the patient has very good standing balance.

Reclining platform chairs

A patient with minimal hip and knee flexion, or with a rigid spine, may find using an 'Arthrodeeze' platform chair is the only way to stand up unaided. These platforms are mechanically or electrically controlled and move from the horizontal to the vertical, until the patient is standing up in the chair. Someone with extended fixed knees and mobile hips can have a platform that accommodates hip flexion when sitting. These platforms take up considerable space but do provide increased independence.

Reclining chairs

These are indicated for patients who are in constant pain and unable to change their own position spontaneously. The reclining chair allows the user to rest or sleep without having to be moved to a bed by a helper. It also shifts pressure from the ischial tuberosities to the spine, and may thus be helpful in preventing presure sores. Patients are usually more comfortable sleeping in the reclined position than in the upright one (where they very often slide down the chair). The better chairs tilt the front of the seat up and raise the leg rests as well as reclining the back. This tilting from the front effectively lowers the buttock area and prevents sliding out of the chair. Any chair that reclines more than 20 ° will be uncomfortable without leg support.

With mechanically operated reclining chairs the patients must be sitting in just the right position to utilise body weight (as well as pushing hard) to recline the chair. Electrically operated chairs get over this problem, and some have a lifting seat.

Tilting chairs

These are mobile chairs which can be tilted on their back legs and locked in position. They are used by nursing staff to prevent patients sliding down in their chairs. They are contraindicated because they leave the patient trapped, staring up at the ceiling, out of contact with events and people around him.

Mobile chairs

These should be used only by people who are too immobile to get out of a chair and unable to propel a wheelchair or to control an electric chair. It is easier and quicker for nurses and helpers to wheel a patient from one place to another, but it is much better rehabilitation to continue walking as long as possible, however slowly, using a mobile chair only when there is no alternative.

Mobile chairs have fixed wheels or swivelling castors. Wheels go better in a straight line, and castors around corners. A combination of castors on the front and wheels at the back makes manoeuvring easy and also allows the chair to be tilted on its back wheels. Small wheels and castors tend to jam in every obstacle; 13 cm diameter should be sufficient to avoid this. Solid tyres are easier to maintain, but pneumatic tyres give an easier ride. Solid, spongy, semi-rigid tyres are the best compromise.

Patients in mobile chairs will need help to get up, so seat height and brake position are less critical. A footrest which can only be pushed under the chair by an attendant will be quite acceptable, but a fixed footrest makes standing difficult and dangerous because the chair can tip forwards.

Office chairs

These have advantages for more active disabled people. The height and angle of the backrest, and height and sometimes slope of the seat, are all adjustable, so these chairs encourage a more upright sitting posture. The swivelling seat increases reach. A five-pronged base provides good stability; castors are better on carpets and 'glide' on uncarpeted floors. Stability may, however, be a problem when getting up or down; backing the chair against a wall may help. Some chairs have arms; these should not prevent the chair getting close to the work top. Office chairs can be used not only when typing or working at a desk, but also when preparing food or ironing, provided the work surface or ironing board is at a suitable height.

High-seat stools

These are used by disabled people who need to conserve energy by sitting rather than standing, but who need to work at a standing rather than sitting height. Some have backrests and some have armrests. There are also stools with angled seats sloping downwards towards the front, which are used by patients with limited or painful hip flexion or ankylosing spondylitis.

Balans seats

These seats are designed to relieve back pain. They have angled seats and knee rests, but neither backrests nor armrests. The base may be a rocker or it may be fixed. The combination of angled seat and knee rests tends to induce an increased lumbar curve and so encourage a more upright posture, although it is still possible to slump. The rocking base facilitates changing position and redistributing pressure. The seat and knee rests should be well padded but, even so, resting the shins rather than the knees on the knee pads is likely to be uncomfortable. These seats come in various sizes and dimensions from a number of manufacturers under different names. To work from such a seat, the work surface must be a convenient height and preferably sloping slightly upwards.

Moulded seats

Some patients are so severely disabled that even with the most careful assessment and prescription they cannot be adequately supported in a chair, even with extra padding and cushioning. For them, moulded seats may provide the answer. There are various systems. With *vacuum-extracted systems* the patient sits on an envelope filled with polystyrene granules. Air is extracted from this envelope until the seat takes up the shape of the user. This moulded seat can then be fitted into a wheelchair, or it can be used to produce a positive cast on which a moulded plastic seat is shaped. The *matrix body support system* is a series of small plastic units attached together by ball-and-socket joints to form a sheet of material. This is so adjustable that it can take up any shape. It is then covered with foam upholstery, mounted on a tubular frame, or clamped into a wheelchair. Funding for moulded seats to fit into wheelchairs is avaiable from the DHSS. Information about suppliers of moulded seats is available from the Disabled Living Foundation (see Chapter 43, Wheelchairs, Figure 43.7).

Special cushions

Wheelchair cushions increase comfort and can also reduce the risk of tissue ischaemia (Jay, 1984). Everyone who sits in a wheelchair should have a cushion unless there are contraindications. These cushions can also be used in other chairs.

Relief of pressure under the ischial tuberosities can be achieved by sitting on a more conforming cushion, so that pressure is taken over more of the seating area, or by increasing the amount of support in some parts of the sitting area to balance the decrease in support elsewhere, as with alternating pressure cushions. This can also be done by sitting on an ischial cut-out cushion which will redistribute pressure to the thighs, although this may be too uncomfortable for someone with intact sensation. Humidity at the interface can also lead to tissue ischaemia. An absorbent cushion cover or a sheepskin will dissipate perspiration. Cushions with carrying straps are available for arthritics, or people of short stature who always need a high seat. There is also a cushion with a thigh depression to accommodate an arthrodesed hip or knee. More information about wheelchair cushions is given in Chapter 43.

Lumbar support

This must be in the right place. If it is too low in the chair it just pushes the patient forward. Good lumbar support not only provides a more comfortable and upright posture but can reduce pressure under the sacrum.

Lumbar supports are often sold as backrests for use in cars (Bulstrode *et al.*, 1983). Sculptured foam supports come in different shapes which suit different people. Inflatable back supports will mould to fit any back, which is an advantage, but cannot be used for postural control. Lumbar supports covered in vinyl will be hot and sticky. Fabric or sheepskin covers are better.

Lateral support

Side cushions can give support and produce a more upright posture which will equalise pressures over the seating area. Corrective side cushioning, for example for scoliosis, will not be effective unless the pelvis is stabilised first and any pelvic tilt accommodated by a specially designed seat cushion. Side support cushions need to be firm to achieve correction.

Neck support

Bone-shaped neck pillows will provide support when the head is forward-flexed, and they can be removed when lying back. These are small and easy to handle while sitting.

Legrests

These should be stable and height-adjustable to hold the legs in the optimum position. They must be long enough to support the whole lower leg, from ankle to knee, and well padded to spread pressure. Taking weight solely through the calf can restrict circulation; a pillow along the length of the rest can help redistribute pressure.

Many patients prefer a legrest that allows about 20° of knee flexion. If oedema is to be reduced the legrest should be horizontal so that the ankles are at hip height. The end of the legrest adjacent to the chair should be at seat height to support the knee and prevent them hyperextending, which would lead to pain, stiffness and difficulty in rising.

Footstools

These should be high enough to support the feet at a height that prevents pressure under the thighs. Adjustable-height footstools are available or the legs of a wooden stool can be cut to give the desired height. Footstools with ferrules on the legs will give more stability, but patients need telling never to stand up on a footstool. A footstool with castors will be easier to push safely out of the way before getting up from the chair. It can be hooked back with a walking stick. Castors will also encourage leg movement during sitting.

Tables

The height of a table or desk should relate to the height of the chair and the person in it. Elbows should be about table-top height and there should be clearance underneath so that the thighs are not compressed. A strong, solid table will provide support when rising.

Someone who sits mainly in an easy chair may need a cantilevered table which adjusts in height. One with an H-shaped base will be stable, and can be drawn close to the chair. Some have a tilting surface to hold a newspaper or act as a bookrest. The best have a small permanently horizontal section big enough to hold spectacles and a cup of tea.

Trays

A lap desk provides an alternative to a table for someone sitting in an easy chair. It is a tray with a polystyrene bead cushion underneath which moulds itself to fit the shape of the lap. This forms a stable base for writing or taking tea. Some makes of chair have a tray, which attaches to the armrests, as an optional extra.

SOURCES OF SUPPLY AND FINANCE

Social Services departments can often provide special chairs and seating aids on a long-term loan to a disabled client. Both Social Services departments and hospital occupational therapy departments may be able to order chairs at trade price on the understanding that the patient will pay this cost.

Some wheelchair cushions will be supplied free of charge by hospitals or Social Services departments. When the patient must pay, wheelchair cushions, as well as other aids specifically designed for disabled people, including chairs, can be VAT-exempt. Sometimes a standard chair ordered for a disabled person on a doctor's recommendation will be VAT-exempt. The relevent claim form is included in the leaflet *Aids for handicapped people* obtainable from local VAT offices.

MAINTENANCE AND FOLLOW-UP

Chairs wear out, foam degrades and loses its resilience, webbing straps stretch or break. It is not sufficient just to choose a suitable chair. This should be checked at least once a year to make sure it is not worn out. Too many elderly people sit with piles of newspapers under a degraded foam cushion. Upholstery may need cleaning, repairing, or even re-covering.

Mobile chairs, too, need attention. Castors may get clogged up or need lubricating. There should also be a built-in review procedure to check whether the chair is still appropriate for the patient, or whether some other type of seating would now be better.

REFERENCES

Bulstrode, S., Harrison, R.A. and Clarke, A.K. (1983) *Assessment of backrests for use in car seats.* DHSS Aids Assessment Programme

Disabled Living Foundation (DLF) (1987) *Chairs.* Information Sheet no. 2 (revised annually)

Institute for Consumer Ergonomics (ICE) (1983) *Seating for elderly and disabled people.* Report no. 9, *Chair specifications and guidelines for chair selection,* University of Technology, Loughborough (May)

Jay, P.E. (1984) *Choosing the best wheelchair cushion for your needs, your chair and your lifestyle,* RADAR, London

FURTHER READING

Atherton, J., Chatfield, J., Clarke, A.K. and Harrison, R.A. (1980) *Easy chairs for the arthritic,* DHSS Aids Assessment Programme

Atherton, J., Harrison, R.A. and Clarke, A.K. (1982) *Office seating for the arthritic and low back pain patients,* DHSS Aids Assessment Programme

Fire safety in health care premises, furniture, furnishings, bed assemblies, apparel. Health Technical Memorandum 87, DHSS (1983)

Harris, C. and Mayfield, W. (1983) *Selecting easy chairs for elderly and disabled people,* Institute for Consumer Ergonomics, University of Technology, Leicester

Moy, A. (1979) *Assessment of self rise chairs and cushions,* DHSS Aids Assessment Programme

Nelham R.L. (1981) Seating of the chairbound person — a survey of seating equipment in the UK. *J. Biomed. Engng.,* *6,* 267-74

Sitting and seating — a series of articles which include discussion of the Balans seat, personally contoured cushions and moulded seating. *Physiotherapy,* February 1984

Booklet on chairs, available from the Arthritis and Rheumatism Council, 41 Eagle Street, London WC1R 4AR

43

Wheelchairs

John Goodwill

Patients are unable to walk due to a variety of conditions, whose character and severity will determine whether a wheelchair is required for outdoor use only or for use inside the home as well.

Some patients are unable to walk because of tiredness and/or breathlessness due to cardiac or respiratory disease. Others have locomotor disorders which may be due to degenerative arthritis, particularly osteoarthritis of hips or knees, or to inflammatory arthritis such as rheumatoid arthritis or to neurological disease: the most common conditions in the latter group are stroke, multiple sclerosis, cerebral palsy, paraplegia and tetraplegia. It is important that the wheelchair is provided as an aid to increasing the patient's mobility, function and choice in life, and that it is not seen as a sign of disability. This attitude of mind is vital in persuading the patient to accept this new means of mobility. The chair must be prescribed as accurately for the patient as a drug for any medical condition. If the requirement is clear, as for an outdoor transit chair (9L), the general practitioner could order it, but for most other chairs the patient is assessed in a rehabilitation unit, Disabled Living Centre or wherever there is a wide variety of chairs available so that both patient and staff can make an informed choice. Without detailed assessment, including the environment where the chair will be used, the patient may receive the wrong chair, but because he knows that the staff have done their best he will not protest that it could be improved. Clearly a wheelchair is only part of a patient's rehabilitation treatment programme.

PRESCRIPTION

Form AOF5G is used to order a wheelchair from the local Artificial Limb and Appliance Centre (ALAC); requirements must be detailed as on any other prescription. It is signed by a doctor, usually on the advice of an occupational therapist or physiotherapist. For the patient who is totally dependent on a wheelchair for mobility the NHS will provide a more strongly built chair equivalent to the standard range described below. These chairs are supplied by independent companies through the NHS. The chairs look better, have stronger seats and backs but are often heavier than standard NHS chairs.

OUTDOOR USE ONLY

A wheelchair for outdoor use only is required for the patient who can walk sufficiently well indoors, but because of limited exercise tolerance, pain or slowness of movement is unable to move far. The *model 9L transit chair* is suitable for patients weighing up to 100 kg, and will go into most car boots, except very small cars, where the *model 10 chair* can be used. This folds smaller, but is not ideal for the heavier patient. In each case the patient must be pushed by a relative or friend. If the patient can provide some or all of the pushing power a self-propelling *Model 8L, 8BL or 8LJ* as described below can be used. In a hilly area, or over rough terrain or when the attendant has insufficient exercise tolerance to push the patient (as when the husband of the disabled patient is himself arthritic or has dyspnoea due to cardiac or respiratory disease), the *model 28 attendant-operated electric wheelchair may be useful.* This does not fold, and takes up much space in the home or garage, but it will travel a few miles before the battery needs recharging from the mains (Figure 43.1).

In Britain the NHS does not supply patient-operated electric wheelchairs for *outdoor use*, but many types are available (Vessa, Bec, Zimmer, Carter, Newton, Everest & Jennings, etc.). These may be seen at Disabled Living Centres. Purchase of these may be facilitated by a charity or by hire purchase over a two-year period through the Motability scheme using the Mobility Allowance (see Chapter 37). This satisfies the need for local mobility, which is what many patients require.

INDOOR AND OUTDOOR USE

These chairs are for patients who will live all or much of the time in their chair. Many factors will influence those prescribing a wheelchair; the success of this depends on the depth and quality of assessment. *The choice depends on many factors*:

patient's height, weight and body build;
mental attitude and intelligence;
his level of disability, prognosis;
access and egress from the chair;

Figure 43.1: 9L Transit chair: backrest folds down, footrests detach

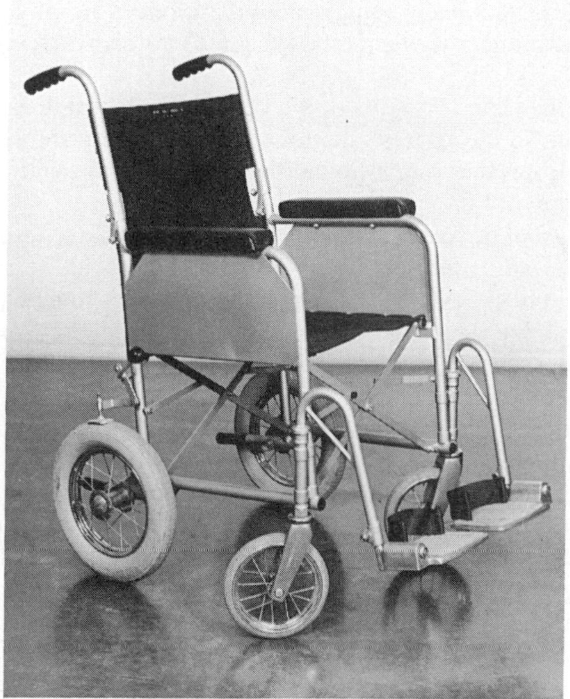

what demands he will make on the chair — heavy or light use;
what he wants to do from the wheelchair;
what special features are required;
where the chair will be stored;
the architectural circumstances in which it will be used at home, at work and for leisure;
the means of transport of the patient and chair.

Disease and disability: one needs to know the diagnosis, the parts of the body affected, whether there is any fixed deformity of a joint, or contracture due to arthritis or neurological disease, whether the patient's limbs or trunk are spastic or subject to flexor or extensor spasms, and whether the patient is intellectually and emotionally normal. This is highly relevant if he is in charge of a powered wheelchair.

The *prognosis* is important; if the patient is expected to decline rapidly it may not be worth struggling to keep him using a self-propelled wheelchair; an electric chair may be more appropriate. If a patient's only exercise for the upper limbs consists of wheelchair propulsion, and he is dependent for transfer on the strength of his arms, one may defer use of an electric chair.

The needs of the helper require consideration: is he physically able to push, fold and manoeuvre the proposed chair, especially over rough ground or steps?

Access to the chair for someone who can walk a short distance is usually from the front, so the armrests do not have to be removable, but for sitting transfer one armrest is removed and the footrest swung out of the way so that the legs are not impeded or damaged.

Environmental factors are important. There may have to be a compromise on chair width; the seat has to be sufficiently wide to accommodate the patient's buttocks but the width of the chair needs to be narrow enough to go through the smallest door in the house, including the bathroom. Frequently houses are small, turning space is limited and storage is a problem both in the house and car. A patient dependent on a chair should have two (although the NHS will not usually provide this); if his only chair breaks down the patient may be unable to follow any of his normal activities, which may be expensive in loss of earnings. Two chairs may be prescribed under the NHS if a lightweight chair is required when travelling alone. Chair design must be related to its like usage; an active 20-year-old paraplegic will bounce his chair up kerbs and use it in an athletic fashion. It needs to be much more robust than the chair for most patients (50 per cent of wheelchairs are supplied to patients over 70 years old). A wheelchair is a seat on wheels, functional rather than beautiful, but its appearance is important as it is seen as an extension of the person. Many doctors forget that the wheelchair provided for severely disabled patients becomes their main chair; many hours are spent in it, and a variety of activities have to be pursued from it. One thus has to ensure that seating is adequate, including provision of suitable seat, back and side cushions as needed.

CHOOSING A WHEELCHAIR — SPECIAL FEATURES AND ACCESSORIES

The figures in Table 43.1 are approximate. Patients vary and there are some patients working or living in a limited space who might prefer an *8L chair* but be reasonably comfortable in the *smaller 8BL*, the latter fitting their circumstances whereas the extra 2 inches (5 cm) of width of the 8L may be too much to turn conveniently from narrow passages through narrow doorways. The *model 7 lightweight* self-propelling chair is available for the patient who has difficulty folding and lifting the chair into his car. Each of these chairs has rear propelling wheels with pneumatic tyres, heel loops to prevent the feet sliding back off the footrests, swinging detachable

Table 43.1: Dimensions of commonly used wheelchairs

Model	Seat size, inches (cm)	Overall width, open	Overall length	Folded width	Rear wheels	Front wheels	Weight, lb (kg)	
Models 9L and 10 (push chairs)								
9L	17 × 17 (43 × 43)	26 (66)	40 (102)	11 (27)	12½ (32)	7½ (19)	34 (15.4)	Folding backrest, alternative seats 18″ × 17″ (46 × 32) 19″ × 18″ (48 × 46)
10	17 × 18 (43 × 45)	24 (61)	43 (109)	10 (25)	11 (27)	7½ (19)	34 (15.4)	Folds small enough for the boot of a mini. Alternative seat size (15″ × 18″) (38 × 45)
Models 7, 8L, 8BL and 8LJ (self propelling)								
7	17 × 18 (43 × 45)	24 (61)	42 (197)	11 (27)	18 (46)	7½ (19)	36 (16.3)	Alternative seat size 15″ × 18″ (38 × 45). Folds smaller than model 8 range
8L	17 × 17 (43 × 43)	25 (63)	43 (109)	10 (25)	22 (56)	7½ (19)	40 (18.1)	For adults up to 16 stone (102 kg). Alternative seat size 18″ × 17″ (46 × 43)
8BL	16 × 16 (41 × 41)	23 (58)	37 (94)	10 (25)	20 (51)	5 (13)	37 (16.8)	For adults up to 10 stone (64 kg)
8LJ	15 × 16 (38 × 41)	23 (58)	43 (109)	10 (25)	22 (56)	7½ (19)	40 (18.1)	Alternative seat sizes 13″ × 15″ (33 × 38) or 16″ × 16″ (41 × 41); for the smaller adult this chair may be better than 8BL for outdoor use because front castors are larger at 7½″ (19) and pass more easily over pavements

footrests and detachable armrests to allow sideways transfer. A pump is provided (Figure 43.2).

Front propelling wheels may be necessary for some patients who cannot extend their shoulders to the standard rear propelling wheels, or who have pain or weakness making pushing in that position difficult. Some patients with muscular dystrophy may find this modification useful but sideways transfer by removing the armrests is then impossible, and the footrests cannot swing out of the way, although the footplates will swing into the vertical positions (Figure 43.3).

Armrests. These are of standard height in NHS chairs but as the distance from elbow to buttocks varies in different people, and the amount of cushioning on the chairs may also vary, it would be better if variable-height armrests were available. Standard armrests may be used by patients to help transfer sideways, or to lean on while getting into an upright position if they walk a short distance. Alternatively desk arms allow close approach to work surfaces. The patient can be provided with *two pairs* of arm-rests: one standard and one desk arm type. A removable tray can be fitted on the

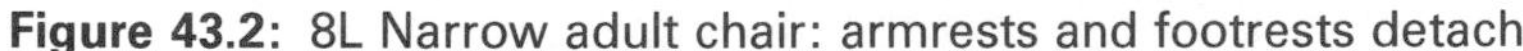

Figure 43.2: 8L Narrow adult chair: armrests and footrests detach

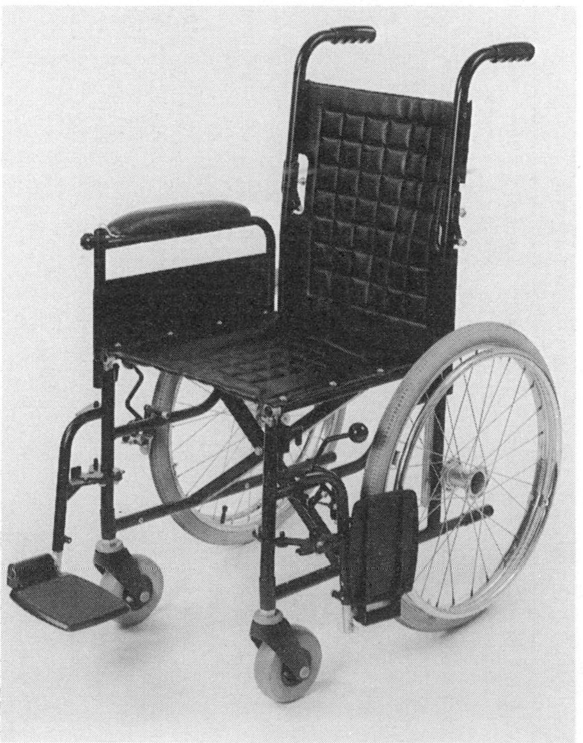

Figure 43.3: Front wheel drive chair; this limits sideways transfer (desk arms can also be seen)

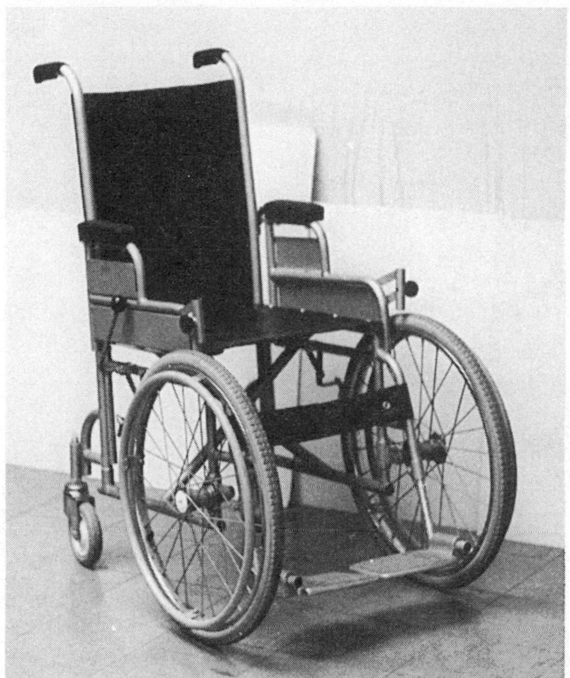

arms. The Bexhill armrest enables the hemiplegic patient to rest his arm in a good position (Figure 43.4).

Backrests slope at different angles on different models, e.g. 15° on the 8L and 8LJ and 10° on the 8BL, and will increase as the back canvas stretches with use — heavier duty canvas is available. Some patients find that a two-inch cushion between their back and the canvas adds to the support and comfort. *A folding backrest* gives less back support and is only used if essential to allow the folded chair to fit into a car.

Headrest extension up to 12 inches (30 cm) is useful where the patient has much neck weakness, as in late multiple sclerosis (MS), motor neurone disease or muscular dystrophy. Those with poor head control are then not in the best position for eating, etc., and may need additional head or neck support at that time. A neck and headrest may also help with extensor spasms; side supports may be fitted on the headrest (Figure 43.5).

Elevating legrests are needed where the knees are fixed in extension, or where ankle oedema is a problem; these greatly add to the length of the wheelchair and the difficulty of manoeuvring in domestic or work environment.

Figure 43.4: Bexhill armrest for hemiplegic patient

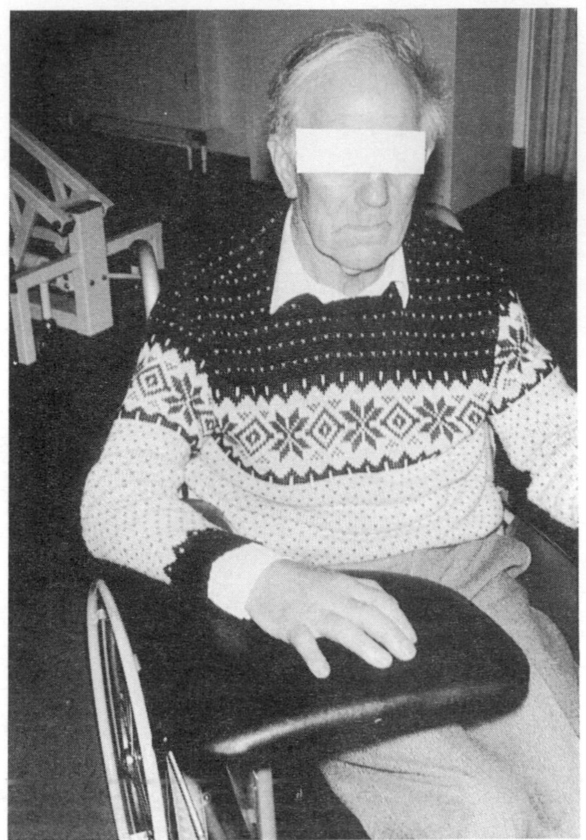

Adjustable semi-reclining or fully-reclining backrests are rarely used except for the patient who wants changes of position, or who is only comfortable in a reclining position. This occurs occasionally with severe ankylosing spondylitis with fixed hips unsuitable for surgery, in high cervical spine injuries above the C6 level and in patients with late progressive neurological diseases, including MS. Where the patient can bend the hips the chair is brought into an upright position for eating or other activities, but when resting the chair is adjusted to recline to the desired angle. A headrest extension and elevating legrests are needed for comfort, but the length of the chair is then 50–60 inches (125–150 cm), depending upon how high the backrest and legrests are positioned. For manoeuvring between rooms the backrest is brought up and the legrests lowered, but still it is a long chair which is very difficult in an ordinary domestic environment.

Figure 43.5: Reclining backrest with extended headrest; elevating legrests are essential if back reclines

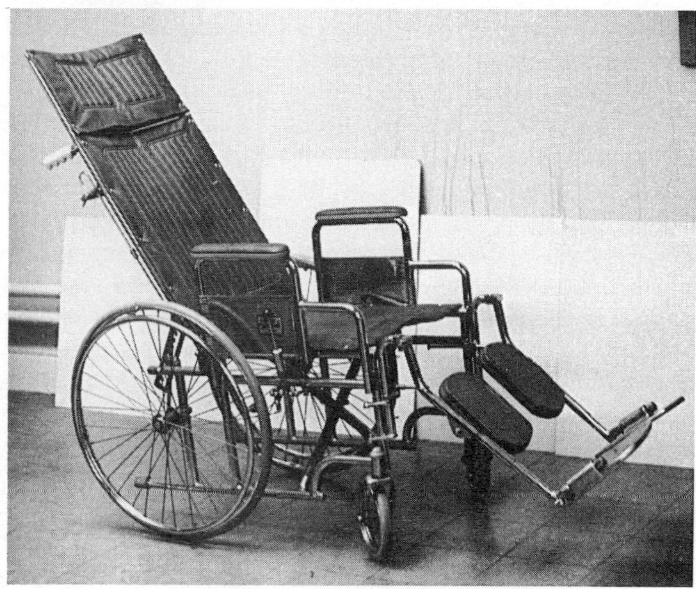

Brakes must be accessible. In hemiplegia the brake handle may need to be lengthened on the weak side so that the good arm can use it, or a cable used to bring the control round to the good arm. In arthritis, lengthened brake handles may aid weak arm function. If an active patient does much moving up or down slopes, one-way brakes may be a useful addition. Brakes work poorly if the tyres are not pumped up.

WHEELCHAIR SEATING AND CUSHIONS (see Jay, 1984)

Attention is needed to ensure comfort and the prevention of pressure sores, especially if the patient is anaesthetic over the weight-bearing areas of the buttocks and hips. The thickness of the cushion will affect the relative height of the armrests, backrest and footrests, and also the reach to propelling wheels and handbrakes. A thick cushion added to an existing chair can prevent feet reaching the floor, making standing and sitting difficult. It can also prevent knees fitting under a table. The cushion (and the chair seat) should extend to within $1^1/_2$ inches (4 cm) of the back of the knee to distribute pressure under the full length of the thighs, as well as under the buttocks. The footrests should be low enough to take weight under the thighs, not just under the buttocks and the soles of the feet. The standard cushion is covered in PVC-coated fabric, which is hard-wearing, flame-retardant and easily cleaned. Some people find this hot and sticky and replace it with a stretch foam cover, which is cooler and more conforming, but flammable; some prefer a corduroy cover. The DHSS will also supply on request a cushion of heavy-duty foam substitute for the more heavily built person, or latex foam, which some people prefer to polyurethane. An incontinent patient needs a cushion with an impermeable cover that is easily cleaned.

When seat sag is a problem a hard base can be incorporated into the cushion. This hard base rests on the horizontal metal tubes of the wheelchair seat. This will stabilise the pelvis and will help someone with an unstable trunk achieve a better sitting position. A hard base makes the patient higher in the chair, since it not only eliminates the sag but has a cushion on top. The cushioning support system is an integral part of wheelchair prescription; different densities of foam seat cushion are available for different weight of individuals. A piece of softer foam may be inset in the firmer material to give relief under areas such as the ischial tuberosities where the skin is at risk.

An alternative is the Gel cushion, which flows to conform to the patient's buttocks but can still give areas of excess pressure, an alternating pressure cushion, or an air support system such as the ROHO cushion, consisting of 72 air-filled cones (9 × 8), one or two of which can be tied off to deflate them under areas of doubtful skin viability. Some high tetraplegic patients feel unsteady on anything but a firm foam cushion (Figure 43.6).

Back cushions help to relieve backrest pressure for those who lack sensation, like tetraplegics, or with partial sensation, like those with MS. A patient with spina bifida, scoliosis or kyphosis may need a back cushion to

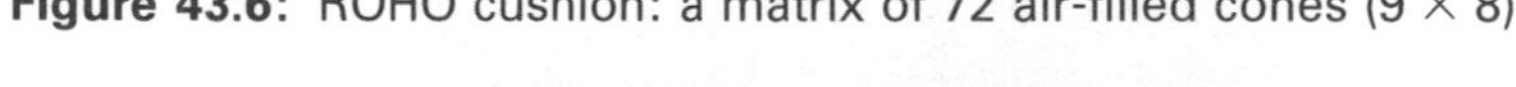
Figure 43.6: ROHO cushion: a matrix of 72 air-filled cones (9 × 8)

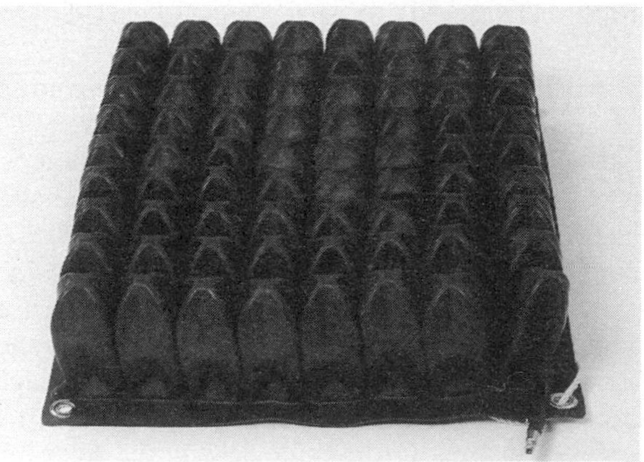

prevent spinal pressure. Underweight elderly patients may need protection too. A back cushion may push the patient too far forward in the chair and make reaching the propelling wheels difficult. Lumbar support cushions can protect the spine and provide a more upright posture without pushing the whole body forwards. The manually inflated Pirelli lumbar cushions, designed for use in a car, will mould to body shape.

Slumping of the trunk to the side may be reduced by side-cushions filling in the armrest(s) or by firm support attached to the armrest or back of the chair and pushing on the thorax. Where the patient needs total support, as for some with severe head injury or cerebral palsy, a moulded seat may be best for the patient, or a matrix seat (Steeper) is used (Figure 43.7). The latter is a sheet of interlinked plastic and metal parts which are moulded to the patient. At the end of the fitting a screw in each part is tightened to make a firm contoured support; this is then covered. Either seat is fixed on a wheelchair chassis. Alternatively a ready-made posture support chair can be used in which the backrest is adjustable for angle and

Figure 43.7: Matrix seat (Steeper): interlinked parts of plastic and metal are moulded to the patient; each part is then tightened with a screw-driver. The whole seat is then covered and mounted on a wheelchair chassis

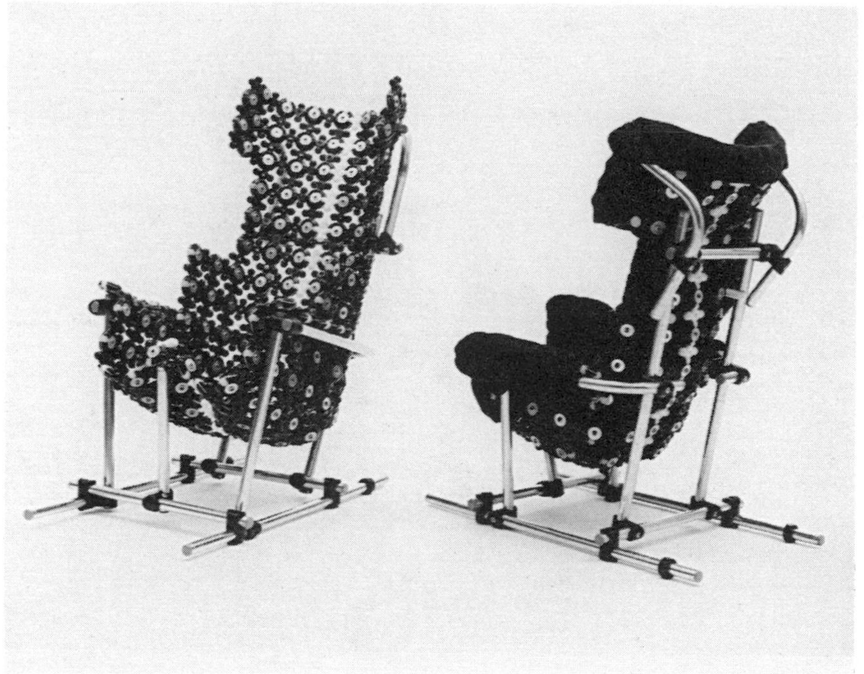

shape, the seat may be angled upwards at the front, side supports are adjustable, the footbox maintains leg position and a pommel between the legs can be fitted to prevent excess adduction (Figure 43.8) (Everest & Jennings, OrthoKinetics, Newton).

Getting the right cushion is not enough. *Cushions wear out*, foam degrades, vinyl covers harden and crease. With air cushions and some water cushions the pressure needs to be checked regularly. Some cushions can be placed in the chair upside-down or the wrong way round. This is particularly a problem in institutions. Patients place things on top of their cushions, such as folded incontinence pads, creased clothing or urine drainage bag straps, or they carry wallets under their cushions, all of which can affect pressure distribution.

Patients needs change. Progressive disability or increasing age add to the risk of pressure sores and the need for a different cushion. New cushions come on the market which may solve old problems.

Restraints are useful if the patient slides forwards, or even out of the wheelchairs. A single strap passes down and back at 45° from the patient's waist behind the junction of the seat and backrest and round the metal of

Figure 43.8: Posture control chair (orthokinetic): adjustable head and pelvic supports with built-in harness, adjustable seat angle and legrest elevation

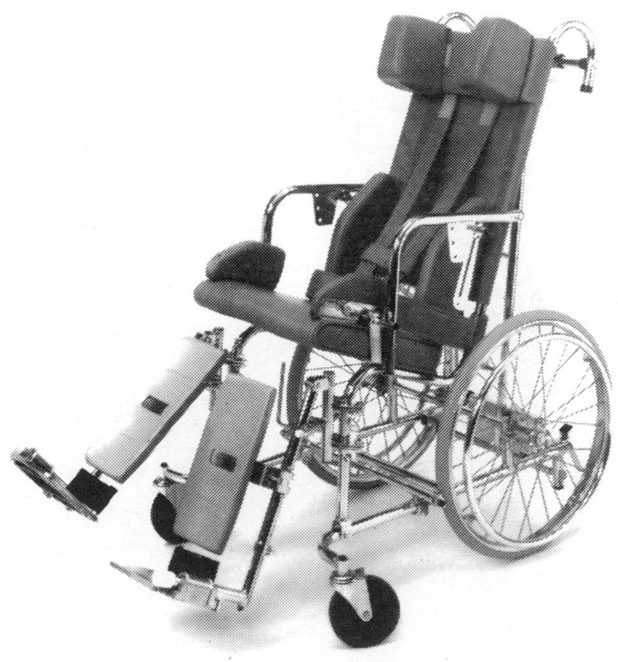

the chair. If this is insufficient a full shoulder harness is used.

Other accessories include detachable tray, footrest extension to prevent spastic legs slipping backwards, or a firm legrest behind the calves which fits onto the foot or legrests. A pump for pneumatic tyres, is supplied. Protective covers against cold and rain are also available.

Sports chairs

Sports chairs are available for private purchase by the fit athletic user; they are light, highly manoeuvrable and very easy to propel. Being less stable than standard chairs they are only used by those with good balance and quick reactions (Figure 43.9) (Cochrane and Wilshere, 1982).

ELECTRIC WHEELCHAIRS FOR INDOOR USE

These are assessed by the technical and medical staff of the ALAC where the patient attends, but it is useful if the patient is first assessed and a detailed prescription prepared by a rehabilitation unit where the therapists will have detailed information about the patient, their needs and circumstances of use of the chair. These chairs are used when the patient is unable

Figure 43.9: Sports chair (Activlite by Bec): lightweight chair, with facility to change rear axle position up–down, fore–aft, to allow greater ease of propulsion

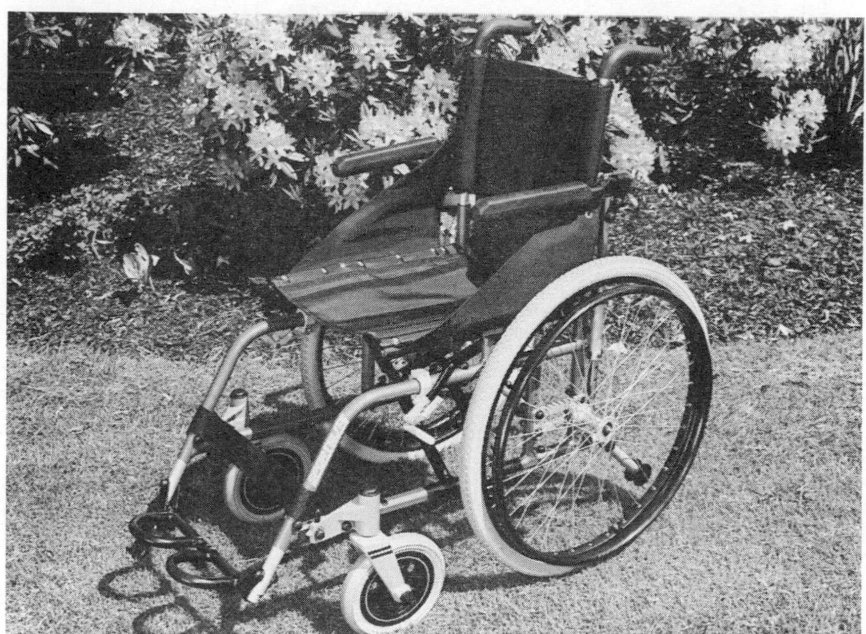

to propel an ordinary wheelchair due to fatigue, breathlessness or motor incapacity. Prescription must consider the factors detailed above including size of chair, cushion support, modifications and accessories. Control is by hand, foot or chin, suck–blow control with the mouth or by head switches in a specially made headrest. The hand control is a short vertical lever or swashplate on the armrest, which may be positioned conveniently on a tray on the wheelchair or centrally on an arm pivoted on the front vertical member of the wheelchair, swinging out of the way to allow access to the chair. *Positioning of the control* is very important for the arthritic who cannot conveniently externally rotate the shoulder to use a control on the armrest, or if there is tremor as in MS, or athetosis as in cerebral palsy, again a more centrally placed control may be easier. Chin control is performed by pushing a lever in the desired direction of travel; pushing downwards accelerates the chair. Exceptionally control is by suck–blow from the mouth or by head switches where other methods are not feasible. It is possible to have separate controls for speed and direction if required.

Proportional control is available on NHS electric wheelchairs for patients in whom jerkiness of the chair causes pain or triggers spasms.

Where space is limited a three-wheeled chair has an advantage: *the model 102* has two 8 inch (20 cm) rear wheels and a single 7 inch (18 cm) front traction/steering wheel. It is 34 inches (86 cm) long by 24 inches (61 cm) wide, comfortable for domestic use but the big footboard has to be folded up for access and egress, at which time a lever on the side of the chair is used to lower a small wheel at each side of the front of the chair to ensure stability — many patients find this awkward. Control is on one armrest, the other being removable to allow sideways transfer. An alternative three-wheeled chair is the *Sleyride (Carter)* which has a small turning circle. Steering is by rotation of the whole control drive unit. This is suitable when the patient can easily control his hands in the midline; the vertical central control bar lifts out for access to the chair.

A better alternative, where reasonable space is available, may be *the model 109*, which is a modified 9L chair which has front castors, each rear wheel being driven by an electric motor (Figure 43.10). The *model 110* is similar, but some patients find the *model 103* with rear castors and front wheel drive more convenient because of greater manoeuvrability when moving forward. It is possible to remove the batteries and fold models 109, 110 and 103, but the model 102 does not fold. A commode fitting is only available on the model 102, which for the incontinent disabled woman may exclude consideration of other powered chairs. Where there are special needs other electric-powered indoor chairs may be supplied under the NHS. Providing the patient can understand the controls, and wishes to use a powered wheelchair, all patients can manage a chair if the detailed prescription, position and type of control is correct. Inability to use the chair is usually due to inadequate prescription.

Figure 43.10: 109 Electrically driven indoor chair; one motor on each rear wheel, control box can be positioned for patient's convenience

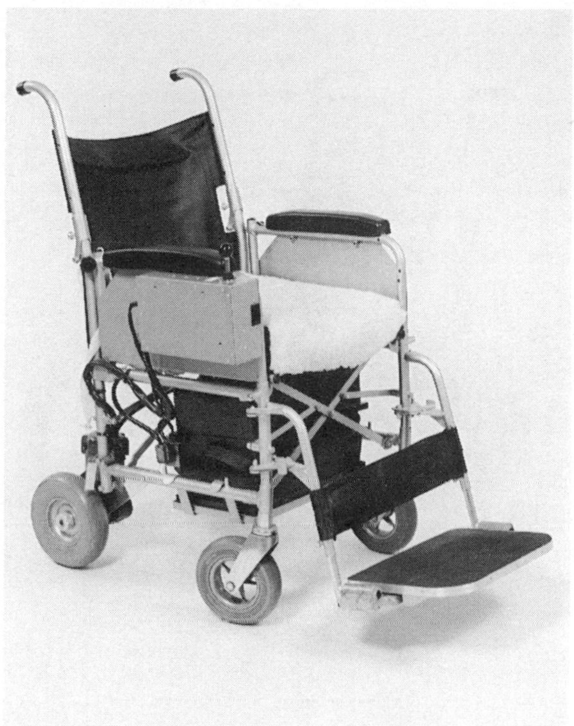

In addition there is a wide variety of electric chairs available for *private purchase* from different companies. If the patient receives Mobility Allowance he can use the Motability scheme to purchase one of a number of these chairs, whether for indoor or for outdoor use. Suitable chairs are made by Carter & Jennings, Dudley, Newton, Vessa, BEC and others, but for efficient outdoor use, including going up and down kerbs easily, a larger chair is needed which is not convenient in the house. Suitable chairs include Ortopedia, made by Everest & Jennings, where the large driving wheels can be at the back or the front; the latter model is more suitable for heavy use outdoors and is similar in style to the chair made by Meyra (Figure 43.11). These are very efficient for outdoor use including over slightly rough ground but some patients may prefer something more substantial such as the Batricar or a scooter such as that made by BEC. There are other outdoor chairs made by other companies listed below (Figure 43.12).

It is very important that the patient tries the wheelchair before purchase. Many suppliers will arrange a free home demonstration, or the patient may attend a centre which has a wide variety available.

Figure 43.11: Outdoor electric chair, will go up and down curbs, and into many shops (Meyra)

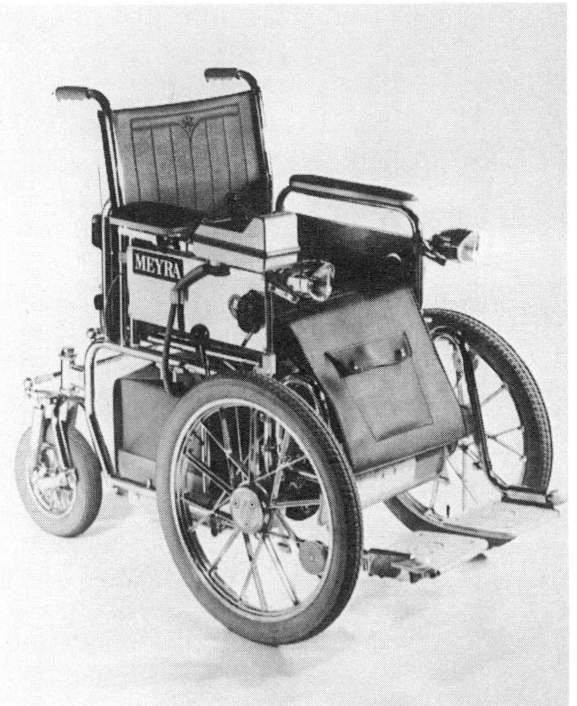

Use and insurance

Powered outdoor chairs can be used on pavements and driven into many shops or public buildings if accessible, but if used on the road at night must be lit as is a bicycle, with a red light and reflector at the rear and a white light at the front. Insurance for these expensive chairs is advisable, as is third party insurance; it is possible to injure a pedestrian.

WHEELCHAIRS IN COMMON CONDITIONS

Arthritis

If outdoor walking is limited a model 9L pushchair is used; for longer distances the patient uses an outdoor powered chair. The best of these are too big to use in the home, which poses no problem if the patient can walk

Figure 43.12: Scooterplus (Bec): cheaper than outdoor chairs and good out of doors, but will not go into shops (weather protection cover is available)

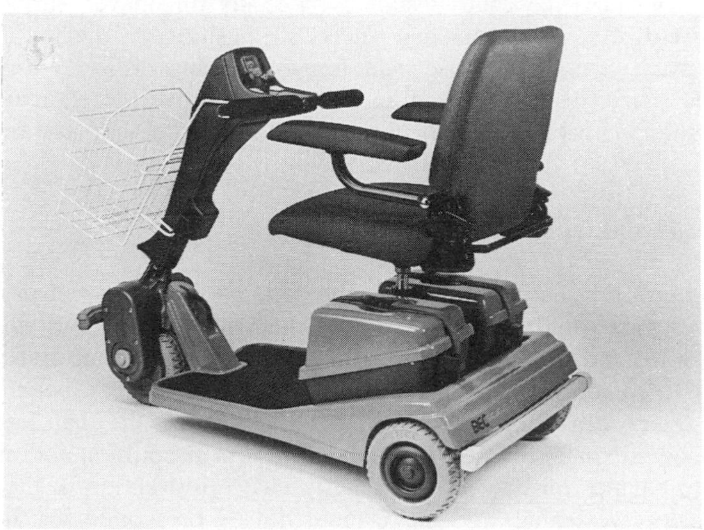

or wheel in the home environment. Where the patient is so disabled by rheumatoid arthritis or ankylosing spondylitis with peripheral joint involvement that an electric wheelchair is needed indoors, outdoor independence may require a second powered chair, or the ability to drive an adapted car.

Inability to flex the hips beyond 65° will require an increased slope of backrest, either fixed or adjustable. Many arthritis patients develop oedema of the ankles, which is reduced by the use of elevating legrests, which are also required if the knees are fixed straight or only comfortable in a relatively straight supported position. Difficulty in propelling a chair due to pain, weakness or joint limitation must lead to early provision of a powered wheelchair to maintain independence. The customary position of the control on the armrest may be difficult if external rotation of the shoulder is limited; then it may be positioned on wheelchair table or on a swivel arm so that it is further towards the middle of the chair within easy reach, but swings out of the way when the patient gets in and out of the chair. Pain in the neck will be helped by a headrest extension.

Leg amputees

The patient may be able to walk short distances in the house but may need a powered outdoor wheelchair for longer distances. Some older amputees may be entirely dependent on a wheelchair indoors. When the arms are normal a self-propelling 8L, 8BL or 8LJ chair is used. If the patient does not wear prostheses the centre of gravity will be displaced backwards, which may make the chair unstable, especially on uneven surfaces. To overcome this the rear propelling wheels are positioned 3 inches (7.5 cm) further back. This makes the chair longer, causing difficulty turning in confined spaces or getting it up kerbs. An alternative is a standard chair with cushioning behind the patient to move the body weight forwards.

Paraplegia and tetraplegia

The width of the chair is dictated by the patient's size. The rear propelling wheels provide good propulsion and the chair must be of robust construction to withstand much heavy use, younger paraplegics being some of the heaviest users of wheelchairs. Young fit paraplegics may benefit from special chairs with the axle moved forward; this makes the chair less stable than standard chairs but provides greater ease of propulsion and makes it easier to balance on the back wheels. Intensive instruction in the use of such chairs is essential, and they should not be prescribed for the older patient.

Armrests are removable for easy transfer, although some patients gain access from the front, especially if they walk a short distance with leg orthoses. Footrests must swing upwards and outwards to prevent damage to the legs on getting in and out.

The patients tetraplegic at C6 level can use a similar chair, but may benefit from capstan hand rims in which there are radial projections from the rims allowing the palm to be used to propel the chair when the patient is unable to grip the hand-rims. They may prefer the latter removed and push on the tyre instead, using *leather hand protectors.* For patients with paralysis above C6 level a powered wheelchair is used.

Stroke

Depending upon the age of the patient, the severity and the subsequent management of the stroke, 15–20 per cent of patients may need a wheelchair much of the time. Others with outdoor mobility problems only may need to be pushed in a transit chair or require a powered wheelchair. For the patient confined to a wheelchair propulsion is usually easiest with a standard 8L or 8BL. Propulsion with the good hand and good foot is slightly erratic, but often preferred by the patient to the alternative, which is a *double hand-rim* on the normal side, the outer smaller rim driving the opposite wheel. This type of propulsion is difficult to learn, especially if the patient has disorder of body image and inattention, which is frequent in severe stroke. An alternative is a foot-steering chair where propulsion is with the good hand only while steering with the good foot, the footplate being linked to both front castors so that steering is by turning a foot (modified 8L chair). This latter type requires good coordination and this modification makes it difficult for helpers to push the chair as the patient must still steer.

The brake on the paralysed side must either have an extended lever for use by the good hand or be brought over to the good side using a cable. Some of the more severely disabled patients like to doze in the chair, for which a headrest is useful, but a reclining chair should not be used because it is too heavy for a hemiplegic patient to propel. A Bexhill armrest for the hemiplegic hand encourages the patient to place it in a functional position.

Multiple sclerosis

Locomotor problems include increasing weakness, spasticity and incoordination, including involvement of the trunk and neck. Elevating legrests may be needed to support spastic and/or oedematous legs and allow a position of comfort for the hips and knees. Late in the disease, when fatigue and/or extensor spasms are a big problem, a headrest extension, possibly with side supports, may be used. As the disease progresses an electric wheelchair may be essential, especially to avoid fatigue. Ataxia may make control erratic, but altering the position of the control from the armrest towards the front of the patient may be helpful. *Proportional control* allows smooth acceleration and deceleration, preventing jerkiness which may trigger spasm and pain. If ataxia of hand or foot prevents control of the powered chair, this may be achieved by use of chin, suck–blow or head control unless the ataxia is too severe there also.

Motor neurone disease

The patient becomes progressively more paralysed, while maintaining sensation and completely normal intellectual function. Outdoor mobility is by a transit chair, electrically driven chair or use of a car. Often if the patient needs an indoor wheelchair the arms are too weak to push it. Some will use a 9L transit chair with the footrests removed, propelling themselves forwards or backwards with their feet. Later an electric wheelchair is required. For the patient who is too weak to stand, a *powered elevating chair* may be useful, with or without powered propulsion. These are expensive and only available by private purchase (Figure 43.13). A headrest extension is used as the neck muscles become weaker, and later the patient

Figure 43.13: Elevating electrically powered chair (Chair–Up): this may be useful at work or at home; armrest lowers or lifts for access.

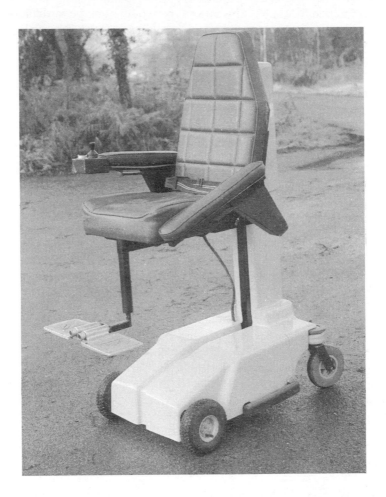

may only be comfortable partially reclining, the legs being supported on elevating legrests. The control for an electric wheelchair must be light, positioned where the hand can reach it, and in these patients certainly one must consider control by chin, suck–blow control on the mouth or even switches in the headrest. The condition may progress rapidly, so it is vital that rapid provision and alteration of the controls is available. This will need close liaison with the ALAC or with a rehabilitation engineer.

Head injury

With severe residual disability a reclining backrest and elevating legrests are often needed, especially in the presence of severe spasticity and contractures, which can occur easily in these patients even with the best care. If position, spasm or intellectual damage causes the patient to slide forward out of the chair a lap strap may be insufficient, satisfactory positioning only being achieved by a *harness.* Where the head flexes on the trunk this may be helped by a headrest, or by use of a firm collar. If there is still difficulty in maintaining the position of the patient in a wheelchair this may be achieved using posture support systems as noted above. Often severe intellectual damage precludes use of a powered chair because of the potential danger to other people.

Cerebral palsy and spina bifida in adults

Children's wheelchairs arc beyond the scope of this book, but disabled children grow into disabled adults. The young adult with spina bifida will be able to propel a standard wheelchair, but the patient's trunk will be short, probably scoliotic, with anaesthetic skin over the supporting areas of the buttocks. Good seating is vital to adequately distribute pressure widely and prevent sores. With a scoliotic spine causing slumping to one side, side cushions on the inside of the armrest or fixed on the back of the chair to support the side of the chest may be needed. Thc lcgs may be underdeveloped, with poor circulation and oedema, so elevating legrests may be needed. If there is severe mental retardation with hydrocephalus a headrest with side supports is of value, as it also may be for the cerebral palsy adult with severe intellectual impairment.

The adult with cerebral palsy, even with athetosis which ocurs in 12–15 per cent, may still be able to walk even if with a very abnormal gait. If a wheelchair is required a standard wheelchair may suffice if there is sufficient arm strength and control to propel it. Propulsion may be with the feet, in which case a transit chair (model 9L) may be used with the footplates removed. To reduce athetosis the patient will sometimes hook an arm around the back of the chair.

If self-propulsion is impossible an electric wheelchair is needed with the control positioned on hand, foot or head. Usually even the most athetoid patient can control an electric wheelchair. Using proportional control prevents jerkiness which triggers spasm: a low gearing will limit the speed of the chair if necessary. Requirements are highly individual and need detailed assessment, which may change over the years.

Muscular dystrophy

The patient with Duchenne pseudohypertophic dystrophy will almost certainly require an electric wheelchair by the time he reaches teenage, but the patient with the Becker type of dystrophy progresses much more slowly. With limb-girdle dystrophy walking is possible for many years, but an outdoor transit chair may be required when walking is limited to short distances; later a self-propelling chair is used. Some of these patients, particularly with limb girdle dystrophy, find front propelling wheels easier than the standard rear propulsion. Some, however, use rear propelling wheels, gaining extra power by hooking their arms round behind the pushing handles on the back of the chair. By the time a wheelchair is used, the need for a powered wheelchair is not far distant.

ACKNOWLEDGEMENT

The author is pleased to acknowledge the help of Miss Peggy Jay in the section on cushioning.

REFERENCES, FURTHER READING AND INFORMATION

Cochrane, G.M. and Wilshere, E.R. (1982) *Equipment for the disabled: wheelchairs.* Nuffield Orthopaedic Centre, Oxford (excellent detailed illustrated list)

Department of Health and Social Security (1982) *Handbook of wheelchairs*, DHSS, London

Fenwick, D. (1977) *Wheelchairs and their users, a survey*, HMSO, London

Garber, S.L. and Krouskop, T.A. (1984) Wheelchair cushion modification and its effect on pressure. *Arch. Phys. Med. Rehabil., 65*, 579-83

Jay, P.E. (1984) *Choosing the best wheelchair cushion for your needs, your chair and your lifestyle*, RADAR, London

Information Service of Disabled Living Foundation, 380-384 Harrow Road, London W9 2HU.

Information and lists of suppliers:
Choosing a wheelchair
Manual wheelchairs
Loading a wheelchair into a car
Electric wheelchairs.

SUPPLIERS

Motability (for lease or hire-purchase of car or electric wheelchair)
Boundary House, 91-93 Charterhouse Street, London EM1M 6BT

W. & F. Barrett Ltd,
22 Emery Road,
Bristol BS4 5PH

Batricar Ltd
Griffin Mill, Thrupp, Stroud, Glos GL5 2AZ

BEC Wheelchairs BEC Mobility
Fennspool Avenue, Wollows Industrial Estate,
Riley Hill,
West Midlands.

Carters (J. & A.) Ltd
Alfred Street, Westbury, Wilts BA13 3DZ

Chair-Up Ltd
Building 75,
Bournemouth Hurn Airport,
Christchurch, Dorset BH23 6ED

Everest & Jennings Ltd
Princewood Road, Corby, Northants NN17 2DX

Meyra-Rehab (UK) Ltd
Millshaw Park Ave, Leeds LS11 0LR

N. V. Distributors Ltd (Dudley)
Soothouse Spring, Valley Road Industrial Estate, St Albans, Herts AL3 6PF

Ortho-Kinetics (UK) Ltd
24 South Hampshire Industrial Park, Totton, Southampton SO4 2ZZ

Spastics Society (Newton)
Meadway Works, Garretts Green Lane, Birminghan B33 0SQ

SML Aids Ltd (Levo)
Bath Place, High Street, Barnet, Herts EN5 5XE

Hugh Steeper Ltd
237-239 Roehampton Lane, London SW15 4LB

Vessa Ltd
Paper Mill Lane, Alton, Hants GU34 2PY

44

Patient Transfers: Hoists and Stairlifts

Christine Tarling and Janet Stowe

Where physically disabled patients require assistance with transfers it is often quicker and easier for staff to lift them manually or otherwise physically assist them. Current teaching of rehabilitation techniques, and the need to prevent back injuries amongst nurses due to lifting and carrying, are changing attitudes towards patient transfers. Current thought is leading to the decision to use a hoist or lifting aid on all but the lightest of dependent patients. For those who are less dependent, transfer techniques must be taught by the whole team and practised as an important part of rehabilitation.

MANUAL LIFTING

The comfort of the patient, the avoidance of pressure on painful areas and joints, the sureness of the lifters' grip and the weight of the patient are the main factors of importance in using various manual lifts. Recent research has shown that the 'orthodox lift' and the 'drag lift' are both extremely stressful to the lifter and uncomfortable for the patient. Many of the manual techniques will be difficult to use successfully when assisting patients with painful shoulder or elbow joints. Modifications of manual lifts can be used on the lighter-weight adult patients, and such items as draw sheets or commercially available lifting sheets offer both comfort to the patient and a firm grip for the lifter.

However, using manual lifting methods implies that there will always be a carer available to assist the patient. If rehabilitation is to be as complete as possible, independent forms of mobility and transfer must be discussed and tried. Elderly patients often return home to the care of an equally elderly and frail relative, and the physical stresses of manually handling a disabled relative contribute to many breakdowns in caring partnerships.

SEATING

There are many small items of equipment available that will either assist with transfers or alleviate the need to move the patient. Correct seat height of furniture is important in allowing the patient to rise from the seated position without assistance. Beds, too, need to be sufficiently high to allow patients to get in and out on their own. There are a number of ways in which bed and chair legs can be extended to make sure that the seat height is right. For those patients who have difficulty in getting their legs *into* bed, there are now electrically operated leg-raisers which can be attached to beds, apart from the use of an adapted simple pulley system. The electrically controlled 'sit-up' beds may help some people into a seated position when they are at their most immobile in the early morning. Once seated, the independent sideways transfer becomes possible. For those patients who have arthrodesed hips and knees, who find sitting almost impossible, there are 'stand-up' beds that put the patient on his feet, and similarly designed chairs. Chairs with riser seats are available whether electrically or mechanically operated (Figure 44.1). Some are adjustable to the weight of the user, while others have the spring mechanism set in the factory as they are made. Choosing the right chair, particularly for its seat height, is a most important aid to independence (see Chapter 42).

BATHING AND TOILET

The bathroom and toilet present problems early in many disabilities. Transfers on and off the toilet seat are some of the earliest goals in rehabilitation planning. The toilet seat must not be so high that feet cannot rest firmly on the floor, nor so low that the patient requires a great effort to rise from it. Rails securely fastened on the wall or adjacent to the toilet will help the patient to pull up to transfer. Plastic rails are warmer to touch than metal, and the use of plastic also prevents additional safety wiring having to be provided. The rail should usually be fastened at a height that is just below the seated person's elbow, and should rise from a point level with the centre of the toilet pan to a point 20 cm (8 inches) in front of the pan and at an angle that rises slightly up and away from the seated person. Where the toilet seat is too low, raised seats may be provided in 5 cm (2 inch), 10 cm (4 inch) or 15 cm (6 inch) depths. There are many designs of these, some incorporating a dip in the front of the seat which allows patients to clean themselves while still seated. For people who are too severely disabled to manage transfers on and off the toilet from a wheelchair, there are modified cushions that fit inside the wheelchair with a gap where a small hand-held urinal can be fitted between the legs and under the patient. Provided that the patient is wearing adapted clothing, where the crotch of

Figure 44.1: Patient rising from an electric tip-up chair

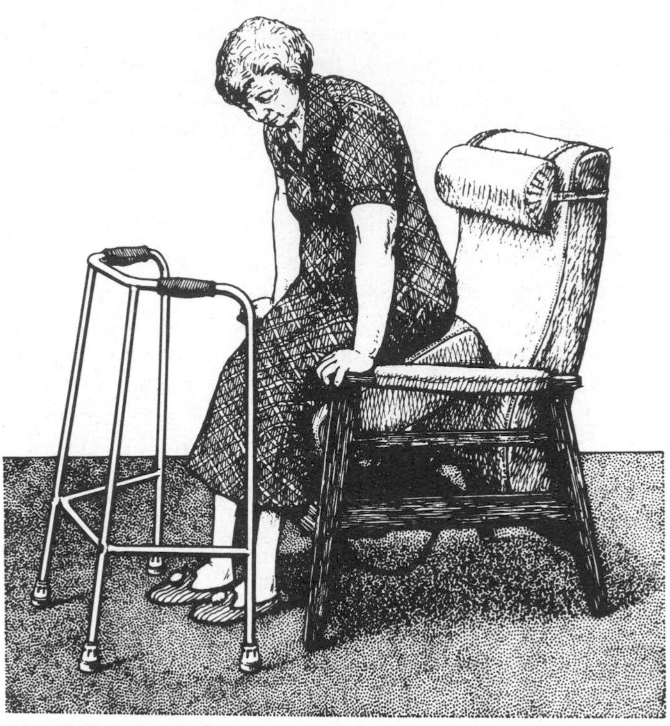

the pants can be opened, then a urinal or simple funnel and tube can be placed in position, and the patient can use the toilet without transferring.

Getting out of the bath presents problems. The simple bath board across the top of the bath, and a bath seat inside the bath, make it easier for someone to sit on the side of the bath (providing it is not too low) and then swing the legs over the edge before moving into the middle of the board and then down on to the seat. Patients need to have reasonable strength and movement in the upper limbs in order to pull themselves upwards on to the seat or board when getting out. The design of lightweight acrylic baths mean that wedging bath seats cannot be used.

If it is decided that a shower is the answer to personal hygiene, then the base of the shower unit needs to take into account that wheeled shower chairs might be used, and the disabled person may not be able to step over ledges into the shower tray. There is a variety of wall-mounted shower seats available with slatted, solid or holed seats. A stool may be used, or a wheeled shower chair which will also act as a mobility aid between the bedroom and the shower, as well as being pushed over the toilet to eliminate the need for yet another transfer.

As long as the patient has good use of his upper limbs, small aids to transfers will be the most that are needed. Once the upper limbs as well as the lower limbs lose their power, then transfers become increasingly difficult. Many more severely disabled patients will require a hoist to enable them to transfer either independently or with the assistance of a carer. Most disabled people now have high expectations of a rewarding and full life within their own home and in the community to which they belong. The use of a hoist may be the only way in which these expectations can be fulfilled. However, the family of the disabled person has already had to accept many alterations to its way of life, and many items of complex-looking equipment. Whatever is chosen to solve lifting and transfer problems must cause as little disturbance as possible to the family. Members of the rehabilitation team will know how difficult it can be to persuade patients that the use of a wheelchair, even for part of the day, can increase mobility. The same is true of using a hoist, which is seen as a symbol of dependency, but can offer the freedom to transfer when and where the patient wants without relying on community nursing staff, care attendents or frail relatives.

The majority of disabled people living in private dwellings do not live in houses that have been designed for the use of a wheelchair. For many years to come, 'normal' housing will need alterations and extension to accommodate a disabled person. The most common sites for hoists are in the bathroom and the bedroom, but there are many other areas where transfers may be difficult and a hoist helpful. Hoists may be used to pick fallen people up from the floor, get people in and out of cars, or on and off a soft, deep easy chair.

HOISTS

The following review of types of hoists will outline the choice available in order that detailed assessments and decisions can be made:

Mobile hoists

These can be divided into three main classes:

larger models suitable for hospitals;
mobile electric models;
smaller models suitable for the domestic environment.

Larger mobile models

Hoists such as the Mecanaids Ambulift (Figure 44.2) are commonly used in hospitals and residential care homes. They are larger in size, and incor-

Figure 44.2: Mecanaids Ambulift model D, with seat and leg extension

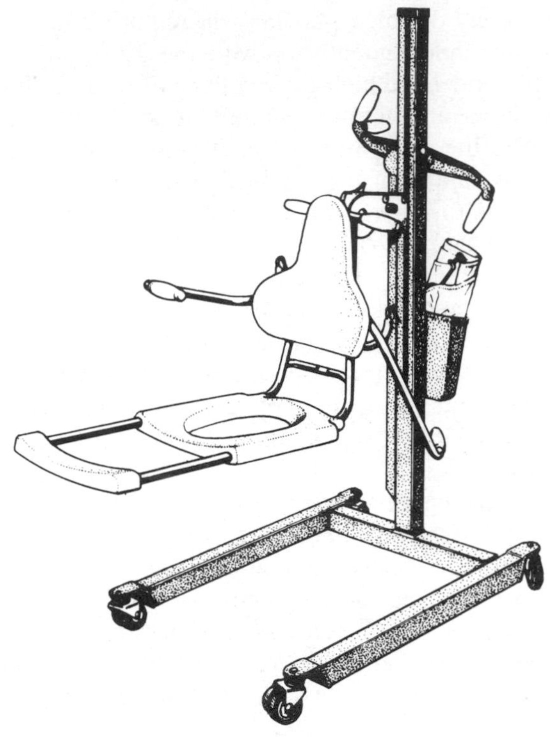

porate either slings or a static seat (which can be detached from the hoist and placed on a mobile chassis). The static seat may not offer enough support to the severly disabled person. The larger models can lift a heavier load, usually up to 160 kg (25 stone) with some manufacturers offering a hoist that will lift 190 kg (30 stone). However, it is important that the equipment chosen for use on the hospital ward is the same as that the patient will use at home; it is confusing to the patient and relatives if they have to learn how to use one hoist in hospital and then quite a different model in their own home.

Electric mobile hoists

These have recently become available on the UK market. Most of these models tend to be of the larger size as the batteries have to be carried on the base chassis. They are of most use on long-stay, high-dependency units where patients are not generally on rehabilitation programmes.

Smaller mobile hoists (Figure 44.7)

There is a range of these small mobile hoists available both in hospitals and

Figure 44.3: Overhead track hoist with traversing motor unit

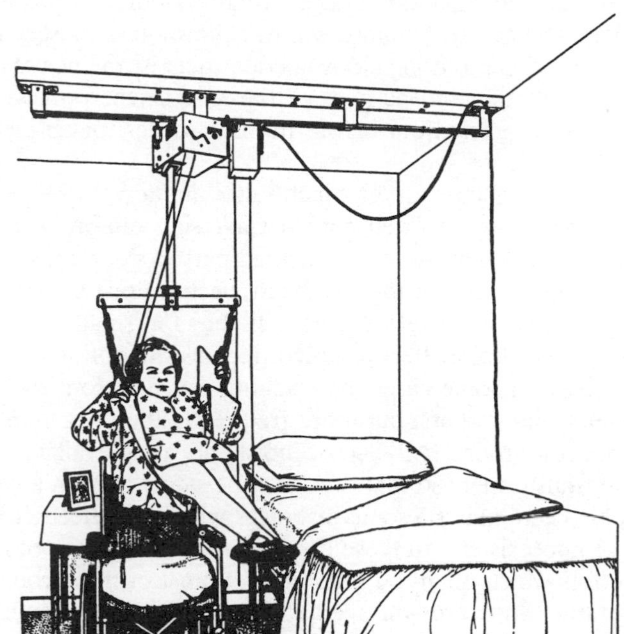

in the community. The Mecalift, Isis, Compact and MobyImp are some of the smaller models that will lift a 127 kg (20 stone) person, and are appropriate for the domestic environment. These models may be taken apart for storage or for transportation in a car, and they all have a variety of slings to cope with different disabilities.

Mobile hoists can usually be used at any site, either inside or outside the home, so that if there are transfer problems at more than one site then a mobile hoist may be the answer. If the patient travels, or does not have a fixed routine, then this type of hoist gives great flexibility. However, none of these mobile models can be operated by the patient independently.

Overhead track hoists (Figure 44.3)

The majority of these overhead hoists are electric, and run on a fixed track which may be supported at each end by an A-shaped metal frame resting on the floor or fastened to the ceiling in a predetermined place. The former is used where the person is waiting to be rehoused, or is in privately rented accommodation where the landlord will not allow alterations, or in the case of terminal care where a lifting aid is needed to assist the heavy load of the carers. It can also be used as part of the assessment process where an electric hoist is to be tried out before the final order for an installation is made.

The hoist has an electric motor which raises and lowers the person in the sling(s). The hoist can be fitted with a traversing motor, or a system of pulleys may be used to move the suspended person sideways.

One of the advantages of the overhead electric hoist is that it takes up no floor space and is therefore very suitable for small bathrooms and toilets. This type of hoist offers disabled persons the option to operate the hoist themselves. In some cases the tracking can run from room to room and be taken round corners, but more frequently the track runs from wall to wall within one room. All electric hoists are now available in 24 volt models with transformers so that they may be safely used in a room with a water supply. There may be some instances where the electricity supply is unreliable or non-existent. In these cases there are a number of mechanical overhead hoists which might be suitable, but most of these come from the industrial market and care will need to be taken when selecting slings to match with them.

Bath hoists

This is the area of most frequent hoist provision and there are many varieties. There are two basic types:

(a) those that fit inside the bath, and move up and down;

(b) those that fit outside the bath and swing over the bath before going up and down in the bath.

Those bath hoists that fit inside the bath require the bath base to be checked for strength. With a lightweight type of bath there may be a need to strengthen points beneath the bath to take the stresses of the weight of the hoist and user. When using the hoist the patient will usually need to be able to lift his legs over the side of the bath, requiring hip and sometimes knee flexion, as well as reasonable balance. Because they require little fitting, they can be used as a short-term hoist where the patient's circumstances may change. Nearly all bath hoists have an upright seat on which the patient remains seated. This type of hoist is not for those patients who wish to lie back and luxuriate in a bath.

There is a range of bath hoists that take the form of a seat attached to a pillar mounted in the bathroom floor (Figure 44.4). They may be used independently by the patient. Some models are designed so that the carer can move the seat on to a chassis so that it can act as a mobility aid between the bathroom and bedroom, and may also be pushed over a toilet. Many of these types of bath hoists will have a leg bar as an extra attachment to the seat, so that the patient's legs can be raised as they are swung over the rim of the bath.

Car access

Mobility and freedom of movement are important aims of rehabilitation. Many disabled people own and/or drive their own cars, and access to the outside world is a normal expectation. Transferring in and out of a car may be achieved by: a sliding or transfer board, a car-top-mounted hoist, a mobile hoist or alterations to the design of the car.

Figure 44.4: P&L bath lifter Model BS216: a bath hoist mounted on a pillar which swings over the bath

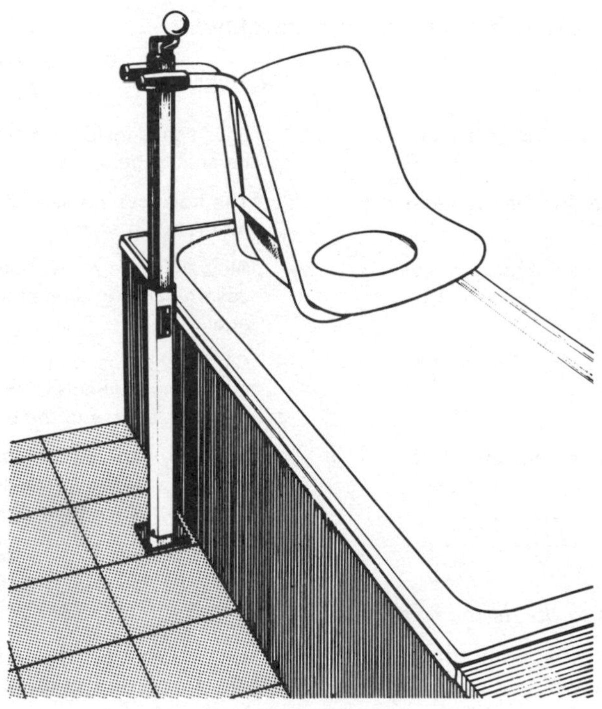

Sliding board

Because of the awkward body positions in which the carer will have to try and assist the patient in and out of the car, the use of a small lifting aid will ensure that the transfer is achieved with little physical stress. A sliding board can be used by removing the nearside arm of the wheelchair and placing the wheelchair next to the driver or passenger seat. The patient's feet are lodged on the car sill ready to slip into the footwell as the transfer takes place. The board is slipped part way under the seated patient's hips and the lifter goes around the car and kneels on the other car seat facing the patient. Getting hold of a belt around the patient's waist, or grasping the material of his trousers where maximum weight is on them, the lifter then pulls the patient towards him and the patient will slide over the board and into the seat. In this way the lifter is not lifting in a twisted or bent position, and the patient is not subjected to the discomforts of manual handling.

Car-top hoist

A car top hoist is fixed to the roof of the car and works with a hydraulic pump system operated by the carer. Table 44.1 lists the points which need to be taken into consideration when choosing between a car top or mobile hoist for car transfers:

Table 44.1: Comparison between types of hoist

Car top hoist	Mobile hoist
Space is left free inside the car	Less space inside the car if the hoist is to be carried
The hoist can only be used for car transfers	The hoist can be used in many different situations
Quick to use as the hoist is always in position	Slower to use as the hoist has to be assembled and then stored away again
Can be used on the front or back seats of the car	Can only be used on the front seat as the back wheels of the car usually obstruct access to the back seat
Can be used on a variety of surfaces	Can only be used on relatively smooth surfaces because of the wheels of the mobile chassis

Alterations to the design of the car

One of the most common adaptations of a car is to alter the passenger seat so that it swivels out from the side of the car, thus creating greater space for a transfer. The person is seated as he is swung back into the car, thus avoiding the need to duck the head while transferring (Figure 44.5). For a totally dependent person a van's roof can be raised, and a ramp created at the back so that the person may be pushed up into the van and travel whilst remaining seated in their wheelchair. The wheelchair *must* be clamped to the floor of the van (Chapter 47).

This is not an exhaustive description of the hoists available. There are now models which will cope with a wide range of lifting and transfer problems, as varied as getting in and out of a swimming pool, to on and off a horse and trap.

SLINGS

There are five main types of support used on hoists: the static seat; two-piece band slings; divided leg sling; full-body hammock sling; one-piece sling.

The static seat

This may be used on a mobile hoist such as the Ambulift, or on a bath hoist such as the Autolift. If used on a mobile hoist then the seat may be detached from the main hoist and the patient may be rolled on the bed, the seat placed beneath him and then, with the patient on the seat, it is reconnected to the hoist and raised off the bed. If the seat is on a fixed floor bath

Figure 44.5: Swivel sliding car seat (ELAP Ltd)

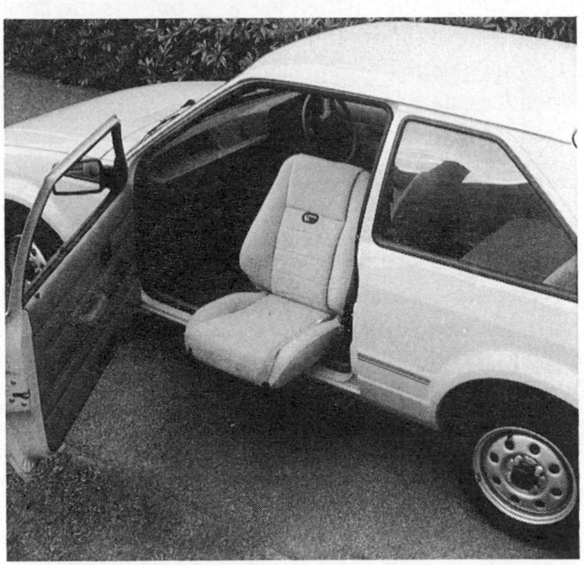

hoist then the patient must be able to effect the transfer with minimal assistance. Since the use of a hoist is to obviate the need to lift, unless the patient can be rolled, or can effect a transfer himself, then the use of a static seat on a hoist should be questioned.

Two-piece band slings

Although these have been commonly used until recent years, they are only used by those people who are experienced hoist users. The narrower band goes around the chest wall, *under the axillae with the arms outside the sling*, the wider band goes under the thighs as close to the hip joints as possible. In lifting with the hoist, unless the slings have been carefully positioned the chest sling will rise, and can cause uncomfortable pressure through the shoulder joints, while the thigh sling may slip towards the knees, thus causing the patient to 'jack-knife' through the slings. This design may be used by the hoist user who does not have a carer to assist in placing the slings, and who has considerable experience in hoisting himself.

Divided leg sling

Most manufacturers now produce a divided leg sling to fit their own hoist. These have developed so that there are now no chains or metal parts in the sling. The sling is in one piece with a deep backpiece that supports up to the shoulder joints, and two longer sidepieces which are slid beneath the patient's legs. It is a quick and simple task for a carer to place the sling around the patient and to remove it after the transfer is completed.

The full-body hammock sling (Figure 44.6)

This is similar in shape to the divided leg sling but has the additional height at the back to offer head support to those patients with little or no head control. These slings are also useful when the patient is semi-conscious or in a highly dependent state while in hospital.

One-piece sling (Figure 44.7)

The patient is rolled on to this type of sling while in bed and then hoisted to a commode or wheelchair, but he must then remain sitting on the sling as it cannot be removed without lifting. This sling is often used by frail carers who need to assist with a transfer but who cannot get a divided leg sling on and off easily. If the patient is to remain seated on the sling, and particularly if the sling has a commode aperture, then a sheepskin liner to the sling might help in maintaining good skin care. The one-piece sling may also be used by an independent hoist user when a carer is not available.

Figure 44.6: Hammock sling with commode hole in use

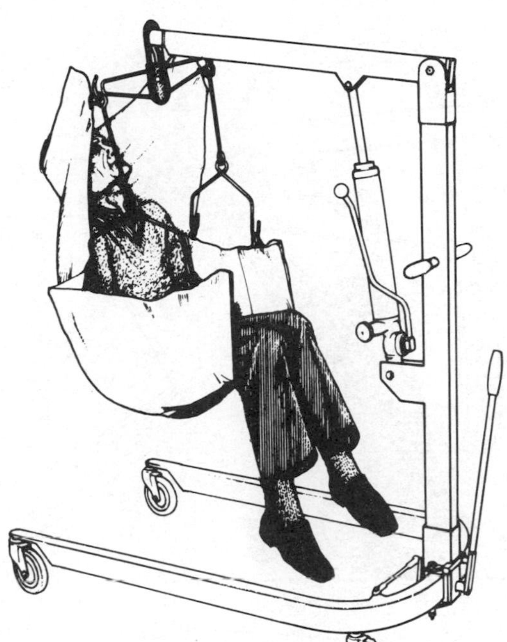

Conclusion

Whichever sling and hoist is used, training will be needed for all those concerned with its use. Most manufacturers will provide training sessions to ensure that the users of their equipment are competent, and that the hoist does all that is required. Where hoists are to be supplied through a centralised loan equipment store, then it is desirable that the hoist is not delivered to the patient's home long before the staff member is informed or available to teach its use and check its installation. These training sessions may need to be repeated from time to time, especially if there are changes in the staff members using the hoist or in the circumstances of the patient and his family. Follow-up check visits are also necessary to maintain the hoist and its slings in safe working order.

The use of a hoist or small transfer aid can open up a wide range of activities and freedom of movement to many disabled people. While some patients may have to accept the assistance of a carer to operate the hoist, it still leaves him the ability to choose the timing and method of his transfer. For those patients able to self-operate an electric overhead or bath hoist the independence is invaluable, and a most important part of the rehabilitation process.

Figure 44.7: The S/5 car sling being used with an Isis hoist for a car transfer

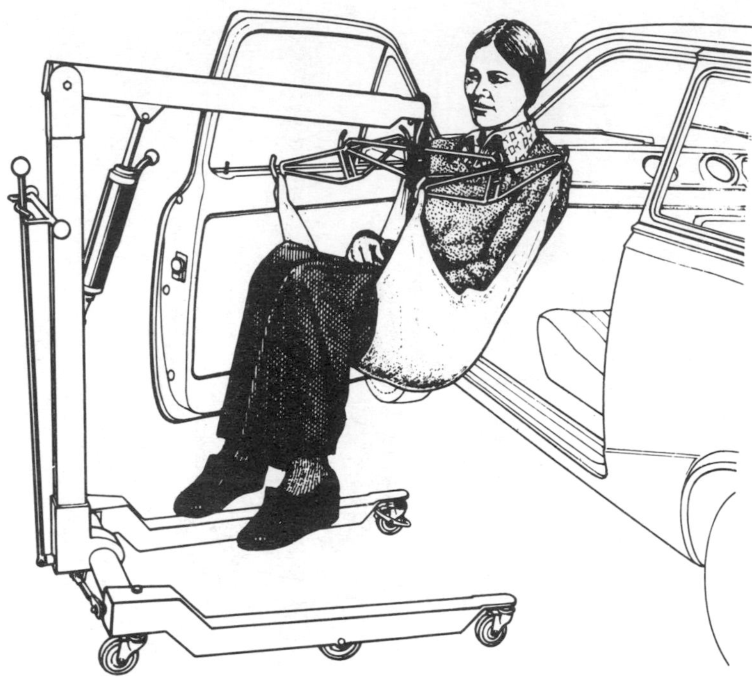

STAIRLIFTS IN THE HOME

To the home dweller, access to all parts of the house is extremely important, especially sleeping, bathing, toileting and living areas. When a patient has problems with mobility, and lives in a house of two or more storeys, access to the higher levels is often difficult and painful, and sometimes impossible. A number of solutions are therefore available.

(1) *Move the bed downstairs* — this is only practical when few people live in the house and there is more than one living room. There must also be a toilet available downstairs, as constant use of a commode is disagreeable to most people. Few people find this the ideal solution. Where there is a family, the bed downstairs causes undue stress, due in part to lack of privacy.

(2) *Build an extension* — this necessitates enough space outside to accommodate a bedroom, and if necessary WC and bathroom. Very often there is not the land available. It is also a costly undertaking, and few authorities are willing to bear the cost in full, especially as there are usually cheaper alternatives.

(3) *Move house* — this solution is often totally unacceptable to the client. Long-standing relationships have often been established with neighbours, especially where the client lives alone. Neighbours help with shopping, frequently do a bit of cooking, and keep the client company for many a long afternoon or evening. Such relationships are almost impossible for a disabled person to initiate after a move, and consequently to move to a new environment can bring loneliness, isolation and subsequent depression.

(4) *Install a stairlift or through-ceiling lift* — this solution is usually the most acceptable, being the least expensive and also maintaining the use of all areas of the home. Life is therefore as normal as possible.

Stairlifts

A stairlift is a seat and/or platform mounted onto a drive unit, running up a track which is superficially mounted onto the staircase. These are usually made to cope with a straight staircase, with alteration often possible where there is a half-landing and two or three steps round a corner at the top. There are a few made to cater for curved staircases, but these are much more costly (Figure 44.8).

Through-ceiling lift

Where the patient is confined to a wheelchair, or finds it very difficult to transfer from the wheelchair to the seat, and would therefore need another wheelchair at the top of the stairs, a through-ceiling lift is now more frequently being installed. These are also being installed when the staircase configuration is costly or impossible to negotiate. It transports the client seated either in his wheelchair, or on a seat in the lift, or even standing, from one floor through the ceiling to the next floor. The lift runs on two tracks fitted to the wall, and when out of use is neatly stored away on the upper floor, out of sight, to be called down again when needed by the push of a button.

Method of selection

It is best practice to call in the local community occupational therapist who will, in some authorities, work together with an engineer. Between them they will assess the patient. This calls for much skill and accurate observation. The client's medical condition and prognosis need to be taken into consideration, as do mental abilities; physical ability; the needs of the rest of the family, especially children where applicable; type of house; physical

Figure 44.8: Patient operating stairlift; pushbuttons on the front of the arm of the seat

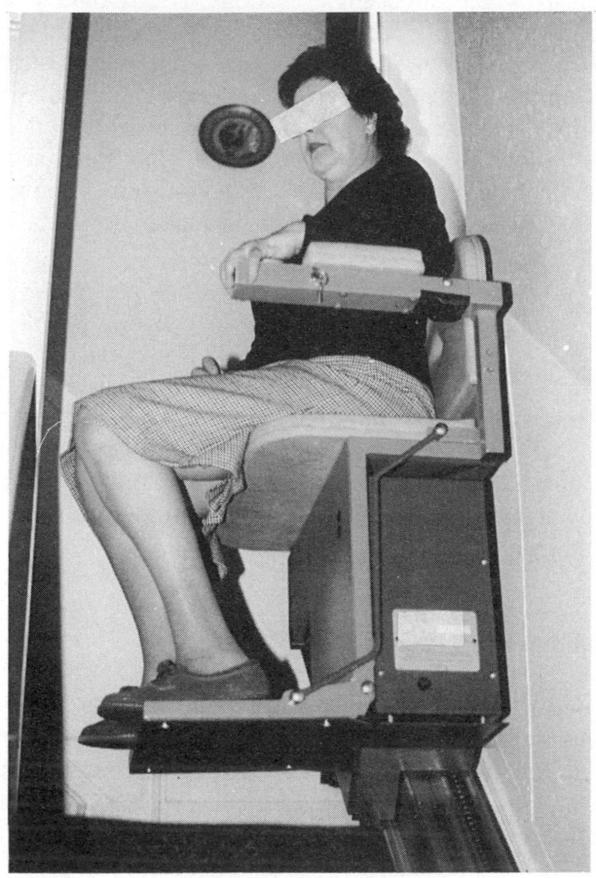

characteristics of the staircase; headroom available; positioning of doors, electrical points, windows and any other relevant details. A selection can then be made from the many choices available.

Many months may elapse between the initial request for equipment and the final delivery and fitting, mainly because agreement on funding usually has to be sought.

In the case of the stairlift, the *track* must be suitable for the staircase, and must not protrude any further than necessary. Some tracks need to extend a long way past the bottom step, depending on the angle of the rise of the staircase. The height of the *footplate* varies considerably. A footplate which is high off the ground when the stairlift has come to rest at the top or bottom of the staircase is a disadvantage. The client usually needs to stand on the footplate in order to get onto the seat. Not all are weight-bearing.

The footplate should be sufficiently deep in order to take the feet securely, without the risk of them slipping off. It should be so positioned that the knees need only be bent up to 90°.

The relationship between the *seat* and the *footplate* dictates the amount of knee flexion required, and one needs also to consider how far back on the seat the client is able to sit comfortably. Usually a gap between the backrest and seat enables the user to sit right at the back of the seat, thus putting minimal pressure on the knees as they do not have to be tucked well under.

The *harness* or seat belt, if required, needs to be easy to fit, fasten and release. The user must feel secure, and this applies particularly to children and all people with poor muscular control.

Stairlifts can be operated in a number of ways — the most common being by continuous pressure on a pushbutton located on or near the armrest. When this cannot be manipulated, modified controls such as a rocker switch or joy-stick can be used. These modifications are usually available at an extra cost, and the additional outlay required must be checked.

Stairlifts vary in levels of *noise*; whether this is acceptable depends on where they are situated, for example on a party wall in a pair of semi-detached houses.

Servicing arrangements need to be organised — either through the social services or privately. Each area in the UK has its own policy on servicing, and information regarding this needs to be sought locally. Some authorities operate a 24-hour call-out service; others rely solely on the stairlift company.

Insurance needs to be taken out, and its provisions clearly understood.

Training the clients in the use of the stairlift should be thorough, and a telephone number where the therapist, lift engineer, or lift company can be reached in case of emergency needs to be available.

When selecting a stairlift a few patient-related points need to be considered. For example: Will the client sit or stand? If he/she sits, how far can the knees be bent? As most stairlift seats face sideways, those patients with limited knee flexion need to be looked at carefully, and perhaps a forward-facing stairlift installed. Can the patient operate the control buttons, which are usually constant-pressure ones? If not, do they simply need to be relocated or are other types of switch needed, such as a rocker, joy-stick or wobblestick? If the patient cannot operate the controls at all, as is the case with some, especially children, a wander lead can be installed for the patient/carer to use. Call switches are usually installed at both top and bottom of the stairs.

Access to the stairlift or into the through-ceiling lift needs to be looked at carefully. Most stairlifts have some sort of a step up onto the footplate:

can the patient cope with this? Sometimes the footplate does not take the weight of a person, and thus the patient has to be able to sit on the seat and bring the legs up after him. Access to a through-ceiling lift can be either up a small raise of 2–3 cm (1 inch), or a ramp may be lowered to ensure a smooth ride into the lift.

Conclusion

The provision of a stairlift or through-ceiling lift may not only be of direct benefit to a patient in terms of access: it may enable him to keep his or her family intact and close, giving the disabled person help and independence but also allowing the latter to contribute to the family's well-being.

ACKNOWLEDGEMENT

Figures 44.1, 44.2, 44.3, 44.4, 44.6 and 44.7 are reproduced from *Hoists and their Use*, by Christine Tarling (Disabled Living Foundation/Heinemann, London, 1980) with permission.

FURTHER READING

Equipment for the Disabled (1985) *Hoists and Lifts*, Mary Marlborough Lodge, Nuffield Orthopaedic Centre, Oxford OS3 7LD

Hollis, M. (1985) *Safer lifting for patient care*, 2nd edn, Blackwell Scientific Publications, Oxford

Tarling, C. (1980) *Hoists and their use*, Disabled Living Foundation, London

Lloyd, P., Tarling, C., Wright, B. and Troup, D. (1987) *The handling of patients — a guide for nurse managers*, Back Pain Association and Royal College of Nursing, London

Stowe, Janet (1988) *Guide to the selection of stairlifts*, Rheumatism and Rehabilitation Research Unit, School of Medicine, University of Leeds, 36 Clarendon Road, Leeds LS2 9PJ

Equipment for the Disabled (1986) *Housing and Furniture*, Mary Marlborough Lodge, Nuffield Orthopaedic Centre, Headington, Oxford OX3 7LD

Goldsmith, Selwyn (1976) *Designing for the disabled*, Royal Institute of British Architects, London

Department of Health and Society Security (1978) *Stairlifts for the Disabled and Infirm People*, DHSS, London

45

Orthotics (Callipers and Appliances)

John Goodwill

DEFINITION AND USE

Orthotics is the science of selecting, making and fitting the correct appliance to improve function in an individual patient. The orthotist is the trained professional who can advise on the choice and construction of orthoses and supervise the fitting and adjustment.

Orthoses are used to *redistribute load*, as in the foot; to *support* an unstable or painful arthritic joint; or to *provide a mechanical means of compensating for weak or absent muscle function*, and may also have to resist spastic antagonistic muscles. They may be made of leather, metal or plastic, the particular properties of different plastics and the other materials allowing for different degrees of strength, support and flexibility in the orthosis (see normal and abnormal gait, Chapter 8).

Insoles and other foot orthoses are known as foot orthoses (FO), those extending above the ankle as ankle–foot orthoses (AFO), those extending from the foot to above the knee as knee–ankle–foot orthoses (KAFO) and those extending above the hip as hip–knee–ankle–foot orthoses (HKAFO). *This terminology* was introduced by the American Academy of Orthopedic Surgeons, and allows a more concise description of the appliance, reminding the prescriber which joints are being treated with the orthosis. As well as those used on the leg (also called callipers or braces), orthoses include those used on the arm or hand as well as collars, corsets and spinal braces.

Orthoses may be static or dynamic

Static orthoses are used to support an arthritic joint, to prevent joint contracture in paralysis or for serial splinting of a joint to correct contracture.

Dynamic orthoses are used to apply forces to a joint which is damaged by arthritis, or when the muscles that normally control it are weak. A dynamic orthosis has joint(s) which may be free-moving or lockable to prevent movement.

PRESCRIPTION

This must include:

- the aims of the orthosis;
- what joint(s) are being treated;
- what materials are to be used;
- which pressure points must be avoided, e.g. scars, thin skin, bony prominences;
- how the patient will don and doff it;
- how the patient will fasten it in position;
- how the best cosmetic appearance will be achieved.

Prescription of an orthosis is best done by the doctor jointly with the orthotist, with advice from the occupational therapist or physiotherapist who is treating the patient.

Usually the patient requires an individually made orthosis, and where a plastic is used this is produced from a mould taken from the patient, on which the material is then formed, so the finished plastic is then in total contact with the skin. Clearly this type of orthosis cannot be used where there is variation in limb size due to oedema, or where pressure on the skin is inadvisable because of thinning of the skin or ulcers. Metal orthoses are made from measurements taken from the patient's leg, arm or spine.

BIOMECHANICS IN LEG ORTHOSES

The ankle and foot

Correct prescription of an orthosis requires understanding of how the patient's gait deviates from the normal (Chapter 8). To which joints and in what direction must the forces be applied to compensate for the disability in gait? To apply a *dorsiflexion force to the ankle* for dropped foot, the posterior calf band *pushes forward* and so should be firm. *The upward force* on the foot and ankle comes from the sole of the shoe, which needs to be firm from the heel to the ball of the foot; if necessary a spring steel shank is built into the shoe. These two forces must be as far from the ankle axis as possible to dorsiflex the ankle. Acting together, they produce a resultant force which will lift the patient's heel out of the shoe unless *resisted by a force from the shoe-fastening pushing down and back* as close to the ankle as possible. An inadequate shoe fastening, or poorly constructed shoe, will negate the action of the orthosis. If the patient cannot tie laces one must use a strap and buckle fastening, as elastic laces are not firm enough to provide a counteracting force (Figure 45.1).

The knee

The axis of flexion–extension traverses the femoral condyles, being near the front in extension and moving backwards in an arc as the knee flexes. This movement of the anatomical knee axis does not occur when the patient walks with a fixed extended knee, but its changing position must be considered if the patient is walking with a free knee on the orthosis. *A backward force over the front of the knee* is required to maintain the weak knee in extension so that the leg can support the body weight for walking. Alternatively this force may be applied over the lower thigh and/or upper tibia over the patellar tendon. This force needs to be directed backwards as near to the knee axis as possible, to achieve maximum effect with least local pressure. The backward force at or near the knee is resisted by *forces pushing forward* as far from the knee axis as possible. *Above the knee* this is provided by a wide firm posterior thigh band with a soft but unyielding

Figure 45.1: Forces to produce dorsiflexion at the ankle joint: the shoe fastening must be firm or the heel will lift out of the shoe

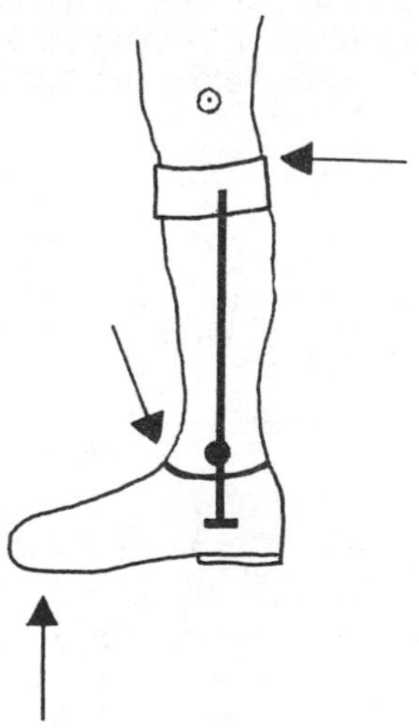

front fastening, or by a plastic quadrilateral ischial-weight-bearing socket. *Below the knee* forward pressure is derived mainly from the heel of the shoe, which must be of firm construction. The firm posterior calf band maintains the alignment of the metal uprights, and is not intended to apply a forward force to the back of the calf. The orthotic knee axis is aligned with the centre of the femoral condyles 2 cm above the joint line; if it is too low the posterior calf band presses into the patient on flexing the knee, if too high the posterior part of the thigh band presses in on flexing the knee for sitting (Figure 45.2).

The different sites of application of these forces are discussed with a biomechanical analysis by Lehmann and Warren (1976).

FOOT ORTHOSES

These are used for painful foot conditions. A patient will neither need nor accept an orthosis prescribed because of the appearance of the foot alone, such as a mobile painless flat foot. The exception is the anaesthetic foot of diabetes (or Hansen's disease), which is considered later. Orthoses are used where there is painful abnormal loading of the foot, particularly where the joints do not move normally, such as in painful stiff flat foot, in pes cavus, in arthritic conditions including osteoarthritis and rheumatoid arthritis, and where there is muscle imbalance as after poliomyelitis.

Calluses indicate abnormal pressure (weight-bearing) on the foot, and their gradual reduction after supply of an orthosis is a sign that it is correct.

Figure 45.2: To maintain knee extension in stance phase forces push forwards behind the thigh and the heel, and to a lesser extent behind the calf. These are resisted by force(s) pushing backwards as near to the knee joint as possible, above and/or below the knee, or over the front of the knee

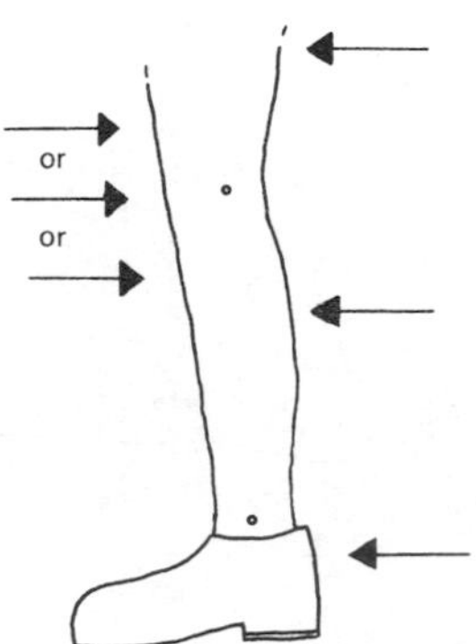

Reduction of pain is achieved by:

(1) redistribution of forces through the foot;

(2) support of painful areas;

(3) weight relief round these areas;

(4) sometimes by alteration of the gait pattern.

Prolonged abnormal weight-bearing, either in valgus due to arthritis or in varus due to spastic dropped foot, causes further damage to the foot structure. Where pain arises in the ankle or hindfoot it will be felt mainly at heel-strike and the beginning of stance phase of gait, but if the pain is from the metatarsal region it will be felt later in stance phase and at push-off (see Gait, Chapter 8).

Hallux rigidus due to osteoarthritis of the first metatarsophalangeal (MTP) joint causes limitation of the normal dorsiflexion at this joint in late stance phase of gait, making it difficult to lift the heel normally without causing pain. An outside rocker bar on the sole of the shoe allows the toes to move down as the heel rises, reducing the movement at the MTP joints needed to achieve normal pain-free gait (Figure 45.3).

Pain at the MTP joints due to rheumatoid arthritis, hallux valgus or other conditions is reduced by shifting some of the thrust of the body weight *behind* the metatarsal heads with a *metatarsal support* on an insole. This support lies under the necks of the metatarsals curving laterally and backwards following their line. If this relieves the pain only partially an *outside rocker bar* may be used in addition. A biomechanical analysis of the use of rocker bars has been done by Petersen *et al.* (1985).

Figure 45.3: Outside rocker bar, shifts weight further back in the foot and reduces the amount of MTP dorsiflexion required for heel-off

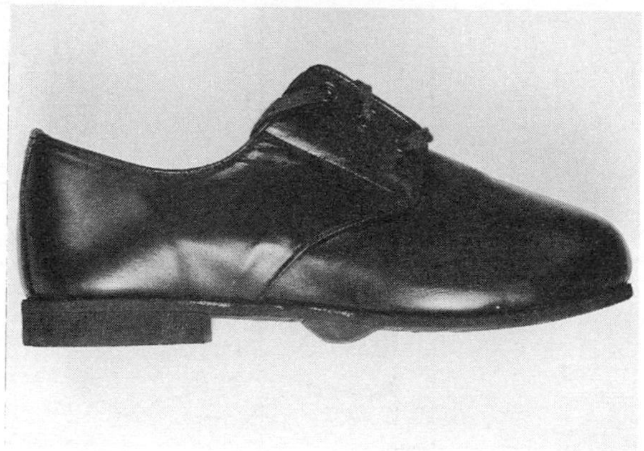

Where the foot goes into *valgus on weight-bearing*, as in rheumatoid arthritis or osteoarthritis of the tarsal joints, a *valgus support* may be built up under the medial arch of the foot to reduce the dropping of this arch and to spread the load of weight-bearing. Where pain is particularly pronounced on heel-strike arising from arthritis of the ankle or tarsal joints, or due to plantar fasciitis, a *cushion heel* is provided by inserting a wedge of energy-absorbing material into the heel of the shoe; energy-absorbing pads inside the shoe under the patient's heel are used, but are less effective. No shoe modification will produce its required effect unless the shoe is of firm construction and the foot held firmly in it by suitable laces or other fastening.

Firm leather medial and lateral heel counters built into the shoe resist deformities, whether valgus or varus, and for the valgus foot the medial counter can be extended forward to provide additional support in conjunction with support built into the insole. Alternatively moulded poly-propylene heel cups can be inserted in the shoes; these support the medial arch of the foot extending forward to the metatarsals. In order to correct some of the abnormal mechanical stresses in the valgus foot a wedge can be built into the medial side of the heel of the shoe tapering towards the middle, and also under the side of the sole if needed, the heel can also be extended medially (heel float) (Figure 45.4). For the varus foot these are built into the lateral side of the shoe. These shoe modifications tilt the foot slightly towards the normal position.

Figure 45.4: Valgus rheumatoid foot. Medial heel wedge, medial float. These shoe modifications with supporting insole are usually sufficient. If more support is needed a double-upright ankle–foot orthosis with free ankle joints may be added, together with a T-strap (or Y-strap) attached between the upper and the sole of the shoe, pulling up and out to a metal loop which maintains its position on the metal upright

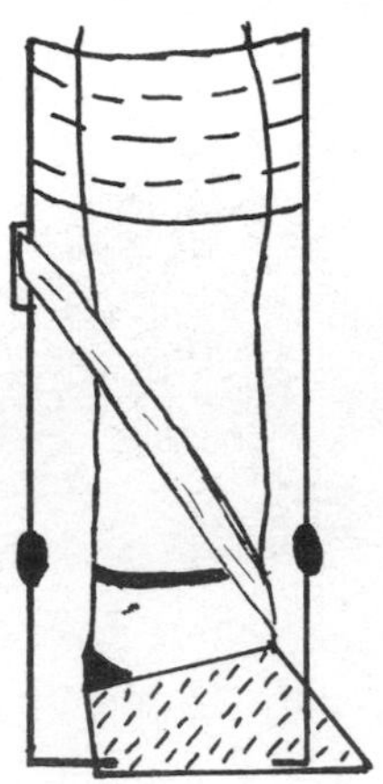

If the patient will accept boots with the above features built in, the support at and above the ankle helps to relieve discomfort on heel-strike and throughout stance phase. Lacing may have to extend down to the toes if oedema occurs. If the situation is temporary a felt or Plastazote boot is cheap, quickly delivered and may encourage acceptance of a more serviceable leather boot or shoe. Where the foot is misshapen by arthritis, pes cavus or other conditions shoes may be made to measurements or preferably to casts of the patient's feet, allowing not only enough length and width but also enough depth, particularly where there is clawing of the toes as in rheumatoid arthritis, or in some neurological conditions such as Charcot–Marie–Tooth disease. This makes the shoe less easily acceptable to women patients. The higher the heel the more of the body weight is borne by the forefoot. Most standard women's shoes provide very little support for the feet, and are frequently narrow and shallow at the toes. Made-to-measure footwear is extremely costly, and patients with less extreme deformities may be accommodated by deeper ready-made shoes (Tuck, 1972) either of leather or synthetic materials (Figure 45.5).

Insoles may be made from measurements, but better from casts of the soles of the feet with the above features moulded into them. They are of cork with a thin leather covering, or of combinations of material such as soft and high-density Plastazote or microcellular rubber. Where a combination of materials is used the firmer is underneath, the less dense in contact

Figure 45.5: Ready-made soft shoe made from a strong felt-like material, lightweight, it can be fitted with a Plastazote insole (Cumbria Orthopaedic, London SE6)

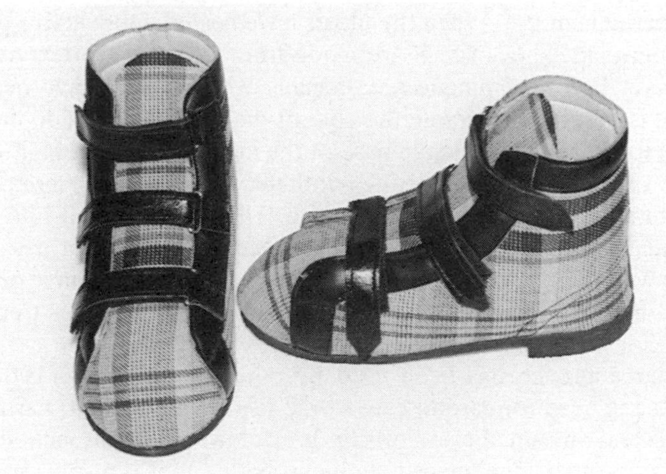

with the patient's foot. Other firmer thermoplastics are also available for foot orthoses, again covered above in a softer material (Doxey, 1985).

THE DIABETIC FOOT

In diabetes foot ulcers are a common condition due to ischaemia or neuropathy. Adequate footwear is an important part of their prevention and treatment. Edmonds *et al.* (1986) reported treatment of 239 patients with foot ulcers, whom they divided into 148 with neuropathy who had absent ankle reflexes, palpable foot pulses and normal Doppler ultrasound arterial readings, and 91 with ischaemia who had absent foot pulses — some of the latter also had neuropathy. The neuropathic group had ulcers particularly on the plantar surface of the big toe, over the ends of the other toes and under the metatarsal heads, while in the ischaemic group they occurred more often over the dorsum of the big toe, over the ends of all the toes and over the heel. In 181 patients narrow shoes were a major cause, the problem being worsened by oedema or by toe deformities such as claw toes or pes cavus. Eighty-six per cent of the neuropathic ulcers and 72 per cent of the ischaemic ulcers were healed by a regime of dressings, antibiotics, chiropody and provision of footwear. The causes of diabetic foot ulcers are fully reviewed by Edmonds (1986).

Footwear

While the ulcer is healing the patient is provided with ready-made extra-depth shoes made from synthetic material and lined with Plastazote on the soles and uppers; patients who move around little may be content with these for permanent use. When the ulcers have healed, more active patients need custom-made shoes which are made from a cast of the feet avoiding pressure over bony prominences, especially where ulcers have occurred. The insole is moulded to cradle the sole of the foot, with cushioning (e.g. neoprene) used at these sites; the base of the insole is made of high-density Plastazote or other firm supporting synthetic, and this is covered with a softer material such as ordinary Plastazote. This insole is built into a shoe with adequate width and depth, which will accommodate foot deformities such as claw toes, etc. An outside rocker bar is used if ulcers have occurred under the metatarsal heads. It is clear that ulcers heal with this treatment, and the incidence of amputation also drops.

A similar approach has been used by others, and Tovey (1986) also emphasises the need for careful care of the feet by the patient, particularly of the nails and any small areas of skin breakdown, daily inspection of the soles being essential. The anaesthetic neuropathic foot is also at risk from foreign bodies in the shoe, so the patient must learn to check for these, as his feet will not feel them and pressure ulcers will result.

ORTHOSES USED IN HINDFOOT ARTHRITIS

(1) When rheumatoid or osteoarthritis affects the talar and/or ankle joints, pain on weight-bearing is felt mainly at heel-strike and the beginning of stance phase. If shoe modification does not relieve the pain, subtalar fusion or triple arthrodesis may relieve talar joint pain, but fusion is not usually indicated for the ankle. An orthosis may be used to reduce the pain on weight-bearing in which the foot is frequently forced into some degree of valgus; reducing this lateral deforming force often reduces the pain (Figure 45.4). The orthosis consists of *medial and lateral metal uprights* extending from the heel to 2–3 cm below the neck of the fibula, supported by a rigid posterior calf band covered in soft leather and fastened by a strap and buckle or by a velcro fastening going through a loop and back on itself. The orthosis has *freely moving ankle joints* positioned at the anatomical ankle axis which passes through the malleoli; no stops or springs are needed as there is no muscle weakness. Heel attachment is into rectangular sockets built into the heel of the shoe. Clearly the shoe must be of firm construction gripping the foot, but if the arthritic patient has poor hand grip and cannot cope with laces, a strap and buckle, or velcro fastening, may be substituted on the shoe.

(2) An alternative for the arthritic hindfoot which will not only reduce some of the lateral force on these joints but also relieve some of the weight-bearing thrust, is a similar orthosis with *two metal uprights,* but this does not have a calf band. Instead it is attached above to a moulded *patellar–tendon–bearing* (PTB) socket, the socket extending two-thirds of the way down the calf. This socket is *bivalved behind the metal uprights* with rigid metal fastenings to close it. This PTB orthosis works better if the socket is flexed by about 10° on the uprights, enabling more thrust to be taken on the pateller tendon, and it is similar to a prosthetic socket (Chapter 11) (Lehmann *et al.*, 1971).

(3) An alternative design is made entirely of a plastic, being moulded to go round the malleoli and under the foot (Demopoulos and Eschen, 1977).

ORTHOSES FOR KNEE JOINT CONDITIONS

The simplest support is made of elasticated or non-stretchable material closely fitting the knee, closed in front with velcro, and having hinged metal side-members slotted into pockets in the fabric (Cinch orthosis). These may have a multicentric joint to approach more nearly to knee flexion motion. For the knee joint that is painful due to potential or actual instability during weight-bearing, whether due to arthritis or injury, an above-knee orthosis extending down to the shoe may be too bulky, so that one extending from mid-thigh to mid-calf is preferred. These shorter orthoses work on shorter moment arms about the knee, and so may be less effective. For knee injury and sports use only the types discussed in (3) below are used.

The object of the orthosis is to relieve pain by applying correcting forces to the knee: anteroposterior, valgus–varus, medial–lateral, or to limit hyperextension or rotation (Beets *et al.*, 1985; Butler *et al.*, 1983).

There are many types of metal and/or plastic orthosis available:

(1) TVS (telescopic valgus–varus support);

(2) moulded plastic thigh and calf parts;

(3) rigid frame metal providing firm fixation for supporting straps. [(1), (2) and (3) extend from mid-thigh to mid-calf, the knee joint flexes freely]

(4) Single metal upright knee–ankle–foot orthosis;

(5) double metal upright knee–ankle–foot orthosis;

(6) plastic thigh and calf–foot parts; 'cosmetic' or 'conforming' orthosis. [(4), (5) and (6) extend from thigh to foot; the patient walks with the knee locked in extension, unlocks it for sitting]

Which knee orthosis (KO) or knee–ankle–foot orthosis (KAFO) should be used?

For mild pain in osteoarthritis (OA) or rheumatoid arthritis (RA) the TVS orthosis is light and useful. For more severe *weight-bearing pain* the all-plastic type is usually less useful than the rigid metal frame types. A KAFO should only be used occasionally: if knee surgery is contraindicated, or if a knee orthosis alone will not control the pain and the patient will tolerate a relatively large and heavy orthosis.

(1) TVS brace

A TVS brace (telescopic valgus–varus–support) extending from mid-thigh to mid-calf may be used for the osteoarthritic or rheumatoid knee where there is little active synovitis, only moderate pain; the varus or valgus is less than 15° and fixed flexion is less than 15°. Pressure on the thigh and calf is applied with moulded plastic ovals (14 × 12 cm) fixed with velcro straps and held apart by a flexible plastic rod, with a pivoted telescopic metal tube to give support and allow flexion–extension of the knee. From these plastic ovals straps extend in front to the points of a triangular leather cuff from the third point of which a strap extends behind the knee to be clipped on to the telescopic metal tube separating the thigh and calf pieces of the orthosis (Figure 45.6). The orthosis for the *valgus* knee applies a force pushing *medially* over the lateral calf and thigh from each plastic oval and pushing *laterally* from the triangular leather cuff pulling on the medial side of the knee. Careful fitting and adjustment is required to relieve some of the valgus or varus force on weight-bearing, but this orthosis is light and unobtrusive and so very acceptable for moderate pain and deformity (Cousins *et al.*, 1977). The painful osteoarthritic knee with mild *varus* may be helped by a TVS brace, this time applied with the thigh and calf pieces on the medial side and the leather cuff on the lateral side of the knee to pull it medially during weight-bearing. Jawad and Goodwill (1986) obtained relief of knee pain in 14 out of 18 patients with osteoarthritis but in only five out of 13 with rheumatoid arthritis.

Figure 45.6: Telescopic valgus–varus support (TVS)

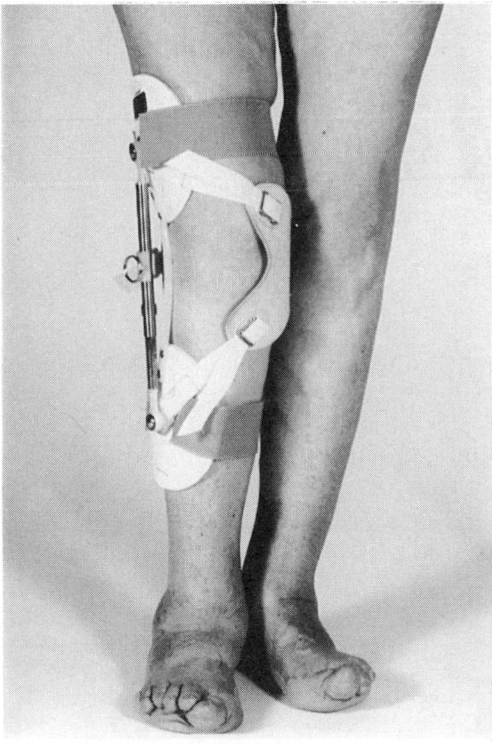

(2) Moulded plastic thigh and calf parts

These are made from a plaster cast and hinged at the knee (alternatively separate metal hinges can be moulded into the plastic). The orthosis is padded over the area of the medial or lateral femoral condyle to resist valgus or varus respectively. This orthosis is probably less satisfactory than the next types of knee orthoses described.

(3) Rigid frame metal knee orthoses

These provide firm fixation for supporting straps. Many types are available, but there is an absence of sufficient comparative trials of their merits and demerits in patients with different conditions. The author has used the Can-Am orthosis successfully for painful OA or RA of the knee and it is also used for ligamentous sports injuries. It is a semi-rigid, custom-made knee brace providing lateral stability and rotational control, while maintaing full flexion–extension through polycentric knee joints, and preventing hyperextension (Figure 45.7). For the sports person with a ligamentous knee injury the Lennox–Hill brace may be used (Hanswyk and

Figure 45.7: Can-Am knee orthosis

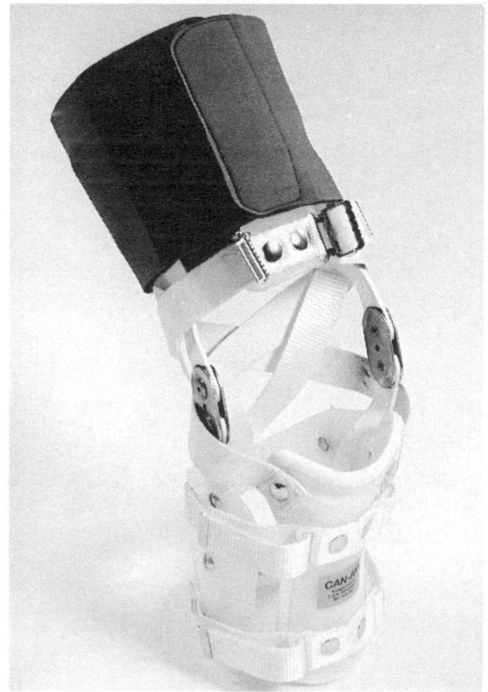

Baker, 1982) and to prevent hyperextension alone, the Swedish knee cage may be useful.

KNEE–ANKLE–FOOT ORTHOSES (KAFO) FOR KNEE ARTHRITIS

These have the advantage of a longer lever arm to resist valgus or varus but are more bulky and less acceptable cosmetically. As with other orthoses for the knee they will only help mechanical *weight-bearing pain, not resting pain.*

(4) Single-upright knee–ankle–foot orthoses

For the valgus knee a single above-knee outside metal upright is used with a knee hinge. This extends down through a free orthotic ankle joint to fit into a rectagular heel socket. The patient walks with the orthotic knee locked in the extended position, releasing the knee for sitting; up to 15° of fixed flexion can be built into the orthosis if the knee does not go straight. The rigid posterior calf and thigh bands have soft antcrior fastenings and a *broad leather cuff extends from the metal upright round the medial* side of the knee pulling outwards. The support is less than with double uprights but adequate for some patients. This cuff also presses back on the knee holding it in extension. *For the varus knee* an inside metal upright is used with the leather cuff round the outside of the knee pulling medially.

(5) Double-upright knee–ankle–foot orthosis

This is similar to (4) but with medial and lateral uprights, again with free ankle joints. A leather knee cuff is used as for (4). It is rarely indicated, but may be useful for a heavy patient.

Knee-locks for (4) and (5). These can be simple drop lock(s), or spring-loaded to lock automatically as the knee is extended. With or without spring-loading the two locks can be connected together in front by a metal hoop. Pulling up on this releases both locks at the same time for sitting; this hoop can be hinged to allow easier application of the orthosis.

(6) Plastic thigh and calf-foot parts; 'cosmetic' or 'conforming' orthosis

The below-knee part is made of ortholon moulded to the calf, extending behind the heel and under the foot to the metatarsal heads (as used for flaccid drop foot). If hindfoot pain is present due to arthritis the plastic can be moulded forward round the malleoli to give support there also. Medial and lateral metal uprights attached to the ortholon extend upwards through knee hinges to a plastic quadrilateral ischial-weight-bearing socket, of the same design as for a prosthesis (Chapter 11). The socket can be left intact or have a front closure if needed; the latter gives less support. There is a wide velcro band attached to the metal uprights, fastening in front above the knee, or the fastening may be just below the knee; either is near the knee axis, pushing backwards to hold the knee extended for walking. Release of knee locks is by pulling up on a cord in front of the patient's thigh, the cord being chanelled through a plastic tube attached to the thigh socket (Figure 45.8).

Which KAFO should be used? (if a knee orthosis alone does not give sufficient pain relief)

The single-upright (4) may help the patient who only wishes to walk a little inside the home. The double-upright (5) is heavy, unsightly and seldom used. For the active patient one or even both knees may usefully be supported by the moulded plastic orthosis (6), with the added advantage of

Figure 45.8: 'Cosmetic' orthosis: fastening is in front above the knee

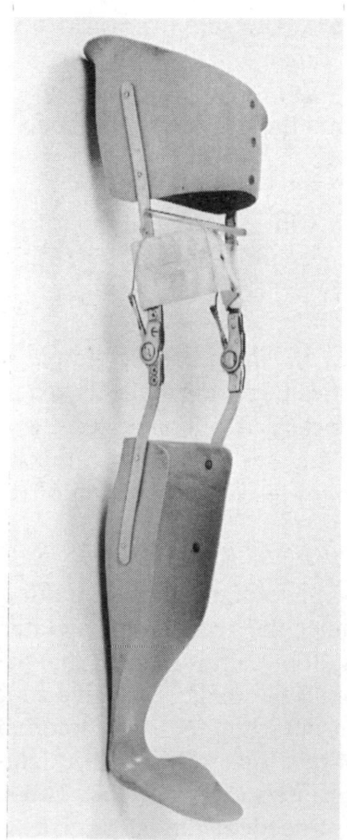

supporting the hindfoot where needed. Whichever KAFO is used, walking with the knee locked in extension will usually require the use of walking aids (Chapter 46).

ORTHOSES FOR FLACCID DROP FOOT

Flaccid drop foot causes dragging of the toes on the floor during swing phase of gait, requiring increased elevation of that side of the pelvis with excess flexion of knee and hip for the toes to clear the floor. This abnormal gait pattern can be rectified with an orthosis (Lehmann *et al.*, 1986). The commonest cause of this is a common peroneal nerve palsy due to pressure at the neck of the fibula, sometimes on a background of a generalised peripheral neuropathy such as in diabetes. These orthoses may also be used in muscular dystrophy or in Charcot–Marie–Tooth disease. Nerve root lesions due to a disc or tumour are usually relieved by surgery, but some cause persistent foot drop. When appropriate, tendon transfer of the tibialis posterior to produce active dorsiflexion may be used, but in many patients an orthosis is appropriate, particularly where recovery is expected. Oedema may be a contraindication to a total contact plastic appliance, but whatever is used the object is to produce a dorsiflexion force at the ankle, not to pull up the toes; a toe-raising appliance is entirely inappropriate.

(1) *An ankle foot orthosis moulded from ortholen* or polypropylene extends upwards to 2–3 cm below the neck of the fibula, being closed with a strap or velcro fastening in front. The orthosis is moulded round behind the malleoli and under the heel, moulded under the foot extending forwards to just behind the metatarsal heads. It fits under the sock or stocking so that for some patients a slightly larger shoe is needed. The further the plastic is cut back at the malleoli the more mobility is obtained; the further forwards the plastic is extended the more stability is achieved, reducing inversion of the foot as well as foot drop (Figure 45.9).

Polypropylene can be flexed and extended many times without breaking. Ortholon will lose its function rather sooner, but it can more easily be given a softer, more cosmetic finish.

(2) An alternative is a *single inside metal upright* with a piston ankle joint containing a coil spring pushing down behind the axis of the ankle joint; the dorsiflexion force may be increased by tightening this spring by turning the hollow hexagonal screw above the spring (Figure 45.10). If inversion is to be prevented a broad outside T-shaped (or Y-shaped) strap is attached to the outer part of the heel and instep of the shoe between the upper and the sole; the strap narrows as it passes medially in front and behind the ankle to go through a metal sleeve fixed to the outer side of the metal upright (Figure 45.4). Only in a very heavily built person with much

Figure 45.9: Ortholon ankle–foot orthosis for flaccid dropped foot. For a mildly spastic dropped foot this may be made of polypropylene. For more support and prevention of varus the trim line of the plastic may be brought further forward; if needed it can even be in front of the malleoli

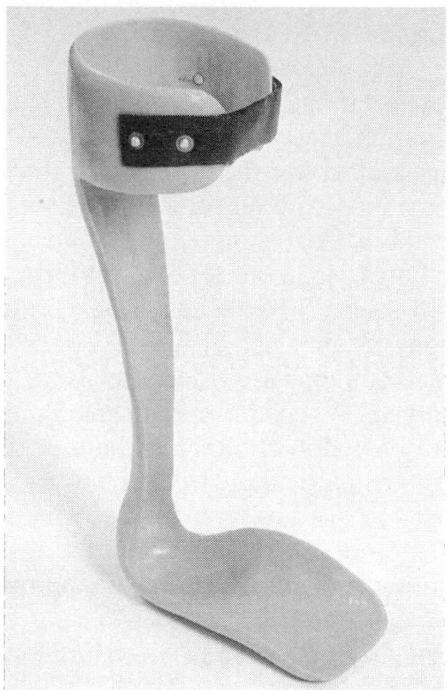

inversion force would a double-upright below-knee orthosis be required with similar features.

(3) Sometimes a single inside upright without an ankle joint, but with a round heel socket, is used; planter flexion during swing phase being prevented by the back of the upright hitting the *heel stop fitted into the shoe.* However, this shifts the orthotic ankle axis away from the anatomical axis and moves it down the heel, causing movement of the metal upright in relation to the ankle during walking.

(4) There are other ankle–foot orthoses which are usually less satisfactory, such as a metal leaf spring passing down the back of the calf and held with a calf band above, and with a shoe clasp at the lower end gripping the back of the heel of the shoe; this does not give firm support and soon the back of the shoe breaks down. In another type two below-knee metal uprights extend below to a coil spring; these are connected together under and round the heel of the shoe, gripping it to provide dorsiflexion force. This orthosis may be useful as a temporary measure to determine whether one of the above orthoses would be useful. The biomechanics of ankle–foot orthoses are discussed by Lehmann (1979).

ORTHOSES IN FLACCID CALF MUSCLE PARALYSIS

These have been studied by Lehmann *et al.* (1985) and it is clear that the excess dorsiflexion, the delayed heel-off towards the end of stance phase and the reduced step length can be greatly improved by a double-upright ankle–foot orthosis with *anterior* stops set at 5° plantar flexion. This prevents excessive dorsiflexion by the unopposed action of the dorsiflexor muscles. If plantar flexion is also weak, posterior stops are also needed, and the sole of the shoe must be firm, if necessary strengthened with a rigid sole plate (Lehmann *et al.*, 1980).

ORTHOSES FOR SPASTIC DROP FOOT

Spastic drop foot is more difficult to treat. Not only is there dragging of the foot during swing phase of gait but also spastic equinovarus causes instability in stance phase, the calf muscles providing the main inverting force at the subtalar joint. The gait abnormalities are discussed in Chapter 8. The most common indication for an orthosis is for a spastic hemiplegia due to stroke, although some patients with other intracranial pathology may have a similar problem. The spasm may be reduced by physiotherapy directed not only at the spastic muscles but at the whole pattern of limb and body use and movement. If spasticity in the calf muscles is a persistent severe problem injection of 5 per cent phenol into motor points of gastrocnemius may reduce it. Some patients will walk better, and in particular be more stable during stance phase, with the aid of an orthosis. Where the predominant leg weakness is of abduction and extension of the hip the use of an *ankle–foot orthosis* might just tip the balance to enable the patient to walk safely. An *above-knee orthosis* (KAFO) is inadvisable even if the knee is weak. It is better to try to stabilise the involved knee in stance phase by adjusting the ankle position on a below-knee orthosis (AFO) so that it is in slight plantar flexion; this helps to keep the body weight in front of the knee axis in stance phase, although it may make initiation of swing more difficult.

There are four main types of AFO in use:

(1) double metal uprights with piston ankle joints;

(2) double metal uprights with double-stop ankle joints;

(3) polypropylene or ortholon;

(4) functional electrical stimulation.

(1) To control twisting of the hindfoot into equinovarus during stance phase *medial and lateral metal uprights* are needed which fit into rectangular sockets in firmly built and fastened shoes. The posterior calf band is made of leather-covered metal to give firm support. It is closed in front with a strap and buckle, or with velcro attached on the medial side going through a metal loop on the lateral side of the front of the calf band and back onto itself for fastening. This can be achieved with one hand, and is invaluable for the stroke patient. *An orthosis is of limited value if the patient cannot put it on and off himself. At the ankle joints* piston ankles are used with stops behind the axis preventing foot drop during swing phase, as springs are insufficient to resist the spastic antagonist muscles (Figure 45.10).

(2) A double-piston ankle with stop in front and behind the ankle axis. This *double-stop ankle joint* can be used to control the knee as well as the ankle joint (Figure 45.11). The stops are set at about 90° in a position that prevents clonus on weight-bearing which is sometimes a problem in stroke.

Figure 45.10: Double-upright ankle–foot orthosis with piston ankles with stops inside to prevent plantarflexion during swing phase (*single* inside metal upright with piston ankle with coiled spring inside is used to provide dorsiflexion force for *flaccid* drop foot)

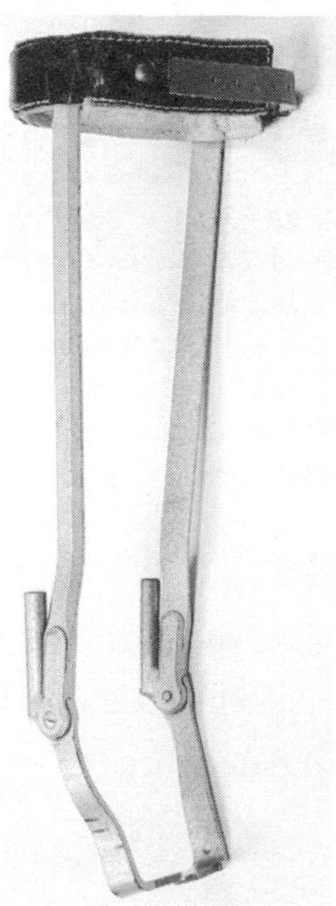

Figure 45.11: Double-stop ankle joints to limit dorsiflexion as well as plantarflexion

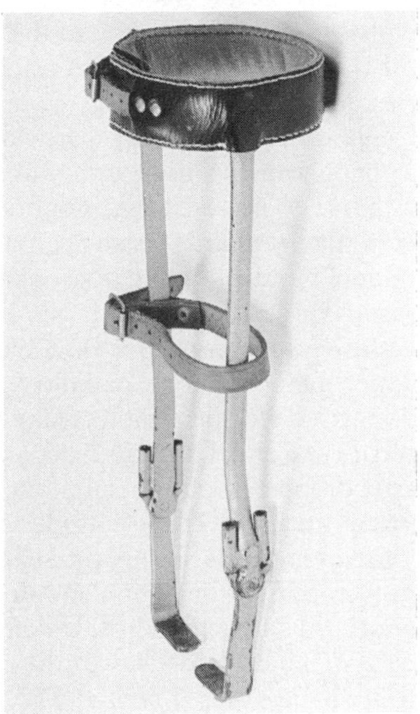

If a few degrees dorsiflexion is allowed or the ankle set slightly dorsiflexed the slight forward tilting of the tibia will help to prevent knee hyperextension in stance phase. If too much dorsiflexion is allowed the increased knee-bending may allow the joint to give way. Often these patients begin stance phase with the foot flat, but if there is an initial heel-strike the line of body weight from the point of the heel may pass up too far behind the knee axis with excess bending moment on the knee. This line of body weight may be moved forward nearer to the knee axis by using a cushion heel or a 45° cut-off at the back of the heel (Lehmann, 1979).

Medial and lateral metal uprights may be used *without ankle joints.* These uprights pivot in round heel sockets; plantarflexion is prevented by heel stops fixed in the heel behind the metal uprights. These allow rotation below the anatomical axis of the ankle. They cannot be adjusted, as can stops at the ankle joints, and so are less satisfactory. With either of these ankle–foot orthoses persisting inversion may be reduced by an outside T-strap extending from the outside of the shoe across and round the medial metal upright of the orthosis. Sometimes a lateral heel float may be useful, this may be combined with a lateral wedge on the sole and heel.

(3) *With moderate spasticity* a moulded polypropylene orthosis will

prevent foot drop (Figure 45.9). It may need to extend further forward to the front of the malleoli both medially and laterally than the orthosis used for flaccid drop foot; in this way it also produces some medial–lateral stability during stance phase. The further forward the plastic extends at the ankle the more support is obtained (Lehmann *et al.*, 1982). Polypropylene may be strengthened with carbon fibre inserts.

Multiple sclerosis with drop foot causes particular problems, as the patient is frequently a young woman who does not like the appearance of a metal orthosis below the knee on each leg. For these patients the best solution may be ortholen if there is little spasticity, or polypropylene if it is moderate, reserving double-upright ankle–foot metal orthoses for the patient with severe spasticity with equino-varus.

(4) *Functional electrical stimulation* (FES). Stimulation of the intact peripheral nerve in upper motor neurone pathology, as after a stroke of partial spinal cord lesion, is a developing subject and programmed stimulation is being developed (Turk and Obreza, 1985). It may be applied to correct the mildly spastic dropped foot in hemiplegia by stimulation of the common peroneal nerve at the knee. Two electrodes stimulate the nerve to produce dorsiflexion of the foot during swing phase; during stance phase a cut-off switch in the heel stops the stimulation and dorsiflexion action. Not only does the stimulation provide active dorsiflexion allowing the foot to clear the ground, but it also inhibits spasticity in the plantarflexor muscles. *This orthosis should only be used for a patient who is able to walk relatively well* but where there is a problem with foot drop, possibly with mild plantarflexion spasticity (Liberson *et al.*, 1961; Lee and Johnston, 1976). FES is used for training or for long-term treatment.

The electrodes are placed over the common peroneal nerve — one in the popliteal fossa and one near the neck of the fibula. The patient feels some mild discomfort at first but very rapidly adjusts to this. The amplitude and duration of the train of electrical impulses to the nerve, and the exact position of the electrodes, must be adjusted by the physiotherapist during gait training. The patient must learn how to position the electrodes and maintain them in position (Figure 45.12).

Conclusions

In stroke patients there is increasing use of plastic orthoses rather than those with metal uprights (Offir and Sell, 1980) although the energy consumption is the same with either type when used on the same patient (Corcoran *et al.*, 1970). In the patient who starts stance phase with toe-strike instead of the normal heel-strike, this can be corrected in some of the less spastic patients by the use of an orthosis (Lee and Johnston, 1973).

Figure 45.12: Functional electrical stimulation (FES): the electrodes are placed over the common peroneal nerve at the neck of the fibula and in the popliteal fossa; the heel cut-out switch (on the left) functions during stance phase. The control unit (centre) controls duration and amplitude of stimulation

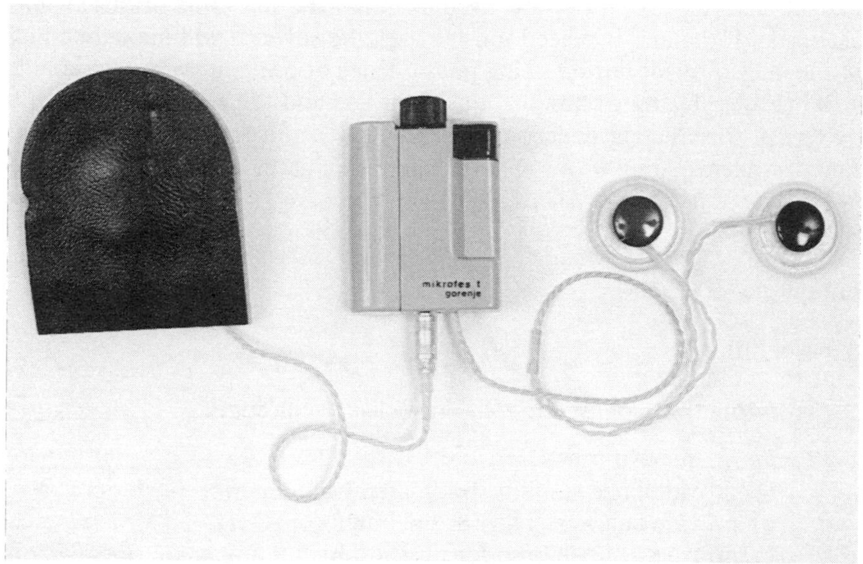

NEUROLOGICAL CONDITIONS REQUIRING KNEE BRACING

Multiple sclerosis and stroke

For the patient with a knee that is so weak that bracing appears necessary it is almost always inadvisable to provide an above-knee orthosis (KAFO). The associated weakness of the hip muscles and sensory loss, as well as the weight of the orthosis, usually prevent any improvement in gait. If knee *hyperextension* is a problem, a Swedish knee cage, or similar plastic orthosis, may be used.

Flaccid weakness of one leg

This is usually due to poliomyelitis, and the orthosis will be as described below for paraplegia. *If the hip extensors are preserved* the patient may be able to walk with a free knee, by placing the orthotic knee axis further back behind the anatomical knee axis, possibly with the addition of hydraulic damping at the ankle and posterior heel advancement to bring the line of body weight (ground reaction force) further forward.

During stance phase of gait this allows the line of body weight to pass in front of the orthotic knee axis, locking the knee in extension to support the patient. The hip extensors are used to force the leg (and orthosis) into extension. If the axis is placed too far back, however, it will make bending of the knee difficult during swing phase. Knee bending in swing phase aids walking by reducing circumduction of the leg and the need to 'hitch' the pelvis up, so reducing energy requirements. This 'free-knee' KAFO may cause problems going *down* a slope when the line of body weight may be *behind the orthotic knee axis.*

Paraplegia

Aims of orthosis:

(1) *during swing* phase the foot must clear the ground;

(2) *during stance* it must:
  (a) provide knee stability, both lateral and anterior–posterior;
  (b) provide lateral stability at the hindfoot;
  (c) provide a stable base for push-off by limiting ankle dorsiflexion and by having a firm sole to the shoe to aid heel lift. This will also provide firm support for weight-bearing in stance phase.

(Knee–ankle–foot orthoses (KAFO) will be discussed first — those extending above the hip will be mentioned briefly at the end.)

Some patients with flaccid paraplegia will be able to walk with plastic KAFO, as described above for knee arthritis (No. 6 in that section), but most will need metal orthoses.

In the usual KAFO two metal uprights extending from the upper thigh down to the ankles are connected by rigid posterior calf and thigh bands, which keep the uprights in their correct position and are closed in front with soft fastenings.

An older type of KAFO that is still in common use (Figure 45.13) relies on a leather cuff over the front of the knee to stabilise the joint in extension, and only has stops behind the ankle axis, which is less effective in aiding heel-off than those discussed below.

For effective function the following features need to be considered.

(1) *Each ankle joint* needs a posterior stop to prevent footdrop in stance phase and an anterior stop to limit dorsiflexion during heel-off; the

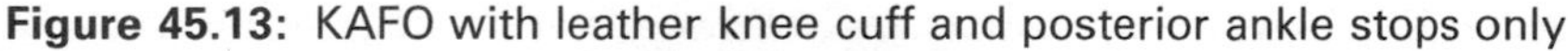

Figure 45.13: KAFO with leather knee cuff and posterior ankle stops only

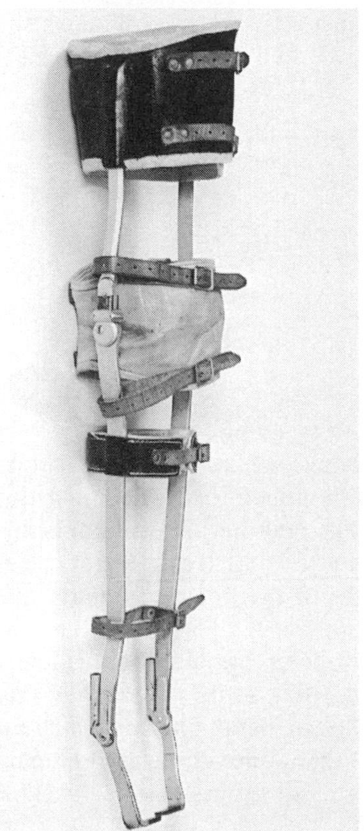

latter works best if combined with a sole stiffener, usually a flexible metal shank extending from the heel to the metatarsal necks (Figure 45.14) (Lehmann *et al.*, 1969). A posterior stop alone may work even with a slightly flexible shoe, but only if the patient has a flaccid paraplegia, e.g. cauda equina level.

(2) *The knee is stabilised* by a force pushing forward behind the thigh and at the heel of the shoe, while the forward pressure from the calf band should be low as it is nearer the knee and so has a shorter lever arm. The backward-directed force in front of the leg to complete the knee stabilisation is applied by a flexible band over the lower thigh or below the knee over the upper tibia and/or the patellar tendon; the latter may be of plastic similar in shape to the anterior part of a PTB prosthesis (see Figure 11.6).

(3) *Sheer force* at heel-strike tends to move the femur forward on the tibia, while later in stance and at heel-off this is reversed (Lehmann and Warren, 1976). These forces are best resisted by pressure over the patellar

Figure 45.14: (a) With anterior as well as posterior stops at the orthotic ankle joints and a rigid sole, the heel lifts off with bending at the front of the foot. (b) With double-stop ankles and a soft shoe the foot bends at the instep. (c) With posterior stop only and a soft shoe, the heel may not rise at all unless the whole leg is lifted

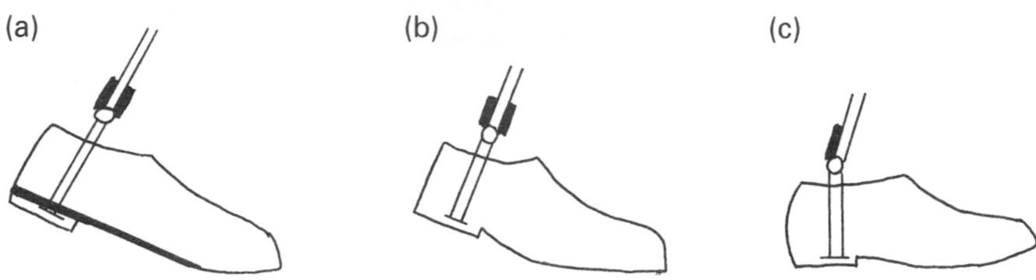

tendon, preferably with an additional force over the supracondylar area. It is mainly in the very active walker that these factors need to be considered.

(4) *Knee locks* as described for KAFO in arthritis may be used, or the two orthotic knee locks may be joined behind by a metal ring. Pressure upwards on this ring releases the locks, either done manually or by upward pressure from the seat of the chair on which the patient is about to sit down.

The Scott–Craig orthosis combines many of these features including anterior and posterior ankle stops, a steel sole plate, set-back knee joints and a solid anterior tibial band for knee stabilisation. This latter band applies a higher force than other closures (Lehmann *et al.*, 1976) and may usefully be changed to an anterior tibial shell bearing on the patellar tendon, possibly with the addition of a supracondylar strap. Energy consumption with the Scott–Craig orthosis is 25–30 per cent less than using conventional orthoses without anterior ankle stops (Merkel *et al.*, 1984). In a follow-up study of 247 paraplegic patients only 18 (7 per cent) were functional walkers, but four of these had no working abdominal muscles and five had upper abdominals only, so clearly they have an advantage for some patients (O'Daniel and Hahn, 1981).

In a retrospective study of 98 paraplegic patients (Coghlan *et al.*, 1980) at a mean of $6\frac{1}{2}$ years after injury, only twelve patients were functional walkers, all of these having strong abdominal, back extensor and hip-hiking muscles, *but the types of orthosis were not stated.* Other patients found them useful for standing or exercise only.

Which patients with paraplegia should use orthoses?

Those with cauda equina lesions can walk relatively efficiently, whereas lesions from T10 to L2 cause more difficulty (except for the young traumatic paraplegic). Although orthoses are supplied to patients with lesions above that level it is only the young, strong and determined who will use them functionally. For walking the patient uses two elbow crutches, and in standing depends on extending the hips and increasing the lumbar lordosis to obtain stability. Others may benefit by the standing and exercise that they allow, but a standing frame is easier to use, without the need to don and doff the orthoses (Chapter 23).

Orthoses extending above the hip (in adults)

These provide support for the hips and the lower trunk. It is usually only the young patient who is suitable for a trial of one of these orthoses. For lesions between T6 and T12 the *hip-guidance orthosis* may be tried. This consists of two leg orthoses attached through hip joints to a metal frame spinal support reaching up to the chest (Rose, 1986; Patrick and McClelland, 1985) (Figure 45.15).

Functional electrical stimulation (FES)

FES may be added to this to give a programmed stimulation of muscles to achieve gait; this is discussed above, and by Turk and Obreza (1985).

An alternative approach is the *reciprocating gait orthosis*, in which plastic KAFOs are attached above to a metal spinal support, but in this method the leg components are interconnected so that as one hip flexes the other extends and supports the body weight (McCall *et al.*, 1983).

Pneumatic orthoses are of one piece, enclosing the legs and trunk up to the axillae, support being provided by vertical inflatable tubes in the material of the orthosis. These are experimental but some favourable results have been reported in thoracic paraplegia (Strachan *et al.*, 1985).

CERVICAL ORTHOSES

Collars

Aims

To reduce pain, e.g. cervical spondylosis, and *to limit movement* (particularly flexion) in rheumatoid arthritis, in cervical spine injuries, or in destructive lesions due to malignancy or infection or in vertebro-basilar insufficiency.

Use

(1) *For spondylosis* the support and moderate limitation of movement from a Plastazote collar is sufficient, and the patient can still move his head against the restriction of the collar if he wishes (Figure 45.16). For night pain a softer plastic foam is used, covered in stockinette. To produce more neck support and limitation a polythene collar is used; this is circular and

Figure 45.15: Hip guidance orthosis

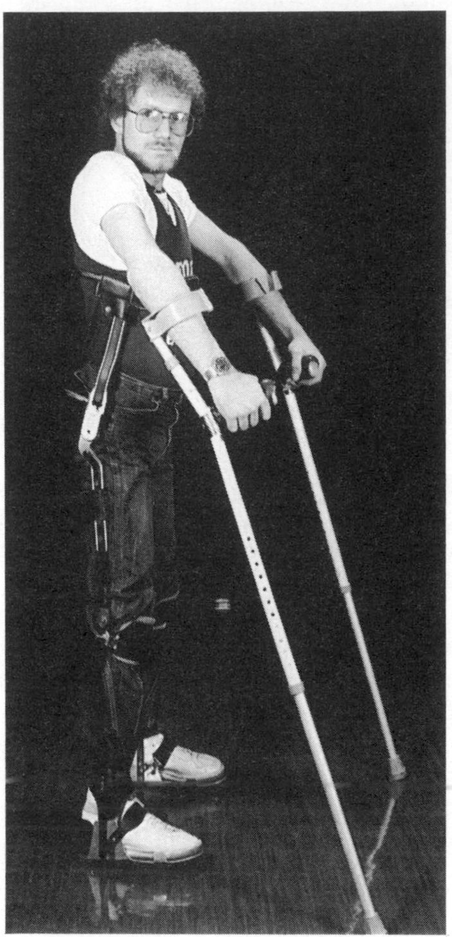

flared out at the top and bottom, particularly over the sternum and under the chin.

(2) *To control cervical spine instability much firmer support is required.* All these will limit mouth-opening, and so interfere with eating, but are used where prevention of cervical movement is essential to prevent spinal cord damage.

The Minerva Collar is made of polythene and is in two parts: the back part is moulded up over the occiput and down over the back of the shoulders, while the front part is moulded up under the chin and down over the upper sternum. The two parts are joined by flexible material on one side and closed by straps on the other side.

Figure 45.16: A relatively soft plastic foam collar (*left*) and a firmer plastic collar with screw adjustment at front (*right*)

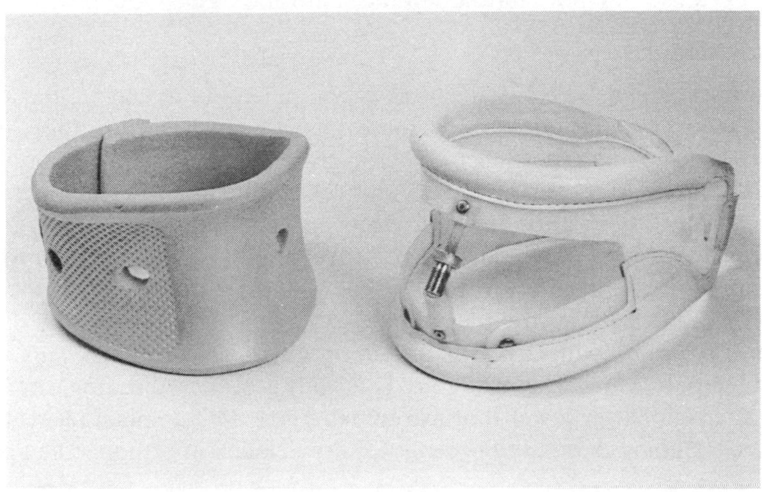

The four-poster collar consists of four adjustable uprights, pushing up on chin and occipital plates above, and on sternal and upper thoracic plates below. For greater limitation of movement the orthosis must extend lower round the trunk. These orthoses are not discussed further here, but producc substantial limitation of movement (Fisher *et al.*, 1977). This group found that the four-poster or the sternal–occipital–mandibular immobilisation orthosis (SOMI), produced the most efficient cervical immobilisation, as judged by goniometry and flexion-extension X-rays. Other orthoses to maintain control of the cervical spine in neck injuries are detailed in orthopaedic texts.

Corsets

Aims

To support the lumbar spine, to relieve pain; to limit movement of the lumbar spine; to prevent the patient bending the spine (attempted bending will cause the corset to dig into the tissues over the lower ribs and pelvis).

Use

A corset should only be used for a clear reason in a patient with low back pain. In acute pain due to a disc or ligament injury it will rest the back, and may enable the patient to continue at work. For the painful collapsed vertebra in the older patient (e.g. due to osteoporosis) it may be used for two to three months while healing occurs. Long-term use of a corset should only be advised where no other treatment will relieve the pain, as prolonged use will inevitably stiffen the spine and weaken the muscles.

Prescription

The corset extends below to the bony pelvis and above to enclose the lower ribs. Some women find the upper part digs into the flesh, but this can be helped by extending the corset higher in front as a brassière. The corset is closed in front with several velcro or buckle fastenings, and two or four vertical spring-steel strips are inserted in pockets in the back of the corset to provide support and limitation of movement. These should follow the contour of the back closely to be effective. A shorter corset without steels is sometimes used, but gives little support. Any pain relief is probably due to the warmth and comfort that it produces. For really firm back support a moulded polythene jacket is required and this is also used during mobilisation after lumbar or lower thoracic spinal injury. Other spinal jackets and braces, including those used in scoliosis, are detailed in orthopaedic texts.

ARM ORTHOSES

Static

For the patient with a *painful rheumatoid wrist* a supporting splint may reduce pain and increase function. This may be ready-made of fabric with a metal volar insert extending to the palm, or moulded from a plastic material, many types being available. The thumb is left free. Polypropylene is light and rigid, whilst other plastics are slightly more flexible but are often thicker, but have the advantage that modifications are easier than with polypropylene. However any support that covers the palm has the disadvantage of reducing the sensation of the object being grasped. For the relief of *carpal tunnel* symptoms at night the ready-made support is adequate, the wrist again being held in a neutral or slightly dorsiflexed position.

For painful osteoarthritis of the first carpometacarpal joint the support does not have to extend so far up the forearm, but the first metacarpal is included in the support, to limit movement of the painful joint.

Dynamic

In hemiplegia due to stroke the shoulder is frequently subluxed and painful; several types of support for this are available but none really seem to achieve their object. However the functional shoulder orthosis (FSO) described by Brudny (1985) shows some promise of helping these patients. A metal ball-and-socket joint attached to pelvic and thoracic bands is placed between the chest and the upper arm. From this orthotic joint a rod extends down to a cuff round the upper arm. This in turn is attached to a forearm cuff through medial and lateral orthotic elbow joints. In a small study three out of eight patients found this functionally useful, and even in the others shoulder subluxation was reduced.

The flail elbow may be supported by an orthosis consisting of metal or plastic upper arm and forearm cuffs, joined medially and laterally by metal hinges. The orthotic elbow can be moved by the patient into one of four or five positions, and locked to give the flexion that is required for different activities.

In a brachial plexus lesion with a flail arm an orthosis can help to improve function. However, the orthosis is complicated, skilled fitting and training is essential, and some preservation of sensation is needed for good use. Many patients prefer to function one-handed. Their use is reviewed by McKenzie and Buck (1978).

In tetraplegia due to cervical spine injury or other conditions the weak hand can be made more functional by a dynamic hand orthosis, the details of which are well described by Malick and Meyer (1978) and Bender (1982). These orthoses work best where elbow flexion is retained (C5–6 level) and need to be much more complex where this function also must be substituted with an orthosis.

MOBILE ARM SUPPORTS (MAS)

Indications

These are used to counterbalance the weight of the arm when any disease causes muscle weakness (grade 2), preventing useful arm movement against gravity. They are used where weak shoulder and elbow muscles limit *hand placement*, but are only useful if there is residual *hand function*, or when useful items such as typing stick or a spoon can be gripped by, or fixed to, the hand. Most commonly this occurs with motor neurone disease, progressive muscular atrophy, muscular dystrophy and sometimes in tetraplegia or multiple sclerosis. The patient must be firmly supported in a functional position, if necessary by special cushioning in the wheelchair (Chapters 42 and 43).

Contraindications

(1) Spasticity

(2) Tremor or involuntary movements.

(3) Limitation of joint movement due to arthritis or contracture. *The shoulder* needs to: abduct 60°, flex 50°, extend 20°. *The elbow* needs to: flex 120°, and have not more than 30° fixed flexion, *supination/pronation* should be nearly full. *Wrist movement* is less important, although preferably the wrist should extend 20° and flex 30°.

(4) Lack of understanding of their function by the patient.

(5) Lack of staff to adjust and balance the MAS (this is done by an OT over a period of a few days).

Fitting

The supporting adjustable clamp is fixed round the metal backrest support, which should not usually be angled back more than 12°. If the patient has weak neck muscles the backrest may have to be angled back further to allow a headrest to support the head, then a *universal clamp* is used, which allows the MAS to be positioned correctly. The wheelchair must *not* have a folding backrest, or the hinge will get in the way of the clamp. Occasionally the clamp may be fixed to an upright firm armchair instead of to a wheelchair. *The proximal metal arm* pivots in this clamp, and extends out to provide another socket for pivoting of the *distal metal arm*, into the end of which the *forearm trough* fits with a swivel attachment. For weaker patients *this swivel may be offset* to allow greater adjustment (Figures 45.17 and 45.18).

Adjustment

(1) *Height of the clamp* on the wheelchair is adjusted for the patient's natural forearm position when well supported in the wheelchair.

(2) *Rotation of the clamp inwards or outwards* will assist adduction or abduction of the shoulder.

(3) *Tilt of the bracket* on the clamp will alter the angle of support of the MAS, tilt upwards will aid flexion, or downwards will aid extension, of the elbow.

(4) *The anterior–posterior position of the forearm trough* on the distal

Figure 45.17: Mobile arm supports (MAS) showing supporting clamp on wheelchair upright, pivoting of proximal and distal arms, the latter supporting standard forearm troughs

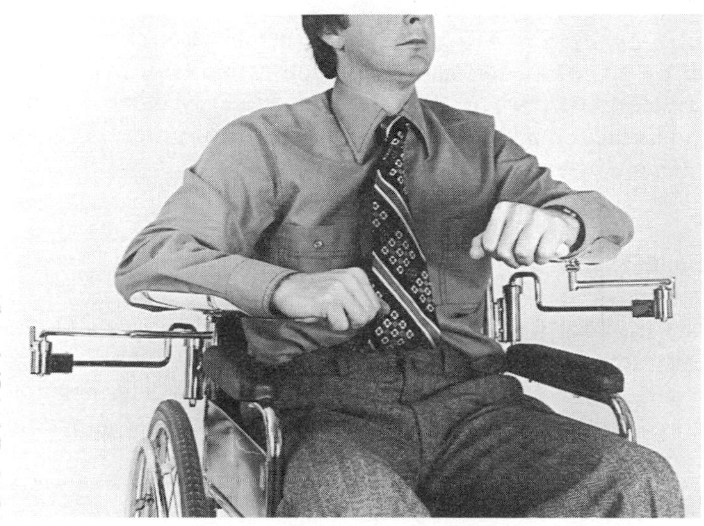

Figure 45.18: MAS with universal clamp to allow correct positioning and tilt when used on a reclining backrest. The offset swivel on the forearm trough allows finer adjustment and easier vertical arm movement

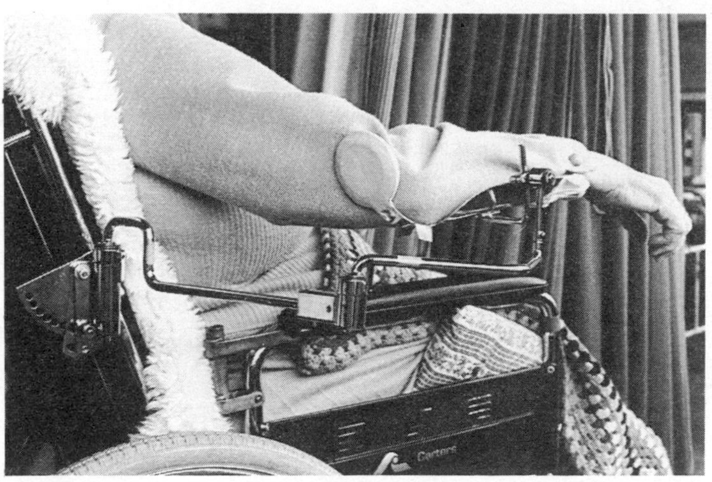

arm will not only aid flexion or extension of the elbow, but also influence rotation at the shoulder.

(5) *The offset swivel support* for the forearm allows a greater range of vertical movement of the hand, especially if the patient is very weak.

(6) *A T-bar extension* to the forearm trough is used to support the hand if the wrist extensors are weak, and a *supinator assist* can be used under the trough to provide supination (Nichols, 1971). Further adjustment may be needed as the condition progresses, and *regular review is essential.*

Use of mobile arm supports

These are used for feeding, writing/typing, turning pages and other work and hobby activities. About half of the patients fitted with MAS continue to use them, and in the author's experience the determination of the patient, and the acceptance of the orthosis, are the most important factors in achieving useful function once they have been correctly prescribed and adjusted (Haworth *et al.*, 1978; Yasuda *et al.*, 1986).

ACKNOWLEDGEMENT

I am grateful to my in-house artists Miss Anne-Marie Goodwill and Mr Mark Goodwill for the line diagrams, and to Gordon Rose FRCS and Robin Luff FRCS for helpful comments on the script.

REFERENCES

Beets, C.L., Clippinger, F.W., Hazard, P.R. and Vaughn, D.W. (1985) Orthoses and the dynamic knee: a basic overview. *Orthot. Prosthet. 39*, 33-9

Bender, L.F. (1982) Upper extremity orthotics. In F.J. Kottke, G.K. Stillwell and J.F. Lehmann (eds), *Handbook of physical medicine and rehabilitation*, W.B. Saunders, Philadelphia, pp. 518-29

Brudny, J. (1985) New orthosis for treatment of hemiplegic shoulder sublaxation. *Orthot. Prosthet., 39*, 14-20

Butler, P.B., Evans, G.A., Rose, G.K. and Patrick, J.H. (1983) A review of selected knee orthoses. *Br. J. Rheum., 22*, 109-20

Coghlan, J.K., Robinson, C.E., Newmarch, B. and Jackson, G. (1980) Lower extremity bracing in paraplegia — a follow-up study. *Paraplegia, 18*, 25-32

Corcoran, P.J., Jebsen, R.H., Brengelmann, G.L. and Simons, B.C. (1970) Effects of plastic and metal leg braces on speed and energy cost of hemiparetic ambulation. *Arch. Phys. Med. Rehabil., 51*, 69-77

Cousins, S.J., Lusby, D.L.V. and Chodera J. (1977) Assessment and field trial of the Canadian Arthritis and Rheumatism Society–University of British Columbia orthosis for valgus/varus knee instability (CARS-UBC brace). Annual report of the biomechanical research and development unit, Roehampton

Demopoulos J.T. and Eschen, J.E. (1977) Experience with an all-plastic patellar tendon bearing orthosis. *Arch. Phys. Med. Rehabil.*, *58*, 452-6

Doxey, G.E. (1985) Clinical use and fabrication of molded thermoplastic foot orthotic devices. *Phys. Ther.*, *65*, 1679-82

Edmonds, M.E. (1986) The diabetic foot: pathophysiology and treatment *Clin. Endocrinal. Metab.*, *15*, 889-916

Edmonds, M.E., Blundell, M.P., Morris, M.E., Thomas, E.M., Cotton, L.T. and Watkins P.J. (1986) Improved survival of the diabetic foot: the role of a specialised foot clinic. *Quart. J. Med.*, *60*, 763-71

Fisher, S.V., Bowar, J.F., Awad, E.A. and Gullickson, G. (1977) Cervical orthoses effect on cervical spine motion: roentgenographic and goniometric method of study. *Arch. Phys. Med. Rehabil.*, *58*, 109-15

Hanswyk, E.P. and Baker, B.E. (1982) Orthotic management of knee injuries in athletics with the Lennox-Hill orthosis. *Orthot. Prosthet.*, *36*, 423-7

Haworth, R., Dunscombe, S. and Nichols, P.J.R. (1978) Mobile arm supports an evaluation. *Rheum. Rehabil.*, *17*, 240-4

Jawad, A.S.M. and Goodwill, C.J. (1986) TVS brace in patients with rheumatoid arthritis or osteoarthritis of the knee *Br. J. Rheum.*, *25*, 416-17

Lee, K.H. and Johnston, R. (1973) Bracing below the knee for hemiplegia: biomechanical analysis. *Arch. Phys. Med. Rehabil.*, *54*, 466-70

Lee, K.H. and Johnston, R. (1976) Electrically induced flexion reflex in gait training of hemiplegic patients. *Arch. Phys. Med. Rehabil.*, *57*, 311-14

Lehmann, J.F. (1979) Biomechanics of ankle–foot orthoses: prescription and design *Arch. Phys. Rehabil.*, *60*, 200-7

Lehmann, J.F. and Warren, C.G. (1976) Restraining forces in various designs of knee ankle orthoses: their placement and effect on the anatomical knee joint *Arch. Phys. Med. Rehabil.*, *57*, 430-7

Lehmann, J.F., DeLateur, B.J. Warren, C.G., Simons, B.C. and Guy, A.W. (1969) Biomechanical evaluation of braces for paraplegics. *Arch. Phys. Med. Rehabil.*, *50*, 179-88

Lehmann, J.F., Warren, C.G., Pemberton, D.R., Simons, B.C. and DeLateur, B.J. (1971) Load bearing function of patellar tendon bearing braces of various designs. *Arch. Phys. Med. Rehabil.*, *52*, 367-70

Lehmann, J.F., Warren, C.G., Hertling, D., McGee, M., Simons, B.C. and Dralle, A. (1976) Craig–Scott orthosis: a biomechanical and functional evaluation. *Arch. Phys. Med. Rehabil.*, *57*, 438-42

Lehmann, J.F., Ko, M.J. and DeLateur, B.J. (1980) Double-stopped ankle-foot orthosis in flaccid peroneal and tibial paralysis: evaluation of function. *Arch. Phys. Med. Rehabil.*, *61*, 536-41

Lehmann, J.F., Esselman, P.C., Ko, M.J., Craig-Smith, J., DeLateur, B.J. and Dralle, A.J. (1982) Plastic ankle-foot orthoses: evaluation of function. *Arch. Phys. Med. Rehabil.*, *64*, 402-7

Lehmann, J.F., Condon, S.M., DeLateur, B.J. and Smith, J.C. (1985) Ankle–foot orthoses: effect on gait abnormalities in tibial nerve paralysis. *Arch. Phys. Med. Rehab.*, *66*, 212-18

Lehmann, J.F., Condon, S.M., DeLateur, B.J. and Price, R. (1986) Gait abnormalities in peroneal nerve paralysis and their corrections by orthoses: a biomechanical study. *Arch. Phys. Med. Rehabil.*, *67*, 380-6

Liberson, W.T., Holmquest, H.J., Scott, D. and Dow, M. (1961) Functional electrotherapy: stimulation of the peroneal nerve synchronised with the swing phase of gait of hemiplegic patients. *Arch. Phys. Med. Rehabil.*, *42*, 101-5

Malick, M.H. and Meyer, C.M.H. (1978) *Manual on management of the quadriplegic upper extremity*, Harmaville Rehabilitation Centre Pittsburgh, PA 15238
McKenzie, M.W. and Buck, G.L. (1978) Combined motor and peripheral sensory insufficiency. Management of spinal cord injury. *Phys. Ther.*, *58*, 294-303
McCall, R.E., Douglas, R. and Righters, N. (1983) Reciprocal gait orthosis. Its use in neurologic deficient patients. *Orthop. Trans.*, *7*, 565-9
Merkel, K.D., Miller, N.E., Westbrook, P.R. and Merritt, J.L. (1984) Energy expenditure of paraplegic patients standing and walking with two knee-ankle-foot orthoses. *Arch. Phys. Med. Rehabil.*, *65*, 121-4
Nichols, P.J.R. (1971) Mobile arm supports in P.J.R. Nichols (ed.) *Rehabiliation of the severly disabled.* Butterworths, London, pp. 266-78
O'Daniel, W.E. and Hahn, H.R. (1981) Follow-up usage of the Scott-Craig orthosis in paraplegia. *Paraplegia, 19*, 373-8
Offir, R. and Sell H. (1980) Orthoses and ambulation in hemiplegia: a ten year retrospective study. *Arch, Phys. Med. Rehabil.*, *61*, 216-20
Patrick, J.H. and McClelland, M.R. (1985) Low energy cost reciprocal walking for the adult paraplegic. *Paraplegia*, *23*, 113-17
Peterson, M.J., Perry, J. and Montgomery, J. (1985) Walking patterns of healthy subjects wearing rocker shoes. *Phys. Ther.*, *10*, 1483-9
Strachan, R.K., Cook, J., Wilkie, W. and Kennedy, N.S.J. (1985) An evaluation of pneumatic orthoses in thoracic paraplegia. *Paraplegia*, *23*, 295-305
Tovey, F.I. (1986) Care of the diabetic foot. *Pract. Diabetes*, *3*, 130-4
Tuck, W.H. (1972) A new approach to orthopaedic footwear problems. *Proc. Roy. Soc. Med.*, *65*, 15-16
Turk, R. and Obreza, P. (1985) Functional electrical stimulation as an orthotic means for the rehabilitation of paraplegic patients. *Paraplegia*, *23*, 344-8
Yasuda, Y.L., Bowman, K. and Hsu, J.D. (1986) Mobile arm supports: criteria for successful use in muscle disease patients. *Arch. Phys. Med. Rehabil.*, *67*, 253-6

FURTHER READING

Redford, J.B. (ed.) (1980) *Lower limb orthotics*, Williams & Wilkins, Baltimore
Rose, G.K. (1986) *Orthotics: principles and practice*, Heinemann, London

46

Walking Aids

Jill Fisher and Mary Jackson

INTRODUCTION

Walking aids are used by many people, principally to provide stability in the event of muscular weakness or incoordination, or to reduce the load being transmitted by painful and damaged joints. After trauma to the lower limbs they allow the patient to become ambulant with no weight or only partial weight being taken through the injured limb.

Though the load through the lower limbs is decreased, that through the arms is increased. The joints of the arms are not designed for this and in inflammatory arthritis, for instance, may respond with synovitis. When the arms are used to propel the body the muscles of the arms and shoulder girdle have to become stronger. A variety of walking aids is illustrated, and some mention made of their uses and limitations. The type of gait obtainable is stated.

Skilled assessment is required to ensure the patient is provided with the appropriate aid for his needs. Instruction is necessary for the patient to receive the maximum benefit from this aid, and safety has to be considered at all times. In more complex cases assessment and training is most appropriately carried out by a physiotherapist.

ASSESSMENT

When selecting the most appropriate walking aid and the type of gait to be used the physiotherapist will consider the following factors: (1) physical, (2) psychosocial, (3) environmental.

Physical

(a) One should know the specific problem for which the aid is required, e.g. how much does the condition limit weight-bearing?

(b) One should know the age and general level of fitness of the patient, e.g. axillary crutches are rarely appropriate for elderly or frail patients.

(c) The musculoskeletal system of the patient should be assessed, especially weight-bearing joints, including upper limbs.

(d) Neurological factors should be taken into account, e.g. an elderly patient with a moderately severe injury to the leg and poor balance may require a walking frame, where normally walking sticks would be appropriate.

Psychosocial

(a) Psychological: these include intelligence, anxiety and motivation, e.g. an intelligent well-motivated patient may learn to use elbow crutches where a less motivated patient would require axillary crutches or a frame.

(b) Attitude to the aid: a patient's self-image may be adversely affected when using a walking aid, although this can be minimised by the careful choice (and presentation) of aid.

(c) Support available, e.g. when a patient has a relative who can give assistance and supervision at home an aid can be provided that is less stable but that with practice will be more appropriate for the patient.

(d) Hazard caused by aid, e.g. in psychogeriatric homes use of aids may be restricted if the residents are at risk: some may fall over an aid; and others have been known to use their aids as weapons!

Environmental

(a) Living accommodation: homes are frequently small and conditions cramped. The arrangement of furniture, distances to be walked, position and other features of stairs, width and position of doorways, access to the house, etc., are all factors which require consideration: a home visit may be necessary.

(b) Non-domestic environments: other areas that the patient visits should be considered, including workplace. The geography of outside areas, hills, distance to shops, etc., is important.

(c) Transport requirements, e.g. ordinary frames are very difficult to place in most cars, so a folding frame may be more appropriate for a patient who will be travelling in a car. Frames are rarely allowed in buses and ambulances, thus limiting the mobility of their users.

Walking aids are used for two main purposes: (a) to reduce weight-bearing through the legs; (b) to assist balance. Whether the indication is (a) or (b), or a combination of both, one of the main considerations in the selection of an aid, and walking pattern with the aid, is the maintenance of as near normal a gait pattern as possible. This will minimise secondary problems caused by abnormal use of joint musculature, etc., and also facilitate, where possible, return to normal gait pattern without the use of aids.

It should be remembered that in many situations the patient will be reluctant to bear weight on a weak or painful limb, and will require encouragement to progress from non-weight-bearing, to partial weight-bearing, and finally to full weight-bearing through the limb. As a general rule, therefore, the minimum required support should be provided, though there are some important exceptions to the rule. Careful instruction in the use of the aid is also important to avoid the problem of overdependence.

Examples in selection of aids

(1) Soft tissue injury to the knee (e.g. partial tear medial ligament)

The patient may initially be non-weight-bearing with axillary crutches, but when weight-bearing is allowed it may well be advisable to exchange the axillary crutches for walking sticks, first two and then one, to encourage the patient to take an increasing amount of his weight through the affected leg.

(2) Hemiplegic patient

In the early stages of treatment the patient may be given assistance by a trained helper during walking, to encourage recovery of the affected side. Walking aids tend to promote dependence on the sound side. Later a long walking stick may be the aid of choice, as this will assist balance whilst discouraging excessive weight-bearing through the stick. Gait training as part of a treatment programme is very important (Chapter 35).

(3) Rheumatoid arthritis

Here the patient may benefit from using an aid at a relatively early stage. Reduction of weight-bearing through a damaged joint may slow the progression of the condition and reduce eventual damage. Careful consideration must be given to the involvement of upper limb joints, not putting pressure through involved joints as far as possible, in selecting the most appropriate aid (Chapter 10).

Various types of gait using walking aids

(1) Three-point gait

The three-point gait is used when the patient is non-weight-bearing through one leg and is using crutches. The crutches are moved forward together while the body weight is borne through the good leg. Weight is then taken through the arms and crutches as the weight-bearing leg is brought forward to a point either in front or behind the line of the crutches to avoid the instability of a linear base. When ascending stairs the good leg goes up the stairs first, followed by the crutches; on descending, the crutches move down on to the lower step first. Patients are advised that this manoeuvre is not safe without some assistance unless a good stair rail is available, in which case the crutches are used together as one crutch and the patient uses the free hand to grasp the rail.

(2) Four point gait

This may be used when weight can be borne through both legs. The pattern is — right crutch (or stick), left leg, left crutch, right leg.

(3) Swing-through walking

This system is used when both legs are very weak. The patient balances on both legs whilst the crutches are moved forward together. The weight is then taken through the arms whilst the legs are swung through the crutches. The abdominal muscles may be used to tilt the pelvis to assist weak hip flexors to bring the legs forward, and must be strong.

(4) Swing-to walking

This is an adaptation of swing-through. The legs are brought forwards towards the crutches but not through them. When one stick or elbow crutch is used it is carried in the opposite hand to the weak or painful leg so that the pattern of walking resembles the normal pattern where the opposite arm and leg move forward together.

Patients are always encouraged to walk with a gait which is as normal as is possible, for them to relieve strain on weight-bearing joints and facilitate their full rehabilitation where this is possible.

WALKING AIDS

Axillary crutches (Figure 46.1a)

Measurement should be made from the shoe heel to 5 cm below the posterior axillary fold. The position of the handpiece should be adjusted as for a

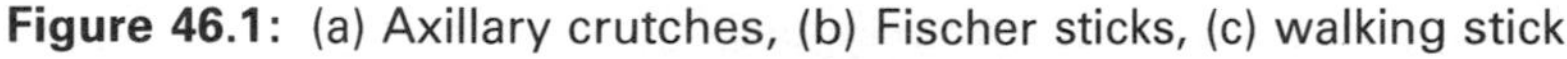
Figure 46.1: (a) Axillary crutches, (b) Fischer sticks, (c) walking stick

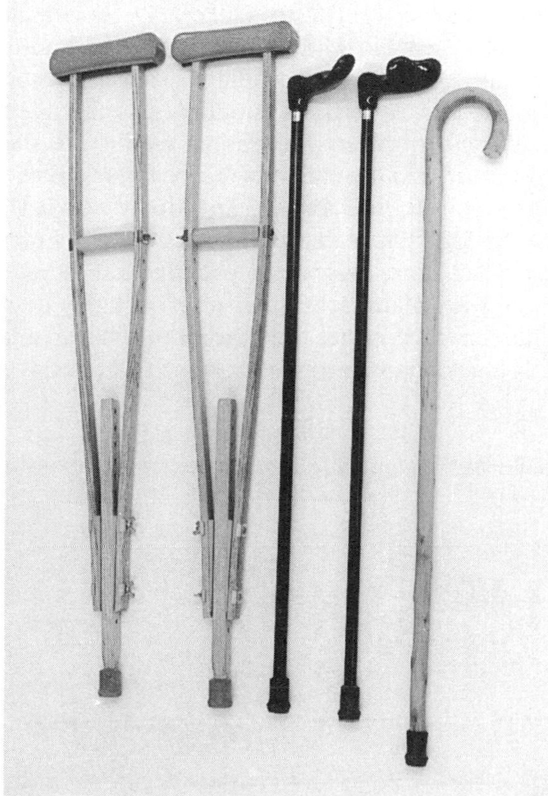

pair of sticks, i.e. allow 15° flexion of the elbow when the crutch is held to the side and resting 15 cm out from the front of the shoe toe.

It is important that the crutches are not too long, as this can cause pressure on nerves and vessels in the axilla and a consequent paresis in the hand. If the hand-grip is too low it can have the same effect, and if too high the crutches slip out from under the axilla and cause instability.

During walking the patient's weight is taken through the shoulders, arms and hands, and transferred to the floor through the lower part of the crutches. Axillary crutches are used when one leg is non-weight-bearing with or without a plaster cast, in partial weight-bearing and in swing-through walking when the arms are weak.

Forearm support (gutter) crutches (Figure 46.2a)

These can be used as an alternative to axillary or elbow crutches, or with one elbow or axillary crutch when there is some abnormality of the patients' arm or arms, e.g. the elbow is held in fixed flexion or the arm in a forearm cast. The length of the crutch is adjusted so that the forearm rests in the gutter comfortably without the patient raising the shoulder girdle. The handpiece is adjusted to the patient's grasp. These crutches are heavier and less stable to walk with than axillary and elbow crutches; the patient's weight is taken through the forearm to the crutch. Forearm support crutches may be fixed on a trolley for patients with severe rheumatoid arthritis. For those with milder arthritis it may be highly desirable to take weight through the forearms rather than the elbow and wrist joints.

Figure 46.2: (a) Forearm support (gutter) crutches, (b) elbow crutches

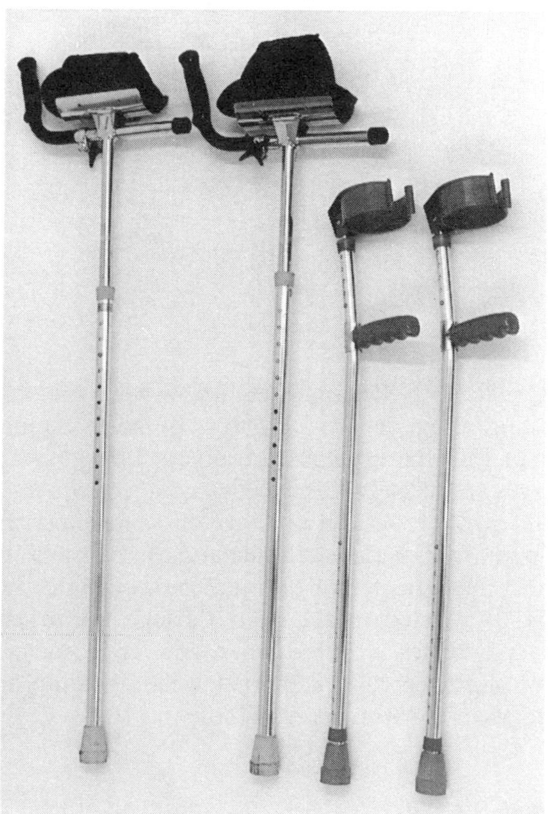

Elbow crutches (Figure 46.2b)

These can be used as an alternative to axillary crutches but are less stable and need stronger arms if the patient is non-weight-bearing. They are adjusted so that the handpiece is grasped with the elbow at 15° and cannot be used if there is more than some 40° of fixed flexion at the elbow. The upper part of the crutch may not be adjustable, and should rest round the upper third of the forearm.

Walking stick (Figure 46.1c)

These may be wooden, in which case they have to be cut to the length required for each patient, or metal, and adjustable. When the patient stands upright and grasps the handle of the stick the elbow should be at 15°. However, stroke patients may require slightly longer sticks to aid balance without taking weight through the stick.

When two sticks are used, four-point walking is preferable, otherwise the painful or weak leg is placed with the foot between the sticks, and is followed by the good leg. The patient is encouraged to take even paces.

When only one stick is required it is carried in the hand opposite the affected leg. Some weight is transferred through the stick from the hand, and by increasing the size of the patient's base it aids balance and, therefore, confidence. Elderly patients may prefer to use furniture to hold on to in the home but find a stick helpful outside, particularly on uneven pavements.

Walking sticks are simple and extremely useful, even if they do no more than alert other pedestrians to the fact that the person using the stick requires a little consideration and space.

Fischer sticks (Figure 46.1b)

Patients with rheumatoid arthritis may find a normal stick difficult or painful to grip. The hook may be padded but if this is still not satisfactory they may find a stick with a moulded handpiece, such as the Fischer stick, more comfortable. These give a larger platform for the transference of weight from the hand to the stick. *Right-hand and left-hand sticks are not interchangeable.* Moulded hand-grips can be used on other walking aids for those with severely deformed hands.

Tripod (Figure 46.3)

The tripod is more stable than a stick and may be used by patients with severe problems of balance. *Quadripods* may be used for additional stability.

Frame (Figure 46.4)

A frame may be used in non-weight-bearing walking, e.g. Potts fracture, and is particularly useful for elderly patients. The patient lifts the frame forwards and then hops into it. It is much more stable than crutches. Crutches may fall on to the floor out of reach when the patient is carrying out functions in the home, and the elderly may have difficulty in recovering them. The frame remains where it is put, and within reach. However, walking with a frame is slow and cannot be used on stairs or transported unless it will fold. It can also be used for partial weight-bearing and full weight-bearing with frail or unsteady elderly patients. Frames may be set on wheels; they may be reciprocating or they may be triangular.

Gutter frame (Figure 46.5)

This gives more support than the ordinary frame because patients take weight through both forearms. It is particularly useful on orthopaedic

Figure 46.3: Tripod

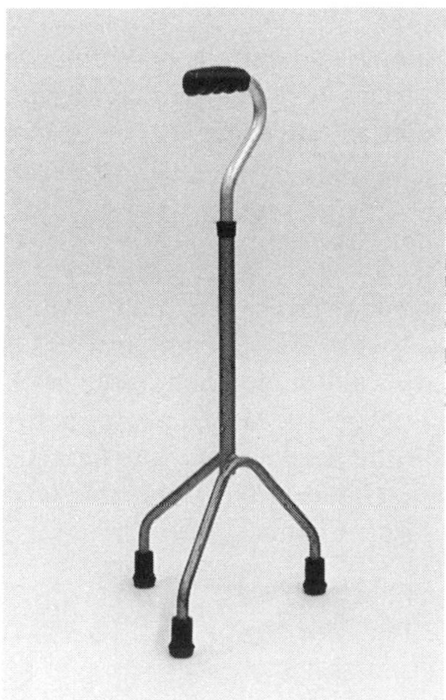

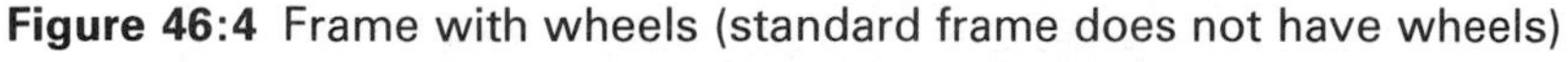
Figure 46:4 Frame with wheels (standard frame does not have wheels)

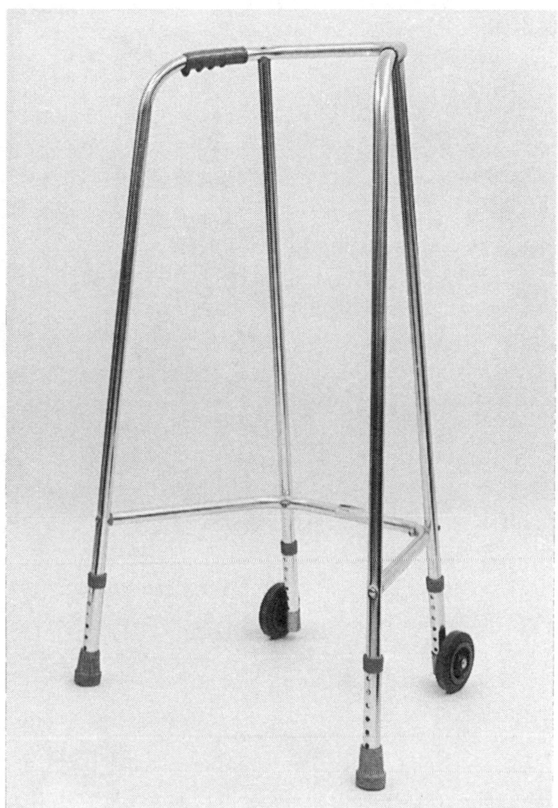

wards for early ambulation after fractures of the lower limbs, and for patients with rheumatoid arthritis, where it is desirable to protect the joints. It is rarely suitable for use in the home, because of its size and poor manoeuvrability, but occasionally can be of use to young neurological patients.

Bond frame (A frame) (Figure 46.6)

This is an adaptation of the gutter frame, which was developed for the use of stroke patients. The forearms rest in gutters which are slightly angled in towards each other and there is a single hand grip for both hands. The rollators (Figures 46.7 and 46.8) and the frame with wheels (Figure 46.4) are used occasionally for neurological patients.

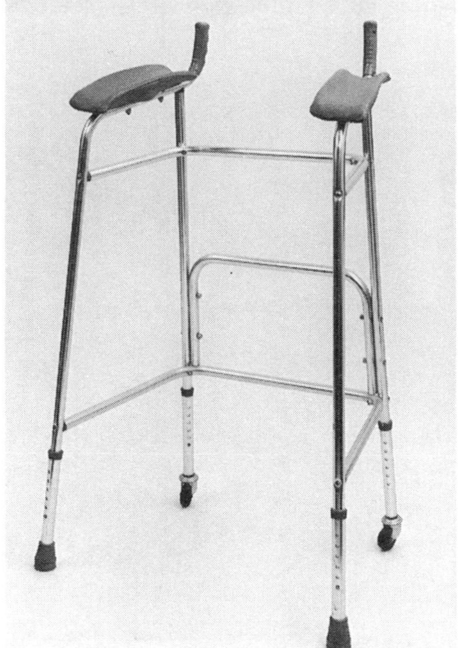

Figure 46.5: Gutter frame

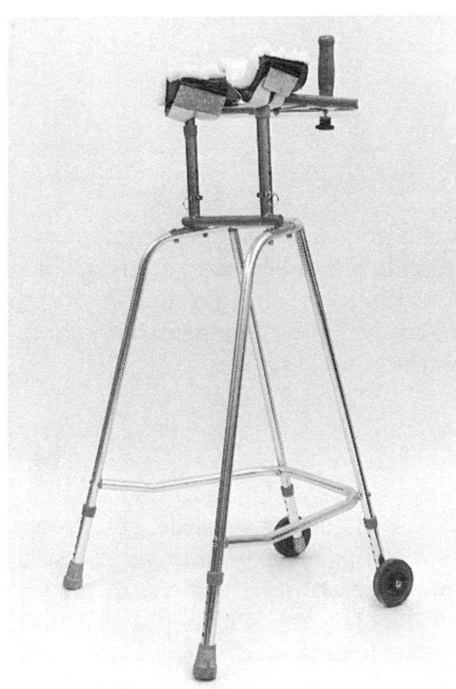

Figure 46.6: Bond frame

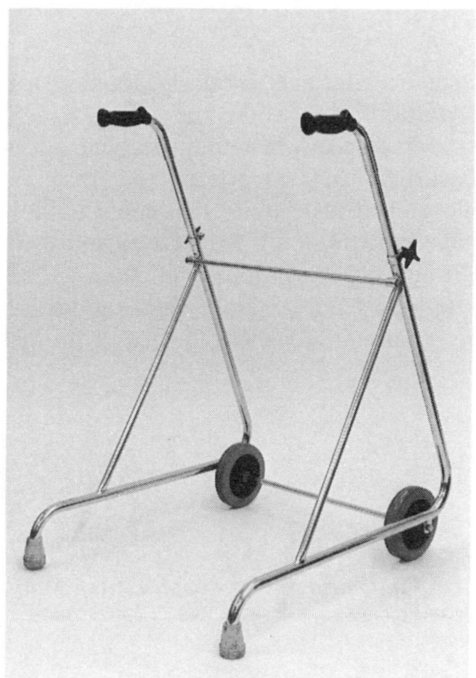

Figure 46.7: Rollator

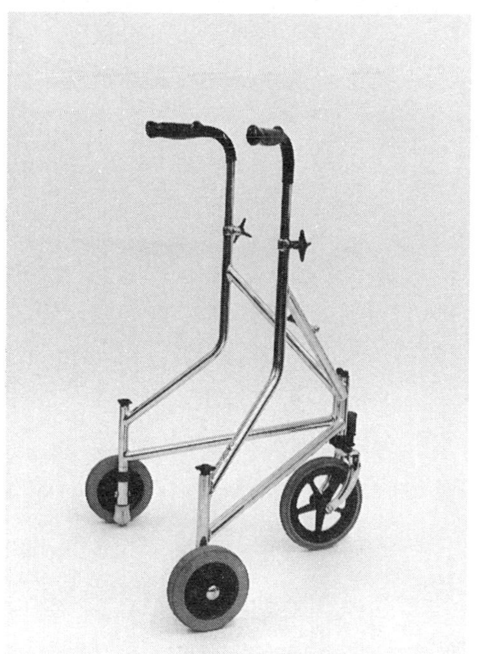

Figure 46.8: Folding rollator

CARE OF AIDS AND GENERAL ADVICE

Patients should be advised to inspect walking aids regularly, looking for signs of wear-and-tear including splintering of wood and wear of any mechanical parts. Ferrules should be replaced when they become worn (they should always have a metal washer inside to prevent the tip from piercing the ferrule). Bolts on axillary crutches require tightening if they work loose. When using walking aids patients should be advised to avoid slippery and irregular surfaces, e.g. uneven paving stones and slopes. The floor should be kept clear in the patient's home; loose rugs should be removed; holes in carpets should be repaired. Shoes should be well-fitting, have low heels and non-slip soles.

FURTHER READING

Hollis, M. (1981) *Practical exercise therapy*, Blackwell Scientific Publications, Oxford

Walking Aid booklet (1985) in series on *Equipment for the disabled*, from Mary Marlborough Lodge, Nuffield Orthopaedic Centre, Oxford OX3 7LD

47

Car Driving for the Disabled

John Goodwill

Independent mobility is taken for granted by able-bodied people, but for those with a locomotor handicap or severe dyspnoea access to public transport is limited in spite of efforts by some transport authorities. Disabled people are frequently unable to negotiate the steps up to buses or trains, stairs or escalators to platforms, have difficulty in moving from one mode of transport to another (e.g. rail and bus stations are rarely adjacent), and in cities there is the hazard of crowds.

Independent mobility is important as it helps to keep the person at work, maintains leisure interests and family life, and with the disabled person doing more there is less demand on carers and statutory services. The current European Situation is well reviewed by Haslegrave (1985).

The following discussion applies only to the driving of private cars and not to taxis, public service vehicles (PSV) or heavy goods vehicles (HGV), to which more stringent conditions attach.

This is not a definitive legal document; it is the present situation as seen by the author, but regulations change. If there is any doubt reference must be made to the licensing authority.

Before considering the patient as a driver it is reasonable to ask how much he/she will actually use the vehicle. Costs of motoring are high and if the patient's requirements are limited it may be more convenient and more economic to use taxis, hire cars, dial-a-ride or similar Social Services schemes. However, there is no doubt that independent mobility is preferred by many people, disabled as well as able-bodied. Full independence is often only achieved by those who can not only drive, but also are able to fold and transfer the wheelchair into the vehicle and out at the destination. Inability to drive is seldom due to locomotor problems only, for these are usually soluble. Thus most arthritics should be able to drive, but many with neurological disability cannot do so.

ASSESSMENT

Initial assessment is done by the doctor treating the patient, who needs to consider the patient's driving needs, and to determine that there is no bar to driving due to physical or mental illness. Providing the patient is fit to drive, and wishes to do so, a practical assessment may then be done at a school of motoring with experience of disabled drivers; but if the situation is complicated it is often helpful for the patient to attend an assessment centre for disabled drivers, which will provide a detailed report (see list at end of chapter), and then be referred for driving tuition. If the problem is complex, particularly if there is brain damage from injury or illness, or if there is severe arthritis, an appropriate consultant opinion should be sought and/or advice obtained from DVLC (see below) (Raffle, 1985; Darnborough and Kinrade, 1985).

Assessment must include:

(1) *the driver*: physical and mental function, fitness to drive;

(2) *the car*:

  (a) the type most suitable for work/social needs;
  (b) how the disabled driver (or passenger) will get in/out of the car;
  (c) seating, comfort, vehicle control and safety;
  (d) primary controls: steering, brakes, accelerator (? clutch);
  (e) secondary controls: lights, horn, seat belt, etc.

  What modifications are needed to any of these controls, to the seating or for ease of access?

(3) How will the car and modifications be *financed*, e.g. Mobility Allowance is a tax-free allowance paid to those 'unable or virtually unable to walk'; this may be used for the Motability scheme to hire-purchase or rent a car (Chapter 37).

THE DRIVER: FITNESS TO DRIVE

Each applicant or possessor of a driving licence is required to inform the Driving and Vehicle Licensing Centre in Swansea (DVLC) if they have a 'relevant disability', such as epilepsy, liability to sudden attacks of disabling giddiness or faintness, mental retardation or inability to meet the visual requirements, or *any disability which could be a danger when driving.* When in doubt the licensee should declare the disability to the Medical Advisory Branch at Swansea for decision by the medical staff there. This includes a 'prospective disability' which may in time become a relevant disability'. Clearly there is room for variation in opinion on this, except for specific disabilities. Therefore any doctor treating a patient has a *duty to advise that patient* if his/her condition affects, or is likely to affect the ability to drive. This would not apply to temporary conditions such as a fracture of a leg bone where the disability is not expected to last more than three months. The Medical Advisory Branch at Swansea will normally communicate with the doctors treating the individual patient for any required information, and may require a medical examination and a report. *The duty is with the patient to inform the licensing bureau*, not for the doctor to do so, but where the patient clearly has a disability that may cause him to be a danger on the road he must be firmly persuaded to inform the Licensing Centre. Only in extreme circumstances should the doctor consider breaking professional confidence to inform against the patient's wishes. It is better to persuade the patient to give you written signed permission to write to the Centre yourself but, if in spite of persuasion the patient refuses and the risk to the public is great, the doctor would be wise to discuss the situation with his medical defence organisation before proceeding further.

Ordinary driving licences are issued from age 17, a full licence being valid up to the age of 70, but only for periods of three years after that age. Patients who are receiving Mobility Allowance may be granted a licence to drive a car from the age of 16 years, which will often help them in their education or work. Where a driving test is required for a licence this is carried out in the usual way by an ordinary driving examiner.

CAR MODIFICATIONS

Access and seating

Before buying a car it is important for the disabled driver to know what adaptations, if any, are required. Is the seat giving support where it is needed? Is there sufficient leg room, especially if prostheses or orthoses are worn? Can the seat be moved to allow easy access and egress from the driver or passenger side of the car? A two-door car with wider front doors may be more convenient and can also ease stowing of the wheelchair. The driving seat may need to be modified to allow it to move further forward and/or backwards, or to allow alterations in height. If the patient is of small stature it may have to be individually built for him. Is the safety belt fastening manageable or can it be modified? Investigation has shown problems with fastening and unfastening seat belts (Bulstrode *et al.*, 1985). The driver may get in on the passenger side, pulling the folded wheelchair into the space in front of the passenger seat. Alternatively access is from the driver's side with the wheelchair brought in behind the driver's seat. To allow enough space a two-door car, with a driver's seat which can be moved well forward, is generally needed, the seat then being moved back into the driving position (Figure 47.1). An alternative is to fold the wheelchair, and hook it to a pulley system which electrically lifts the chair so that it lies folded flat on top of the car in an enclosed compartment (Figure 47.2). For the patient who can walk a few steps from the boot round to the driver's door, the chair may be folded and lifted into the boot either manually or using a small hoist driven off the car battery. Some patients cannot manage to lift their own wheelchair into the car but still benefit by driving. With special modifications to a car or light van it is possible for a person to *move into the vehicle still sitting in the wheelchair* and to drive with the chair firmly anchored in the driving position; travelling sitting in the wheelchair may also be best for some heavily disabled passengers (Figures 47.3 and 47.4). Usually the latter can transfer into the car direct, or with the use of a sliding board, but occasionally a swivel-sliding seat is used, in which the seat slides out of the car for ease of transfer without the helper having to bend under the car roof. The seat is then pushed into position in the car (Chapter 44).

Controls

The patient's use of the main controls of steering, brake and accelerator is looked at first. Automatic transmission removes many problems, and use of a hand clutch should be strongly discouraged. Brake and accelerator can

Figure 47.1: Transfer to car from driver's side: wheelchair armrest removed, car seat pushed back (Photo: Mr M. Venables)

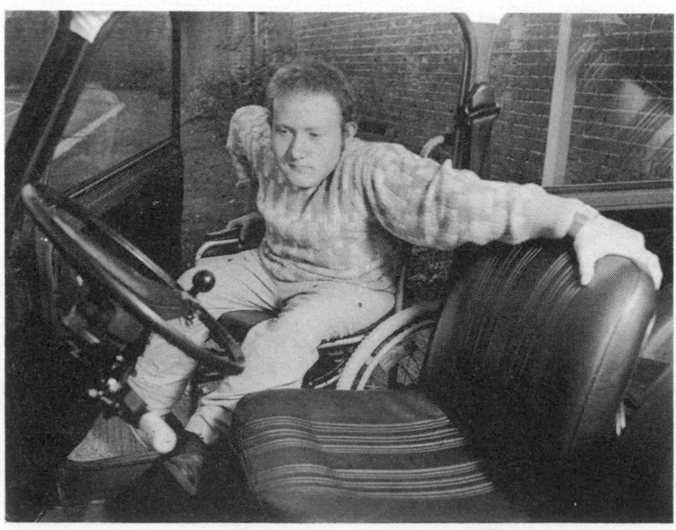

Figure 47.2: Chair-Up wheelchair storage system: the chair is lifted and lowered using power from the car (Photo: Mr M. Venables)

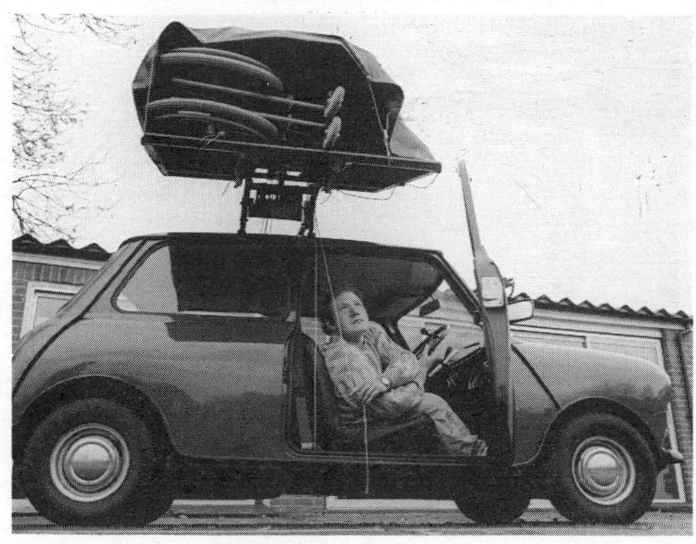

Figure 47.3: Demonstration car with Car Chair in the passenger side; it can also be used in driver's side. Single combined lever hand control (brake–accelerator), instructor's dual-control lever, and electronic testing equipment on dashboard (Ford Motor Company)

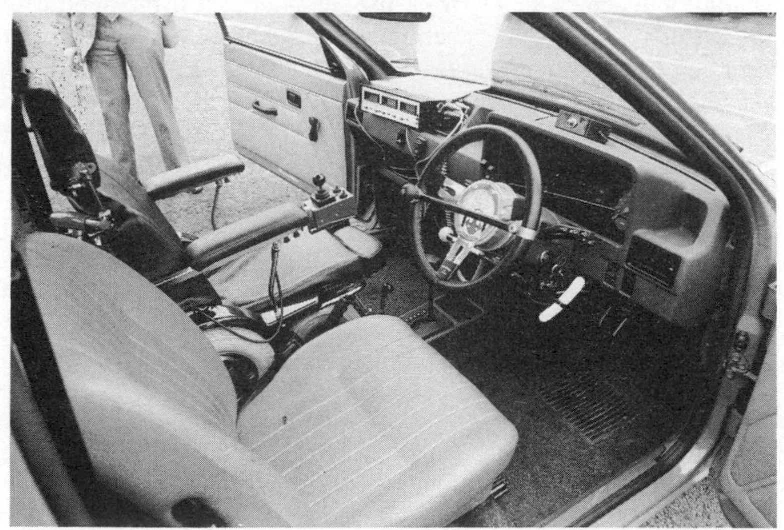

Figure 47.4: Astra conversion. Raised roof, rear ramp with rear suspension lowering for access, wheelchair anchorages and seat belt for occupant of wheelchair (Gowrings Mobility International)

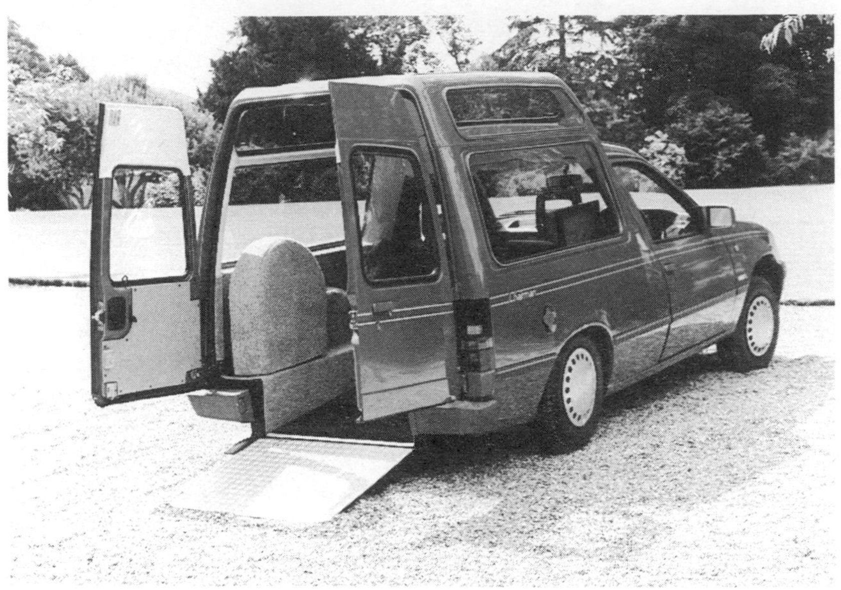

be used by either foot, or are easily brought up under the wheel for operation by either hand. They can be on one lever or separate, and other positions for these are possible.

Steering force comes mainly from the shoulder, but if the hand cannot grip the wheel a steering ball, steering peg or other attachment is fitted to the wheel so that the arm power is transmitted to the steering. Power steering helps, but only comes as a manufacturer's option on larger cars. However, smaller cars can be fitted with it at reasonable cost. Other steering modifications are possible, including steering by footplate, joy-stick between fingers or toes or other methods, which are particularly useful for the multiple limb-deficient patient (Figure 47.5).

The handbrake requires at least three distinct hand movements to release it. If weakness or joint limitation prevents this it can be converted to an overthrow cam type with a vertical lever for knock-off/knock-on action. Secondary controls such as lights, wipers, etc., must be brought within reach of a controllable limb action, on hand, shoulder, leg or foot; controls may be positioned on the door if required. The ignition key, door key, inside and outside door handles and seat belts must be manageable, but all these are usually only a problem with severe arm disability.

If the arms cannot move actively above shoulder height due to arthritis

Figure 47.5: Left-hand steering peg and right-hand combined single lever unit (British School of Motoring)

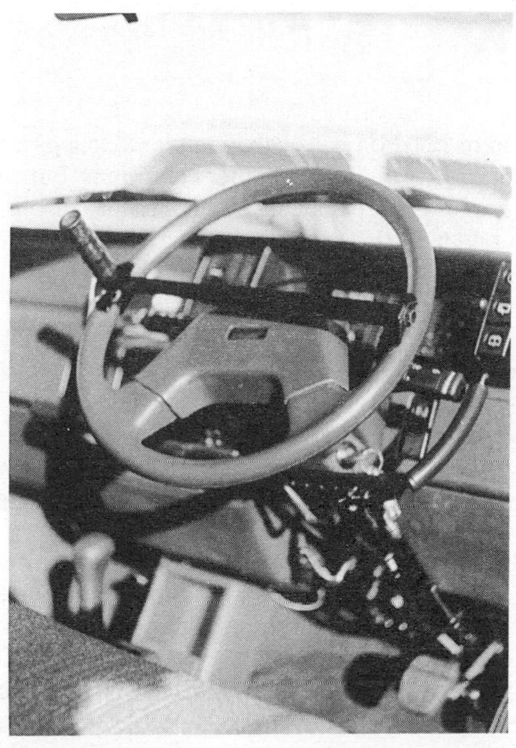

or muscle weakness so that the sun visor cannot be rotated down, a tinted strip across the top of the windscreen is required.

The following is a more detailed discussion of some diseases which commonly affect driving ability:

Epilepsy
Transient ischaemic attacks
Vertebrobasilar insufficiency
Vision, hearing defects
Stroke, multiple sclerosis
Paraplegia
Parkinson's disease
Muscle weakness due to other causes
Disorder of movement control
Diabetes
Heart and lung conditions
Mental disorders

The older driver
Amputation and limb deficiency
Arthritis

HEAD INJURY

The resulting loss of function is usually complex. Epilepsy, visual loss and motor loss are discussed below under other conditions, but with head injury it is the sensory impairment, behavioural changes and disorders of perceptual/cognitive functioning that often prevent a return to driving (Sivak *et al.*, 1981).

EPILEPSY (Chapter 25)

This must be declared to the licensing authority. A licence may be issued when the patient has been free of attacks for two years, with or without drug treatment. Where the attacks only occur during sleep, they should *only* have occurred *during sleep* for three years. Therefore a patient with recent attacks during sleep, but a history of attacks occurring while awake between two and three years ago would not receive a licence. Where there is organic brain disease or psychological disturbance the issue of a licence may have to be delayed further.

It is extremely important that the diagnosis of epilepsy is confirmed by a neurologist, for to label a person erroneously as epileptic may result in the loss of driving licence and have severe effects on work and family life. The diagnosis is not always straightforward and epilepsy is not a single disease — there are different causes and varieties of epileptic attacks. A problem may arise once the patient has been free of fits for two years while taking drugs, because reduction or cessation of treatment, if followed by even a single fit, would require the loss of a licence for a further two years. Clearly also the drug treatment must not be causing side-effects that impair ability to drive.

The occurrence of a *single fit* while awake or asleep in a person without a history of epilepsy, and with no evidence of underlying brain disease, gives rise to difficulties, particularly if the nature of the attack is uncertain. It would be hard to label the patient epileptic in these circumstances, and therefore to cause loss of licence for two years. The patient should inform the driving licence centre, and it may be possible for driving to be resumed after one year if there is no recurrence of the event. Follow-up is essential.

Where there is clear *intracranial pathology* such as residua of head injury, tumour, abscess, or if there has been surgery for intracranial vascular lesion, the occurrence of a *single fit* requires loss of licence for two years. Where *no fit* has occurred the doctor will have to judge the likelihood of these occurring, and also the possible requirement for prophylactic antiepileptic drug treatment. The patient should be advised not to drive for six months after *craniotomy for aneurysm* of the anterior or posterior communicating systems or the subarachnoid portion of the internal carotid artery, but after surgery for aneurysm of the middle cerebral artery driving should not be allowed for one year. *If an attack occurs* two years must elapse from the date of the last one before driving is restarted. Advice should be sought from the Medical Advisory Branch at Swansea (*Lancet* editorial, 1980; Jennett, 1983).

Attacks should be regarded as *provoked* if occurring *for the first time* while the patient is on a drug that is known to cause attacks occasionally, e.g. psychotropic drugs, baclofen. If the drug can be stopped and no more attacks occur the patient may keep his licence, providing the underlying physical or mental condition does not prevent driving. If the patient has had *previous attacks* then two years off driving is needed, unless there have been no attacks for the previous five years, when the patient may resume driving after one year only.

TRANSIENT ISCHAEMIC ATTACKS (TIA)

These cause impairment of mental functions as well as motor and/or sensory deficits, so the patient should not drive for six months. TIA may be the prelude to a major stroke, and so always require investigation. If there is only a single TIA driving is permitted after three months, but as with other conditions which might affect ability to drive, there is an obligation on the driver to inform the Licensing Centre.

VERTEBROBASILAR INSUFFICIENCY

This may cause faintness or vertigo on sudden turning of the head — not usually unconsciousness as occurs with epilepsy or cardiac causes. If the symptoms are easily controlled with a collar while driving it is reasonable to continue driving providing adequate external and internal mirrors are provided to allow clear all-round vision. Careful diagnosis is required for these patients, as some with this label are actually suffering from paroxysmal disturbances of cardiac rhythm.

VISION (spectacles may be worn)

In the UK a driver must be able to read a number plate with letters $3^1/_2$ inches high at 25 yards; this is *visual acuity* of approximately 6/12. Visual standards vary in other countries. Monocular vision on its own is acceptable providing the patient is accustomed to it, for which six months should be allowed after the loss of binocular vision. A recent cataract extraction is a bar to driving until the patient has readjusted, which will be rapid with a contact or intraocular lens, but will take longer with glasses (over three months) where peripheral vision may be distorted. There is a *visual field requirement* of between 120° and 140°. Hemianopia after stroke may be a bar to driving; e.g. with a right-sided stroke there may not only be some left visual field loss, but, more important, there may be left *visual inattention.* On formal testing the patient sees objects in the left visual field, but when tested simultaneously on the two sides with a moving object he invariably points to the object on the right, ignoring that on the left; the potential hazard of this is obvious in driving.

It is the lower quadrants of vision that are largely used in driving; therefore defects there are more important than those in the upper field of vision. Lack of *colour vision* is not a practical problem in driving, but dark adaptation decreases slightly with age, and the elderly driver should plan any long journeys in daylight as far as possible. *Double vision* is clearly a bar to driving, whether it is continuous or episodic; fatigue, as in myasthenia gravis, must be controlled with drug treatment before driving is permitted.

HEARING

Deafness on its own can be compensated for by mirrors although, if combined with other disabilities, it might prevent driving. When driving on motorways or other main roads hearing is used very little anyway, and even at other times a loud radio in the car is legal and clearly will greatly reduce the hearing of any audible warnings from other drivers. As with all disabilities related to driving, it is the combination of different factors that must be considered. Severe deafness combined with slowness of thought and movement would clearly rule out driving.

STROKE

The stroke patient may be barred from driving by intellectual loss, lack of concentration, poor judgement or perceptual problems. There may be hemianopia or inability to read and understand road signs; less obvious may be the left-sided body image and inattention problems mentioned previously due to right parietal damage. A few patients develop epilepsy after a stroke. It is often the combination of mild loss of several functions that prevent driving, and anyway the patient should not drive for three to six months after a stroke.

Providing none of these bars to driving is present the patient may drive with the remaining good arm and leg, using automatic transmission with the good foot. If necessary the accelerator is transferred to the left foot. A steering ball is used with the good hand, and secondary controls are placed within reach of residual function (Wilson and Smith, 1983; Legh-Smith *et al.*, 1986).

MULTIPLE SCLEROSIS

This causes many of the most difficult problems related to driving, especially in the younger person. Muscle weakness can usually be accommodated by the use of power on brakes and/or steering with automatic transmission. A severely spastic or ataxic limb should not be used for driving although mild intention tremor may be acceptable. For the patient who is mainly paraplegic the solution is easy, using hand controls.

Any significant tremor of head and neck makes driving dangerous; epilepsy may also occur in MS. Visual acuity may be temporarily lost due to optic neuritis, at which time driving must temporarily cease. Providing vision improves again to the required standard of acuity and visual fields driving can be resumed when the attack has subsided. Intellectual loss is not usually a problem as more obvious physical deficits will have already prevented driving in most of these cases. MS, being a common relapsing condition, may cause temporary inability to drive due to limb involvement and individual assessment is required by thc physician to advise each patient.

PARAPLEGIA

This is no problem with hand controls. A hand clutch is available but automatic transmission is much more satisfactory (Figure 47.5). *A low tetraplegic* (at C8 or T1 level) can drive with brake and accelerator controlled by circumferential or up–down movement of a single lever under the steering wheel. Usually the patient is limited by the inability to get the wheelchair in and out of the car independently. Steering may require a steering ball attachment on the wheel, but the actual power of steering in all people comes largely from the shoulder, which is functioning in these tetraplegics.

PARKINSON'S DISEASE

This condition usually progresses slowly, but significant slowness of movement due to rigidity will prevent driving, although mild tremor at rest is not usually a problem. Episodic akinesia causes episodes of immobility which may occur without warning. Patients with this condition are unfit to drive.

MUSCLE WEAKNESS

Muscle weakness due to residual paralysis from nerve injury or poliomyelitis can be compensated for mechanically. Even if both arms are not functioning, driving with the legs only is possible using a steering footplate. Limb-girdle dystrophies can be accommodated with automatic transmission, power brakes/steering and moving secondary controls within reach of residual function. The same almost always applies to limb-deficient patients, where major modifications may be required, and for the most severe disability a small joy-stick between fingers or toes wired to motors can be used to control the steering (drive-by-wire system); special seating may be needed.

Peripheral neuropathy would have to be unusually severe and persistent to cause difficulties due to persistent sensory loss and weakness, as one would expect hand controls still to be usable.

DISORDERS OF MOVEMENT CONTROL

Disorders of control due to athetoid or choreiform movements usually prevent driving for this group of *cerebral palsy* patients, but in those without these problems, and with good intellectual function, driving may be possible. Incoordination due to cerebellar tumours or vascular cause must preclude driving, but when due to a slowly progressive degeneration driving may continue for a long time.

DIABETES

Diabetes itself does not give rise to difficulties in driving unless complications such as myocardial infarction occur. However, the diabetic on insulin may be at risk of hypoglycaemia causing rapid impairment of cerebral function. Before this occurs the driver should have taken note of the usual symptoms of cold sweating, feeling of hunger and nervousness, which allow oral glucose to be taken before symptoms impair thinking and decision-making. While driving, the delay of a meal or sudden exertion such as changing of a wheel may cause hypoglycaemia, preventable by taking glucose. The appearance of a hypoglycaemic driver may be similar to drunkenness, so the potential problems are not only those of injury to self or others.

HEART

Ischaemic heart disease can occur suddenly, causing accident or damage to others, but these occurrences are rare, and often the patient will have sufficient warning to allow him to stop safely even if the attack proves fatal. Following uncomplicated myocardial infarction the patient should not drive for two months, and even then the occurrence of angina on driving, or with the tension of driving, must be treated by medical or surgical means before driving is safe. Drugs used in cardiac conditions or hypertension, particularly beta blockers, may cause symptoms of faintness which impair concentration with consequent reduction of driving skills. Hypertension itself is not a bar to driving.

Cardiac dysrhythmia can usually be adequately controlled by drugs. If there is more severe dysrhythmia, with faintness or even unconsciousness due to heart block, this will need to be controlled with a pacemaker for at least a month before driving can be resumed. A certificate from a cardiologist is required, and the DVLC must be informed, as with any other relevant or prospective disability.

Valve disease in the heart will usually only cause difficulty in the case of aortic valve disease, particularly stenosis, where sudden loss of consciousness may be provoked by effort or emotion. After surgical replacement of any valve there is usually no objection to driving, except in the few who develop attacks of cerebral ischaemia causing giddiness or faintness.

RESPIRATORY CONDITIONS

A car is often vital to the mobility of a severely dyspnoeic patient. The only potential problem would be attacks of uncontrolled coughing causing loss of vehicle control. Only in the late stages of respiratory failure would cerebral anoxia cause difficulty in concentration and thinking.

MENTAL DISORDERS

Gross mental handicap clearly bars driving as well as many other activities, but there are degrees of this disability blending upwards to normality. Psychotic and neurotic illness causes more difficulty in deciding fitness to drive. Clearly aggressive or suicidal behaviour at the wheel has obvious dangers, especially if combined with a grudge against others or life in general, but stopping a patient driving may make work difficult and aggravate the condition. If the mental illness is at all significant a psychiatrist should be asked to advise on suitability for driving.

THE OLDER DRIVER

We all slow mentally and physically as we get older. The population is ageing so more elderly drivers will be on the road, needing their car to maintain independence. Experience, knowledge of their regular routes and some degree of extra caution will usually compensate for the slowing of physical and mental reactions until these are very marked. Only the driver over the age of 70 is required to make a declaration of health every three years. Drivers over 65, as well as those between 17 and 24, have a higher accident rate than others, although this is not sufficient to stop the elderly (or the young) from driving.

AMPUTATION AND LIMB DEFICIENCY

In patients with above-knee or below-knee amputation that limb is not used for driving. With automatic transmission clearly loss of the leg is no problem. Loss of the right leg is compensated by provision of a second accelerator on the left of the brake pedal, retaining the usual accelerator position for others to drive. If manual transmission is used either the clutch or the brake/accelerator is brought up to the wheel for hand use. Amputation or loss of use in one arm is compensated for by using automatic transmission, and a steering ball on the wheel. A bilateral arm amputee can drive like this, the prosthesis having an attachment for fitting to the steering wheel. In all cases of arm disability the secondary controls such as lights, windscreen wipers, horn, etc., must be brought within reach of residual motor function.

High bilateral arm amputation, congenital limb deficiency or severe paralysis of both arms with good leg function requires automatic transmission using the right foot for brake and accelerator. Steering may be possible with residual arm function using power steering and modified steering control, or the left foot used on a steering footplate. These modifications may appear unusual, but are safe with training. If limb deficiency involves the legs as well as the arms, driving is still usually possible with further modifications to the vehicle, cost is the limiting factor (Figures 47.6–47.8).

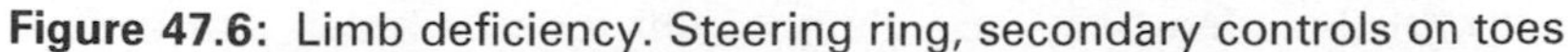

Figure 47.6: Limb deficiency. Steering ring, secondary controls on toes

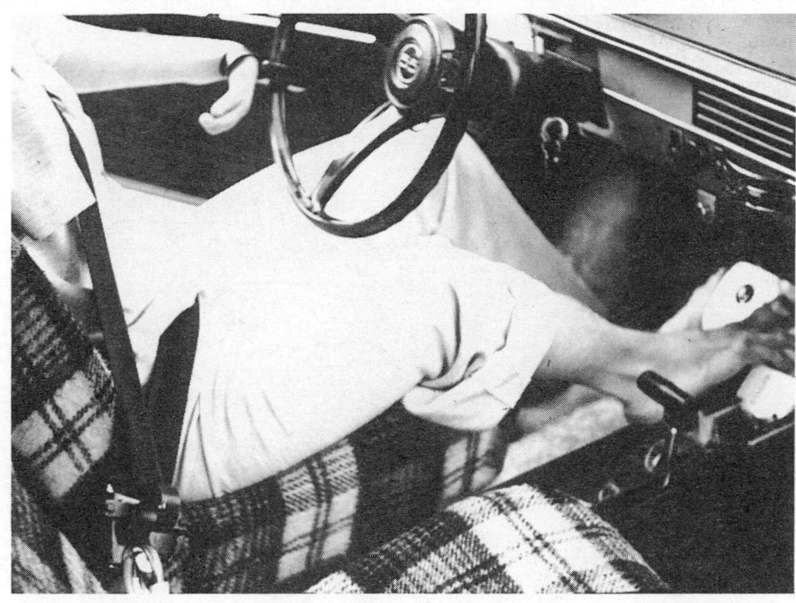

Figure 47.7: Limb deficiency, insufficient arm length for steering, so a steering footplate is used, in which the driver's shoe slips into a metal 'shoe' pivoted on the footplate. Secondary controls on door activated by the short upper limb

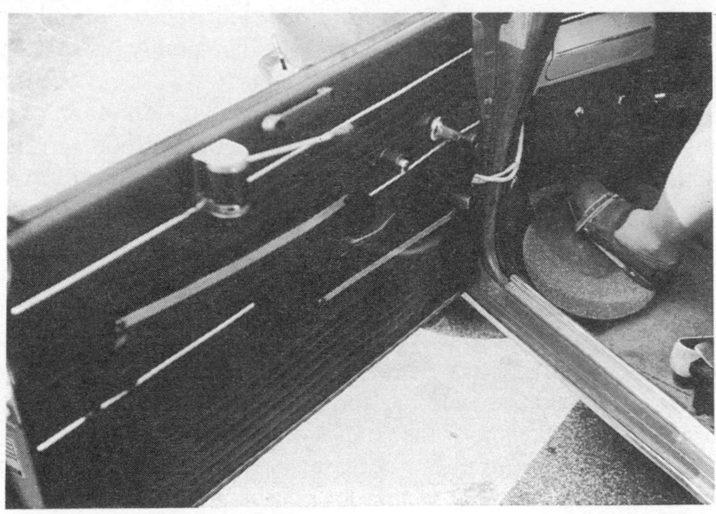

Figure 47.8: Steering from the right shoulder for a limb-deficient patient. Right foot controls brake/accelerator, left foot for secondary controls (Steering Developments Ltd)

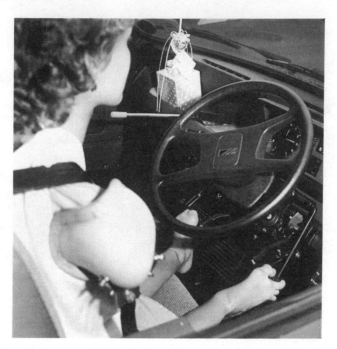

ARTHRITIS

There are very few patients so severely disabled due to juvenile chronic arthritis, adult rheumatoid disease or ankylosing spondylitis that they are unable to drive. Difficulty in driving can almost always be overcome by modification of the vehicle or surgery for the patient! Limitation of cervical spine movement can be compensated for by adequate door mirrors and a panoramic rear-view mirror. An adequate head restraint is important with any *cervical spine condition* and for all rheumatoid patients, because this limits cervical spine and head movement in an accident which may cause tetraplegia due to fracture of the rigid spine in ankylosing spondylitis or subluxation of the unstable rheumatoid cervical spine. *The elbow or knee* only needs to move 30–40° in mid-range during driving, but more than 65° fixed flexion of either causes difficulty. If this is in one knee or elbow it can be compensated as for an amputee, but if the patient has gross bilateral fixed flexion of the elbows driving may be impossible unless successful surgery is achieved on at least one elbow. With a fixed straight knee, as after arthrodesis, use of that leg is usually unsafe. The presence of two very stiff straight knees requires the use of hand controls.

The hip joint moves only about 30° in the mid-range in driving, from about 45° to 75°, so it is only if there is inability to flex beyond about 45° that there will be a problem, otherwise having the driving seat inclined slightly backwards will usually be comfortable and safe. With severe hip joint limitation the steering wheel may have to be brought back within reach of the patient, but it is usually better to do hip arthroplasty. Limitation of *shoulder* movement is seldom a problem; the common loss of abduction and external rotation causes little difficulty when driving, but with severe rheumatoid arthritis the sudden occurrence of pain in the shoulder may cause equally sudden relaxation of grip on the wheel and attention to the road. Poor *hand-grip* due to arthritis rarely impedes driving, but with swan-neck deformity of all fingers it may be difficult to curl the fingers round and grip the wheel, and enlarging the wheel rim or possibly providing a steering ball may be required. In all arthritic conditions it is not only the joint limitation and pain which cause difficulty in driving, but the simultaneous occurrence of muscle weakness, either due to the arthritis itself or due to associated peripheral neuropathy or cervical myelopathy that must be considered. Frequently automatic transmission with power on brakes and possibly on steering will solve the difficulty of the arthritic patient driving. These patients are frequently not employed and earning to their full potential, so the limitation on driving may be more financial than physical. Seat belts may be a particular problem for arthritic patients (Arie, 1986).

ACKNOWLEDGEMENT

Figures 47.1–47.3 are reproduced with permission of Banstead Place Mobility Centre.

REFERENCES

Arie, E. (1986) Car safety belts; a study of two models adapted for people with arthritis. *Br. J. Rheum.*, *25*, 199-205

Bulstrode, S.J., Clarke, A.K. and Harrison, R.A. (1985) *Assessment of car seat belt adaptations*, DHSS, London

Darnborough, A. and Kinrade, D. (1985) Motoring and mobility for disabled people, in *Directory for the disabled*, Royal Association for Disability and Rehabilitation, 25 Mortimer St, London W1N 8AB

Editorial (1980) Epilepsy after head trauma and fitness to drive. *Lancet*, *23*, 401-2

Haslegrave, C. (1985) *Car conversions for disabled drivers*, Vehicle Engineering Division, Transport and Road Research Laboratory, Crowthorne, Berks

Jennett, B. (1983) Anticonvulsant drugs and advice about driving after head injury and intracranial surgery. *Br. Med. J.*, *286*, 627-8

Legh-Smith, J., Wade, D. T. and Langton Hewer, R. (1986) Driving after a stroke. *J. Roy Soc. Med.*, *79*, 200-3

Raffle, A. (1985) *Medical aspects of fitness to drive*, Medical Commission on Accident Prevention, London

Sivak, M., Ohlson, P.L., Kewman, D.G., Won, H. and Henson, L.H. (1981) Driving and perceptual/cognitive skills: behavioural consequences of brain damage. *Arch. Phys. Med. Rehabil.*, *62*, 476-83

Wilson, T. and Smith, T. (1983) Driving after stroke. *Int. Rehabil. Med.*, *5*, 170-7

DISABLED DRIVERS' ASSESSMENT CENTRES

Banstead Place Mobility Centre
Park Road, Banstead, Surrey SM7 3EE

BSM Disability Training Centre
81 Hartfield Road, London SW19

Derby Disabled Drivers' Assessment Centre
Derwent Hospital, Derby DE2 4BB

Mobility Advice and Vehicle Information Service (MAVIS)
Department of Transport, TRRL, Crowthorne, Berks RG11 6AU

Mobility Information Service
Copthorne Community Hall, Shelton Road, Shrewsbury, Salop

Northern Ireland Council for the Handicapped (NICH)
2 Annadale Avenue, Belfast BT7 3JR

Rookwood Hospital
Llandaff, Cardiff CF5 2YN

Stoke Mandeville Hospital
Mandeville Road, Aylesbury, Bucks HP21 8AL

Tehidy Mobility Centre
Tehidy Hospital, Camborne, Cornwall TR14 0SA

Vehicles for the Disabled Centre
Astley Ainslie Hospital, 133 Grange Loan, Edinburgh EH09 2HL

Welsh Disabled Drivers' Assessment Centre
Briardene, North Road, Cardiff

This list is not exhaustive; some car conversion firms do their own assessments.

Driving and Vehicle Licensing Centre (DVLC)
Department of Transport, Medical Advisory Branch, Oldway Centre, Orchard Street, Swansea SA1 1TU

INFORMATION

Transport (1986) published by Disabled Living Foundation, 380 Harrow Road, London W9 2HU (Includes addresses for car conversions, lifting systems for wheelchairs, garage doors, transport information for the disabled driver or passenger. etc.)

Outdoor Transport, Equipment for the disabled (1982) Mary Marlborough Lodge, Nuffield Orthopaedic Hospital, Headington, Oxford OX3 7LD

Disabled Drivers Association, Ashwellthorpe Hall, Ashwellthorpe, Norwich, Norfolk NR16 1EX

Disabled Drivers Insurance Bureau, 292 Hale Lane, Edgware, Middx, HA8 8NP

Disabled Drivers Motor Club, 1a Dudley Gardens, Ealing London W13 9LU

Disabled Motorists Federation, Unit 2A, Atcham Estate, Upton Magna, Shrewsbury SY4 4UG

Ins and outs of car choice (A guide for disabled people), Transport and Road Research Laboratory, Crowthorne, Berks

Steering Developments Ltd, 3 Eastman Way, Hemel Hempstead, Herts HP2 7HF

48

Environmental and Telephone Controls

John Goodwill

The patient with severe locomotor handicap causing limited function in hands or arms may find difficulty in controlling all the switches and knobs in the home that the able-bodied take for granted. There are many solutions to such problems: light switches may be repositioned, changed to rocker or touch-switches, or to a pull-switch hanging from the ceiling. A door lock can be changed to an entryphone system with an electronic lock-release, the control placed accessible for the patient, and an intercom/alarm provided. The patient can wear a control which remotely triggers an alarm or dials a series of telephone numbers previously stored by the owner until a response is obtained; it then repeats a taped emergency message. There are many types of alarm and call systems, illustrated and described in *Equipment for the disabled, communication* (see 'Information', at end of chapter). However if the patient is too disabled for simple modifications such as these to suffice, then he can control entry to the house and electrical appliances such as light, room heater, etc., by having a bank of six switches (e.g. Possum PSU2), in a unit placed within easy reach. All these aids may be supplied by Social Services.

Some patients are too heavily disabled to use simple aids. Patients with high tetraplegia, in the later stages of multiple sclerosis, motor neurone disease and some with stroke are the commonest patients requiring major *environmental controls* such as described below. Providing the patient can trigger a switch, control is possible for alarm, intercom, radio, television, light, heater, page-turner, electric bed and other electrical equipment operated by that switch. Telephone control is also included for outgoing and incoming calls. Control of a computer, word processor and printer is also possible, though these are rarely supplied by the statutory services. They may be essential to allow continued employment, in which case the Manpower Services Commission (Department of Employment) may be able to help, or if the computer, etc., is wanted for home use, money may be found from a charity.

CONTROL MECHANISM FOR ENVIRONMENTAL CONTROLS

Control by the patient is achieved by whatever voluntary muscle power is available, e.g. by using a finger, foot or special switches mounted in the headrest of the wheelchair, or by eyebrow switches on special spectacles. Over 60 per cent of patients use suck–blow on a mouthpiece. The switches may be as light in action as the patient requires. These patients will usually be using an electric wheelchair so that the suck–blow control may be fixed in a convenient position for the patient to drive up to it.

If the patient is static in bed or a chair a suck–blow switch is positioned so as to be accessible on turning the head slightly, or the switch is on a moulded hand splint and moved by a finger. All these switches are basically two-position switches, on–off, so it cannot be long before remote control is developed, eliminating the wire from the control to the display unit.

The patients rapidly learn to use the equipment if they have the incentive to use it, although initially they may require encouragement from family and professional staff, with home visits by the occupational therapist. There are two commonly used units, made by Steeper or by Possum. With either system the telephone has a loudspeaker and microphone (Servophone from British Telecom).

Steeper (Figure 48.1)

Before use the light remains on at the top of the display panel. When the equipment is triggered the light moves down successive boxes indicating the different functions, and a bleep is heard as it moves from one to the next function. The speed at which this occurs is kept low when the patient is learning about the equipment, and may be speeded up as the patient becomes accustomed to it. The patient ceases triggering the equipment at the function required, which is then switched on. Further triggering brings the equipment back to the stand-by position at the top of the display panel. Equipment is switched off by repeating the process. Electrical appliances are plugged into the back of the control box using ordinary 13-amp plugs.

With the Steeper equipment the patient may dial out any of ten preselected numbers by selecting telephone, and then the particular number required. Alternatively dialling out may be done by selecting each digit in turn.

Television and radio may be turned on or off only, but facility for channel and volume change is being developed for this unit. The unit contains batteries that charge off the mains. In the event of a power cut the Steeper unit will maintain essential functions for four hours; the Possum unit will maintain alarm, intercom, telephone and door lock.

Figure 48.1: Steeper: the indicator light moves down the line of square boxes in the centre of the indicator board. The Servophone is seen in front, and the control box on the left has 13-amp sockets behind, into which the different items may be plugged

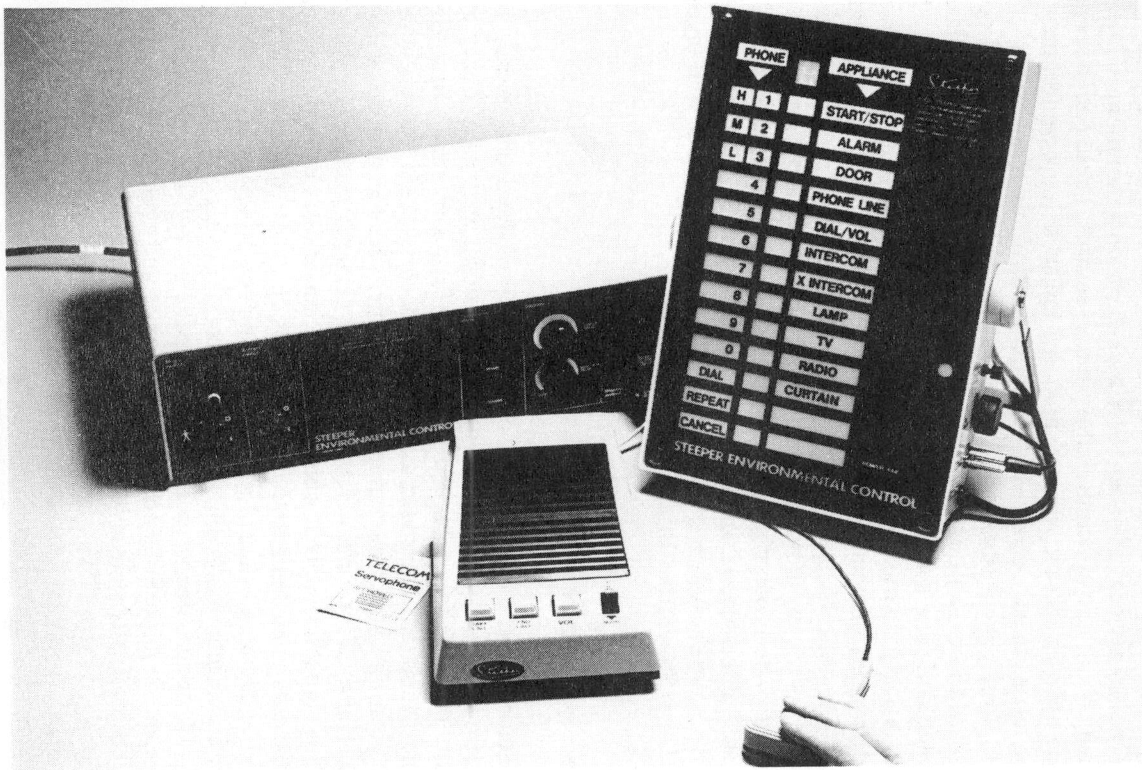

Possum (Figure 48.2)

Possum (PSU3) has similar functions, but here the display board is a matrix, the indicator light moving *down* the left-hand column. The light is stopped at the appropriate function, after which triggering the equipment again moves the light *horizontally*. The patient stops the light at the appropriate box to turn the equipment on/off or to achieve other indicated function. Controls of radio and TV include a facility for channel and volume change, so that if these are particularly needed by the patient the Possum equipment is preferred to the Steeper equipment. If channel change on radio only is needed, either equipment may be used with several small portable radios each tuned to the preselected station and plugged in separately, to be activated by different points on the control panel. The telephone control on the Possum panel gives three preselected numbers; dialling-out of other numbers is done by triggering the telephone control, after which a successive digital display from 0 to 9 appears in the top right-hand corner of the control panel. The equipment is triggered when the first digit of the desired phone number appears, successive digits being 'caught' in the same way. The numbers are serially stored in the equipment and dialled out automatically once the number is complete. There is no limit on the number digits that may be dialled using this or the Steeper equipment.

In 1979 Sell and colleagues evaluated eight different environmental control equipment on 52 high-level quadriplegic patients; each had some advantages and disadvantages but as equipment changes so much in this field their results are not really applicable to the two units discussed above. However, it was clear that patients like to have audio as well as visual feedback from the machine, and it was important that the patient could use the machine not only in one room but also when lying down in bed. These features are both possible with the Possum or Steeper units.

In a follow-up study of 48 patients with PSU3 environmental control equipment by Bell *et al.* (1987) 60 per cent were still using it nine months after supply, although four were having problems using their second unit in the bedroom because the visual indicator board was in the other room (with the Steeper equipment this board is moved so this would not be a problem). Fifteen per cent did not want the equipment, 10 per cent died and a further 15 per cent preferred not to use it after it was supplied. Non-use was not related to age, sex, disability or disease progression of the user, nor to the availability of an attendant, or even to patients' knowledge and expectations before supply. In the whole group 65 per cent had progressive neurological conditions, but the usage rate was the same as in those with static conditions. One must conclude that use or non-use depends on the patient's psychological attitude rather than any physical factors.

Figure 48.2: Possum: suck–blow control of all functions; the control box is housed below the display panel

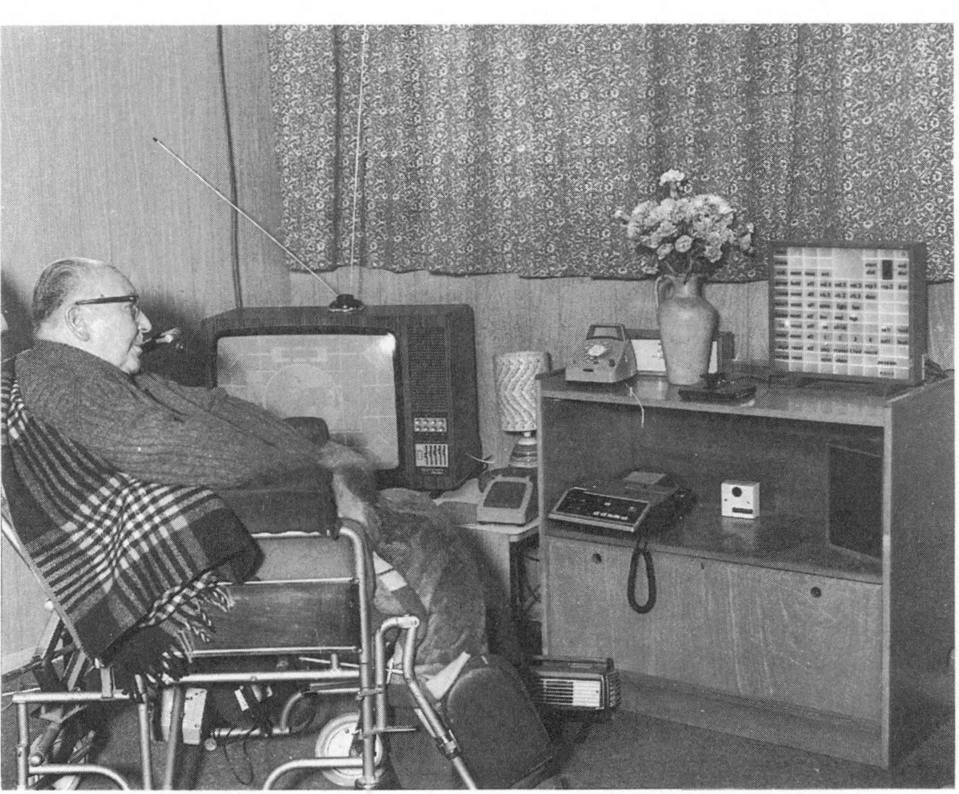

SUPPLY OF ENVIRONMENTAL CONTROL IN THE UK

Possum or Steeper equipment is supplied free under the National Health Service in the UK to those who need it. The patient's doctor applies to the Regional or District Medical Officer, arrangements are made for a consultant environmental control assessor (ECA) to visit the patient at home, preferably with the domiciliary OT who knows the patient, so that his needs for control of equipment are fully appreciated; the functions that need controlling and the particular type of equipment can be decided. The order is then passed to the manufacturer, who supplies and maintains the equipment thereafter. Either a general practitioner or hospital doctor may initiate the request for an assessment visit, and if another health or Social Services professional realises the patient has such needs she should speak to the patient's doctor to initiate supply of the equipment. Some patients will be found to be unable to control the equipment, usually because of lack of mental ability or severe receptive speech problems. Occasionally the assessor may decide that the patient will be equally well helped by simpler and cheaper aids which will achieve the same control of the environment in the home. Such aids would normally be supplied by Social Services and not centrally from the DHSS. During the assessment visit other needs of the disabled patient are frequently found, relating to many aspects of the disability, from management of spasticity, incontinence or skin care to the need for detailed wheelchair assessment or home modifications. Appropriate assessment and management is then arranged.

Telephone

In order to achieve greater independence at home the person with severe locomotor disability may need full environmental control equipment including telephone control (Servophone), but others often require only simple aids. Detailed information can be obtained in a *36-page booklet from British Telecom Offices,* at some of which equipment may be inspected. The domiciliary OT should be able to advise in detail on requirements, if necessary with a BT engineer.

The visually handicapped may have raised and/or enlarged numerals round the outside of the dial or use a push-button phone, the latter having large buttons. A large-print booklet or braille version of STD codes is available. Most BT switchboards can be suitably modified. Those with *hearing disability* can have an amplifying handset, a loud-speaking telephone or a second earpiece so that the user may listen with both ears; outside noise is reduced. A loud bell and/or flashing light signal indicates when the phone rings. An inductive couplet may be fitted in the telephone earpiece and used with a hearing aid, the switch on the latter being moved to the 'T' position, this facility is also available on public payphones and in those public buildings fitted with an induction loop system. Other more complex communication aids using the telephone line are available; basically these use small computers (see B.T. booklet). Those with a *very soft voice* may be helped by an amplifier on the telephone or worn on the neck. For these patients, or for those with *severe* dysarthria, unless the problem is easily solved, the patient should see a speech therapist and may need assessment for communication aids (Chapter 15) (Figures 48.3 and 48.4).

For those having *difficulty with finger and hand movement or control* such as in multiple sclerosis, Parkinson's disease or rheumatoid arthritis, it may suffice for the telephone to be firmly fixed at the correct angle and position; with *ataxia* a pushbutton telephone with a key guard may be required. Those with *more limited hand use* may be helped by a pushbutton telephone with an on/off control that does not require lifting a handset. On some phones the handset is fixed on an adjustable stand and positioned conveniently, or the telephone incorporates a microphone and loudspeaker. A single button is pressed to use one of ten previously stored

Figure 48.3: Large-number dial for visual disability, lamp signal on handset in addition to telephone bell and second earpiece for a deaf person (Yeoman-Plus phone)

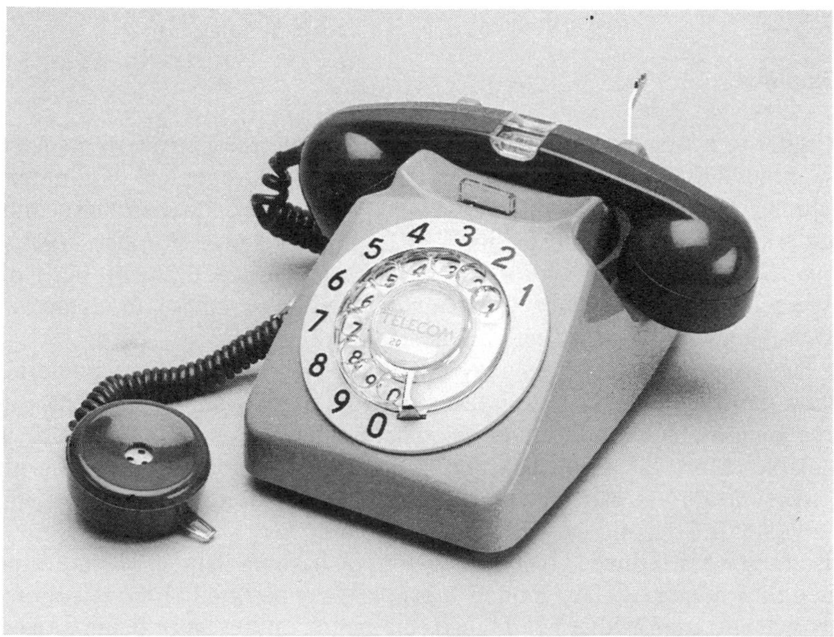

Figure 48.4: Sceptre 120 phone with ten-number memory, last number re-dial, visual display, call-timer and clock

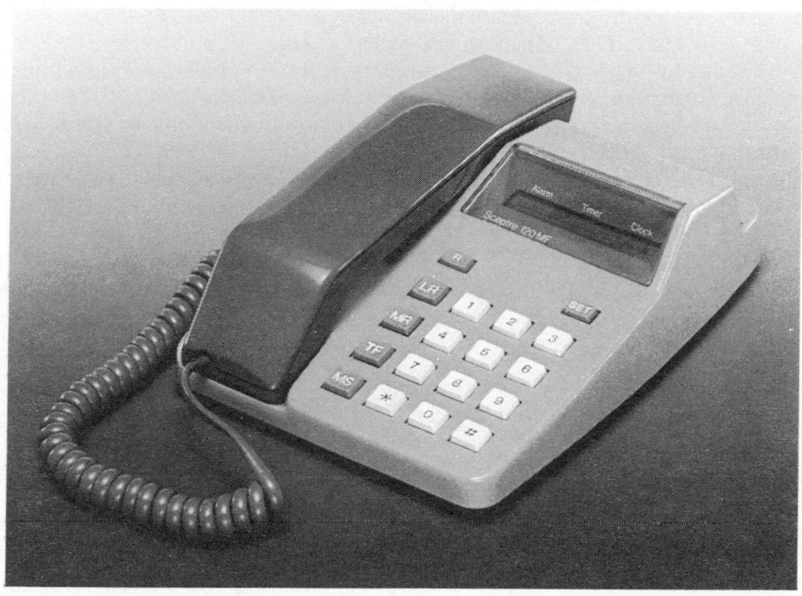

numbers, the particular number then being selected by pressing only one of the 0 to 9 buttons on the telephone. Other phones will store up to 50 numbers. Other features available on different models of telephone include: display of number dialled (to prevent errors); last number re-dial, and cordless operation up to 100 metres. For severely disabled patients the telephone is usually included with the environmental control unit, but some prefer to have a separate single on/off switch for outgoing calls. The caller is connected direct to the operator, requesting special assistance, following which the operator dials the number; the caller pays at operator telephone rates. If only a single switch is used this may be on a pushbutton telephone, but it can be a lever or any other type of switch to control on/off in the electrical circuit. The patient has either a normal handset, which is positioned with a clamp and arm so that he can drive his electric wheelchair up to it, or has a microphone–loudspeaker phone. A cordless telephone is preferred by some patients, one model having a nine-number memory.

REFERENCES AND FURTHER READING

Arroyo, R. (1976) Control and communication devices for severely disabled. *Bull. Prosthet. Res.*, *10*, 55-68

Bell, F., Whitfield, E. and Rollett, R.P. (1987) Investigation of Possum users in Scotland. *Int. Rehabil. Med.*, *8*, 105-12

Kelly, S.N. (1983) Adaptations for independent use of cassette tape recorder/radio by high-level quadriplegic patients. *Am. J. Occup. Ther.*, *37*, 766-7

Sell, G.H., Stratford, C.D., Zimmerman, M.E., Youdin, M. and Milner, D. (1979) Environmental and typewriter control systems for high-level quadriplegic patients. Evaluation and prescription. *Arch. Phys. Med. Rehabil.*, *60*, 246-52

Staros, A. and Peizer, E. (1976) Evaluation of environmental control systems. *Bull. Prosthet. Res.*, *10*, 220-3

Symington, D.C., Lynwood, D.W., Lawson, J.S. and MacLean, I. (1986) Environmental control systems in chronic care hospitals and nursing homes. *Phys. Med. Rehabil.*, *67*, 322-5

INFORMATION

Possum Controls Ltd
Middlegreen Trading Estate, Middlegreen Rd, Langley, Slough, Berks SL3 6OF

Hugh Steeper Ltd
237-239 Roehampton Lane, London SW15 4LB

British Telecom
Action for Disabled Customers, Room B 4036, B.T. Centre, 81 Newgate Street, London EC1A 7AJ; Linkline, local call charge from anywhere in the UK

Equipment for the Disabled: Communication (speech aids, callsystems, telephones, environmental controls, page-turners and other reading aids, typing, blind and deaf aids), Mary Marlborough Lodge, Nuffield Orthopaedic Centre, Headington, Oxford OX3 7LD

Many of these aids and information may be seen in hospital rehabilitation departments and at Disabled Living Centres (Chapter 49).

Part 8

Delivery of Services

49

Resources Available

Elizabeth Fanshawe

(1) INTRODUCTION

The onset of a disabling condition, the birth of a handicapped child, or the consequences of a serious accident, are shattering occurrences. The people involved may need to re-think their lives entirely; they may need to learn a completely new set of techniques for carrying out activities of daily living; they may need to know about new benefits, new facilities, and/or new legislation; they may need to adapt the fabric of their homes, use new equipment, perhaps change their employment or leisure activities, and even adjust their relationships with other people. The effects of permanent disability are present throughout the day and night, and will have a bearing on all activities. However, many of the problems can be solved by appropriate rehabilitation — in its widest sense — and by the provision of information on resources available.

Because the long-term support of disabled people is a complex matter, it is unlikely that any single member of the care team will know all there is to know about the practical and emotional problems caused by disability. It is important for any practitioner to know of the skills of local colleagues in other professions, and local facilities, in order to provide the disabled person with a full coverage of support.

(2) TYPES/ORGANISATION IN PROVISION OF RESOURCES

Some of the main sources of information about services, aids and equipment, and other facilities, are described in the following sections. Addresses for organisations, publishers, etc., are given in a final section (with the exception of central government and other statutory bodies, where local offices will be the first point of contact). It should also be noted that references to local statutory agencies relate to authorities in England,

Scotland and Wales — departments and arrangements will vary in Northern Ireland.

Resources and information are available from statutory or voluntary agencies, at national or local level as follows:

(a) Statutory agencies

Government departments — such as Department of Health and Social Security, the Scottish Home and Health Department, Manpower Services Commission, the Department of Transport — produce documentation on facilities, benefits and aids available through their particular offices, and most of these are available in leaflet form suitable for patients' waiting rooms. In addition, local authorities will provide information on equipment and facilities available from — for example — Social Services or Housing Departments.

(b) National voluntary bodies

These can give information on different aspects of disability, for example the Disabled Living Foundation (DLF) provides information on any matter (with the exception of the purely medical) to do with problems caused by disability; the Royal Association for Disability and Rehabilitation (RADAR) is the UK representative of Rehabilitation International, and supplies information on many subjects, including housing, legislation, and holidays, and the Scottish Council on Disability is the major source of information in Scotland. Other national voluntary organisations are concerned with particular problem areas — such as building design, Centre on Environment for the Handicapped (CEH) — and the financial benefits, Disability Alliance. Others are concerned with particular disabilities, Association for Spina Bifida and Hydrocephalus, the Multiple Sclerosis Society, and many more.

(c) Local voluntary bodies

Many of the national organisations have local groups, which not only form a source of information, but also provide a basis for mutual support and, in some cases, will act as pressure groups. DIAL (UK) (Disabled Information and Advice Lines) is a network of local information providers; a list of groups can be obtained from their head office. Most areas of the country will also have a county or some other 'umbrella' association for disabled people — a national list of these is available from RADAR, or individual addresses should be available from local authorities. The 'Yellow Pages' section of local telephone directories will include useful national and local addresses in a section 'Disabled — amenities and information'. The following is an attempt to give a point of contact in the major problem areas: it cannot be comprehensive, but the subsequent list of books and other publications can be used for more complete reference, as can the national information sources such as DLF and RADAR.

(3) AIDS AND EQUIPMENT (GENERAL)

Some problems can be solved by the use of 'aids to daily living', such as bathing aids, aids for getting in and out of bed, coping with housework, mobility aids, furniture with special features or aids to leisure activities.

The type of equipment, or the reason for its use, will dictate the source of supply, and some specific areas are covered below. Meanwhile, the following can give general information.

Statutory agency: local Social Services Department or regional Social Work Departments in Scotland — contact the occupational therapist, or local hospital Department of Rehabilitation — contact the occupational therapist or physiotherapist.

National voluntary body: The Disabled Living Foundation answers letter/telephone enquiries on all types of equipment, and also runs an Aid and Equipment Centre where items on display can be seen and tried out. The Scottish Council on Disability fulfils a similar function to DLF in Scotland.

Aids and equipment can be seen (usually by appointment) at the following aids centres, which can also answer letter/telephone enquiries. The aids centres listed are exhibitions where a selection of aids for disabled people can be seen and tried out. They provide information to those professionally concerned, disabled people and their friends and relatives (as Centres vary considerably in size, content and the kind of service they offer, it is wise to check that the purpose of the visit can be fulfilled).

Visitors should always telephone or write to make an appointment before they visit an aids and equipment centre

Disabled Living Centres offering a comprehensive service

Belfast
Prosthetic Orthotic and Aids Service, Musgrave Park Hospital, Stockman's Lane, Belfast BT9 7BR

Birmingham
Disabled Living Centre, 260 Broad Street, Birmingham B1 2HF

Caerphilly
Aids and Information Centre, Wales Council for the Disabled,

Figure 49.1: A member of the Disabled Living Centre team demonstrating wheelchairs to a visitor at the Disabled Living Foundation

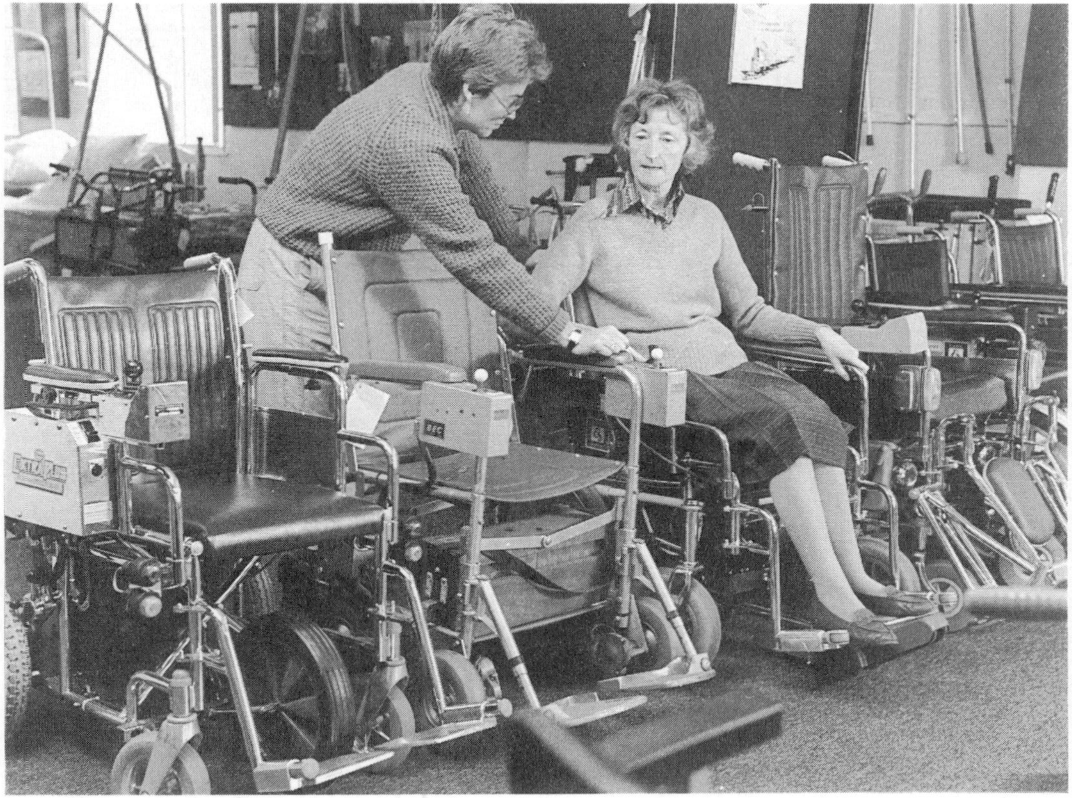

Caerbragdy Industrial Estate, Bedwas Road, Caerphilly CF8 3SL Mid Glamorgan

Edinburgh

S. Lothian Aid Centre, Astley Ainslie Hospital, Grange Loan, Edinburgh EH9 2HL

Leeds

The William Merritt Disabled Living Centre, St Mary's Hospital, Greenhill Rd., Armley, Leeds LS12 3QE

Leicester

TRAIDS (Trent Region Aids, Information and Demonstration Service), 76 Clarendon Park Road, Leicester LE2 3AD

Liverpool

Merseyside Aids Centre, Youens Way, East Prescott Road, Liverpool 14 2EP

London

Disabled Living Foundation, Equipment Centre, 380/384 Harrow Road, London W9 2HU

Manchester

Disabled Living Services, Disabled Living Centre, Redbank House, 4 St Chad's Street, Cheetham, Manchester M8 8QA

Newcastle upon Tyne

Newcastle upon Tyne Council for the Disabled, The Dene Centre, Castles Farm Road, Newcastle upon Tyne NE3 1PH

Sheffield

Sheffield Independent Living Centre, 108 The Moor, Sheffield S1 4PD

Southampton

Southampton Aids and Equipment Centre, Southampton General Hospital, Tremona Road, Southampton SO9 4XY

Stockport

Aids/Assessment Unit, Stockport Area Health Authority, St Thomas's Hospital, Shawheath, Stockport SK3 8BL

Swindon

Swindon Centre for Disabled Living, The Hawthorn Centre, Cricklade Road, Swindon, Wilts SN2 1AF

Disabled Living Centres offering a limited service

Blackpool

Aids Centre, 8 Queen Street, Blackpool, Lancs FY1 1PD

Dudley

Dudley Aids and Assessment Centre, 1 St Giles Street, Netherton, Dudley

Paisley

Disability Centre, Community Services, Queens Street, Paisley PA1 2TU

Portsmouth
Disabled Living Centre, Prince Albert Road, Eastney, Portsmouth PO4 9HR

Mobile aids centres
The following are travelling exhibitions which tour the country. Contact the organisation for details of the places to be visited. An appointment is preferable.
Mobile Advice Centre
Scottish Council on Disability, Princes House, 5 Shandwick Place, Edinburgh EH2 4RG
Visiting Aids Centre
The Spastics Society, 16 Fitzroy Square, London W1P 5HQ

Other places where aids and equipment can be seen by appointment
Local Occupational Therapy Departments in hospitals; local Social Services Departments (some have assessment centres). Addresses in your local phone book.
Play Matters/The National Toy Libraries Association, 68 Churchway, London NW1 1LT. National toy library, loan scheme. Advice and information centre.
The Spastics Society, 16 Fitzroy Square, London W1P 5HQ (in addition has an assessment centre for children).

For details of proposed new centres in other parts of the country, please contact the Disabled Living Centre Council, c/o TRAIDS (Trent Region Aids, Information and Demonstration Service), 76 Clarendon Park Road, Leicester LE2 3AD

REFERENCES

DLF and the Scottish Council on Disability Information Service, lists and bulletins (available on subscription or individual purchase). Disabled Living Foundation. Scottish Council on Disability.

Equipment for the disabled: a series of 13 booklets on different ranges of equipment: *Communication, Clothing and dressing for adults, Home management, Outdoor transport, Wheelchairs, Leisure and gardening, Disabled mother, Personal care, Incontinence and cystoma care, Hoists and lifts, Walking aids, Disabled child, Housing and furniture*; Oxfordshire Health Authority, Nuffield Orthopaedic Centre, Oxford.

Jay, P. (1984) *Coping with disability*, Disabled Living Foundation, London.

(4) PERSONAL CARE/NURSING AT HOME

A disabled person may not be able to manage housework or cooking. However, a more severely disabled person might need not only aids and equipment but also personal assistance with bathing, toileting and dressing, and if incontinence is present, referral for treatment or help with its management.

Statutory agency: the Community Health Department of local District Health Authorities, or local Health Board in Scotland – contact: general practitioner or the District Nursing Officer for the Community, or Continence Advisor. Local authority Social Services Department should be able to organise 'meals-on-wheels' and home helps. It is not always clear whether equipment or services will be provided by the Social Services Department or the District Health Authority, and sources of supply will vary from area to area; however, the occupational therapist in local Social Services, or community nurse, should be able to advise on the appropriate contact.

National voluntary bodies: Association of Crossroads Care Attendant Scheme coordinates local groups providing trained helpers who can give short-term relief for a disabled person's family. Both DLF and the Scottish Council on Disability run advisory services on incontinence, and the Association of Continence Advisors will know of locally available advice.

REFERENCES

Information sheets: *Personal care, Personal toilet* and *Incontinence*, Disabled Living Foundation, London

Equipment for the Disabled, Personal care

Jay, P. (1984) *Coping with disability*, Disabled Living Foundation, London, Chapter on the lavatory

Mandelstam, D. (ed.) (1986) *Incontinence and its management*, 2nd edn, Croom Helm, London

(5) HOUSING

Most houses will need some adaptation to make them suitable for a severely disabled person, including, perhaps, widening of doors, provision of ramps, a downstairs cloakroom or bathroom, a downstairs bedroom, grab-rails, and lifts or stair-climbing equipment. There are grants from local authorities for such adaptations. In some cases rehousing might be necessary. The local authority occupational therapist or the Housing Department should have information (Chapter 39).

Statutory agencies: Social Services and Housing Departments of the local authority or District Authority Housing Department in Scotland — contact: occupational therapist, social worker, housing officer, environmental health officer or architect.

National voluntary bodies: Centre on Environment for the Handicapped runs an information and advisory service on the environmental needs of all handicapped people. The Access Committee for England can give advice on the design features and statutory regulations for providing access to buildings by disabled people, including doctor's surgeries.

REFERENCES

Goldsmith, S. (1984) *Designing for the disabled*, 3rd edn, RIBA Publications, London

Lockhart, T. (1981) *Housing adaptations for disabled people*, Architectural Press, London

(6) COMMUNICATION

The most basic methods of communication — speech, reading and writing — may be affected by some disabling conditions; but there will usually be some solution — perhaps new techniques such as oesophageal speech for people who have had a laryngectomy, or sign language, or speech replacement aids for others.

Statutory agencies: Local Health Authority for referral — contact: consultant in rehabilitation, district medical officer, district speech therapist or occupational therapist for communication-related problems and for details of local Communication Aid Centre (Chapter 15). If there is no local speech therapist — contact: College of Speech Therapists.

Local Social Services Department — contact: occupational therapist, for provision of communication aids such as page-turners, writing aids, telephone adaptations (and, sometimes, help with telephone expenses), etc. (Chapter 48).

Voluntary bodies: Disabled Living Foundation for information on all types of aids for speech, reading and writing, and other forms of communication. The Royal National Institute for the Blind, and Royal National Institute for the Deaf, for information on communication for people with a sensory impairment.

Other body: British Telecom/BTAID for adaptations to telephone equipment — e.g. enlarged dials, amplifiers, loudspeakers, 'no-hand' sets, etc.

REFERENCES

Disabled Living Foundation Information Service lists: Communication 3A and 3B–DLF

Equipment for the Disabled: *Communication*

Jay, P. (1984) *Coping with disability*, Disabled Living Foundation, London, Chapter 11: Keeping in touch.

(7) WHEELCHAIRS (see Chapter 43)

Wheelchairs are generally available on prescription. The exceptions are outdoor electrically self-operated wheelchairs and high-performance (or sports) wheelchairs, which may become available if the recommendations of the McColl Working Party reviewing the ALAC services are followed.

Statutory agency: local DHSS Artificial Limb and Appliance Centre (referral by consultant or general practitioner). Because of the complexity of assessing the physical and environmental needs of disabled people, most doctors welcome the expertise of local authority or hospital-based occupational therapists or physiotherapists when prescribing wheelchairs. The consumer should also be involved in the choice of chair and, if possible, allowed to try it out before issue or purchase.

Voluntary body: Disabled Living Foundation or Scottish Council on Disability can advise on both DHSS prescription procedures and suppliers of wheelchairs not on prescription.

REFERENCES

Department of Health and Social Security, *Handbook of wheelchairs and bicycles and tricycles* (MHM 408), supplied to general practitioners

Disabled Living Foundation, *Information Service notes: Wheelchairs and Choosing a wheelchair*

Equipment for the Disabled: Wheelchairs

(8) TRANSPORT

For many disabled people (and not only wheelchair users) public transport can be inaccessible; if a car is already owned it might need adapting, or it might be necessary to purchase a car for the first time (see Chapter 47 on Driving). If public transport has to be used, there will need to be very careful forward planning so that special facilities which do exist can be made available.

Statutory agencies: DHSS for Mobility Allowance, a cash benefit for those 'unable or virtually unable to walk' — contact: DHSS Mobility

Allowance Unit. Department of Transport, for Vehicle Excise Duty Exemption and vehicle licensing regulations — contact: local vehicle licensing office or Driver and Vehicle Licensing Centre. Department of Transport's Mobility and Vehicle Information Service (MAVIS) for driving assessment and general information. Local Social Services Department for Orange Badge Parking Scheme, allowing special parking privileges — contact: main Social Services office.

Voluntary bodies: Disabled Living Centres for information on special vehicles, adaptations, etc. Motability, an independent charitable organisation for arranging leasing or hire purchase of vehicles for those in receipt of Mobility Allowance (see Chapter 37), Mobility Information Service for advice on all aspects of outdoor mobility and centres for assessment of adaptations necessary and driving ability (see Chapter 47).

Other bodies: British Rail, for concessionary fares and other special arrangements — contact: local station master, or British Railways Board Special Advisor on the Disabled. Air Transport Users' Committee and Access to the Skies Committee for information on air travel.

REFERENCES

Air Transport Users Committee, *Care in the air — advice for handicapped travellers* (leaflet) Air Transport Users Committee, London

Darnbrough, A. and Kinrade, D. (1985) *Motoring and mobility for disabled people*, 3rd edn, RADAR, London

Department of Transport, *Door to door, 1985.* A guide on all forms of public transport by land, sea and air. Department of Transport, London

Disabled Living Foundation Information Service Sheets: *Transport* (list 8) and *Method of loading a wheelchair into a two-door car.* Disabled Living Foundation, London

(9) FINANCE

The additional costs of living with a disability can be considerable — not only for the purchase of necessary equipment, but perhaps also because of a diminution in earning power. There are State benefits which can be awarded in a variety of circumstances — including awards for very particular special needs (e.g. Supplementary Benefit for heating costs), but finding out what is available, and whether an individual will be eligible, can be an extremely time-consuming and complex exercise. As so much depends on individual circumstances it is not possible to itemise here all the benefits available, but the following should be able to respond to detailed, individual, enquiries.

Statutory agency: DHSS — contact: local Social Security Office.

Voluntary bodies: Disability Alliance, or local Citizens Advice Bureaux, Welfare Rights Officer (National Association of CAB, or telephone directory will give local address). The Scottish Council on Disability and many local voluntary organisations can also give individual advice.

REFERENCES

Department of Health and Social Security, *Which Benefit?* (FB2) and individual leaflets on all benefits from DHSS Leaflets

Disability Alliance, *Disability rights handbook* (annual with quarterly updates)

(10) COUNSELLING

It is natural that there is an emotional response to permanent disability, which is akin to bereavement. Some people will be able to, and prefer to, overcome this by themselves, but many will need help. The skill of counselling may only involve listening to the person, understanding the problems and encouraging him to arrive at his own solutions. Counselling may also be necessary, as well as practical advice on the marital and sexual problems which may arise (Chapter 30).

Statutory agencies: it is possible that some members of the care team in a hospital Rehabilitation Department or Family Practice will have taken an interest, and developed skills in counselling newly disabled people. This is, unfortunately, not very likely, but the suggested contact is the occupational therapist, hospital consultant or general practitioner. Local Social Services Departments might employ specialist counsellors, or social workers who have a particular interest — contact: medical social worker (usually based in local hospital).

National voluntary bodies: those concerned with specific disabilities will usually offer support and be able to put people in touch with 'fellow-sufferers', e.g. Spinal Injuries Association, Multiple Sclerosis Society, Association for Spina Bifida and Hydrocephalus. More generally, Samaritans (see local telephone directory), or British Association for Counselling (a national body providing information about local counselling services and individual counsellors). SPOD offers individual counselling on sexual and personal-relations problems of disabled people, and on sources of local advice. In London there are clubs which provide a meeting point for gay or lesbian disabled people, and their address may be obtained from DLF.

REFERENCES

Davies, B. M. (1982) *The disabled child and adult*, Ballière Tindall, London; Chapter 3: Understanding the physical and emotional problems of disability

Jay, P. (1984) *Coping with disability*, 2nd edn, Disabled Living Foundation, London; Chapter 14: Relationships and attitudes
Oliver, M. (1983) *Social work with disabled people.* British Association of Social Workers, London
Stewart, W. (1985) *Counselling in rehabilitation*, Croom Helm, London

(11) EDUCATION

This book is concerned with the rehabilitation of disabled adults, but it cannot be overstressed that access to the best possible primary, secondary and tertiary education is of the utmost importance. If a person has been disabled since childhood it could be that the need for re-education or training in later years stems from an impoverished early education. The opportunities for further education and training that exist encompass not only standard academic and vocational training, but also areas such as 'social skills' or 'independent living' (see Education, Chapter 40).

As regards the education of disabled children, the Education Act 1981 (which followed many of the recommendations of the 1978 Report of the Warnock Committee) now requires local education authorities to provide facilities in ordinary schools so that all children can be educated together (except in very special circumstances).

Statutory agency: local education authority.

National voluntary bodies: Centre for Studies on Integration in Education, Voluntary Council for Handicapped Children.

REFERENCES

Book lists about children with particular handicaps or learning difficulties can be obtained from the Department of Education and Science Library, and from DLF

Further education

Mainstream

Although it is the legal duty of local education authorities to provide education at school or college for all 16–19-year-olds who require it (under the Education Act 1944) the actual provision is patchy. Many disabled people will attend 'ordinary' courses (in many cases it is only poor access to buildings or special equipment which debars disabled people from integration). Some universities and colleges or technology have special accommodation and provide physical help with personal care. The Open University welcomes disabled students (see Chapter 40).

Statutory agency: local education authority, Open University.

Voluntary bodies: National Bureau of Handicapped Students.

Specialist colleges or training establishments

These are set up solely for disabled students and are usually residential, giving an opportunity for training in personal independence. They provide vocational guidance and training.

Statutory agency: MSC for details of major establishments (in Durham, Mansfield, Leatherhead and Exeter).

Voluntary bodies: contact DLF for list of other residential colleges. Some national bodies representing specific disabilities have establishments for their own members.

Vocational guidance

In addition to the local careers advisory services, the National Bureau of Handicapped Students can advise.

REFERENCES

Brennan, W.K. (1982) *Special education in mainstream schools: the search for quality*, National Council for Special Education, Stratford-upon-Avon

National Bureau for Handicapped Students (1984) *After 16 — what next?*, NBC

Newell, P. (1983) *Special education handbook: the new law on special educational needs*, Advisory Centre for Education, London

Pappenheim, K. (1982) *Special school leavers: the value of further education in their transition to the adult world*, Greater London Association for the Disabled, London

Queen Elizabeth's Foundation for the Disabled (1984) *Directory of opportunities for school leavers with disabilities*, Queen Elizabeth's Foundation for the Disabled, Leatherhead, Surrey

Spastics Society (1984) *A statement on students with special needs — the right to education after 16*, Spastics Society, London

A reading list can be obtained from the DLF.

(12) EMPLOYMENT

Disability can affect the ability to get, or keep, employment; not only because of physical and/or mental limitations, but also sometimes because of poor access to places or work and negative attitudes of some employers (Chapter 41).

Statutory agencies: Manpower Services Commission (MSC), Employment Division, runs the network of Jobcentres; specialist services include advice on, and placement in, open or sheltered employment, rehabilitation services, and the provision of special work aids or adaptations to work equipment and accommodation; the MSC's Training Division aims to provide training suited to individual need — contact: the Disablement

Resettlement Officer, Blind Persons Resettlement Officer, or occupational therapist (see Chapter 34).

Voluntary body: the Association of Disabled Professionals keeps a register of practising members who can advise (but does not act as an agency).

REFERENCES

Fallon, B. (1979) *Able to work*, Spinal Injuries Association, London

Manpower Services Commission, series of leaflets on most special disability services, available from local Jobcentres

Right to work, produced by Films of Today, sponsored by Remploy Ltd, distributed by Centre Film Library

Royal National Institute for the Blind, series of leaflets.

(13) LEISURE ACTIVITIES (including holidays and sports)

If the onset of disability reduces the opportunity for employment, the need to fill leisure time in a constructive and fulfilling way is extremely important. Many aids are available to allow a disabled person to continue with an existing interest — e.g. special garden tools, playing-card holders. There are hobby and sports organisations specially for disabled people, but many 'ordinary' clubs encourage membership by disabled people. The trend to include access features in buildings (now mandatory in many types of new buildings used by the general public — e.g. new cinemas and theatres) is seen also in sporting and leisure complexes, countryside parks, and nature reserves. Many theatres also now install loop systems for deaf people.

With careful planning, even a very severely disabled person should be able to enjoy a break away from the daily routine and environment, and this may be equally important for the carers. References given in the section on Transport are relevant to travel, and this section gives references for accommodation.

Statutory agency: local Social Services Department, for provision of group holidays for disabled people — contact: occupational therapist or social worker, who should also know of services available through other departments — e.g. Libraries and Museums Department (housebound library service), Parks and Recreation Department (access to local amenities).

National voluntary bodies: British Sports Association for the Disabled is the national coordinating and development organisation, and can give information on all types of sporting activities. The Sports Council can also advise on specialist and general sporting organisations and activities. Royal Association for Disability and Rehabilitation (RADAR) has a Holiday

Officer, who can advise on all aspects of holidaying both here and abroad, as can the Scottish Council on Disability. The Winged Fellowship is one organisation which provides 'interest' or general holidays for very severely disabled people with or without their families.

REFERENCES

Disabled Living Foundation, Information lists, Leisure activities (6) and Sport and physical recreation facilities for disabled people (6A). Latter compiled by Sports Council, both available from Disabled Living Foundation.

(14) PUBLICATIONS FOR PATIENTS' WAITING ROOMS (AND STAFF REST ROOMS)

The following publications are highly recommended for patient waiting rooms:

Darnborough, A. and Kinrade, D. (1985) *Directory for the disabled*, 4th edn, Woodhead Faulkner, Cambridge

Department of Health and Social Security, *Help for handicapped people*, leaflet HB1, available from: DHSS Leaflets

Disability rights handbook, published annually with quarterly updates, by Disability Alliance

Jay, P. (1984) *Coping with disability*, Disabled Living Foundation, London

Mental Health Foundation (1985) *Someone to talk to: a directory of self-help and community support agencies in the UK and Republic of Ireland*, Routledge & Kegan Paul, London

There are also 'access guides' to many towns throughout the country: many of these are available from RADAR.

(15) ADDRESSES

(Addresses of specific disability organisations not listed here can be obtained from the Disabled Living Foundation. Addresses correct at January 1987 but subject to change.)

ACE Aids to Communications in Education Centres, Ormerod School, Headington, Oxford

Air Transport Users Committee, 129 Kingsway, London WC2B 6NN

Association of Continence Advisors, 380–384 Harrow Rd, London W9

Association of Crossroads Care Attendant Schemes, 94a Coton Road, Rugby CV21 4LN (addresses for local schemes will be available)

Association of Disabled Professionals, The Stables, 73 Pound Road, Banstead, Surrey

Association for Spina Bifida and Hydrocephalus, 22 Upper Woburn Place, London WC1H 0EP

Banstead Place Assessment Centre, Park Road, Banstead, Surrey SM7 3EE

British Association for Counselling, 37a Sheep Street, Rugby CV21 3BX

British Railways Board, 222 Marylebone Road, London NW1 6JJ

British Sports Association for the Disabled, Hayward House, Barnard Crescent, Aylesbury HP21 8PP

British Telecom/BTAID, Room B5049, British Telecom Centre, 84 Newgate Street, London EC1A 7AJ

CEH — see Centre on Environment

Central Film Library, Chalfont Grove, Gerrards Cross, Bucks SL9 8TN

Centre on Environment for the Handicapped, 35 Great Smith Street, London SW1P 3BJ

Centre for Studies on Integration in Education — see Spastics Society

Child Poverty Action Group, 1 Mackling Street, London WC2 5NH

College of Speech Therapists, Harold Poster House, 6 Lechmere Road, London NW2 5BW

DIAL UK, Dial House, 117 High Street, Claygross, Chesterfield, Derbyshire SL5 9DZ

DIG (Disablement Income Group), Attlee House, Toynebee Hall, 28 Commercial Street, London EC1

Disablement Advisory Service (Employment), Consult DRO at local Jobcentre

DHSS Leaflet Store (for leaflet HB1), Honeypot Lane, Stanmore, Middx

DHSS Mobility Allowance Unit, North Flyde Central Office, Blackpool FY5 3TA

DHSS Store (for Wheelchair Manual), No. 2 Site, Manchester Road, Heywood, Lancs OL10 2PZ

Department of Transport, Door-to-Door Guide, Freepost, Victoria Road, South Ruislip HA4 0NZ

Disability Alliance, 25 Denmark Street, London WC2 8NJ

Disabled Living Foundation (DLF), 380–384 Harrow Road, London W9 2HU

Driver and Vehicle Licensing Centre, Swansea SA6 7JL

Equipment for the Disabled, Mary Marlborough Lodge, Nuffield Orthopaedic Centre, Headington, Oxford OX3 7LD

HMSO, The Government Bookshop, Her Majesty's Stationery Office, PO Box 276, London SW8 5DT

Mencap — see Royal Society for Mentally Handicapped Children and Adults

Mental Health Foundation, 10 Hallam Street, London W1

Methuen & Co Ltd, Publishers, EXPs, 11 New Fetter Lane, London EC4

Mobility Information Service, Copthorne Community Hall, Shelton Rd, Shrewsbury, Salop

Motability, Boundary House, 91-93 Charter House Street, London EC1M 6BT

Motor Neurone Disease Association, 38 Hazelwood Road, Northampton NN1 1LN

Multiple Sclerosis Society, 25 Effie Road, Fulham, London SW6 1EE

Muscular Dystrophy Group of Great Britain, Nattrass House, 35 Macauley Road, London SW4 0QP

National Association of Citizens Advice Bureaux, Middleton House, 115/123 Pentonville Road, London N1 9LZ

National Bureau for Handicapped Students, 48 Brunswick Square, London WC1N 1AZ

National Council for Special Education, 1 Wood Street, Stratford-Upon-Avon, Warwickshire CV37 6JE

Northern Ireland Information Service, 2 Annandale Avenue, Belfast BT7 3JF

PHAB (Physically Handicapped and Able Bodied), Tavistock House North, Tavistock Square, London EC1H 9HX

RADAR (Royal Association of Disability and Rehabilitation), 25 Mortimer Street, London W1N 8AB

RIBA Publications Ltd, Finsbury Mission, Moreland Street, London EC1V 8VB

Remploy Ltd, 415 Edgwarc Road, London NW2 6LR

Routledge & Kegan Paul Ltd, Broadway House, Newtown Road, Henley-On-Thames, Slough, Bucks

Royal National Institute for the Blind, 224 Great Portland Street, London W1N 6AA

Royal National Institute for the Deaf, 105 Gower Street, London WC1E 6AH

Royal Society for Mentally Handicapped Children and Adults, 123 Golden Lane, London EC1Y 0RT

Spastics Society, 12 Park Crescent, London W1N 4EQ

SPOD (Sexual and Personal Relationships of the Disabled), 286 Camden Road, London N7 0BJ

Scottish Council on Disability, Princes House, 5 Shandwick Place, Edinburgh EH2 4RG

Spinal Injuries Association, Yeoman House, 76 St James Lanes, London N10 3DF

Sports Council (Central Council for Physical Recreation), 16 Upper Woburn Place, London WC1 0QP

Voluntary Council for Handicapped Children, National Children's Bureau, 8 Wakeley Street, London EC1V 7QE

Wales Council for the Disabled, Caerbragdy Industrial Estate, Bedwas Road, Caerphilly, Mid-Glamorgan CE8 3SL

Winged Fellowship Trust, Angel House, Pentonville Road, London N1 9XD

The carers need support also

Carers Association, Medway Homes, Balfour Road, Rochester, Kent

National Council of Carers and their Elderly Dependents, Mrs A. Gilbourne, 5 Alberta Avenue, Leeds 7

50

Organisation of Rehabilitation Services

John Hunter

Successful rehabilitation involves not only undertaking a thorough assessment of the patient's problems — physical, psychological and social — but also utilising the appropriate resources to deal as effectively as possible with those problems which are amenable to help. Coordination of the work of the various professionals and agencies that may be involved in dealing with patients' problems requires considerable managerial and diplomatic skills, but depends fundamentally on a sound knowledge of the organisation of services. In this chapter I shall summarise the framework of services nationally in the UK, but there are local variations in the pattern of service delivery which obviously cannot be itemised in a book. Professionals working for disabled people must, however, be aware of these local arrangements in order to operate the administrative levers of the system as effectively as possible in the interests of the patient.

OUTLINE OF SERVICE PROVISION

The main providers of services for disabled people are the National Health Service, central government, local government and the voluntary sector; the private sector also makes a small contribution.

The National Health Service

The full range of medical, surgical and other services provided by the National Health Service in district hospitals, regional centres and in the community, may be involved in the successful rehabilitation of a patient. The level of provision of medical, paramedical and nursing services for rehabilitation and long-term care of disabled people varies throughout the country. The problem areas include not only hospital services, but also community-based services, such as community nursing, the provision of domiciliary physiotherapy or arrangements for the optimal management of incontinence. In the field of equipment provision the National Health Service is usually responsible for the supply of mobility and nursing equipment. In Scotland and Northern Ireland the NHS also provides artificial limbs and wheelchairs, but in England and Wales these are supplied through the Artificial Limb and Appliance Centres (ALAC), although the service will soon be administered by the NHS.

In England and Wales the Health Regions have a major planning role and fund certain regional services (e.g. neurosurgical and renal units) directly, but most of their money is passed to Health Districts who have responsibility for providing health care for their population, usually 150,000 to 250,000. In Scotland the Area Health Boards provide an equivalent service, but certain specialised services are provided only by a few boards, and this is reflected in their funding from the Scottish Home and Health Department. Irrespective of geographical location, there is a need for improvement in services to help with the management of disability, a need recognised in many official reports, most recently that of the Royal College of Physicians of London (1986).

Many districts have a planning team for the disabled, charged with the duty of assessing the problems and proposing solutions, remembering that each consultant and GP has the duty of supervising the management of his own disabled patients. A community medicine specialist, who is trained in epidemiology, and an enthusiastic administrator should be included in this team, along with clinical representatives, including a general practitioner; a physician from a specialty, such as rheumatology or neurology, which is involved in caring for disabled people; the district physiotherapist; district occupational therapist; district speech therapist; and representatives of community nursing services. Officials of the Social Services, education, housing, voluntary sector and organisations representing disabled people should be included also. The size of the problem which this planning team has to tackle can be estimated either by extrapolating from existing, but imperfect, studies of disability (making allowance for local variations in age distribution and social conditions) or by undertaking local surveys. Ideally these should cover the whole community, but are more likely to focus on the problems of particular services such as hospital inpatients or outpatients, the disabled school-leaver, etc. The community physician has a major part to play in this work. The views of local general practitioners, who have an important role in maintaining disabled people in the community, must be sought and listened to. Since most consultant appointments relate to particular organs or systems of the body or to 'general' (i.e. acute) medicine or surgery, it is sometimes difficult to find a specialist who can speak with authority on the general problems or management of disability in hospitals. The RCP report (1986) suggested that in each health district there should be ten or eleven sessions shared by two or more consultants practising in a variety of specialities, each consultant having certain specific designated responsibilities for the management of disability. Alternatively some districts might have a full-time consultant appointment in rehabilitation medicine or disability medicine. In practice it seems likely that most future full-time appointments will be at regional centres, probably specialising in the management of particular disabilities, e.g. spinal cord injury or the assessment and management of severely disabled patients, especially those with multiple problems.

The planning process and associated surveys will highlight deficiencies in service provision or areas of inefficiency or ineffectiveness in existing services. These will obviously vary from place to place, but the RCP report (1986) identified 15 specific areas for which provision is required:

(1) Disabled Living Centres;

(2) housing, housing modifications and rehousing;

(3) the physically disabled school-leaver;

(4) support services for younger, severely disabled and handicapped people;

(5) driving for disabled people;

(6) sexual counselling;

(7) head injury services;

(8) visual impairment;

(9) hearing impairment;

(10) communication aids;

(11) wheelchairs;

(12) prosthetics and orthotics;

(13) urinary incontinence service;

(14) stoma care service;

(15) pressure sore prevention and management.

These topics are covered in detail elsewhere in this book, and suggestions on how to make these and other services function as effectively as possible are considered later in this chapter.

The planning team will establish the needs of the disabled, possible solutions and costs, not forgetting to advise the Health Authority of the costs of inaction. Finding out the present costs of patient care in chronic disability is difficult, because methods of cost–benefit analysis of various types of care are only just beginning to be developed.

The report of The Royal College of Physicians also advised a *Disability Centre in each Health Region,* including specialised services for:

(1) assessment of complex disability;

(2) provision of prostheses, specialised orthoses or other equipment which would benefit by the presence of a bioengineering department;

(3) Disabled Living Centre;

(4) spinal unit (may be shared between regions);

(5) the provision of a focus for teaching and research.

(A Health Region has a population of about three million people.)

Central government

Government policy, for example in managing the economy, has an important effect on the lives of disabled people. Although there are specific provisions for disabled people, many of these, such as employment rehabilitation services, are less effective when the general economic climate is harsh than in more prosperous times. The Department of Health and Social Security (DHSS) is the principal government department dealing with the problems of disabled people, but the Department of Employment also plays a small role.

The DHSS is the paymaster of the National Health Service Regions, but it is not concerned with day-to-day provision of health services. A few national services are funded centrally by the DHSS, and new initiatives may receive some 'pump-priming' money for capital and/or revenue direct from the DHSS. In Scotland the Scottish Home and Health Department is the sponsoring agency for the Area Health Boards. The DHSS also provides services directly to disabled people, for example through Artificial Limb and Appliance Centres, and pays for certain pieces of equipment such as hearing aids and environmental control equipment. Its main role, however, is in the provision of pensions and Social Security benefits. The range of benefits is wide (Chapter 37), but the rules and regulations governing them are so complicated that few people understand all their intricacies. The benefits which are contingent on medical adjudication, such as Mobility Allowance, Attendance Allowance and Industrial Injury Benefits, account for only a relatively small proportion of DHSS expenditure.

The *Department of Employment* is responsible for the operation of the

3 per cent quota scheme, and the Disablement Resettlement Officer service. Specific employment initiatives for disabled people such as Employment Rehabilitation Centres, TOPS courses, fares to work and financial assistance for adaptations to workplaces make only a modest contribution to dealing with the employment problems of disabled people (Chapter 41).

Local government

The provision of services which are the responsibility of local authorities is split between district (borough) authorities, who are responsible for *housing*, and regional (county) authorities who provide most other services. There is, however, considerable local variation in the arrangements in different areas.

Social Service (social work) provision has grown greatly over recent years and now includes not only professional staff such as social workers and domiciliary occupational therapists, but others such as home helps. The services which they provide include adaptations to houses, meals-on-wheels (in conjunction with the voluntary sector) and residential homes for elderly and disabled people. The legislation concerning help for disabled people in the Chronically Sick and Disabled Persons Act (1970) is of an enabling nature, i.e. the local authority is encouraged to provide a wide range of services, but there is no legal compulsion for them to provide a particular level of service. This is in contrast to its statutory obligations, for example the provision of social work reports for courts. This will change in the future as the Disabled Persons (Services, Consultation and Representation) Act (1986) begins to take effect. This will impose an obligation on the local authority to assess the needs of a disabled person if requested by the disabled person, a carer or an authorised representative; furthermore the assessment will have to take account of the abilities of the carer. Initially this Act will apply to disabled school-leavers. The rate of implementation of this legislation has still to be fixed by the government but, if and when it is implemented fully, it will have a profound effect on community care of disabled people, particularly those with mental handicap.

Education departments make special educational provisions for disabled and mentally handicapped children, and they are also expected to provide transport and helpers to get them to school. Withdrawal of these statutory provisions when disabled persons leave school magnifies the sense of isolation which they and their parents feel (Chapter 40).

Voluntary sector

The voluntary sector is split into so many agencies that it is possible only to summarise some of the more important services which they provide. Voluntary agencies are active in the building and running of residential homes such as Cheshire Homes, sheltered housing and sheltered workshops for disabled people. They also run day centres, often for sufferers from the specific disease with which they are concerned; provide transport services, holidays and outings for disabled people; and run information services such as DIAL. Most Disabled Living Centres developed as a result of voluntary initiative, although government agencies run some and subsidise others. The variability of provision of services by the voluntary sector is its greatest strength, in that it is capable of developing services in response to changes in the perceived needs of disabled people much more quickly than statutory organisations can, but it is also its weakness because of the precarious nature of the financing of many of these ventures (Chapter 49).

Private sector

The private sector is the supplier to NHS and local authorities of equipment for disabled people. It is the direct source of some items of equipment such as self-controlled powered outdoor chairs which cannot be provided by statutory bodies but are bought by the patients themselves. There has been a recent dramatic increase in the number of residential and nursing homes for elderly and disabled people as a result of changes in DHSS rules.

MAKING THE SYSTEM WORK

Blaxter (1976) showed clearly that one of the principal barriers to achieving optimal rehabilitation was the complexity of the administrative framework of services. Other important barriers include access to buildings; inadequate transport services for disabled people; and ignorance of the range of equipment, benefits and services that are available. While these cannot be overcome without major changes in society, sound professional advice may help individual patients circumvent some of these difficulties.

Listen to the patient and his relatives

Most patients are reluctant to speak about their problems until a good therapeutic relationship has been established, and this usually takes time.

Sometimes a patient's concerns may have been voiced to other patients or to other, perhaps less senior, members of staff, e.g. a student nurse, and the information should then be shared at team meetings. This will not only help to deal more effectively with that patient's problems, but may highlight the need to look into the issue which has been raised, for example discussing the transport of a wheelchair in the ambulance with the ambulance controller.

Discussions with organisations representing disabled people also provide a worthwhile means of enhancing one's understanding and knowledge of disability and handicap.

Develop formal and informal networks within the Health Service

(1) The formal networks include details not only of the administrative structure, but also of the names of the responsible officials who will provide an appropriate lead into their line management. This applies not only in administrative hierarchies, for example the relationship between the hospital therapy departments and the district therapists, but also within medical and surgical divisions which are part of the formal advisory machinery which have an influence on the decision-making process.

(2) Informal networks of knowledge are often much more important. The development of good working relationships with colleagues from other disciplines, and particularly from other hospitals, cannot be over-emphasised. It is always worth trying to make time to visit them, since it allows an opportunity not only to find out how the service works, but also to assess the capabilities and personalities of the people who work there. It is also possible to develop an informal mechanism of team discussion about the management of those disabled patients who are being treated in a unit which does not have time set aside for formal multiprofessional meetings; for example, many important pieces of information can be shared over a cup of coffee in the ward sister's office after the medical ward round is over.

Develop knowledge of outside agencies

Information lists have been developed in some districts which summarise the procedures locally for obtaining the various services and items of equipment. These are important because they give the name and telephone number, as well as the address, of the person to contact. If such a list is not available it should be compiled.

Visits are also an important means of gaining insight and understanding

With local services this usually presents no major problem, but regional and national centres are obviously more remote, and some understanding of their work may be obtained by having a member of their staff come and give a talk.

Operational and financial implications of care for disabled people

There are usually some limited alternatives available in the management of most patients, even the most severely disabled. It is therefore important to have an idea of the relative merits and financial implications of the options. Sometimes there are demarcation disputes between agencies over caring for certain patients who do not fall clearly within defined areas of responsibility; for example, a 63-year-old patient who requires long-term care after a severe stroke may be too young for the geriatric services, too old for the Young Disabled Unit and not eligible for financial assistance towards care in a private nursing home and, therefore, 'blocks' a bed in an acute medical unit pending resolution of the impasse. The fact that this is the most expensive option helps apply pressure to develop less rigid criteria for admission to long-term care. It can, of course, be as expensive, and on some occasions more expensive, to maintain a disabled person in his/her own home within the community if the true cost of care by many different agencies is added up. The fact that the expense is shared between different budgets, however, may facilitate the setting up of these arrangements. The stress on the relatives who shoulder the principal burden of care is not usually measurable in financial terms, and arrangements to provide them with some respite should be made a high priority.

CONCLUSIONS

Rehabilitation requires cooperation between individuals and agencies so that each patient receives optimal care. Future developments in cooperation between agencies, for example between health and social services via joint funding, offer the prospect of breaking down some of the artificial administrative barriers. It will be a long time, however, before the various services become known to each other and become coordinated. It is important for professionals working with disabled people to have a detailed knowledge of the national and local arrangements for the provision of the services that they have to call upon.

REFERENCES

Blaxter, M. (1976) *The meaning of disability*, Heinemann, London

Chronically Sick and Disabled Persons Act (1970) HMSO, London

Disabled Persons (Services, Consultations and Representation) Act (1986), HMSO, London

Royal College of Physicians Report (1986) Physical disability in 1986 and beyond. *J. Roy. Coll. Phys. Lond.*, *20*, 160-94

51

Research and Development in Rehabilitation

Cairns Aitken

Medical rehabilitation has an honourable past, based as it is on need, particularly in wartime. The establishment of employment rehabilitation services was the direct response to the plight of war veterans unfit for work (Tomlinson, 1943). Similarly Bobath therapy arose on the perceived need for an effective physiotherapy treatment of patients with upper motor neurone lesions of the limbs. In both cases the effectiveness of the response to need was not evaluated, and since changes in practice became widespread, the moment passed when scientific evaluation might ethically have been undertaken.

Such assumptions and developments are not unique to rehabilitation. We have seen a complete reversal of the management of patients after heart attacks: at one time they were managed with prolonged bed rest, now emphasis is on regaining physical fitness. The need for research in the management of disease, particularly chronic disease, is thus clear. The difficulties of doing this soon become apparent.

Research is easy to conduct where the benefit of a treatment can be demonstrated by a single measurement (as in early evaluations of the effect of penicillin in acute infections). It is rare that such a simple situation exists in the field of rehabilitation — indeed the complexity of measurement here has been one reason for the delay in tackling many facets of the subjects, such as assessment of mobility. The problem has been further compounded by lack of clarity in definition. Therefore the separation of the concepts of disability and handicap has aided clear thinking (WHO, 1980).

The stimulus for change, or for research into advantageous change, in management has altered. Previously the aftermath of war and infectious diseases exercised doctors' skills: now one might say there is an 'epidemic' of degenerative diseases, which have as yet to claim their fair share of researchers' time and expertise. Nevertheless, pressure groups, politicians and clinicians themselves are coming to realise the desirability of such research to determine the value of new methods of treatment, and to tease out the effective components of present practice. Clinicians are beginning to rise to the challenge, undertaking surverys of need in clinical trials of treatment methods and devising measurement tools which will allow them to do this.

The breakthrough of the 1970s was the appreciation of the complexity of the requirements and the constraints imposed by an inadequate research infrastructure. The research that stimulated the most seminal progress in response can only be a personal choice. For me, the Harris Report (1972) revealed the enormous numbers of handicapped people and the nature of their problems, making clear that most of those affected were elderly. Blaxter's study in Aberdeen (1976), in which she enquired about the adjustment of potentially disabled patients after discharge from hospital, made plain the many matters requiring attention. More and more of the same services would not solve their problems — patients now needed advice simply to ensure that existing help was provided in a coordinated way. Furthermore, the series of studies on outcome after stroke on both inpatients (Garraway *et al.*, 1980) and outpatients (Smith *et al.*, 1981), and on specific treatments like speech therapy (David *et al*, 1982) have revealed only marginal gains from other than routine treatment. The principal advantage from introducing a special management or procedure seemed to be reducing the tendency for independence to be lost, rather than to enhancing what already had been achieved.

Studies on amputees drew attention to the poor standard of their rehabilitation except in certain centres (Van de Ven, 1981). Observations of many disabled patients in hospital have shown clearly that the outcome has been less than optimal.

AVAILABILITY OF REHABILITATION KNOWLEDGE

Medical rehabilitation has been notorious for its knowledge being hidden in reports that were often irretrievable. The 1970s saw a radical change. Two new scientific journals were launched devoted to disability and handicap, namely *International Disability Studies* and the *International Journal of Rehabilitation Research.* Therapist journals have endeavoured to increase the number of reports concerning research and innovations, though these journals in Europe still contain fewer such articles than those published in North America. Many studies relevant to rehabilitation are to be found in other specialised journals such as those for geriatric medicine, psychiatry, mental handicap, paediatric medicine or rheumatology.

Another growth in the past decade has been in 'journalist'-type articles about disability. Several such publications are distributed free and targeted directly towards disabled people and their carers. Voluntary organisations, some for specific disabilities, have contributed greatly to this development which has considerable educational value and encourages self-help. Coverage about handicap on radio and television has increased enormously, and includes information about rights and benefits, new equipment and societies. These publications may be the principal source of knowledge for many professionals, as well as for carers and patients.

During the mid-1970s a small group of doctors met regularly to discuss developments required in medical training for rehabilitation. They realised that the subject lacked a scientific society at which the results of research could be presented and be open to criticism by peers. These doctors appreciated that the need for this existed not only in the medical profession but also for all relevant professions. Funds were obtained from an anonymous donor, and in 1978 the Society for Research in Rehabilitation was launched with its first meeting in Southampton, hosted by the First European Professor of Rehabilitation. Since then the society has met twice yearly.

The topics of research presented have ranged widely, and breadth of interest has been striking, indicative of the heterogeneous needs of disabled people. Abstracts of the proceedings have been published regularly in the *International Journal of Rehabilitation Research.*

Meetings of new multiprofessional groups have been held, often to discuss a special subject, such as the Tissue Viability Society, the Incontinence Task Force or the Motor Club. Therapists have formed special interest groups such as for hand disorders. Those working in Disabled Living Centres meet regularly, as do those working in Young Disabled Units in certain parts of the UK. These groups have helped to disseminate knowledge by discussion on how best to tackle difficult clinical and service problems.

PURPOSE AND PROBLEMS OF SCIENTIFIC RESEARCH

Scientific research is undertaken to confirm or deny a hypothesis; for those engaged in the care of patients the questions posed will usually relate to the needs of patients rather than being basic scientific investigations. In this situation the researcher may have to tolerate much 'background noise' in his experiment, and on many occasions a compromise will have to be reached between what is scientifically desirable and what is humanly possible. Such research is not easy, but there are spin-offs from such discipline and skill as are required to complete scientific work and to read it to a learned society. The process is stimulating; it usually leaves the worker asking more questions and the chance to present work to an interested, sympathetic and constructively critical audience is challenging. Rational discussion about the cost-effectiveness of various proposed changes becomes possible, although this is only just beginning to develop in rehabilitation. The priority for attention remains to improve the tools for measurement of disability and handicap status. Both Wright (1985) and

Clarke (1985) confirmed this for rheumatic diseases despite considerable research on the benefits of treatment in these common conditions.

SUPPORT FOR RESEARCH

Most research in rehabilitation is done by clinicians actively engaged in the practice of rehabilitation. In a sense their involvement in research is a by-product of their clinical duties and one very much to be welcomed. This encourages observations on series of patients, though often only during a short time period. Patients are generally assessed cross-sectionally, and few studies of a longtitudinal nature are done. Rehabilitation tends to be a slow process and even to measure outcome and status at follow-up may require a long-term commitment.

There is more opportunity nowadays for research to be undertaken by staff employed directly for that purpose. This requires someone to obtain the funds for their support, which in turn depends on the formation of a clear statement about what is to be done. To develop such good ideas is one of the most difficult aspects of rehabilitation research. To design an experiment to test a hypothesis may be appropriate for the topic. The most common research is to make observations in a way that describe in quantitative terms the matter of interest. For instance Bookis (1983) describes vividly the plight of disabled adolescents after a survey conducted with remarkable rapidity. Whatever research is to be done, clear ideas are necessary both about the purpose and how it is to be achieved.

Rehabilitation research, like any other research, requires certain skills. These need not involve sophisticated knowledge of any technique or of statistics, but rather the discipline to stick rigorously to an experimental design while collecting the data. Hence it is essential to obtain statistical and other technical advice when *planning* a study. Thereafter the analysis and display of the data are simplified and the conclusions can be drawn straightforwardly.

To write an application to obtain research funds is a skill in itself. The objectives have to be precise and the methods to be used clear. There are many sources of funds; some governmental through Departmental Chief Scientists, others charitable with interests relating to disability. Each has its own rules for application which must be strictly followed.

TYPES OF RESEARCH UNDERTAKEN

As rehabilitation may be appropriate to almost any clinical condition, certainly any chronic one, and with any aspect whether physical, psychological or social, the spectrum for relevant research is broad. Three topics can be considered in illustration of certain principles — equipment, environment and information.

Equipment and aids

The marketplace has been flooded with devices for a wide variety of purposes. Many have been designed with ingenuity and have found an established place in solving a problem for a particular disability. Few have been evaluated and a 'best buy' recommended.

Some items of equipment such as lifting devices (hoists) have been studied in detail (Bell, 1984). Standards of safety have been adopted, particularly in prosthetics. The use of equipment by certain types of patient, as after a stroke, has been investigated. Advances are being made in the application of computers, which could have dramatic impact such as with functional electrical stimulation on the mobility of paraplegic patients.

Design and engineering of equipment is only part of the requirement. The remainder relates to assessment, prescription, supply, training, suitability and effectiveness.

The system should begin with correct assessment of the patient's problem and correct prescription of an aid for its solution. In terms of the efficiency of supply, studies have shown (e.g. Chamberlain *et al.*, 1978) that the need for an aid was identified, but that it usually arrived many weeks after the patient was discharged home. Further study (Chamberlain *et al.*, 1981) showed that the involvement of an occupational therapist, specifically to prescribe early for a patient's needs, led to improvement. Few patients received instruction in the use of the aid prescribed, or had the opportunity of seeing the range of equipment available. Training in the use of the equipment is necessary for both patient and carer in order to maximise effectiveness (and cost–benefit) of the aid for that patient. Systems for maintenance and replacement also require to be arranged.

Attention to these matters could bring about as much improvement as attention to deficiencies in design of equipment. The latest technology may not be required, but simply efficient availability of what has been around for some time. Sadly, it seems to be more difficult to bring about improvement in the system than it does in design. It seems to be less glamorous and attractive to be involved in research on supply and delivery care than in research on equipment itself.

Factors in the environment

There has been greater attention in the past decade or so on factors in the environment that disadvantage disabled people. Access for wheelchairs into buildings is an obvious example. Planning the environment to be convenient is obviously a challenging task, involving as it must architects and other professionals. Sensitive thought about the needs, and listening to advice from disabled people themselves, is essential. Many buildings have been inappropriately designed and require extensive modification to be suitable. Even most basic requirements may not be available in the most vital places. Their lack simply discourages independence in personal care. Toilets and bathrooms are the notorious blackspots; ease of use by patients in wheelchairs has rarely been contemplated (Chamberlain *et al.*, 1978). Attention to these matters has low priority; however, the difficulties are sometimes formidable, requiring considerable alteration of structure to become ideal. Access to various forms of transport can produce comparable difficulties.

The research on such topics should not only identify deficiencies but suggest solutions. Questions of how to obtain improvement are challenging. Politicians, local and national, are becoming more responsive to disabled people and their requirement for allocation of specific resources, and some of the pressure that has brought this about has resulted from effective publicity of the relevant research.

Information services

Many patients fail to receive the services they require because they, their carers or treating professionals do not know about them. There has consequently been considerable endeavour to develop information services, but as yet little to evaluate their effectiveness. Existing rehabilitation services seem to be fully used, and so it is assumed that they are beneficial and reaching those who require them. Yet still a gap exists between what can be done and what is made available to many disabled people. Hence much thought and enquiry are required on how best to bring about improvement. That is easier said than done, partly because of insufficient expertise about the topic amongst those in professional rehabilitation services.

Reasons for such failures in communication are many and complex, and not unlike those in health education in general. Despite certain modifications of behaviour being essential to improve health, such as stopping smoking or reducing alcohol intake, there is considerable resistance to change, particularly in lower socioeconomic groups. The same is true of information about disability. Those likely to have the greatest need are probably those least likely to use whatever information service is available. Similar problems require to be tackled to ensure that professional staff can obtain the information required; these relate to their education and training, and many considerations apply.

The development and greater availability of Disabled Living Centres where information and equipment can be examined is one response to this difficulty. Some are renowned and sophisticated, such as that at the Disabled Living Foundation in London. Others are simpler but effective for local circumstances; for instance one in Scotland is in a van visiting local areas — Mobile Aids Centre (MAC). There appears to be a need for more exploration of how best to ensure that necessary information (a) reaches those who need to know, and (b) is acted upon appropriately, whether by patient or carer, whether professional or relative.

PRIORITIES FOR THE FUTURE

To accelerate the desired improvement in the standard of rehabilitation, the policy to build up the number of staff engaged in research should continue to be pursued with vigour. This could be facilitated by therapists and nurses being trained to graduate level, with more of them having the opportunity for postgraduate research training. Indeed all professional staff involved in rehabilitation services require more in-service continuing education. University and other special Departments of Rehabilitation should be catalytic in promoting such activities.

It is to be hoped that therapy schools and academic departments interested in rehabilitation will foster enquiries and promote teaching based on their findings. The aim is to widen involvement by imparting an appreciation of the value of research. Only by involving many clinicians in tackling a difficulty such as comprehensive assessment, will the quality of the enquiry improve. The priority is to improve the reliability and validity of any method used to measure disability, handicap and the outcome of rehabilitation in specific disorders. Simplified methods are required that produce not only consistent and meaningful results, but ones that are sensitive to change and specific in its detection.

There is an urgent need to evaluate existing clinical procedures and methods of clinical management. Questions need to be answered about the most appropriate way to tackle many problems, and thus improve overall the system of response.

More classical clinical trials are required whereby the constituents of a rehabilitation programme are examined. In stroke, for instance, more needs to be known about the most appropriate time for intervention, and about the optimal amounts of differing kinds of treatment within the total clinical care. We need to ascertain the value of any equipment used in patients' therapy, and how to improve its usefulness.

Rehabilitation is labour-intensive and therefore expensive. Hence research into cost–benefit is important. Surveys are required to develop a greater awareness amongst staff and funding authorities about the nature of needs. It is beginning to be realised that, by supplying more and more of the same, the remedial problems of disabled people will not be solved. What may be suitable for one patient in one setting may be inappropriate for another.

Developments in services generally do not occur as a result of some master-plan. They occur more as a result of increments here and there. Fertile soil must be present for seeds of ideas to germinate and flourish. Pressure for developments usually arises from ideas starting in the periphery supported by evidence, which then receives a welcome at the centre. To obtain evidence requires the research being discussed in this chapter.

CONCLUSION

To do research is a way of life. To pose a question, to design how to answer it and then to obtain information that when analysed will do so, requires discipline and faith — faith that improvements in standards of care will result. Such faith is not always rewarded. Some good ideas remain unused; some are ahead of their time; but there is much to encourage new researchers. The work done in the past decade is already bearing fruit: attitudes have improved; the situation is no longer static. Many clinical workers are now receptive to change and are eager for developments. More rehabilitation research is the way to a better future for patients with disability — certainly that is the belief of a Professor of Rehabilitation Studies and the editors of this book.

REFERENCES

Bell, F. (1984) *Patient-lifting devices in hospitals*, Croom Helm, Beckenham

Blaxter, M. (1976) *The meaning of disability*, Heinemann, London

Bookis, J. (1983) *Beyond the school gate: a study of disabled young people aged 13–19*. Royal Association for Disability and Rehabilitation, London

Chamberlain, M.A. Thornley, G. and Wright, V.B. (1978) Evaluation of aids and equipment for bath and toilet. *Rheumatol. Rehabil.*, *17*, 187-94

Chamberlain, M.A., Thornley, G., Stowe, J. and Wright, V. (1981) Evaluation of aids and equipment for the bath: II. A possible solution to the problem. *Rheumat. Rehabil.*, *20*, 38-43

Clarke, A.K. (1985) Measuring outcome. *J. Roy. Soc. Med.*, *78*, 981-2

David, R.M., Enderby, P. and Bainton, D. (1982) Treatment of acquired asphasia: speech therapists and volunteers compared. *J. Neurol. Neurosurg. Psychiatry*, *45*, 957-61

Garraway, W.M., Akhtar, A.J., Hockey, L. and Prescott, R.J. (1980) Management of acute stroke in the elderly: follow-up of a controlled trial. *Br. Med. J.*, *281*, 827-9

Harris, A. (1972) *The handicapped and impaired in Great Britain*, HMSO, London

Smith, D.S., Goldenberg, E., Ashburn, A. *et al.* (1981) Remedial therapy after

stroke: a randomised controlled trial. *Br. Med. J.*, *282*, 517-20
Tomlinson Committee (1943) *Rehabilitation and resettlement of disabled persons.* Report of the inter-departmental committee, HMSO, London
Van de Ven, C.M.C. (1981) Investigation into the management of bilateral amputees. *Br. Med. J.*, *282*, 707-10
Wade, D.T., Langton Hewer, R., Skilbeck, C.E. and David, R.M. (1985) *Stroke: a critical approach to diagnosis, treatment and management,* Chapman & Hall Medical, London
World Health Organization (1980) *International classification of impairments, disabilities and handicaps,* WHO, Geneva
Wright,V. (1985) Measurement of outcome in rheumatic diseases. *J. Roy. Soc. Med.*, *78*, 985-94

Subject Index

Name Index